PEDIATRIC EMERGENCY MEDICINE

Just the Facts

Gary R. Strange, MD, FACEP

Chairman
Department of Emergency Medicine
University of Illinois at Chicago
Chicago, Illinois

Valerie A. Dobiesz, MD

Associate Professor of Clinical Emergency Medicine and Education Director
Department of Emergency Medicine
University of Illinois at Chicago
Chicago, Illinois

William R. Ahrens, MD

Associate Professor of Clinical Emergency Medicine
Department of Emergency Medicine
University of Illinois at Chicago
Chicago, Illinois

Kemedy K. McQuillen, MD

Medical Director, Pediatric Emergency Center
Christ Hospital and Medical Center
Oak Lawn, Illinois

Patricia Lee, MD

Medical Director
Department of Emergency Medicine
Advocate Illinois Masonic Medical Center
Chicago, Illinois

Heather M. Prendergast, MD

Assistant Professor of Emergency Medicine
Department of Emergency Medicine
University of Illinois at Chicago
Chicago, Illinois

McGraw-Hill

Medical Publishing Division

New York   Chicago   San Francisco   Lisbon   London   Madrid   Mexico City
Milan   New Delhi   San Juan   Seoul   Singapore   Sydney   Toronto

Pediatric Emergency Medicine: *Just the Facts*

1 2 3 4 5 6 7 8 9 0   CUS/CUS   0 9 8 7 6 5 4 3

ISBN 0-07-140086-9

This book was set in Times New Roman by Macmillan India.
The editors were Andrea Seils, Michelle Watt, and Mary E. Bele.
The production supervisor was Richard Ruzycka.
The cover designer was Aimee Nordin.
The index was prepared by Andover Publishing Services.
Von Hoffmann Graphics was printer and binder.

This book is printed on acid-free paper.

Library of Congress Cataloging-in-Publication Data

Pediatric emergency medicine : just the facts / edited by Gary R. Strange... [et al.].
    p. ; cm.
  Includes bibliographical references and index.
  ISBN 0-07-140086-9
    1. Pediatric emergencies—Examinations, questions, etc. 2. Pediatric intensive care—
Examinations, questions, etc. I. Strange, Gary R., 1947-   .
    [DNLM: 1. Emergencies—Child—Examination Questions. 2. Pediatrics—Examination
Questions.   WS 18.2 P369945 2004]
RJ370.P45324 2004
618.92´0025—dc21
                                                    2003048793

CONTENTS

CONTRIBUTORS

Thomas J. Abramo, MD, Emergency Center, Children's Medical Center of Dallas, Dallas, Texas

Thomas J. Abrunzo, MS, MPH, MD, FAAP, FACEP, Co-Medical Director, After Hours Pediatrics, Inc., Clinical Associate Professor of Pediatrics, University of South Florida College of Medicine, Tampa, Florida

William R. Ahrens, MD, Associate Professor of Clinical Emergency Medicine, Department of Emergency Medicine, University of Illinois at Chicago, Chicago, Illinois

Steven E. Aks, DO, FACEP, FACMT, Department of Emergency Medicine, Mercy Hospital and Medical Center, Chicago, Illinois

Yona Amatai, MD, Section of Clinical Toxicology, Cook County Hospital, Chicago, Illinois

Tanya R. Anderson, MD, Assistant Professor of Psychiatry, University of Illinois, Chicago, Illinois

Grace Arteaga, MD, Attending Physician, Pediatric Intensive Care Unit, Assistant Professor of Pediatrics, University of Illinois at Chicago, Chicago, Illinois

Joilo Barbosa, MD, Department of Emergency Medicine, Emory University, Atlanta, Georgia

Roger Barkin, MD, Division of Emergency Medicine, University of Colorado Health Sciences Center, Denver, Colorado

Brian A. Bates, MD, Methodist Children's Hospital of South Texas, San Antonio, Texas

Elizabeth E. Baumann, MD, Instructor of Pediatrics, Section of Endocrinology, Department of Pediatrics, University of Chicago, Chicago, Illinois

Kenneth Bizovi, MD, Department of Emergency Medicine, Oregon Health Science University, Portland, Oregon

Ira J. Blumen, MD, Division of Emergency Medicine, University of Chicago, Chicago, Illinois

Mary Jo A. Bowman, MD, Emergency Medicine, Columbus Children's Hospital, Columbus, Ohio

Kathleen Brown, MD, Department of Emergency Medicine, Upstate Medical University, Syracuse, New York

Richard M. Cantor, MD, Central NY Poison Control Center, Department of Emergency Medicine, SUNY University Hospital, Syracuse, New York

Andrea Carlson, MD, Department of Emergency Medicine, Christ Hospital and Medical Center, Oak Lawn, Illinois

Stephen A. Colucciello, MD, Department of Emergency Medicine, Carolinas Medical Center, Charlotte, North Carolina

D. Mark Courtney, MD, Division of Emergency Medicine, Northwestern Memorial Hospital, Chicago, Illinois

Michael Cowan, MD, Children's Medical Center of Dallas, Emergency Center, Dallas, Texas

Ronald A. Dieckmann, MD, Pediatric Emergency Medicine, San Francisco General Hospital, San Francisco, California

Valerie A. Dobiesz, MD, Associate Professor of Clinical Emergency Medicine and Education Director, Department of Emergency Medicine, University of Illinois at Chicago, Chicago, Illinois

Timothy Erickson, MD, Associate Professor of Emergency Medicine, Department of Emergency Medicine, University of Illinois, Chicago, Illinois

Susan Fuchs, MD, Division of Pediatric Emergency Medicine, Children's Memorial Hospital, Chicago, Illinois

Marianne Gausche-Hill, FACEP, FAAP, Department of Emergency Medicine, UCLA School of Medicine, Harbor-UCLA Medical Center, Torrance, California

Michael J. Gerardi, MD, Pediatric Emergency Services, St. Barnabas Medical Center, Livingston, New Jersey

Jill Glick, MD, Medical Director Child Protective Services, University of Chicago, Chicago, Illinois

Collin S. Goto, MD, Children's Hospital and Health Center, San Diego, California

Michael Green, MD, Department of Emergency Medicine, Mercy Hospital and Medical Center, Chicago, Illinois

Russell H. Greenfield, MD, Carolinas Integrative Health, Charlotte, North Carolina

Geetha Gurrala, MD, Attending Physician, Department of Emergency Medicine, University of Illinois at Chicago, Chicago, Illinois

Leon Gussow, MD, Department of Emergency Medicine, Cook County Hospital, Chicago, Illinois

Suchinta Hakim, MD, Department of Emergency Medicine, Hinsdale Hospital, Hinsdale, Illinois

Brenda N. Hayakawa, MD, Emergency Department, Foothill Presbyterian Hospital, San Dimas Community Hospital, Arcadia, California

Bruce E. Herman, MD, ED, Primary Children's Medical Center, Salt Lake City, Utah

Daniel Hryhorczuk, MD, Director, Cook County Hospital, Great Lakes Center for Environmental Health and Safety, School of Public Health, University of Illinois at Chicago, Chicago, Illinois

William B. Ignatoff, MD, Carondelet St. Joseph's Hospital, Tucson, Arizona

David M. Jaffe, MD, FAAP, FACEP, Department of Pediatrics, Washington University School of Medicine, St. Louis Children's Hospital, St. Louis, Missouri

Shabnam Jain, MD, Assistant Professor of Pediatrics, Emory University School of Medicine, Attending Physician, Emergency Department, Children's Healthcare of Atlanta at Egleston, Atlanta, Georgia

Alan E. Jones, MD, Department of Emergency Medicine, Carolinas Medical Center, Charlotte, North Carolina

Susan A. Kecskes, MD, Director, Pediatric Intensive Care Unit, Department of Pediatrics, University of Illinois at Chicago, Chicago, Illinois

Katherine M. Konzen, MD, Department of Pediatric Emergency Medicine, Children's Hospital, San Diego, California

Jane E. Kramer, MD, Associate Professor of Pediatrics, Director, Section of Pediatric Emergency Medicine, Department of Pediatrics, Rush Medical College, Chicago, Illinois

Ann Krantz, Pharm D, Division of Occupational Medicine, Cook County Hospital, Chicago, Illinois

John D. Lantos, MD, Associate Professor of Pediatrics and Medicine, Associate Director, Center for Clinical Medical Ethics, Co-Director, Robert Wood Johnson Clinical Scholars Program, Chief, Section of General Pediatrics, University of Chicago, Chicago, Illinois

Patricia Lee, MD, Medical Director, Department of Emergency Medicine, Advocate Illinois Masonic Medical Center, Chicago, Illinois

Jerrold B. Leikin, MD, Department of Occupational Medicine & Clinical Toxicology, Rush North, Glencoe, Illinois

Steven Lelyveld, MD, FACEP, FAAP, Associate Professor of Clinical Pediatrics and Medicine, Chief, Section of Pediatric Emergency Medicine, Pritzker School of Medicine, University of Chicago, Chicago, Illinois

Marshall Lewis, MD, Department of Pediatrics, University of Illinois Hospital, Chicago, Illinois

Jordan D. Lipton, MD, FACEP, Carolinas Emergency Physicians, Department of Emergency Medicine, Mercy Hospital South, Charlotte, North Carolina

Wendy Ann Lucid, MD, Director and Section Chief, Pediatric Emergency Services, Good Samaritan Regional Medical Center, Phoenix, Arizona

John Marcinak, MD, Section of Infectious Disease, Department of Pediatrics, University of Illinois, Chicago, Illinois

Diana Mayer, MD, Department of Pediatrics, University of Illinois, Chicago, Illinois

Bonnie McManus, MD, Toxicology Fellow, Department of Emergency Medicine, University of Illinois at Chicago, Consultant, Toxicon Consortium, Chicago, Illinois

Kemedy K. McQuillen, MD, Medical Director, Pediatric Emergency Center, Christ Hospital and Medical Center, Oak Lawn, Illinois

Rustin Morse, MD, Phoenix Children's Hospital, Phoenix, Arizona

Mark Mycyk, MD, Department of Emergency Medicine, Northwestern University, Chicago, Illinois

Thomas T. Mydler, MD, Pediatric Emergency Medicine, Children's Medical Center of Dallas, Dallas, Texas

Margaret Paik, MD, Department of Pediatric Emergency Medicine, University of Chicago, Wylers Children's Hospital, Chicago, Illinois

Frank P. Paloucek, Pharm D, DABAT, Director, Residency Programs, Clinical Associate Professor in Pharmacy Practice, Department of Pharmacy Practice, College of Pharmacy, University of Illinois at Chicago, Chicago, Illinois

Barbara Pawel, MD, Section of Emergency Medicine, Philadelphia, Pennsylvania

Nattasorn Plipat, MD, Pediatric Infectious Diseases Fellow, Division of Infectious Diseases, Children's Memorial Hospital, Chicago, Illinois

Elizabeth C. Powell, MD, MPH, Attending Physician, Pediatric Emergency Medicine, Children's Memorial Hospital, Chicago, Illinois

Heather M. Prendergast, MD, Assistant Professor of Emergency Medicine, Department of Emergency Medicine, University of Illinois at Chicago, Chicago, Illinois

Patricia Primm, MD, Emergency Center, Children's Medical Center of Dallas, Dallas, Texas

Kimberly S. Quayle, MD, Division of Pediatric Emergency Medicine, St. Louis Children's Hospital, St. Louis, Missouri

Veena Ramaiah, MD, Department of Pediatrics, Division of Pediatric Emergency Medicine, University of Chicago Children's Hospital, Chicago, Illinois

Rebecca R. Reamy, MD, Pediatric Emergency/Critical Care, MUSC Children's Hospital, Charleston, South Carolina

Sally L. Reynolds, MD, Assistant Medical Director, Pediatric Emergency Medicine, Children's Memorial Hospital, Chicago, Illinois

Timothy J. Rittenberry, MD, FACEP, Department of Emergency Medicine, Illinois Masonic Medical Center, Chicago, Illinois

Jaime Rivas, MD, California Emergency Physicians Medical Group, Oakland, California

Howard Rodenberg, MD, Medical Director, Volusia County EMS, Adjunct Professor of Human Factors, Embry-Riddle Aeronautical University, Daytona Beach, Florida

Simon Ros, MD, Department of Pediatrics, Loyola University Medical Center, Maywood, Illinois

Julia A. Rosekrans, MD, Head, Section of Pediatric Emergency Services, Director, Pediatric Residency, Department of Pediatrics, Mayo Medical Center, Consultant in Pediatric and Adolescent Medicine, Mayo Graduate School of Medicine, Rochester, Minnesota

Robert L. Rosenfield, MD, Division of Pediatric Endocrinology, University of Chicago, Chicago, Illinois

Alfred Sacchetti, MD, Emergency Physician, Department of Emergency Medicine, Our Lady of Lourdes Medical Center, Voorhees, New Jersey

John P. Santamaria, MD, Director, Pediatric Emergency Services, Director, Wound and Hyperbaric Center, St. Joseph's Hospital, Clinical Assistant Professor of Pediatrics, School of Medicine, University of South Florida, Tampa, Florida

Robert W. Schafermeyer, MD, FACEP, FAAP, Department of Emergency Medicine, Carolinas Medical Center, Charlotte, North Carolina

Susan M. Scott, MD, Assistant Professor, Emergency Center, Children's Medical Center of Dallas, Dallas, Texas

Ghazala Q. Sharieff, MD, FACEP, FAAP, Clinical Assistant Professor, Department of Emergency Medicine, University of Florida, Jacksonville, Director of Pediatric Emergency Medicine, Palomar-Pomerado Health System, San Diego, California

Kimberly Sing, MD, Fellow in Toxicology, Toxicon Consortium, University of Illinois at Chicago, Chicago, Illinois

Jonathan Singer, MD, Department of Emergency Medicine, Wright State University, Kettering, Ohio

Tulika Singh, MD, Department of Pediatrics and Emergency Medicine, Illinois Masonic Medical Center and University of Illinois, Chicago, Illinois

Edward P. Sloan, MD, MPH, Department of Emergency Medicine, University of Illinois at Chicago, Chicago, Illinois

David F. Soglin, MD, Chairman, Pediatric Emergency Medicine, Department of Pediatrics, Cook County Children's Hospital, Chicago, Illinois

Gary R. Strange, MD, FACEP, Chairman, Department of Emergency Medicine, University of Illinois at Chicago, Chicago, Illinois

Todd B. Taylor, MD, Attending Emergency Physician, Banner Good Samaritan Medical Center, Phoenix, Arizona

Frank Thorp, MD, Department of Pediatrics, University of Chicago, Chicago, Illinois

William C. Toepper, MD, Department of Emergency Medicine, Illinois Masonic Medical Center, Chicago, Illinois

David A. Townes, MD, Division of Emergency Medicine, University of Washington, Seattle, Washington

Timothy Turnbull, MD, Pinnalle Emergency Medical Consultants, Morrow, Georgia

Dennis T. Uehara, MD, Chairman, Department of Emergency Medicine, Rockford Memorial Hospital, Rockford, Illinois

Michael Van Rooyen, MD, Department of Emergency Medicine, John Hopkins University, Baltimore, Maryland

Robert A. Wiebe, MD, Children's Medical Center of Dallas, Emergency Center, Dallas, Texas

Kelly D. Young, MD, Harbor-UCLA Medical Center, Department of Emergency Medicine, Torrance, California

Michele Zell-Kanter, Pharm D, Division of Occupational Medicine, Cook County Hospital, Chicago, Illinois

PREFACE

Pediatric Emergency Medicine: Just the Facts is a distillation of the material provided in *Pediatric Emergency Medicine: A Comprehensive Study Guide, 2nd Edition*, which was published in 2002. *Just the Facts* has been developed as a resource for pediatric emergency physicians, general emergency physicians, pediatricians, and others who regularly provide pediatric emergency care or who only occasionally are called upon to care for sick or injured children. Following the same topical organization as the larger *Study Guide*, this work provides the essential information needed in the emergency care of children in a readily accessible manner. In order to do this, we have omitted much information that is of a supporting or enhancing nature. The current work is not intended to be comprehensive but is designed to be a quick reference, an overview for the first-time user or a refresher course for the experienced clinician. By virtue of its smaller size, the work is more affordable and more portable than its larger companion. We have included multiple choice questions with each chapter to facilitate the use of the material as a self-test and as a review for those preparing for in-training, board certification, or recertification examinations.

We would like to express our gratitude to the authors of the chapters in the *Second Edition*. In this work, the editors and question-writers have, to a significant degree, used that work as the basis of this much more concise piece. We are pleased to acknowledge their contributions and the many contributions of individuals who have assisted us including Andrea Seils at McGraw-Hill whose wonderful support and encouragement has been so helpful. In addition, the support of Bailet Wright at the University of Illinois has allowed us to move through the publication process smoothly.

So with a final word of appreciation to our families, friends, and colleagues who have tolerated our withdrawal from them for the past several months, we present this work for your consideration and use. Your feedback will be most appreciated.

Gary R. Strange, MD, FACEP

PEDIATRIC EMERGENCY MEDICINE

Just the Facts

Section 1
RESUSCITATION

1 INTRODUCTION TO PEDIATRIC RESUSCITATION

Robert A. Wiebe
Susan M. Scott
William Ahrens
Valerie A. Dobiesz

EPIDEMIOLOGY

- Most pediatric cardiac arrests occur in infants less than 1 year of age.
- Pediatric cardiac arrest results from tissue hypoxia that is the end-result of respiratory failure or shock. In the arrest phase, hypoxia-induced bradycardia progresses to pulseless electrical activity, to asystole.
- The specific causes of pediatric cardiopulmonary arrest are diverse and vary with age (Table 1-1).

PROGNOSIS

- By the time cardiac arrest has occurred, hypoxia has virtually always caused significant end-organ damage, especially to the central nervous system. Consequently, the prognosis for full cardiopulmonary arrest in infants and children is very poor.
- Resuscitations requiring more than two doses of epinephrine or lasting more than 10 to 15 min rarely result in intact neurologic survival.

TABLE 1-1 Epidemiology of Cardiopulmonary Arrest in Children

AGE	ETIOLOGY
Less than 1 year	Respiratory disease
	Pneumonia
	Bronchiolitis
	Upper airway obstruction
	Central nervous system disease
	Seizures
	Meningitis
	Hydrocephalus
	Cardiac disease
	Congenital heart disease
	Cardiomyopathies
	Myocarditis
	Sepsis and shock
	Sudden infant death syndrome
	Congenital anomalies
	Metabolic disease
1 to 2 years	Injuries
	Drownings
	Falls
	Electrical shock
	Pedestrian/bike/motor vehicle crashes
	Congenital anomalies
	Malignancies
	Homicide
	Cardiac disease
	Asthma
Adolescence	Injuries
	Asthma
	Suicide, toxic ingestions
	Homicide
	Cardiac disease
	Hypertrophic cardiomyopathy

BIBLIOGRAPHY

Hazinski MF, Chahine AA, Holcomb GW, et al: Outcome of cardiovascular collapse in pediatric blunt trauma. *Ann Emerg Med* 23:1229–1235, 1994.

Hickey RW, Cohen DM, Strausbaugh S, et al: Pediatric patients requiring CPR in the pre-hospital setting. *Ann Emerg Med* 25:495–501, 1995.

Kuisma M, Suominen P, Korpela R: Pediatric out-of-hospital cardiac arrests: Epidemiology and outcome. *Resuscitation* 30:141–150, 1995.

Mogayzel C, Quan L, Graves JR, et al: Out-of-hospital ventricular fibrillation in children and adolescents: Causes and outcomes. *Ann Emerg Med* 25:484–491, 1995.

Pitetti R, Glustein JZ, Bhende MS: Prehospital care and outcome of pediatric out-of-hospital cardiac arrest. *Prehosp Emerg Care* 6:283–290, 2002.

Ronco R, King W, Donley DK, et al: Outcome and cost at a children's hospital following resuscitation for out-of-hospital cardiopulmonary arrest. *Arch Pediatr Adolesc Med* 149: 210–214, 1995.

Schindler MB, Bohn D, Cox PN, et al: Outcome of out-of hospital cardiac or respiratory arrest in children. *N Engl J Med* 335:1473–1479, 1995.

Sirbaugh PE, Pepe PE, Shook JE, et al: Outcome of out-of-hospital pediatric cardiopulmonary arrest. *Ann Emerg Med* 33: 174–184, 1999.

Young KD, Seidel JS: Pediatric cardiopulmonary resuscitation: A collective review. *Ann Emerg Med* 33:195–205, 1999.

QUESTIONS

1. Which of the following is correct regarding pediatric cardiopulmonary arrests?
   A. Most arrests occur in adolescent patients.
   B. The majority are caused by cardiac dysrhythmias.
   C. The prognosis for full cardiopulmonary arrest is very poor.
   D. Pediatric patients surviving prolonged resuscitation generally have no neurologic deficits.
   E. Cardiopulmonary arrest is always caused by sudden infant death syndrome.

2. The most common progression of cardiac dysrhythmia in pediatric cardiopulmonary arrest is:
   A. Bradycardia to pulseless electrical activity to asystole.
   B. Supraventricular tachycardia to ventricular fibrillation to asystole.
   C. Ventricular tachycardia to ventricular fibrillation to asystole.
   D. Atrial flutter to ventricular fibrillation to asystole.
   E. Atrial fibrillation to asystole.

ANSWERS

1. C. Most pediatric cardiopulmonary arrests occur in infants less than 1 year of age and are the result of tissue hypoxia that is the final consequence of respiratory failure or shock. The specific causes of pediatric cardiopulmonary arrest are diverse and vary with age. The prognosis for full cardiopulmonary arrest in infants and children is very poor.

2. A. In the arrest phase, hypoxia-induced bradycardia progresses to pulseless electrical activity, to asystole.

2 RESPIRATORY FAILURE

Thomas A. Abramo
Michael Cowen
William R. Ahrens
Valerie A. Dobiesz

ANATOMY AND PHYSIOLOGY

- Respiratory failure is usually preceded by respiratory insufficiency, characterized by impaired exchange of oxygen and carbon dioxide despite an increase in the work of breathing.
- Infants and young children have relatively narrow airways, highly elastic and collapsible chest walls, and limited alveolar space, all of which create vulnerability to respiratory failure from many causes.
- Due to limited lung reserve, an increased respiratory rate is required to augment minute ventilation and facilitate elimination of carbon dioxide. The increased work of breathing can lead to muscle fatigue, especially in young infants, who have limited metabolic reserve.

HISTORY AND PHYSICAL EXAMINATION

- Most patients with respiratory difficulty will present to the emergency department with a history of difficulty breathing. Coughing and wheezing are common complaints. In infants, difficulty bottle feeding can indicate respiratory compromise—it signifies dyspnea on exertion.
- Patients with a past medical history of prematurity with bronchopulmonary dysplasia, asthma, or cystic fibrosis are at increased risk for respiratory compromise.

- Mental status is an important indicator of respiratory status. Restlessness, anxiety, and irritability may indicate significant respiratory insufficiency. Extreme agitation and lethargy are ominous signs of potential impending respiratory arrest.
- An increased respiratory rate is virtually always present in patients with respiratory distress. In infants and children, however, normal respiratory rate is age dependent, and is influenced by factors such as mental status and body temperature.
- Retractions result from the use of accessory muscles of respiration and imply significant respiratory distress. They can result from both upper and lower airway disease.

LABORATORY STUDIES

- Pulse oximetry is a rapid and useful way to assess a patient's oxygen status. It does not give any information about P_{CO_2} or acid–base status, and can be unreliable in low perfusion states.
- Measurement of arterial blood gas provides a relatively comprehensive picture of respiratory and acid–base status. Strictly speaking, respiratory failure occurs when Pa_{O_2} is less than 60 mm Hg despite supplemental oxygen of 60%, or Pa_{CO_2} of greater than 60 mm Hg.
- Arterial blood gas measurement must be viewed in the context of a patient's baseline respiratory status; patients with underlying lung disease may have chronic hypoxia and CO_2 retention.

ASSISTED VENTILATION

INDICATIONS

- Progressive muscle fatigue (common in infants and young children)
- Apnea
- Inability to maintain a patent airway (common in patients with altered mental status)
- Refractory shock (to decrease the work of breathing)
- Controlled ventilation (as in increased intracranial pressure)
- Progressive hypoxia or hypercarbia despite maximum therapy

BAG-VALVE-MASK VENTILATION

- Prior to establishing an artificial airway, it may be necessary to provide artificial ventilation via bag-valve-mask (BVM) ventilation.

- The two types of bags available for artificial ventilation are the anesthesia bag and the self-inflating bag. The anesthesia bag maintains filling by a constant inflow of oxygen. It has the advantage of supplying a very high concentration of oxygen, but requires a very tight mask-face seal and takes considerable expertise to use it correctly.
- Self-inflating bags require less training, and can provide 60 to 90% inspired oxygen when used with a reservoir and an oxygen flow rate of 10 to 15 L/min. Three sizes are available: 250 mL for neonates, 450 mL for infants and young children, and 1000 mL for adults.
- Circular masks, as opposed to triangular shaped, are utilized for infants and young children.
- Ventilatory assistance begins with establishing a patent airway. If a cervical spine injury is suspected, stabilize the head and neck. Open the airway with the jaw-thrust maneuver. If no cervical spine injury is suspected, the head-tilt chin-lift maneuver may be utilized (see Fig. 4-1 for details).
- Clear the airway of secretions.
- An oropharyngeal airway can bypass obstruction from the tongue; it should span the distance from the central incisor to the angle of the mandible. It can induce vomiting in conscious patients. A nasopharyngeal airway can also bypass the tongue; its diameter should approximate that of the patient's nostril.
- Infants are ventilated at a rate of 20 to 30 breaths per min; older children at a rate of 16 to 20 breaths per min. Adequate ventilation is assured by the presence of chest expansion and bilateral breath sounds on auscultation.
- Prolonged BVM ventilation can produce gastric distension, which can impede ventilation. This can be alleviated by decompression with nasogastric suction.

ADVANCED AIRWAY MANAGEMENT

- Endotracheal intubation and rapid sequence intubation are discussed in Chapter 5.

BIBLIOGRAPHY

Berry AM, Brimacombe JR, Verghese C: The laryngeal mask airway in emergency medicine, neonatal resuscitation and intensive care medicine. *Int Anesthesiol Clin* 36:91–109, 1998.

Cardoso MM, Banner MJ, Melker RJ, et al: Portable devices used to detect endotracheal intubation during emergency situations: A review. *Crit Care Med* 26:957–964, 1998.

Gausche M, Lewis RJ, Stratton SJ, et al: A prospective randomized study of the effect of out of hospital pediatric endotracheal intubation on survival and neurological outcome. *JAMA* 283:783–790, 2000.

Hirschl RB: Support of respiratory failure in the pediatric surgical patient. *Curr Opin Pediatr* 14:459–469, 2002.

Richman PB, Nashed AH: The epidemiology of cardiac arrest in children and young adults: Special considerations for ED management. *Am J Emerg Med* 17:264–270, 1999.

Saugstad OD: Practical aspects of resuscitating asphyxiated neonates and infants. *Eur J Pediatr* 157(suppl):S11–S15, 1998.

Sullivan KJ, Kissoon N: Securing the child's airway in the emergency department. *Pediatr Emerg Care* 18:122–124, 2002.

Ward KR, Yearly DM: End-tidal carbon dioxide monitoring in emergency medicine, clinical applications. *Acad Emerg Med* 5:637–646, 1998.

QUESTIONS

1. Which of the following findings does not typically indicate respiratory difficulty in pediatric patients?
   A. Coughing
   B. Wheezing
   C. Difficulty in bottle feeding
   D. Tachypnea
   E. Vomiting

2. A 5-year-old boy with a history of asthma presents in severe respiratory distress. Which of the following may be an indication for assisted ventilation in this patient?
   A. A Pa_{O_2} less than 70 on arterial blood gas measurement on room air
   B. Progressive hypoxia or hypercarbia despite maximum therapy
   C. A respiratory rate greater than 60 on arrival
   D. An allergy to steroids
   E. A history of multiple prior intubations for respiratory failure

3. Which of the following is true regarding bedside tests used in determining respiratory status?
   A. Pulse oximetry has replaced the need to obtain arterial blood gas measurements.
   B. Pulse oximetry can help to determine acid–base status.
   C. Arterial blood gas measurements help to determine the respiratory and acid–base status.
   D. Respiratory failure occurs when the Pa_{O_2} is less than 60 mm Hg.
   E. Pulse oximetry is highly reliable in low perfusion states.

4. A 3-year-old boy presents to the ED after being struck by a car while running across the street. The father is carrying the boy in his arms. The patient is brought to the resuscitation area and is noted to be unresponsive and has no gag reflex. Which of the following is correct regarding management of his airway?

   A. Triangular-shaped masks for bag-valve-masks are used in infants and young children.
   B. A patent airway should be established using a head-tilt chin-lift maneuver.
   C. The head and neck should be stabilized while establishing a patent airway.
   D. An oropharyngeal airway should be placed and should span from the central incisor to the hyoid bone.
   E. The patient should be ventilated at 10 to 12 breaths per min.

5. Which of the following is true regarding respiratory failure in pediatric patients?
   A. Respiratory failure is usually sudden without any preceding respiratory symptoms.
   B. Infants and young children have relatively narrow airways making them susceptible to respiratory failure.
   C. Patients with a history of cystic fibrosis have a decreased risk of respiratory compromise.
   D. Mental status changes, such as anxiety, are indicative of a good response to therapy.
   E. Retractions indicate lower airway disease.

ANSWERS

1. E. Respiratory difficulty may present in pediatric patients with coughing, wheezing, and an increased respiratory rate. In infants, difficulty in bottle feeding may indicate respiratory compromise as it signifies dyspnea on exertion.

2. B. In this patient, progressive hypoxia or hypercarbia despite maximum therapy may be an indication for assisted ventilation. Generally, the need to use assisted ventilation is a clinical decision and is not based on arterial blood gas measurements or pulse oximetry alone. This decision is made based on the patient's response to therapy. Although a patient with a history of multiple prior intubations is at considerable risk, this alone is not an indication for assisted ventilation.

3. C. Pulse oximetry assesses a patient's oxygen status but does not give any information about P_{CO_2} or acid–base status and can be unreliable in low perfusion states. Arterial blood gas measurements provide a comprehensive picture of respiratory and acid–base status. Respiratory failure can be defined as $Pa_{O_2} < 60$ mm Hg despite supplemental oxygen of 60% or $Pa_{CO_2} > 60$ mm Hg, but it must be viewed in the context of a patient's baseline respiratory status as a patient with chronic lung disease may have chronic hypoxia and hypercarbia.

4. C. This patient needs ventilatory assistance and treatment should begin by establishing a patent airway. The patient is at risk for cervical spine injury and needs his head and neck stabilized with subsequent jaw-thrust maneuver to establish a patent airway. The head-tilt chin-lift maneuver should only be used if no cervical spine injury is suspected. Circular masks are used for infants and young children for bag-valve-mask ventilation. An oropharyngeal airway may be a useful adjunct to maintain a patent airway in this patient but should span from the central incisor to the angle of the mandible. Infants are ventilated at rate of 20 to 30 breaths/min, older children at a rate of 16 to 20 breaths/min.

5. B. Respiratory failure is usually preceded by respiratory symptoms indicating an increase in work of breathing. Infants and young children have relatively narrow airways, highly elastic and collapsible chest walls, and limited alveolar space, all of which create vulnerability to respiratory failure. Patients with a history of cystic fibrosis are at increased risk for respiratory compromise. Mental status is an important indicator of respiratory status and changes may indicate significant respiratory insufficiency. Retractions from accessory muscle use can result from both upper and lower airway disease.

3 SHOCK

Robert A. Wiebe
Susan M. Scott
William R. Ahrens
Heather M. Prendergast

INTRODUCTION

- Shock is characterized by insufficient delivery of vital nutrients to the tissues and inadequate removal of the waste products of cellular metabolism. The clinical manifestations of shock result from both the metabolic consequences of cell dysfunction and the compensatory mechanisms activated to preserve metabolic integrity.
- Shock can be classified clinically as:
  - Compensated—tissue perfusion is maintained and blood pressure is generally preserved
  - Decompensated—compensatory mechanisms are unable to maintain organ perfusion, and blood pressure may fall

  - Irreversible—a devastating physiologic cascade refractory to the most aggressive treatment
- The major etiologies of shock are:
  - Hypovolemia
  - Sepsis
  - Cardiac disease
  - Illness resulting in maldistribution of intravascular volume

PATHOPHYSIOLOGY

- Shock affects all organ systems. Tissue perfusion is disrupted fundamentally.
  - The work of breathing increases.
  - Cardiac output and blood pressure are altered.
  - Decreased renal perfusion results in oliguria and in severe cases, can cause renal failure.
  - Shunting of blood to the heart and brain leaves the gastrointestinal tract vulnerable to ischemic injury.
  - Activation of the coagulation cascade can result in disseminated intravascular coagulation.
  - Hypoxia, hypercarbia, and hypoperfusion of the brain can result in variable degrees of neurologic injury.
- Many of the systemic manifestations of shock result from chemical mediators that affect myocardial function, pulmonary and systemic vasomotor tone, vascular integrity, and platelet function. In this sense, shock behaves as a systemic inflammatory disease. Specific inflammatory mediators include many metabolites of arachidonic acid, including leukotrienes, thromboxanes, prostaglandins, and platelet-activating factor. Cytokines produced by macrophages and other cells are the principle mediators of septic shock. Activation of the complement system can lead to increased vascular permeability and hypotension.

HYPOVOLEMIC SHOCK

- Hypovolemic shock results from a decrease in circulating intravascular volume. Common causes in pediatric patients include:
  - Severe gastroenteritis
  - Acute hemorrhage
  - Fluid loss secondary to burns
- Severely decreased intravascular volume associated with hypovolemic shock results in decreased cardiac output and impaired peripheral perfusion. If there is delayed or inadequate volume replacement, compensatory mechanisms can fail and decompensated shock can result.

SEPTIC SHOCK

- Sepsis is a response to invading microorganisms and the toxins they produce. Current terminology refers to the systemic inflammatory response syndrome (SIRS) that can occur in infection, resulting in derangement in temperature, heart rate, respiratory rate, and white blood cell count; in severe cases, hypotension, organ dysfunction, and death can result.
- The early, or hyperdynamic, phase of septic shock is characterized by normal or high cardiac output. Blood pressure may be normal, though pulse pressure may be widened. Systemic vascular resistance is increased, pulses are bounding, and the extremities are pink and warm. Patients may be tachypneic.
- Cardiac dysfunction and poor peripheral perfusion characterize the late phase of septic shock. Mental status is usually impaired, and the extremities are cool, with diminished or absent pulses. Hypotension may be present, and is an ominous sign.

DISTRIBUTIVE SHOCK

- Distributive shock results from disruption in the integrity of the intravascular compartment.
- In anaphylactic shock, an acute allergic reaction resulting from the interaction of an allergen with specific IgE antibodies can cause respiratory difficulties or profound hypotension. Common causes of anaphylaxis include foods, bee and wasp stings, drugs, and latex rubber.
- Neurogenic shock can result from severe spinal cord injury. It is caused by a complete loss of sympathetic vasomotor tone and consequent vasodilatation.

CARDIOGENIC SHOCK

- Cardiogenic shock results from a primary disruption of the heart as a pump. In infants and young children, cardiogenic shock most commonly results from:
  ○ Arrhythmias
  ○ Congenital lesions that obstruct the left-ventricular outflow tract
  ○ Myocarditis

RECOGNITION AND MANAGEMENT

- In infants and young children, the early phase of shock is notoriously difficult to detect. This is largely because compensatory mechanisms can preserve perfusion until late in the disease course, when sudden collapse can occur.
- In severe cases, patients may present with a complaint of "not acting right" or difficulty breathing.
  ○ Hypovolemic shock is usually accompanied by a history of vomiting and diarrhea.
  ○ In septic shock, there is usually a history of febrile illness.
  ○ In anaphylaxis, there is almost always a history compatible with an acute allergic event.
  ○ Cardiogenic shock is generally preceded by a period of increasing respiratory distress due to pulmonary congestion.
- Infants and young children rely on increased heart rate to maintain cardiac output, since they have limited ability to increase ejection fraction. Tachycardia is the most sensitive sign of circulatory compromise in children. It is, however, relatively nonspecific.
- In early, or compensated shock, blood pressure can be normal or elevated due to increased systemic vascular resistance. However, peripheral pulses may be diminished compared to central pulses, and distal extremities may be cool. Hypotension is a late and ominous sign. It may be accompanied by mottling of the skin.
- In the early phase of septic shock, peripheral pulses may be increased and the extremities pink and warm. Hypotension eventually results.
- Hypoperfusion of the brain can result in irritability or lethargy. Babies in shock may fail to recognize their parents, or have a diminished response to pain.

LABORATORY DATA

- Elevation of the white blood cell count or an increased percentage of immature neutrophils supports the diagnosis of bacterial infection. Neutropenia in the context of fever and shock suggests overwhelming infection.
- In early shock, arterial blood gas may reveal respiratory alkalosis. In the later phases, metabolic acidosis generally results from anaerobic metabolism due to impaired tissue perfusion. Serum lactate may also be elevated.
- Hypocalcemia is common in shock.
- Elevation of blood urea nitrogen and creatinine indicate prerenal azotemia due to hypoperfusion.

TREATMENT

- Treatment of the patient in shock strives to restore perfusion and oxygenation to the brain, heart, and kidneys. The underlying etiology is also addressed.

- Oxygen is administered immediately, and the adequacy of ventilation assured. Intubation and assisted ventilation are indicated in cases of fulminant shock or when hypotension and acidosis are not quickly corrected by fluid resuscitation. In septic and cardiogenic shock, assisted ventilation may decrease the work of breathing and restore metabolic balance.
- Immediate fluid resuscitation is necessary in patients with hypovolemic and septic shock. Isotonic crystalloid, either 0.9 normal saline or lactated Ringer's solution, is administered in a bolus of 20 mL/kg, as rapidly as possible. Perfusion is reassessed by evaluating heart rate, peripheral pulses, color, mental status, and blood pressure. If there is little or no improvement, another 20-mL bolus is administered, and perfusion is reassessed. In severely dehydrated or septic patients, further 20 mL/kg boluses may be necessary. Patients in septic shock can require particularly massive amounts of fluid to restore perfusion. In ideal settings, invasive monitoring may be necessary.
- Patients with anaphylactic shock require the emergent administration of 1:1000 epinephrine. Current literature suggests that it is most effectively administered intramuscularly. Rapid infusion of crystalloid is also indicated, as are antihistamines. A delayed or biphasic reaction can occur after the initial insult in up to 3 to 6% of patients, requiring delayed administration of epinephrine. Steroids may ameliorate the delayed reaction.

PHARMACOLOGIC AGENTS

- Pharmacologic therapy is indicated in patients who do not achieve adequate perfusion despite sufficient volume replacement.
  - Inotropic agents increase myocardial activity.
  - Chronotropic agents increase heart rate.
  - Most agents possess both characteristics in a dose-dependent fashion.
- The most commonly used drugs are the sympathomimetic amines, which include:
  - Endogenous catecholamines: epinephrine, norepinephrine, and dopamine
  - Synthetic catecholamines: dobutamine and isoproterenol
- At lower doses, epinephrine has a predominantly inotropic effect, with an increase in stroke volume and cardiac index.
  - At higher doses, alpha stimulation predominates, causing vasoconstriction and increased vascular resistance.
  - Some clinicians prefer epinephrine in refractory septic shock because of possible depletion of endogenous catecholamines.

- Norepinephrine has predominantly alpha effects and produces profound vasoconstriction.
  - It is used predominantly in shock refractory to other vasoactive agents, especially for septic shock.
- Dopamine is an endogenous catecholamine with cardiac adrenergic, peripheral adrenergic, and renal dopaminergic effects.
  - At low doses, it may increase renal blood flow and glomerular filtration.
  - In moderate doses, its effect is predominantly inotropic.
  - At high doses, it causes peripheral vasoconstriction.
  - Response to dopamine in septic shock may be poor.
- Dobutamine is a synthetic catecholamine that increases cardiac contractility and decreases systemic vascular resistance.
  - It is useful in the treatment of myocardial dysfunction associated with shock.
  - Higher doses may cause dysrhythmias.
- Isoproterenol is used primarily in the treatment of bradycardia and hypotension associated with heart block refractory to atropine. Its use is associated with tachydysrhythmias and myocardial ischemia.
- Phosphodiesterase inhibitors, such as amrinone and milrinone, are a newer and useful category of inotropic agents.
  - They enhance myocardial contractility by preventing the metabolism of cyclic AMP.
  - There is a concomitant decrease in systemic vascular resistance.
  - Beneficial characteristics of these agents include decreased tendency to cause tachydysrhymias and no increase in myocardial oxygen consumption.
  - They are used primarily in volume-resuscitated patients as adjuncts to sympathomimetics in an effort to improve myocardial function.

BIBLIOGRAPHY

Carcillo JA, Fields AI, American College of Critical Care Medicine Task Force Committee Members: Clinical practice parameters for hemodynamic support of pediatric and neonatal patients in septic shock. *Crit Care Med* 30:1365–1378, 2002.

Lee JM, Greenes DS: Biphasic anaphylactic reactions in pediatrics. *Pediatrics* 106:762–766, 2000.

Qwan P: ABC of allergies: Anaphylaxis *BMJ* 316:1442–1446, 1998.

QUESTIONS

1. A 5-year-old is brought to the emergency department for evaluation of several days of intense vomiting and diarrhea. On examination, you find a moderately dehydrated child. You are concerned that the child is in early shock. Which of the following findings would be expected in this child?
   A. Mottling of the skin
   B. Respiratory alkalosis
   C. Hypotension
   D. Elevated lactate levels
   E. Prerenal azotemia

2. You are informed by EMS dispatch that a 7-year-old child is being brought to your emergency department for an allergic reaction. On arrival, the child is clearly in anaphylactic shock. The management priority in this patient would be which of the following?
   A. Antihistamines
   B. Assisted ventilation
   C. Fluid resuscitation
   D. Epinephrine
   E. IV steroids

3. A 10-year-old child with leukemia is brought to the emergency department for fevers and altered mental status. The patient is hypotensive and not responding to fluid resuscitation. Which of the following pharmacologic agents would **NOT** be recommended in this patient?
   A. Epinephrine
   B. Norepinephrine
   C. Dopamine
   D. Vancomycin
   E. Broad spectrum antibiotics

ANSWERS

1. B. In early shock, the arterial blood gas may reveal respiratory alkalosis. As the tissue perfusion worsens, metabolic acidosis develops, lactate levels begin to increase, and patients can demonstrate a prerenal azotemia. Hypotension is a later finding and is associated with mottling of the skin.

2. D. Patients with anaphylactic shock require the emergent administration of 1:1000 epinephrine intramuscularly. Rapid infusion of crystalloid is also indicated. Steroids are useful in preventing the delayed or biphasic reaction commonly seen in these patients. Oxygen should be administered immediately, and the adequacy of ventilation assessed prior to assisted ventilation.

3. C. Pharmacologic therapy is indicated in patients who do not achieve adequate perfusion despite sufficient volume replacement. The most commonly used drugs are the sympathomimetic amines. Dopamine is an endogenous catecholamine; however, the response to dopamine in septic shock may be poor. In a patient with presumed septic shock, it is advisable to begin broad spectrum antibiotics after cultures have been obtained. Due to the potential for antibiotic resistance of pneumococci in some regions, it is reasonable to add vancomycin to the antibiotic regimen when treating infection due to an unknown agent.

4 CARDIOPULMONARY RESUSCITATION

Patricia A. Primm
Rebecca R. Reamy
William R. Ahrens
Heather M. Prendergast

PEDIATRIC BASIC LIFE SUPPORT

- The primary goal of basic life support (BLS) is to provide oxygenation and ventilation to children in cardiopulmonary arrest. Prompt initiation is important, since most cardiac arrests in children result from asphyxial processes.
- The sequence of pediatric BLS differs from adult BLS in the timing of EMS notification, which is delayed until rescue breathing is initiated.

THE SEQUENCE

- Determine unresponsiveness
  ○ If the patient is unresponsive, call for help.
  ○ Do not move a patient who may have suffered a cervical spine injury; if necessary, an assistant can provide in-line-traction to minimize movement of the neck.
- Open the airway
  ○ In most cases, the airway is opened using the head-tilt chin-lift maneuver.
  ○ If a cervical spine injury is suspected, open the airway using the jaw-thrust maneuver (Fig. 4-1).
- Provide rescue breathing
  ○ In an infant, the rescuer places his or her mouth or mouth-to-mask device over the patient's nose and mouth.
  ○ In a larger patient, the rescuer makes a mouth-to-mouth seal, pinching the patient's nose closed with

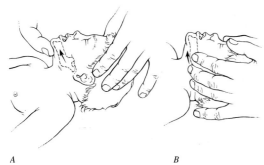

A   *B*

FIG. 4-1. *A*. The head-tilt chin-lift maneuver. To open the airway, place one hand on the patient's forehead and tilt the head back into a neutral or slightly extended position. Use the index finger of the other hand to lift the patient's mandible upward and outward. *B*. the jaw-thrust maneuver. To open the airway while maintaining cervical spine stabilisation, place two or three fingers under each side of the lower jaw angle and lift the jaw upward and outward. Maintain the neck in a neutral position manually to prevent craniocervical motion.

the forefinger of the same hand used to maintain the head tilt.
- Two slow, 1- to 1.5-s rescue breaths are provided.
- Adequate volume will cause the chest to rise.
- Rescue breathing then continues at 20 breaths per min.
- If ventilation is difficult, consider an airway obstruction, either from malpositioning or a foreign body.
• Assess the pulse
- In infants, feel for a pulse over the femoral or brachial arteries.
- In children, palpate a pulse over the carotid artery.
- If no pulse is appreciated, begin chest compressions.
• Chest compressions
- Chest compressions are performed to provide some circulation to vital organs.
- Figure 4-2 demonstrates appropriate techniques in infants and children. Note that for infants, Fig. 4-2 B demonstrates the preferred technique when there is more than one rescuer.
- In infants, compressions should achieve a depth of 0.5 to 1 inch; for children a depth of 1 to 1.5 inches is desirable.
- For all ages, the rate is 100 compressions per min.
- After every fifth compression, allow a 1- to 1.5-s pause for ventilation.
- After 20 cycles of compressions/ventilation, recheck for a pulse.
• Notify Emergency Medical Services (EMS)
- When performing CPR on children less than 8 years of age, activate the EMS system after 1 minute of resuscitation.

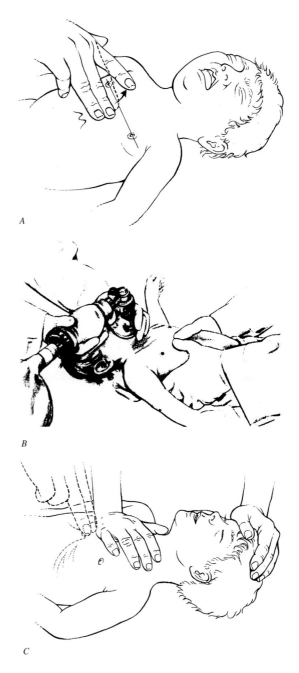

A

B

C

FIG. 4-2. *A*. Proper finger position for chest compressions in infants less than 1 year of age: use two fingers to perform compressions one finger width below the intermammary line. *B*. Proper technique for two-thumb encircling hands technique over lower third of sternum. *C*. Proper finger position for chest compressions in children from 1 to 8 years of age: use the heel of one hand to perform compressions two finger widths above xiphoid.

FOREIGN BODY ASPIRATION

• Foreign body aspiration is possible in infants and children who develop sudden respiratory distress associated with coughing, gagging, or stridor. Do not intervene if the patient has spontaneous coughing, can speak, and has adequate ventilation. If the cough becomes ineffective, respiratory distress worsens, or the patient loses consciousness, intervention is necessary.

○ Treat infants with foreign body obstruction with a combination of back blows and chest thrusts.
  ▪ The baby is placed face down over the rescuer's forearm, supported on the thigh, with the head lower than the trunk.
  ▪ Five blows are delivered between the scapula with the back of the rescuer's hand.
  ▪ The baby is then turned over and five thrusts are delivered to the chest over the mid sternum.
  ▪ If the foreign body is observed, it is removed but blind finger sweeps are not advised.
  ▪ If the obstruction persists, repeat the process.
○ In the conscious child with an airway foreign body, the Heimlich maneuver is performed.
  ▪ The rescuer stands behind the victim, with his or her arms around the chest and the thumb side of one fist placed above the umbilicus and below the xiphoid, and grasped by the other hand.
  ▪ Five upward thrusts are delivered in succession.
○ The unconscious victim with an airway foreign body is placed on his or her back.
  ▪ The rescuer straddles the patient's hips and places the heel of one hand above the umbilicus and below the xiphoid, and grasps it with the other hand.
  ▪ Five quick upward thrusts are then delivered.
  ▪ If the foreign body is dislodged and visualized, it is removed and if necessary, rescue breathing is begun.
  ▪ If the obstruction remains, the abdominal thrusts are repeated.

PEDIATRIC ADVANCED LIFE SUPPORT

• The focus of pediatric advanced life support (PALS) is on the delivery of:
  ○ Oxygen
  ○ Fluids
  ○ Medication
  ○ Cardioversion or defibrillation
  ○ Basic CPR
• Oxygen is the most basic and important adjunct in a pediatric arrest. In most patients undergoing CPR, oxygen is administered via bag-valve mask or endotracheal tube.
• Most patients undergoing resuscitation require the delivery of intravenous fluids and medication.
  ○ This can be done intravenously; however, in young infants or in patients in whom venous access cannot

otherwise be obtained, an intraosseous cannula is an acceptable alternative.
  ▪ There is no upper age limit to the use of an intraosseous cannula.
  ▪ Contraindications include osteogenesis imperfecta, osteopetrosis, and, ipsilateral fracture.
  ▪ Complications include extravasation of fluid, fracture, osteomyelitis, and fat emboli (not thought to be clinically significant).
  ○ Some clinicians may be comfortable with inserting central venous catheters in infants and children.
• Lipid soluble drugs, can be administered through an endotracheal tube:
  ○ Epinephrine
  ○ Atropine
  ○ Naloxone
  ○ Lidocaine
  ○ Absorption may be unreliable
• In children who do not respond to oxygenation and ventilation, a fluid bolus of 20 mL/kg of normal saline is appropriate in an attempt to achieve a perfusing rhythm.
• In infants and children, epinephrine is the drug of choice for asystole and hypoxia-induced bradycardia, both with and without a pulse.
  ○ These are the most common arrest rhythms seen in pediatrics.
  ○ In an arrest situation, epinephrine's α-mediated vasoconstriction may increase aortic diastolic pressure and improve coronary perfusion.
  ○ The use of "high dose epinephrine" has been deemphasized; it has not been found to improve survival.
  ○ See Fig. 4-3 for dosing recommendations.
• Atropine sulfate is a parasympatholytic drug that accelerates sinus and atrial pacemakers and increases atrioventricular node conduction.
  ○ It is much less useful in pediatric resuscitations than epinephrine.
  ○ The primary indication for atropine is the unusual setting of atrioventricular block bradycardia.
  ○ It is also indicated to prevent the vagally induced bradycardia associated with some intubations.
  ○ See Table 4-1 for recommended dosing.
  ○ The minimum recommended dose of 0.1 mg reflects the propensity of atropine to cause paradoxical bradycardia if not given in a vagolytic dose.
• Sodium bicarbonate has been used in the past as a buffer for the metabolic acidosis that usually accompanies arrest situations.
  ○ Currently, there are no data to support its use in pediatric resuscitation.
  ○ The exception to this is an arrest associated with hyperkalemia.

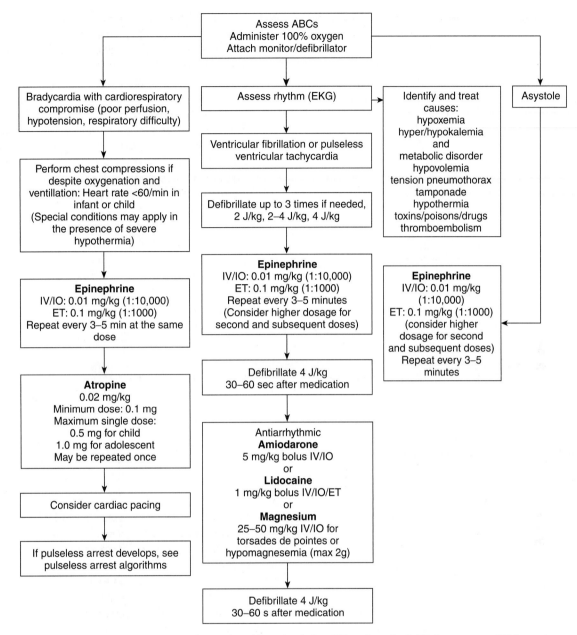

FIG. 4-3 CPR decision tree. ABCs, airway, breathing, circulation; ET, endotracheal; IO, intraosseous; IV, intravenous.

- Complications associated with the use of bicarbonate include:
  - hypernatremia
  - hyperosmolarity
  - metabolic alkalosis
- Although ionized hypocalcemia is common in prolonged arrests, the administration of calcium has not been found to improve outcome, including the scenario of pulseless electrical activity (PEA).
  - Calcium is indicated in cases of:
    - hyperkalemia
    - hypocalcemia
    - hypermagnesemia
    - calcium channel blocker overdosage
  - Calcium chloride is more bioavailable than calcium gluconate.
- Hypoglycemia is very common in stressed in infants and young children, who have high glucose requirements and little glycogen reserve. Glucose must be monitored carefully in critically ill pediatric patients, and hypoglycemia treated aggressively. See Table 4-1 for dose.
- Amiodarone is an antiarrhythmic agent effective in the treatment of both supraventricular and ventricular

TABLE 4-1   Drugs Used in Pediatric Advanced Life Support

DRUG	DOSE	REMARKS
Adenosine	0.1 mg/kg Repeat dose: 0.2 mg/kg Maximum single dose: 12 mg	Rapid IV/IO bolus Rapid flush to central circulation Monitor ECG during dose
Amiodarone	5 mg/kg	Rapid IV bolus Maximum dose 15 mg/kg/day Hypotension may occur Consider for VF pulseless VT
Atropine sulfate	0.2 mg/kg Minimum dose: 0.1 mg Maximum single dose: 0.5 mg in child, 1.0 mg in adolescent	IV/IO/ET Tachycardia and pupil dilation may occur but not fixed dilated pupils
Calcium chloride 10%	20 mg/kg; may be increased	Slowly IV for K, Mg, calcium channel blocker toxicity
Epinephrine for bradycardia	IV/IO: 0.01 mg/kg (1:10,000) ET: 0.1 mg/kg (1:1000)	Be aware of effective dose of preservatives administered (if preservatives are present in epinephrine preparation) when high doses are used
For asystolic or pulseless arrest	All doses IV/IO: 0.01 mg/kg (1:10,000) ET: 0.1 mg/kg (1:1000) Doses as high as 0.2 mg/kg may be effective	Tachyarrhythmia, hypertension may occur
Glucose	0.5–1.0 g/kg 1–2 mL/kg D50W 2–4 mL/kg D25W	IV/IO
Lidocaine	1 mg/kg per dose	Rapid bolus IV, ET
Magnesium	25–50 mg/kg Maximum 2 g/dose	Use for torsades, hypomagnesemia
Naloxone	<20 kg: 0.1 mg/kg >20 kg: 2.0 mg	For total reversal of narcotic effect Use repeat doses
Sodium bicarbonate	1 mEq/kg per dose or 0.3 × kg × base deficit	Infuse slowly and only if ventilation is adequate

ABBREVIATIONS: IV, intravenous route; IO, intraosseous route; ET, endotracheal route.

DRUG	DOSE, μg/kg/min	DILUTION IN 100 mL D5W, mg/kg	IV INFUSION RATE, μg/kg/min
Dopamine	2–20	6	1 mL/h = 1
Dobutamine	2–20	6	1 mL/h = 1
Epinephrine	0.1–1.0	0.6	1 mL/h = 0.1
Lidocaine	20–50	6	1 mL/h = 1

arrhythmias. Its use in pediatrics has been primarily in children with atrial and ventricular ectopy following heart surgery.

○ In a pediatric arrest, amiodarone may be considered after three unsuccessful defibrillations; this recommendation is an extrapolation from the adult experience.

• Lidocaine suppresses ventricular ectopy and raises the threshold for ventricular fibrillation. Lidocaine is indicated in:

○ Ventricular tachycardia associated with a pulse, where it is administered prior to cardioversion

○ Pulseless ventricular tachycardia

○ Ventricular fibrillation, where it is administered after electrical defibrillation

ELECTRICAL THERAPY

• Defibrillation is the unsynchronized depolarization of the myocardium.

○ Defibrillation is the primary treatment of:

▪ ventricular fibrillation

▪ pulseless ventricular tachycardia

○ In children weighing less than 10 kg, pediatric paddles are used for defibrillation and cardioversion.

○ Initial defibrillation is at 2 J/kg; subsequent defibrillation is at 4 J/kg.

• Automated external defibrillators (AEDs) can be used in the out-of-hospital setting in children 8 years of age or older in the extraordinarily rare patient with

TABLE 4-2   Differentiating Types of Tachycardia

	SINUS TACHYCARDIA	SUPRAVENTRICULAR TACHYCARDIA	VENTRICULAR TACHYCARDIA
Rate	Usually < 220	Usually > 220	120–400
QRS complex	Narrow	Usually narrow	Wide
Beat-to-beat variability	Yes	No	No
P waves	Yes (although they may be difficult to see)	No	No

ventricular fibrillation or pulseless ventricular tachycardia. Ideally, the patient's weight should be greater than 25 kg. Even at this weight, the escalating energy doses delivered by a monophasic AED are a cause for concern.
- Transcutaneous pacing may be effective in children with symptomatic bradycardia refractory to medical management.
  - If the child weighs less than 15 kg, small or medium adhesive-backed electrodes are recommended.

MANAGEMENT OF SUPRAVENTRICULAR TACHYCARDIA

- Supraventricular tachycardia (SVT) is the most common cardiac dysrhythmia causing cardiac instability in infants and children.
  - SVT produces heart rates from 220 to 300/min.
  - There is usually no beat-to-beat variation.
  - SVT is usually due to a reentrant mechanism.
- The electrocardiogram usually reveals a narrow QRS complex without discernable P waves.
  - If there is aberrant conduction, the QRS complex can be wide, and SVT becomes difficult to distinguish for VT (Table 4-2).
- The patient with SVT who is in shock or has severe congestive heart failure requires immediate synchronized cardioversion.
  - The initial dose is 0.5 to 1 J/kg.
  - If SVT persists, increase the dose to 1 to 2 J/kg.
- Adenosine is an endogenous nucleoside that interrupts the reentrant pathway.
  - It has a half life of about 10 s.
  - Ideally, it is administered rapidly via a proximal vein.
  - The dose is 0.1mg per kg.
  - If the initial dose is unsuccessful, the second dose is doubled.
  - The maximum dose is 12 mg.
- Stable SVT may respond to vagal maneuvers, such as carotid massage or placing an icebag over the patient's face.
- The use of verapamil in infants and children with SVT is discouraged.

BIBLIOGRAPHY

American Heart Association: Guidelines 2000 for cardiopulmonary resuscitation and emergency cardiovascular care. *Curr Emerg Cardiovasc Care* 11:3, 2000.

American Heart Association: Pediatric basic life support. *Circulation* 102(suppl I):I–253, 2000.

American Heart Association: Pediatric advanced life support. *Circulation* 102(suppl I):I–291, 2000.

Luten R, Wears RL, Broselow J, et al: Managing the unique size-related issues of pediatric resuscitation: Reducing cognitive load with resuscitation aids. *Acad Emerg Med* 9:840–847, 2002.

QUESTIONS

1. You are attending a little league baseball game when a 7-year-old boy collapses on the field and is unresponsive. Which of the following reflects the management priority in this child?
   A. Activation of the EMS system
   B. Assess the child for a pulse
   C. Begin chest compressions
   D. Remove the child from the field
   E. Provide rescue breathing
2. Which of the following represent the primary difference between the sequence of pediatric BLS and adult BLS?
   A. Transport times tend to be shorter in pediatric BLS.
   B. Timing of EMS notification is different in pediatric BLS.
   C. The goal in pediatric BLS is to provide basic transport only.
   D. There are no differences between the sequence of pediatric and adult BLS.
   E. There tend to be less prehospital interventions in pediatric BLS.
3. You are at a restaurant when you observe a child apparently choking. The child is able to cough and can speak. Which of the following describes the **MOST** appropriate intervention?
   A. Activate EMS
   B. Attempt to remove the foreign body if visualized in oropharynx
   C. Administer a combination of back blows and chest thrusts

D. If the cough becomes ineffective, perform the Heimlich maneuver

E. Place the child on the floor and administer five abdominal thrusts

4. Which of the following is a recognized **CONTRAINDICATION** for use of an intraosseous cannula?

A. Age greater than 8 years

B. Fracture involving the ipsilateral leg

C. Previous unsuccessful attempt at placement

D. Multiple traumatic injuries

E. There are no absolute contraindications.

5. Which of the following medications/inventions is no longer recommended in pediatric cardiac arrest situations?

A. Amiodarone

B. Epinephrine

C. Sodium bicarbonate

D. Atropine

E. Defibrillation

6. A toddler is brought to the Emergency Department for evaluation. Per the parents, the child has been ill for 1 week. This morning, the parents noted that the child appeared to have difficulty breathing. Upon examination, you note a rapid pulse but clear lung fields. The cardiac monitor reveals a narrow complex QRS complex at a rate of 240/min. Which of the following statements is **TRUE** regarding management?

A. The patient is symptomatic and requires immediate synchronized cardioversion.

B. The patient is symptomatic and may respond to vagal maneuvers.

C. The patient is dehydrated and requires a fluid bolus at 20 mL/kg.

D. The patient is symptomatic and requires adenosine intravenously.

E. The patient is symptomatic and requires verapamil intravenously.

ANSWERS

1. E. In an unresponsive child, the management priority is to open the airway and provided rescue breathing. Prompt initiation is important since most cardiac arrests in children result from asphyxial processes. If the patient is pulseless, then begin chest compressions. Activate the EMS system after 1 min of resuscitation.

2. B. The primary difference in the sequence of pediatric BLS and adult BLS is the timing of EMS notification. In pediatric cases, notification of BLS should be delayed until rescue breathing is initiated. Rapid transport and oxygenation are common goals of both pediatric and adult BLS.

3. D. In a patient with spontaneous coughing and the ability to speak, no intervention is required. Attempts at visualization and removal in this setting can be harmful. In cases where the patient develops respiratory distress and is conscious, the Heimlich maneuver should be performed. Abdominal thrusts should only be performed on the unconscious victim. Chest and back blows are recommended for infants.

4. B. Recognized contraindications for placement of intraosseous cannula include ipsilateral fracture, osteopetrosis, and osteogenesis imperfecta. There is no upper age limit to the use of an intraosseous cannula. Trauma or unsuccessful previous attempts are not contraindications.

5. C. Sodium bicarbonate has been used in the past as a buffer for the metabolic acidosis in arrest situations. Except in the cases of known hyperkalemia, the use of bicarbonate is not supported in the literature.

6. D. Supraventricular tachycardia is the most common cardiac dysrhythmia in infants and children. Patients in shock or with signs of congestive heart failure require immediate synchronized cardioversion. Adenosine can be used for symptomatic patients. Verapamil is no longer recommended. Only patients with stable SVT should have vagal maneuvers attempted.

5 RAPID SEQUENCE INTUBATION

Rustin B. Morse
Grace Arteaga
William R. Ahrens
Valerie A. Dobiesz

INTRODUCTION

- Rapid sequence intubation (RSI) involves the use of pharmaceutical agents to rapidly produce unconsciousness and paralysis, as well as agents to prevent the physiologic responses to RSI including pain, cardiac instability, and increased intracranial pressure.

- Emergency department patients who require RSI are assumed to have a full stomach, and are at risk for aspiration.

PREPARATION

- The initial assessment of the patient requiring RSI includes:
  ∘ History of present illness
  ∘ Current medications

TABLE 5-1 Congenital Anatomic Features Associated with a Difficult Airway

Macroglossia [trisomy 21 (Down's syndrome)]
Micrognathia (Pierre Robin syndrome)
Midface hypoplasia (Apert's or Crouzon's syndrome)
Cleft lip
Cleft palate
Subglottic stenosis
Tonsillar hypertrophy

- ○ Allergies
- ○ Medical problems that may affect the process of resuscitation
- The physical examination focuses on factors that may impede intubation:
  - ○ Facial trauma
  - ○ Congenital anomalies (Table 5-1)
  - ○ Tonsillar hypertrophy
  - ○ Limitation of cervical spine mobility
- The patient's length is a fast and a relatively accurate method of determining weight, appropriate size of the endotracheal tube, and drug doses. The Broselow tape measure provides the EM physician with this information.
- Children less than 8 years of age are intubated using uncuffed tubes, as their narrow airway prevents air leakage.
- Necessary adjunctive equipment includes:
  - ○ Suction adaptable to rigid and flexible catheters
  - ○ McGill forceps
  - ○ Laryngeal-mask airways
  - ○ Preintubation therapy
- To minimize the risk of aspiration, it is generally desirable to avoid BVM prior to RSI. In some cases, however, this is not possible.
- Patients are "preoxygenated" via a tight-fitting non-rebreather mask to deliver as close to 100% O_2 as possible; this washes nitrogen out of the lungs, and provides a reservoir of oxygen to protect against hypoxemia during laryngoscopy and intubation.
- Atropine is an adjunctive medication used to decrease airway secretions.

TABLE 5-2 RSI Time Course

−5 minutes	Focused history and physical examination
	Provide 100% oxygen; avoid BMV
	Place patient on monitors
	Draw up medication doses
	Assemble airway equipment
−3 minutes	Premedicate (optional)
−1 minute	Give sedative and paralytic
	Apply cricoid pressure
0 minutes	Perform intubation
+1 minute	Confirm placement of endotracheal tube
	Secure endotracheal tube
	Release cricoid pressure

TABLE 5-3 Adjunctive Premedications

MEDICATION	IV DOSE	INDICATIONS
Atropine	0.02 mg/kg Min: 0.1 mg Max: 0.5 mg in child 1 mg in adolescent	Age < 5 years Required if ketamine or succinylcholine are used
Lidocaine	1–3 mg/kg	Head injury Suspected elevated ICP
Fentanyl	2–5 µg/kg	Head injury Suspected elevated ICP Pain control

- ○ Atropine also has vagolytic action that may protect against bradycardia
- ○ Atropine should be considered for patients less than 5 years of age, and in patients who are to receive succinylcholine or ketamine.
- Lidocaine may be useful in head-injured patients to reduce the increase in intracranial pressure associated with intubation.
- RSI time course (Table 5-2)
- Adjunctive premedications (Table 5-3)

SEDATION

- Patients undergoing RSI invariably require sedation. The choice of the agent used depends especially on the patient's hemodynamic status and the suspicion for increased intracranial pressure (Table 5-4).
- Midazolam is a short-acting benzodiazepine with anti-convulsant and amnestic properties.
  - ○ It may produce hypotension in a hypovolemic patient.
- Etomidate is a sedative-hypnotic with a rapid onset of action that:
  - ○ Does not cause cardiovascular instability.
  - ○ Decreases intracranial pressure.
  - ○ Can cause vomiting.
  - ○ Can cause myoclonic activity.
  - ○ May suppress the synthesis of cortisol.
  - ○ Is a useful agent in a head-injured or hypotensive patient.

TABLE 5-4 Sedative Agents for Use in Rapid Sequence Intubation

SEDATIVES	IV DOSE (mg/kg)	ONSET (min)	EFFECTS ON	
			BP	ICP
Midazolam	0.2–0.4	1–2	Minimal	Minimal
Etomidate	0.2–0.4	< 1	Minimal/increase	Decrease
Thiopental	2–5	< 1	Decrease	Decrease
Ketamine	1–2	1	Minimal/increase	Increase
Propofol	2–3	< 1	Decrease	Decrease

- Thiopental is a rapid acting sedative with anticonvulsant properties that:
  ◦ Reduces intracranial pressure.
  ◦ May cause hypotension in hypovolemic patients.
  ◦ May also cause histamine related bronchospasm.
- Fentanyl is an opioid agonist with a rapid onset of action that:
  ◦ Provides both analgesia and sedation.
  ◦ Produces minimal cardiovascular side effects.
  ◦ Is useful as a continuous infusion after intubation to provide sedation.
- Ketamine is a dissociative sedative and analgesic.
  ◦ Sympathomimetic properties can result in:
    ▪ mild increase in heart rate and blood pressure.
    ▪ bronchodilation.
  ◦ Ketamine has potential use as an adjunctive agent in patients with status asthmaticus who require intubation.
  ◦ Side effects include:
    ▪ rise in intracranial pressure
    ▪ increase in airway secretions, which may be prevented by atropine or glycopyrrolate.

PARALYSIS

- Paralytic agents (Table 5-5) are characterized as:
  ◦ Depolarizing—bind to nicotinic receptors and trigger prolonged depolarization of the muscle fiber, rendering it refractory to further acetylcholine stimulation.
  ◦ Nondepolarizing—competitively block acetylcholine from stimulating nicotinic receptors and triggering muscle movement.
- Succinylcholine is a rapid-acting depolarizing agent with a relatively short duration of action commonly used in RSI.
  ◦ It can cause transient muscle fasciculations that can be blocked by premedication with a "defasiculating" dose (generally 1/10 of the paralyzing dose) of a nondepolarizing agent.
  ◦ It can cause hypertension and tachycardia in older children.
  ◦ In younger children and infants, reflex bradycardia may result.

TABLE 5-6   Use of Succinylcholine in RSI

Contraindications
 Muscular dystrophy
 Neuromuscular disease
 Significant burn/trauma that occurred at least 48 hours prior and within the previous 10 days
Personal or family history of malignant hyperthermia
Preexisting hyperkalemia

Considerations
 Defasciculate if >5 years of age
 Premedicate with atropine in children
 Must use atropine prior to a second dose
 Treat malignant hyperthermia with dantrolene

    ▪ the risk of bradycardia may be minimized by pretreatment with atropine.
- In certain clinical scenarios, succinylcholine can cause serious hyperkalemia and is contraindicated (Table 5-6).
- Vecuronium is a nondepolarizing agent with a relatively long duration of action.
- Rocuronium is also nondepolarizing but it induces paralysis more rapidly than vecuronium.
  ◦ It is increasingly used as the agent of choice in RSI.
- The choice of both a sedating agent and paralytic will depend on the clinical situation (Table 5-8).

ENDOTRACHEAL INTUBATION

- After preoxygenation, the patient's head is placed in the "sniffing" position to align the oral, pharyngeal, and laryngeal vectors. Hyperextension is avoided.
- A straight laryngoscope blade is preferred in infants.
- During insertion of the laryngoscope blade and subsequently the endotracheal tube, pressure is placed on the cricoid cartilage to occlude the esophagus and prevent potential aspiration. Cricoid pressure (Sellick maneuver) can also assist in visualizing the vocal cords.
- The appropriate sized endotracheal tube is inserted between the vocal cords (Table 5-7).
- Accurate endotracheal tube placement is confirmed by auscultating bilateral breath sounds. Disposable end-tidal CO_2 detectors also confirm tracheal intubation by changing from purple to yellow in the presence of exhaled carbon dioxide.

TABLE 5-5   Paralytic Agents

MEDICATION	IV DOSE (mg/kg)	TIME TO INTUBATING CONDITIONS (min)	RECOVERY (min)
Vecuronium	0.1–0.2	1–2	At least 20
Rocuronium	1–1.2	< 1	At least 20
Rapacuronium	1.5–2	< 1	5–7
Succinylcholine	1–2	< 1	3–10

TABLE 5-7   Endotracheal Tube and Laryngoscope Sizes for Pediatric Patients

AGE	TUBE SIZE[a]
Endotracheal Tubes	
Newborn	3.0 uncuffed
Newborn–6 months	3.5 uncuffed
6–18 Months	3.5–4.0 uncuffed
18 Months–3 years	4.0–4.5 uncuffed
3–5 years	4.5 uncuffed
5–6 years	5.0 uncuffed
6–8 years	5.5–6.0 uncuffed
8–10 years	6.0 cuffed
10–12 years	6.0–6.5 cuffed
12–14 years	6.5–7.0 cuffed

AGE	BLADE SIZE
Laryngoscopes	
Premature (<2.5 kg)	0 straight
0–3 Months	1.0 straight
3 Months–3 years	1.5 straight
3–12 Years	2.0 straight or curved
Adolescents	3.0 straight or curved

[a] Appropriate depth of insertion can be estimated by multiplying the tube size by 3.

- In some cases, a laryngeal mask airway (LMA) can serve as a bridge to intubation. The LMA is a tube with a deflatable, mask-like projection at the distal end. The LMA is passed through the pharynx and advanced until resistance is felt when the mask is over the tracheal opening. Inflating the cuff occludes the hypopharynx but leaves the distal end open over the glottic opening, providing a patent airway.

SPECIAL SITUATIONS

- If intravenous access cannot be achieved, the clinician may consider using succinylcholine 4 mg/kg IM or rocuronium 2 mg/kg IM to achieve paralysis.

TABLE 5-8   RSI Options for Special Clinical Situations

SCENARIO	PREMEDICATION	SEDATION
Head injury or elevated ICP		
Normal BP	Lidocaine Consider fentanyl	Etomidate, thiopental, midazolam
Decreased BP	Lidocaine Consider fentanyl	Etomidate, midazolam, low dose thiopental
No head injury or elevated ICP		
Normal BP		Etomidate, thiopental, midazolam, ketamine
Decreased BP		Etomidate, ketamine, midazolam
Status epilepticus		Thiopental, midazolam
Status asthmaticus	Atropine Midazolam	Ketamine
Any patient <5 years old	Atropine	
Ketamine used	Atropine Midazolam	

BIBLIOGRAPHY

Berry AM, Brimacombe JR, Verghese C: The laryngeal mask airway in emergency medicine, neonatal resuscitation and intensive care medicine. *Int Anesthesiol Clin* 36:91–109, 1998.

Doobinin KA, Nakagawa TA: Emergency department use of neuromuscular blocking agents in children. *Pediatr Emerg Care* 16:441–447, 2000.

Guldner G, Schultz J, Sexton P, et al: Etomidate for rapid-sequence intubation in young children: Hemodynamic effects and adverse events. *Acad Emerg Med* 10:134–139, 2003.

McAllister JD, Gnauk KA: Rapid sequence intubation of the pediatric patient. *Pediatr Clin North Am* 46:1249–1284, 1999.

Perry J, Lee J, Wells G: Rocuronium versus succinylcholine for rapid sequence induction intubation (Cochrane Review). *Cochrane Database Syst Rev* (1):CD002788, 2003.

Richman PB, Nashed AH: The epidemiology of cardiac arrest in children and young adults: Special considerations for ED management. *Am J Emerg Med* 17:264–270, 1999.

QUESTIONS

1. Which of the following is true regarding rapid sequence intubation in children?
   A. The patient's age is a relatively accurate method of determining weight, appropriate size of endotracheal tube, and drug doses.
   B. All children should have uncuffed endotracheal tubes.
   C. It is reserved for children with empty stomachs (>6 h after last meal).
   D. Children should be preoxygenated prior to intubation.
   E. Lidocaine is used to decrease airway secretions.
2. Which of the following is the optimal choice of sedation agent to use in RSI in a head-injured child that is hypotensive?

A. Etomidate
B. Midazolam
C. Thiopental
D. Ketamine
E. Lidocaine

3. Succinylcholine may be used as a paralytic agent in RSI. Which of the following statements is correct regarding this agent?
   A. It has a relatively long duration of action.
   B. It is a depolarizing agent.
   C. In younger children, hypertension and tachycardia may occur.
   D. It may cause hypokalemia.
   E. It is used without a sedation agent.

4. A 3-month-old child presents to the ED in severe respiratory distress and you determine that intubation is necessary. Which of the following is true in the management of this patient?
   A. The patient's head should be hyperextended.
   B. A curved laryngoscope blade is optimal in this patient.
   C. Accurate ET tube placement may be confirmed using an end-tidal CO_2 detector.
   D. Cricoid pressure (Sellick maneuver) is used to secure the ET tube.
   E. A cuffed tube is indicated in this age group.

5. Which of the following is true regarding the use of a laryngeal mask airway (LMA)?
   A. It has replaced the need for endotracheal tube placement.
   B. It is placed using a laryngoscope blade.
   C. Is only used in the operating room as a temporizing measure.
   D. Is used instead of a nasogastric tube with an endotracheal tube to prevent aspiration.
   E. It occludes the hypopharynx but leaves the distal end patent over the glottis, providing a patent airway.

ANSWERS

1. D. The patient's length is a fast and relatively accurate method of determining weight, appropriate size of ET tube, and drug doses. The Broselow tape measure provides this information. Children less than 8 years of age are intubated using uncuffed tubes, as their narrow airway prevents leakage. Any patient requiring RSI is assumed to have a full stomach and is at risk for aspiration. Children should be preoxygenated prior to intubation to protect against hypoxemia. Lidocaine may be useful in head-injured patients to reduce the increase in intracranial pressure associated with intubation.

2. A. Etomidate is a sedative-hypnotic agent that does not cause cardiovascular instability and also decreases intracranial pressure. Midazolam and thiopental may cause hypotension in hypovolemic patients. Ketamine may cause an elevation of intracranial pressure. Lidocaine is not a sedative agent.

3. B. Succinylcholine is a rapid-acting depolarizing agent with a relatively short duration of action. It can cause hypertension and tachycardia in older children but in younger children and infants, it can cause a reflex bradycardia. This bradycardia can be minimized with pretreatment with atropine. In certain clinical situations, it can cause hyperkalemia. Patients undergoing RSI require sedation.

4. C. The patient's head should be placed in the "sniffing" position and hyperextension should be avoided. A straight laryngoscope blade is preferred in infants. Accurate endotracheal tube placement can be confirmed by auscultating bilateral breath sounds as well as by using disposable end-tidal CO_2 detectors. Cricoid pressure is used to occlude the esophagus and prevent potential aspiration and may help in visualizing the vocal cords. Children less than 8 years of age need uncuffed tubes.

5. E. The laryngeal mask airway (LMA) can serve as a bridge to intubation and can be safely used in the ED. The LMA is a tube with a deflatable mask-like projection at the distal end. The LMA is passed through the pharynx and advanced until resistance is felt when the mask is over the tracheal opening. No laryngoscope blade is needed. Inflating the cuff occludes the hypopharynx but leaves the distal end open over the glottic opening, providing a patent airway.

6 RESUSCITATION OF THE NEWBORN INFANT

Collin S. Goto
Brian A. Bates
William R. Ahrens
Heather M. Prendergast

INTRODUCTION

• At birth, termination of placental blood flow and the onset of respirations trigger a decrease in pulmonary artery pressure and an increase in systemic blood pressure.

TABLE 6-1 Supplies for Neonatal Resuscitation

RESUSCITATION TRAY (STERILE) RESUSCITATION EQUIPMENT

Bulb syringe	Radiant warmer
DeLee suction trap	Wall suction with manometer
Endotracheal tubes	Oxygen source with flow meter
(2.0, 2.5, 3.0, 3.5, and 4.0 mm)	Resuscitation bag (250–500 mL) with manometer
Suction catheters (6, 8, 10, and 12F)	Laryngoscope
Endotracheal tube stylet	Laryngoscope blades (Miller 0 and 1)
Umbilical catheter (3.5, 5F)	Charts with proper drug doses and equipment
Syringes (5, 10, and 20 mL)	sizes for various sized neonates.
Three-way stopcock	Warmed linens
Feeding tubes (5, 8F)	
Towels	
Umbilical cord clamps	
Scissors	

- The ductus arteriosis begins to close and blood that had bypassed the pulmonary circulation begins to flow through the lungs.
- Within days, the pattern of the mature circulation is established.
- Pertinent history of the pregnancy includes:
  - Date of conception
  - Presence of maternal hypertension or diabetes
  - Maternal drug abuse
  - Vaginal spotting or bleeding
  - Duration of rupture of membranes
  - Presence of any meconium in the amniotic fluid
- Prior to deliver, appropriate equipment is readied (Table 6-1).
- After delivery, the physiologic status of the newborn is ascertained by calculating the Apgar score (Table 6-2).
  - Heart rate is assessed by auscultation or by counting the umbilical pulse.
  - Color is best assessed by evaluating the tongue, as virtually all newborns have peripheral cyanosis.
  - The quality of muscle tone is an indicator of the degree, if any, of intrauterine ischemia.
  - Infants with a 1-minute Apgar score of 7 or greater usually require only tactile stimulation and suctioning of the mouth and nose.
  - Infants with Apgar scores of 4 to 6 require more aggressive resuscitation, including vigorous stimulation and probably bag-valve-mask ventilation.

- Patients with Apgar scores less than 3 have suffered severe intrauterine asphyxia and require full resuscitative methods (Fig. 6-1).
- Newborns are placed on their backs in the sniffing position, in a radiant warmer.
  - It is crucial to avoid hypothermia
  - Drying the infant will provide tactile stimulation and prevent evaporative heat loss.
  - A bulb syringe or DeLee suction trap is usually adequate for suctioning the infant's nose and mouth. If wall suction is used, pressure should not exceed 100 mm Hg. Suctioning is discontinued if bradycardia develops.
- Infants with even mild bradycardia are presumed to be hypoxic.
  - Supplemental oxygen can be delivered by "blow-by" at 5 L/min.
    - There is no contraindication to the short-term use of oxygen.
- Bag-valve-mask (BVM) ventilation is indicated in the presence of apnea and bradycardia (heart rate less than 100 beats/min) that does not respond to stimulation.
  - If a self-inflating bag is used, the pop-off valve is bypassed, since the initial pressure required to inflate the newborn's lung can exceed 40 cm H_2O.
  - BVM of the asphyxiated infant has traditionally utilized 100% oxygen; current evidence indicates that

TABLE 6-2 The Apgar Score

PARAMETER	0	1	2
Color	Blue, pale	Body pink, extremities blue	Totally pink
Muscle tone	None, limp	Slight flexion	Active, good flexion
Heart rate	0	< 100	> 100
Respiration	Absent	Slow, irregular	Strong, regular
Reflex irritability (response to nasal catheter)	None	Some grimace	Good grimace, crying

To calculate Apgar score, add numbers for all parameters together.

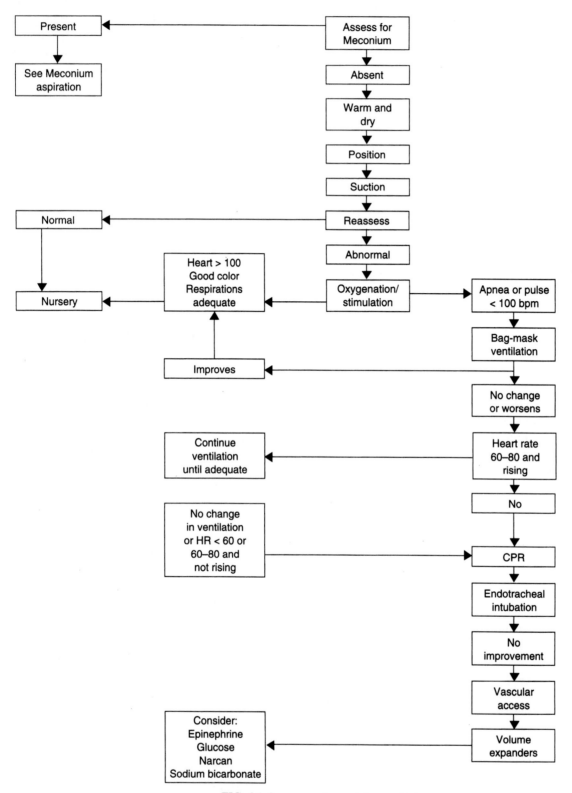

FIG. 6-1 Summary of neonatal resuscitation.

the majority of infants will successfully respond to room air.

- The initial rate of assisted ventilation is 40 to 60 breaths/min.
- After 15 to 30 s, the infant is reassessed.
  - If resuscitation has been successful, the heart rate will increase and the infant will develop spontaneous respirations.
  - If the heart rate is less than 60 beats/min despite 30 s of bvm, intubation is indicated.
- In addition to persistent bradycardia, intubation is also indicated when there is a need for endotracheal suctioning (meconium aspiration) or in severely premature babies.
  - The size of the endotracheal tube depends on the patient's weight:
    - 3.5 mm internal diameter for a 3 to 4 kg newborn
    - 3.0 mm for a 2 kg newborn
    - 2.5 mm for a 1 kg newborn
    - The appropriately sized endotracheal tube is easily inserted and there is no significant air leak.
  - Inadvertent intubation of the right mainstem bronchus is a common occurrence.
    - There is limited data on the use of CO_2 detectors to determine appropriate endotracheal tube placement in newborns.
- Chest compressions in infants may be more effective at providing artificial circulation than in adults. Chest compressions are indicated in newborns for:
  - asystole
  - heart rates that remain below 60 beats/min despite 30 s of adequate BVM
  - The preferred technique for delivering chest compressions is shown in Fig. 4-2B.
  - The ratio of chest compressions to ventilation is 3:1, with 90 chest compressions and 30 artificial breaths per min.
  - The infant's heart rate is reassessed every 30 s and compressions are continued until a sustained rate of 60 beats per min is attained.

VASCULAR ACCESS

- If peripheral access is not rapidly obtained, the umbilical vein is cannulated.
  - The single, thin-walled vein is distinguished from the paired, muscular umbilical arteries.
  - The vein is exposed by trimming the umbilical cord with a scalpel.
  - A 3.5 or 5 French umbilical catheter is then inserted far enough to achieve a free-flowing blood return. Deep catheterization is avoided.
  - The base of the cord is tied off with a ligature, and the catheter sutured in place.

PHARMACOLOGIC AGENTS

- Epinephrine is the drug of choice for asystole and for bradycardia that persists despite effective ventilation and chest compressions for more than 30 s.
  - The dose is 0.1 to 0.3 mL/kg (0.01 to 0.03 mg/kg) of the 1:10,000 solution.
  - It is administered every 3 to 5 min.
  - In newborns, the same dose is administered intratracheally as intravenously.
- Glucose is necessary to correct hypoglycemia in the newborn, defined as blood glucose less than 40 to 50 mg/dL.
  - Hypoglycemia is common in infants of diabetic mothers and in premature infants.
  - Symptoms include hypo- or hypertonia, jitteriness, and seizures.
  - Glucose is administered in a dose of 2 to 4 mL/kg of a 10% solution. A continuous infusion of 6 to 8 mg/kg per min may be necessary.
- Naloxone hydrochloride is a narcotic antagonist indicated to reverse respiratory depression in infants whose mothers received narcotics within 4 h of delivery.
  - The dose is 0.1 mg/kg intravenously, intramuscularly, subcutaneously, or intratracheally.
  - In infants of narcotic addicted mothers, a severe withdrawal syndrome can result.
- Sodium bicarbonate is a buffer that may have a role in cases of prolonged resuscitation associated with metabolic acidosis.

VOLUME RESUSCITATION

- Conditions that produce acute blood loss in newborns include:
  - Placenta previa
  - Abruptio placenta
  - Twin-to-twin transfusion
  - Premature clamping of the umbilical cord
- The detection of acute blood loss in the newborn is extremely difficult.
  - Profound vasoconstriction can preserve pulses and blood pressure despite significant blood loss.
  - The only clinical clue may be that the baby appears inordinately pale.
- The average hemoglobin for a full-term infant is 16.8 mg/dL; however, in acute hemorrhage, hemoglobin does not reflect the severity of blood loss.
- In the setting of suspected acute hemorrhage, volume resuscitation is initiated with normal saline or Ringer's lactate solution administered in aliquots of 10 mL/kg. In some cases, cross-matched packed red blood cells may be necessary.

SPECIAL SITUATIONS

MECONIUM

- Meconium aspiration in the newborn can cause:
  - Airway obstruction
  - Hyperinflation
  - Severe pneumonitis
  - Profound hypoxia
  - Persistence of the fetal circulation
  - Meconium aspiration syndrome is most likely after aspiration of thick particulate material.
- In the presence of meconium-stained amniotic fluid, the infant's nose and mouth are suctioned as the head is delivered, prior to clamping of the cord.
- The vigorous meconium-stained infant usually requires no treatment.
- If, after the delivery, the infant has poor muscle tone and depressed respirations, the trachea is intubated and suctioned to remove particulate material.
  - The endotracheal tube is connected to a meconium aspirator and wall suction.
  - Suction is applied while the tube is withdrawn.
  - The process is repeated until the trachea is free of meconium.
  - Persistent bradycardia may be a limiting factor in instituting BVM ventilation.

PREMATURITY

- The infant is considered premature if the gestational age is less than 37 weeks.
  - However, most complications occur in infants far more premature. These include:
    - perinatal asphyxia
    - pulmonary immaturity
    - intraventricular hemorrhage.
  - In some very premature babies, viability is difficult to determine. In most cases, resuscitation is indicated pending consultation with a neonatologist.

DIAPHRAGMATIC HERNIA

- The vast majority of diaphragmatic hernias occur on the left side.
- The clinical scenario usually includes:
  - scaphoid abdomen
  - cyanosis
  - respiratory distress
- Hypoplasia of the lungs, especially the left, is present.
- BVM is contraindicated as distension of the bowel can worsen pulmonary status.

- The infant is intubated and ventilated.
- A nasogastric tube is placed to decompress the bowel.
- Transfer to a tertiary care facility is arranged.

INFANT OF A DIABETIC MOTHER

- Complications in infants of diabetic mothers include:
  - Macrosomia
  - Birth asphyxia
  - Polycythemia
  - Hyperviscosity syndrome
  - Renal vein thrombosis
  - Hyperbilirubinemia
  - Congenital anomalies, especially affecting the heart
  - Hypocalcemia
  - Severe hypoglycemia

GASTROSCHISIS AND OMPHALOCELE

- Gastroschisis and omphalocele occur when there is herniation of abdominal contents (usually the intestines) through the umbilical ring.
  - An omphalocele is covered by peritoneum.
  - A gastroschisis is not covered.
- The organs are covered with a sterile, saline-soaked dressing and sterile plastic bag.
- A nasogastric tube is placed.
- Volume resuscitation may be required.
- Transfer to a tertiary care facility is arranged.

BIBLIOGRAPHY

American Heart Association in Collaboration with the International Liaison Committee on Resuscitation: Guidelines 2000 for cardiopulmonary resuscitation and emergency cardiovascular care: An international consensus on science. Part 2. Neonatal Resuscitation. *Circulation* 102 (suppl I):I-343, 2000.

Finer NN, Horbar JD, Carpenter JH: Cardiopulmonary resuscitation in the very low birth weight infant: The Vermont Oxford Network Experience. *Pediatrics* 104:428–434,1999.

Saugstad OD: Resuscitation of newborn infants with room air or oxygen. *Semin Neonatol* 6:233–239, 2001.

Shankaran S: The postnatal management of the asphyxiated term infant. *Clin Perinatol* 29:675–692, 2002.

Vento M, Asanel M, Jastar J, et al: Resuscitation with room air instead of 100% oxygen prevents oxidative stress in moderately asphyxiated term neonates. *Pediatrics* 107:642–647, 2001.

Wiswell TE, Gannon CM, Jacob J, et al: Delivery room management of the apparently vigorous meconium stained neonate. Results of the multicenter, international collaborative trial. *Pediatrics* 105:1–7, 2000

QUESTIONS

1. A 17-year-old female presents to the emergency department in premature labor. In obtaining the pertinent history of the pregnancy, which of the following would **NOT** be necessary to obtain immediately?
   A. Maternal drug abuse
   B. Vaginal spotting or bleeding
   C. Date of conception
   D. Presence of maternal hypertension or diabetes mellitus
   E. Obstetric history

2. Which of the following is **NOT** an indication for bag-value-mask (BVM) ventilation?
   A. Apnea
   B. Bradycardia not responsive to tactile stimulation
   C. Heart rate less than 100 beats/ min
   D. Bradycardia induced by suctioning
   E. Bradycardia despite 30 s of BVM

3. Which of the following is a **DEFINITE** indication for intubation of a newborn?
   A. Apnea
   B. Meconium aspiration
   C. Bradycardia not responsive to tactile stimulation
   D. Use of a DeLee suction trap
   E. Mild hypoxia

4. A newborn infant is delivered in the emergency department. Initial Apgar score is 5. Which of the following is the **MOST** appropriate in management of this newborn?
   A. Begin vigorous stimulation and bag-valve-mask ventilation
   B. Begin tactile stimulation by drying the infant
   C. Begin supplemental oxygen by "blow-by" at 5 L/min
   D. Begin chest compressions
   E. Begin endotracheal suctioning

5. A newborn infant is rushed to the emergency department by frantic parents following an unplanned home delivery. On arrival, the infant is cyanotic, has poor muscle tone, and a heart rate of 60 bpm. You immediately intubate the newborn and begin chest compressions. A bedside glucose is 60 mg/dL. Which of the following is the **MOST** appropriate in management of this infant?
   A. Administer dextrose in a dose of 2 mL/kg of a 10% solution

   B. Administer naloxone hydrochloride at a dose of 0.1 mg/kg intravenously or intramuscularly
   C. Administer epinephrine at a dose of 0.1–0.3 mL/kg of the 1:10000 solution
   D. Begin endotracheal suctioning
   E. Begin volume resuscitation

6. Which of the following conditions would **NOT** produce acute blood loss in newborns?
   A. Abruptio placenta
   B. Persistence of the fetal circulation
   C. Placenta previa
   D. Premature clamping of the umbilical cord
   E. Twin-to-twin transfusion

7. A patient presents in active labor at 36 weeks of gestation. Upon delivery of the newborn, you note that the infant is cyanotic and in severe respiratory distress. On physical examination, you note a scaphoid abdomen. You suspect a diaphragmatic hernia is present. Which of the following is **CONTRAINDICATED** in the management of this infant?
   A. Bag-mask ventilation
   B. Intubation
   C. Nasogastric tube
   D. Transfer to a tertiary care facility
   E. Chest compressions for brachycardia

ANSWERS

1. E. Pertinent history of pregnancy includes the following: date of conception, presence of maternal hypertension or diabetes, maternal drug abuse, vaginal spotting or bleeding, duration of rupture of membranes, presence of any meconium in the amniotic fluid. Obtaining this information will help alert the clinician to any potential problems.

2. E. Indications for bag-valve-mask (BVM) ventilation include apnea and bradycardia (heart rate less than 100 beats/min) unresponsive to stimulation. In newborns with persistent bradycardia (heart rate less than 60 beats/min) despite 30 s of adequate BVM, endotracheal intubation is required.

3. B. Meconium aspiration can cause a number of complications in newborns including airway obstruction, severe pneumonitis, profound hypoxia, persistence of the fetal circulation, and the meconium aspiration syndrome. In cases where there is meconium aspiration and the infant exhibits poor muscle tone and depressed respirations, endotracheal intubation is necessary to remove the particulate material.

4. A. Infants with Apgar scores of 4 to 6 require more aggressive resuscitation including vigorous stimulation and probably bag-mask ventilation. Patients with

Apgar scores less than 3 have suffered severe intrauterine asphyxia and require full resuscitative methods.

5. C. Epinephrine is the drug of choice for bradycardia that persists despite effective ventilation and chest compressions for more than 30 s. Glucose is necessary to correct hypoglycemia in the newborn, defined as blood glucose less than 40 to 50 mg/dL.

6. B. Conditions that produce acute blood loss in newborns include placenta previa, abruption placenta, twin-to-twin gestation, and premature clamping of the umbilical cord. Persistence of the fetal circulation is often a complication of meconium aspiration.

7. A. In management of a diaphragmatic hernia, the newborn is intubated and ventilated, bag-value-mask is contraindicated as distension of the bowel can worsen pulmonary status. A nasogastric tube is indicated to decompress the bowel. Transfer to a tertiary care facility is recommended.

7 SUDDEN INFANT DEATH SYNDROME AND APPARENT LIFE-THREATENING EVENTS

Collin S. Goto
Thomas T. Mydler
William R. Ahrens
Heather M. Prendergast

SUDDEN INFANT DEATH SYNDROME

- Sudden infant death syndrome (SIDS) is defined as the sudden death of an infant less than 1 year of age that remains unexplained after a thorough case investigation, including a complete autopsy, examination of the death scene, and review of the clinical history.
- The peak incidence of SIDS is between 2 and 4 months of life.
- The rate is highest among African Americans and American Indians, intermediate among Hispanics and Caucasians, and lowest among Asians.
- The cause or causes of SIDS are unknown. It is likely that there are multifactorial complex interactions between an infant's underlying ability to maintain cardiorespiratory stability and various environmental factors that lead to SIDS. Risk factors for SIDS are listed in Table 7-1.
- Prone sleeping is the environmental risk factor for SIDS with the greatest potential for modification. The rate of SIDS in the United States has decreased

TABLE 7-1 Risk Factors Associated with SIDS

INFANT FACTORS	MATERNAL FACTORS
Male sex	Age < 20 years
Preterm birth	Short interpregnancy interval
Low birth weight	Unmarried
Multiple births	Low socioeconomic status
Low Apgar scores	Low educational level
Treatment in an	Inadequate prenatal care
intensive care unit	Illness during pregnancy
Congenital defects	Smoking during pregnancy
Neonatal respiratory abnormalities	Use of addictive drugs
Recent viral illness	
Previous ALTE	
Sibling who died of SIDS	
Prone sleeping position	
Sleeping on a soft surface	
Bed sharing	
Overheating	

40% since the introduction of the Back to Sleep campaign in 1994.

- Most infants who die of SIDS receive some advanced life support. The usual cardiac rhythm encountered is asystole and the prognosis for a successful resuscitation is extremely poor.
- The vast majority of babies who appear to die of SIDS are not victims of child abuse. The emergency physician and staff must approach the parents of SIDS victims with the utmost sympathy when conducting the necessary interview. Parents must be reassured that they are blameless with regard to the infant's death. Referral to a local SIDS support network may be very helpful.

APPARENT LIFE-THREATENING EVENT

- An apparent life-threatening event (ALTE) is characterized by a combination of:
  ○ Apnea (respiratory pause greater than 15 s)
  ○ Altered mental status
  ○ Pallor or cyanosis
  ○ Alteration in muscle tone
  ○ Choking
- The infant usually requires some form of resuscitation, but may recover from the event spontaneously.
- The relationship between and ALTE and SIDS is unclear, hence the term "near-miss SIDS" is no longer used to describe apparent life-threatening events.
- The differential diagnosis of ALTE is extensive and a probable cause of the event may be found in up to 50% of patients who undergo evaluation (Table 7-2).
- The history focuses on distinguishing an ALTE from common benign events that occur in infants, such as:
  ○ Normal periodic breathing

TABLE 7-2 Differential Diagnosis of an Apparent Life-Threatening Event

Central Nervous System
  Seizure
  Meningitis/encephalitis
  Head trauma (eg, child abuse)
  Increased intracranial pressure (eg, congenital hydrocephalus)
  Apnea of prematurity
  Idiopathic central apnea

Respiratory System
  Upper airway obstruction (eg, nasal congestion)
  Laryngospasm (eg, gastroesophageal reflux)
  Bronchiolitis (eg, respiratory syncytial virus)
  Pneumonia

Cardiovascular System
  Arrhythmia (eg, prolonged QT syndrome)
  Myocarditis
  Severe anemia
  Hemorrhage (eg, child abuse)

Systemic/Metabolic/Other
  Sepsis
  Hypoglycemia
  Inborn error of metabolism
  Toxins/drugs
  Factitious (eg, Munchausen's syndrome by proxy)

- Nonmalignant choking or gagging associated with feeding
- Nonpathologic muscular "jerking"
• Observations consistent with ALTE are:
  ◦ Pallor
  ◦ Cyanosis
  ◦ Hypotonia
  ◦ Persistent muscular rigidity
  ◦ Prolonged cessation of breathing
  ◦ Any infant who required aggressive resuscitation
• The evaluation of the infant with an ALTE is directed by the history, but the usual work-up includes:
  ◦ Complete blood count
  ◦ Urinalysis
  ◦ Cultures of the blood and urine
  ◦ Serum electrolytes
  ◦ Calcium
  ◦ Blood glucose
  ◦ Lumbar puncture (as directed by history and examination)
  ◦ Electrocardiogram (to screen for prolonged QT syndrome)
  ◦ Nasopharyngeal swab for respiratory syncytial virus (RSV)
  ◦ CT scan of the head (if abuse is suspected)
• The ED management of the patient with an ALTE depends on the physiologic status of the patient.
  ◦ Well-appearing patients may require only observation and cardiopulmonary monitoring.
  ◦ If sepsis is suspected, antibiotics are indicated.

• All patients with a history compatible with an ALTE require admission to the hospital.

BIBLIOGRAPHY

American Academy of Pediatrics Task Force on Infant Sleep Position and Sudden Infant Death Syndrome: Changing concepts of sudden infant death syndrome: Implications for infant sleeping environment and sleep position. *Pediatrics* 105:650–656, 2000.

Dancea A, Cote A, Rohlicek C, et al: Cardiac pathology in sudden infant death. *J Pediatr* 141:336–342, 2002.

Schwartz PJ, Stramba-Badiale M, Segantini A, et al: Prolongation of the Q-T interval and the sudden infant death syndrome. *N Engl J Med* 338:1709–1714, 1998.

Williams SM, Mitchell EA, Taylor BJ: Are risk factors for sudden infant death syndrome different at night? *Arch Dis Child* 87:274–278, 2002.

QUESTIONS

1. A 3-month-old infant is brought to the emergency department in cardiac arrest. The mother states the infant was placed in the crib several hours ago after breastfeeding. On arrival, you find no signs of trauma. Resuscitation is unsuccessful. You suspect sudden infant death syndrome (SIDS). Which of the following additional pieces of history would increase your suspicion of SIDS as the cause of death in this child?
   A. Child recently diagnosed as failure to thrive
   B. Child was 4 weeks premature
   C. Child was African American
   D. Child was a twin gestation
   E. Child was placed in supine position

2. An infant is brought to the emergency department by parents for an apparent choking episode. The parents state that during the event, the infant turned "blue" and was unresponsive for several seconds and required stimulation. Which of the following observations are **MOST** consistent with a diagnosis of apparent life-threatening event (ALTE) in this infant?
   A. Duration of symptoms lasting less than 1 min
   B. Nonmalignant choking
   C. Periodic breathing
   D. Hypotonia
   E. Flushed appearance

3. You suspect an apparent life-threatening event (ALTE) in an infant brought to the ED. On examination, the child is well-appearing. The **MOST**

appropriate disposition for this infant would be which of the following?

A. Brief ED observation of 1 to 2 h, if no recurrences then discharge home.

B. Extended ED observation of 4 to 6 h, if infant remains asymptomatic then discharge home.

C. Admit for 23-h observation to general pediatric bed.

D. Admit for 23-h observation to a monitored pediatric bed.

E. Admit to pediatric intensive care unit for continuous monitoring.

ANSWERS

1. C. Sudden infant death syndrome (SIDS) is defined as the sudden death of an infant less than 1 year of age that remains unexplained after a thorough investigation. The rate of SIDS is highest among African Americans and American Indians. The rate is lowest among Asians. Prone sleeping is an environmental risk factor for SIDS.

2. D. An apparent life-threatening event is generally a combination of apnea, altered mental status, pallor or cyanosis, alteration in muscle tone, and choking. It is important to distinguish an ALTE from common benign events that occur in infants, such as normal periodic breathing, nonmalignant choking, and nonpathologic muscular "jerking."

3. D. All patients with a history compatible with an ALTE require admission to the hospital. Well-appearing patients may require only observation and cardiopulmonary monitoring.

8 DISCONTINUATION OF LIFE SUPPORT

Brian A. Bates
William R. Ahrens
Heather M. Prendergast

INTRODUCTION

- Although it is not an "official standard," the failure of a pediatric patient to respond with a perfusing rhythm to 2 standard doses of epinephrine is highly correlated with death. The risk of a more prolonged resuscitation is salvaging a patient who languishes in a persistent vegetative state.

- Cold water drowning is perhaps the most common clinical scenario in which prolonged resuscitation has produced a neurologically viable patient. If the patient is hypothermic, resuscitation may reasonably be continued until the patient has been adequately warmed.

- Terminally ill children may have advanced directives or do-not-resuscitate orders from their attending physicians. Such directives are revocable at any time.

- Patients who suffer brain death and are candidates for organ transplant may be identified in the emergency department, although it is extremely unlikely that brain death will be declared and artificial support withdrawn. In some states, it is preferable to inform the regional organ bank about the patient's status, rather than approaching family members about organ donation.

BIBLIOGRAPHY

American Heart Association and International Liaison Committee on Resuscitation: Ethical aspects of CPR and ECC and pediatric advanced life support, in *Guidelines 2000 for Cardiopulmonary resuscitation and Emergency Cardiovascular Care. Circulation* 102(suppl 1):I-12–I-21 and I-291–I-342, 2000.

QUESTION

1. You are faced with discontinuation of life support for a pediatric patient in your emergency department. In which of the following situations would such a decision NOT be recommended?

A. Traumatic arrest with asystole on presentation and no response to initial resuscitation efforts.

B. Asystolic cardiac arrest unresponsive to repeated doses of epinephrine and atropine.

C. Child with terminal illness and advanced directives in place.

D. Severely hypothermic drowning victim

E. Hypothermic victim warmed to a rectal temp of 37°C

ANSWER

1. D. There are numerous reports of icy water drowning victims undergoing prolonged resuscitation with excellent outcomes. These patients should be adequately warmed before discontinuation of life support.

9 DEATH OF A CHILD

William R. Ahrens
Gary R. Strange
Heather M. Prendergast

INTRODUCTION

- In contrast to patients who die in the hospital or in hospice, the majority of patients who are pronounced dead in emergency departments die suddenly. Survivors are confronted with the loss of a loved one with no prior psychological preparation.

EFFECTS ON PHYSICIANS AND PARENTS

- The majority of emergency physicians feel that managing the death of a child is far more stressful than managing the death of an adult; some physicians feel that it is the most difficult aspect of their job.
- The immediate reaction of family members to the sudden loss of a child is disbelief, even though many say they knew before being told that their child had died. A sense of guilt is probably universal.

THE INTERVIEW

- The process of dealing with the patient's death begins with, and should be considered an important part of, the resuscitation.
- After the patient is pronounced dead, it is the attending physician who is responsible for telling the parents.
- The physician must introduce him- or herself, make eye contact, and address the parents by name. The language used must be direct and nonjudgmental and it cannot be overemphasized that the deceased patient should be referred to by his or her name.

AFTER THE INTERVIEW

- Most, but not all, parents find that spending time with the child is helpful. In certain cases, some family members will want to hold the body, but reluctance to do this is normal for others and is neither a pathologic response nor indicative of abuse.

FOLLOW-UP CARE

- There are many support groups available for parents who have lost children. For many surviving family members, such support groups are extremely helpful.

MANAGEMENT OF GRIEF AMONG EMERGENCY DEPARTMENT STAFF MEMBERS

- Dealing with the effect of the death of a child on the emergency department staff is also problematic. Some emergency physicians and other staff members utilize grief-counseling services, but this service is by no means universally available.
- It is likely that educating physicians and staff about the best way to communicate the death of a child to parents does help to alleviate some of the anxiety that the situation entails.
- At the very least, it creates a mutually supportive culture within the department regarding the management of death.

BIBLIOGRAPHY

Ahrens WA, Hart RG: Emergency physicians' experience with pediatric death. *Am J Emerg Med* 15:642–643, 1997.

Ahrens WA, Hart RG, Maruyama N: Pediatric death: Managing the aftermath in the emergency department. *J Emerg Med* 15:60–63, 1997.

Oliver RC, Fallat ME: Traumatic childhood death: How well do parents cope? *J Trauma* 39:303–306, 1995.

Sachetti A: Acceptance of family member presence during pediatric resuscitations in the emergency department: Effects of personal experience. *Pediatr Emerg Care* 16:85–87, 2000.

QUESTION

1. You are the only attending physician on a busy Saturday night when a 6-month-old infant in cardiac arrest is brought in by paramedics. There are no external signs of trauma. The resuscitation is unsuccessful and you pronounce the child dead. You suspect sudden infant death syndrome (SIDS). You are informed by security that the family has arrived. Which of the following would be **APPROPRIATE** when informing the parents about the death of their child?

A. To avoid having the family wait, ask the charge nurse to speak with the family concerning the child's death.

B. Question and attempt to educate the family about the risk factors for SIDS.

C. Avoid referring to the child by name as this may enhance the parents' grief.

D. Offer the family the opportunity to spend time with the child.

E. Meet the family in the hallway and quietly inform them of the child's death.

ANSWER

1. D. When speaking to a family concerning the death of a child, it is important that it is done in private and in a respectful manner. This includes bringing the family to a private location within the emergency department, introducing yourself, maintaining eye contact, and referring to the child by his or her name. It is important not to be judgmental and lay blame. You can ask the family if they would like to see their loved one. Some family members find it comforting to spend time with the deceased. It is important to contact pastoral care if the family requests.

10 EVALUATION AND MANAGEMENT OF THE MULTIPLE TRAUMA PATIENT

Michael J. Gerardi
Kemedy K. McQuillen
Gary R. Strange

EPIDEMIOLOGY

- Trauma is the leading cause of death in children <1 year of age in the United States and unintentional injury ranks as the leading cause of death from age 1 through age 34 years. Fatality rates are higher for children when compared with adults who have similar injuries.
- Motor vehicle occupant injuries are the leading cause of injury death among children aged 0 to 19 years. Other major causes of death include homicide, suicide, drowning, pedestrian/motor vehicle accidents and burns.
- Blunt injuries account for 87 percent of all childhood trauma, penetrating injuries 10 percent, and drowning 3 percent.
- Children less than 5 years old are at greatest risk from falls and child abuse. They sustain a large number of isolated head injuries.
- Six to 12 year olds are most commonly victims of motor vehicle–related trauma, as pedestrians, bicyclists, or unrestrained passengers. They sustain a large number of closed-head injuries, often in association with other injuries.
- Adolescents engage in many risk-taking behaviors, and are at high risk of homicide and suicide.

UNIQUE ASPECTS OF PEDIATRIC TRAUMA

- The pediatric skeleton and surrounding tissues have greater flexibility and less protective capabilities than does the adult skeleton. The pediatric body is also smaller, resulting in a greater force per volume with external forces being more readily transmitted to the deeper internal structures. Therefore, internal injury must always be considered in the pediatric patient, even in the absence of external signs of trauma.
- The pediatric head is proportionally larger than that of an adult and influences trauma management in the following ways:
  - Head injuries are more common in children than in adults.
  - The head is a major source of heat loss in a child.
  - The occiput is prominent in young children, decreasing in prominence from birth until age 10. This influences head positioning for airway management.
- With more white matter than gray matter, the pediatric brain has greater resilience in withstanding blunt trauma but is more susceptible to axonal shearing forces and cerebral edema. Cranial sutures are open until 18 to 24 months of age and palpation of the fontanels provides useful information regarding intracranial pressure.
- The incomplete development of the bony spine, the relatively large size of the head, and the weakness of the soft tissue of the neck predispose to spinal cord injury without radiographic abnormality (SCIWORA). A younger child's short, fat neck also makes the evaluation of neck veins and tracheal position difficult.
- The pediatric airway is significantly different than the adults:
  - The tongue is proportionally larger.
  - The larynx is more cephalad and anterior and is opposite C2–3

○ The epiglottis is "U" shaped, tilted almost 45 degrees, and more floppy, making manipulation and visualization for intubation more difficult.

○ The cricoid cartilage is the narrowest portion of the child's airway, whereas, in an adult, the glottis is the narrowest part. For this reason, uncuffed tubes should be used in children under 8 years of age.

• With more flexible ribs and less overlying fat and muscle, the child's thorax is quite pliable and allows large forces to be transmitted to underlying tissues. A child's mediastinum is also very mobile and is subject to extreme excursion with tension pneumothorax.

• Children depend on diaphragmatic excursion for ventilation. Aerophagia, with crying, expands the stomach, limits diaphragmatic excursion, and compromises a child's respiratory status.

• Pediatric abdominal organs are more at risk for injury. The liver and spleen are located more caudal and anterior than an adult's. They are pushed below the protection of the ribcage by a diaphragm that inserts at a nearly horizontal angle from birth until approximately 12 years of age and are suspended by compliant ligaments. They have less overlying protection and increased motion at impact.

• Long bones in children have growth plates (epiphyses) and are more flexible than adult bones. The growth plate is the weakest part of the bone making ligamentous injuries uncommon. Growth plates can also "camouflage" fractures on x-ray making the physical examination more sensitive than radiographs for detecting some fractures.

• Children have a high surface area to volume ratio, so they lose heat rapidly when undressed.

PREHOSPITAL CARE ISSUES

• The field care of the traumatized child may include endotracheal intubation, IV access, immobilization, and rapid transport. Care providers who do not treat and transport pediatric patients on a regular basis, though, may have difficulty and delay transport with repeated efforts at intervention. If IV access is not obtained after 2 attempts or 90 s, intraosseous (IO) access should be attempted. It is reasonable that traumatized children can be transported without vascular access or an endotracheal tube if a short transport time is expected and the airway can be temporized with bag-valve-mask ventilation.

• In general, rural systems require more aggressive initial treatment in the field due to transport times that are three to four times greater than those in urban areas.

• The advent of pediatric emergency medicine and emergency medical services for children (EMSC) has led to the development of coordinated systems of care for critically ill and injured children in many parts of the country.

INITIAL ASSESSMENT AND MANAGEMENT GUIDELINES FOR THE INJURED CHILD

• Priorities for caring for the pediatric trauma patient are outlined in Table 10-1.

• It is important to complete the primary and secondary surveys and execute the resuscitation in an orderly fashion to ensure against missing injuries.

• Children with serious injuries require continual reassessment. Repeat vital signs should be performed every 5 min during the primary survey and every 15 min while in the ED awaiting transfer or operative intervention. See Table 10-2 for normal vital signs.

PRIMARY SURVEY

• **A**irway and cervical spine stabilization
• **B**reathing and ventilation
• **C**irculation and hemorrhage control
• **D**isability (neurologic screening examination)
• **E**xposure
• If serious alterations are encountered, resuscitative care is performed prior to moving onto the next system.

AIRWAY

• Secure the airway while stabilizing the neck. Open the airway with the jaw-thrust maneuver and clear the oropharynx of debris and secretions.

• Cervical spine injury should be assumed until a normal examination and radiographs are obtained. Although bony cervical spine injuries are less common in children, the characteristics of the pediatric cervical spine predispose it to ligamentous disruption and dislocations without bony injury.

• Initiate bag-valve-mask ventilation for inadequate respiratory effort. Cricoid pressure must be applied to prevent gastric insufflation.

• Endotracheally intubate the patient for:
  ○ Inability to ventilate the child by bag-valve-mask methods
  ○ The need for prolonged control of the airway
  ○ Prevention of aspiration in a comatose child

TABLE 10-1   Initial Approach to the Pediatric Trauma Patient

1. Before Arrival
Prepare all equipment
Mobilize trauma team and call for assistance (respiratory therapy, nurses, radiology technician)
Have O-negative blood on stand-by

2. First 5 Minutes
Assess respiration, oxygenation; ventilate if necessary
Check pulse oximetry reading
Cardiac and blood pressure monitoring
Consider end-tidal CO_2 monitoring if available
Maintain C-spine immobilization
Perform needle or tube thoracostomy if tension pneumothorax suspected
Intubate or attain surgical airway if indicated
Treat obvious wounds: apply pressure to external hemorrhage; dressing to sucking chest wound

3. Second 5 Minutes
Reassess airway, ventilation, oxygenation, temperature
Assess perfusion
Volume resuscitation: 20 mL/kg with crystalloid and repeat as necessary
Consider uncross matched or O-negative blood
Assess neurologic status
Send laboratory specimens: type and cross, CBC, amylase, liver transaminases, BUN, creatinine, glucose, electrolytes, ABG, urinalysis
Needle pericardiocentesis, thoracotomy, and aortic clamping, if indicated
Nasogastric tube, urinary catheter

4. Next 10 Minutes/Secondary Survey
Reassess airway, ventilation, oxygenation, perfusion, neurologic status, and disability
Assess head, neck, chest, abdomen, pelvis, neurologic examination, extremities
Tube thoracostomy if indicated
Reduce vascular-compromising dislocations
Administer drugs: tetanus toxoid, antibiotics, analgesics, sedatives
Lateral neck, chest, and pelvis radiographs
ECG
Start to make arrangements for transfer, admission, and movement to operating room or ICU

5. Next 10 Minutes
Reassess airway, ventilation, oxygenation, perfusion, neurologic status, and disability
Document resuscitation; talk to family
Splint fractures; dress wounds
IVP, DPL, CT as indicated
Consider more invasive monitoring devices central venous line, arterial line

TABLE 10-2   Pediatric Vital Signs

AGE	WEIGHT,[a] kg	RESPIRATORY RATE	HEART RATE	SYSTOLIC BP[b]
Preterm	2	55–65	120–180	40–60
Term new born	3	40–60	90–170	52–92
1 month	4	30–50	110–180	60–104
6 month– 1 year	8–10	25–35	120–140	65–125
2–4 years	12–16	20–30	100–110	80–95
5–8 years	18–26	4–20	90–100	90–100
8–12 years	26–50	12–20	60–110	100–110
>12 years	>40	12–16	60–105	100–120

[a]Weight estimate: $8 + [2 \times \text{age (years)}] = \text{weight (kg)}$.
[b]Blood pressure minimum $70 + [2 \times \text{age (years)}] = \text{systolic blood pressure}$; $\frac{2}{3} \times \text{systolic pressure} = \text{diastolic pressure}$.
SOURCE: From Fitzmaurice LS. *Pediatric Emergency Medicine, Concepts and Clinical Practice.* St. Louis, MO: Mosby-Yearbook Inc. Modified with permission.

- The need for controlled hyperventilation in patients with serious head injuries
  - Flail chest with pulmonary contusion
  - Shock unresponsive to fluid administration
- Orotracheal intubation is the most reliable means of securing an airway. Use an uncuffed tube in children less than 8 years old. Approximate tube size is estimated by the diameter of the child's nostril or pinky or by adding 16 to the child's age (in years) and dividing by 4.

- Preparation should precede intubation and includes organizing all equipment, drugs, and personnel necessary to adequately manage an acute airway.
- Intubation procedures can lead to increased intracranial pressure (ICP), pain, bradycardia, regurgitation, and hypoxemia. Rapid sequence induction (RSI) can greatly facilitate intubation and reduce adverse effects (see Chap. 5).
- Pediatric surgical airway options include:
  - **Cricothyrotomy:** for patients with extensive central facial or upper airway injury or when there have been unsuccessful attempts at orotracheal intubation. It is not recommended in children under the age of 10 and complication rates are high.
  - **Tracheostomy:** not commonly used in the emergency department because it is time consuming, hazardous, and requires surgical skill.
  - **Needle cricothyrotomy with transtracheal jet ventilation (TTJV):** is the preferred surgical method to secure an emergency airway in children. TTJV provides adequate ventilation for 45 min to 2 h. Prolonged TTJV may result in CO_2 retention. The procedure for needle cricothyrotomy and TTJV is as follows:
    - Attach a 14-gauge angiocatheter to a 5 mL syringe with 3 mL of saline.
    - Stabilize the trachea with the nondominant hand and prep the region.
    - Puncture the cricothyroid membrane in a caudal direction at a 30- to 45-degree angle.
    - Verify placement with aspiration of air.
    - Slide the catheter off the needle and reconfirmed placement with the syringe. Secure the catheter in place.

- Attach the jet ventilation tubing to the O_2 source. The O_2 source *must be a high-pressure* source directly from the wall and not from a regulator valve.
- Start with a low PSI and adjust upward until there is adequate chest excursion. The inspiration:expiration ratio should be 1:3 or 1:4.

BREATHING

- Acceptable ventilation is marked by spontaneous air exchange with normal O_2 saturation and CO_2 levels. Pulse oximetry is mandatory and, when available, end-tidal CO_2 monitoring should also be employed. Children with respiratory insufficiency should have positive pressure ventilation (PPV) with high flow O_2 started immediately. Respiratory function can be compromised by a depressed sensorium, airway occlusion, restriction of lung expansion, and pulmonary injury.
- Severe hypoxemia may be manifested by agitation, altered mental status, cyanosis, poor end-organ function, poor capillary refill, and desaturation on pulse oximetry.
- Hypoventilation is manifested by tachypnea, nasal flaring, grunting, retractions, stridor, and wheezing.
- Place an oro- or nasogastric tube early to alleviate gastric distention and permit improved diaphragmatic excursion and ventilation.
- Evaluate and treat hemo/pneumothorax. The classic findings of absent breath sounds, tympany, hypotension, and jugular venous distention (JVD) are rare in children with pneumothoraces. Needle thoracostomies should be performed for decreased breath sounds, refractory hypotension, hypoxia, or a radiographically confirmed pneumothorax.
- Massive hemothorax may present as absent breath sounds, dullness to percussion, and hypotension. JVD is not commonly seen. Consider operative thoracotomy when the initial drainage is greater than 15 mL/kg or chest tube output exceeds 4 mL/kg/h.
- An open pneumothorax should be occluded on three sides with a dressing of petrolatum gauze or plastic sheet. Tube thoracostomy can be done at the end of the primary survey.

CIRCULATION

- During this phase, hemorrhage is controlled, pulses and perfusion assessed, and vascular access obtained.
  - A palpable peripheral pulse correlates with a blood pressure above 80 mm Hg.

  - A palpable central pulse indicates a pressure above 50 to 0 mm Hg.
  - The capillary refill time of a normovolemic euthermic patient is 2 to 3 s.
- Control external hemorrhage with direct pressure or pneumatic splints. Tourniquets or hemostats should not be used. Trendelenburg position may be of benefit.
- Consider a thoracotomy in children with penetrating chest or abdominal trauma if vital signs are lost in the ED or immediately prior to arrival. Resuscitative thoracotomies are not beneficial in children with traumatic arrest from blunt trauma.
- If chest trauma is present or there has been a deceleration injury, consider the diagnosis of cardiac tamponade. Beck's triad (hypotension, muffled heart sounds, and JVD) is suggestive of cardiac tamponade and echocardiography confirms the diagnosis. Fluid boluses can be temporizing but periocardiocentesis or thoracotomy is lifesaving.
- Obtain vascular access expeditiously through intravenous or intraosseous routes.

DISABILITY

- **Disability** is assessed by performing a rapid neurologic examination addressing level of consciousness (LOC), pupil size, and reactivity. The Glasgow Coma Scale is a quantitative measure of LOC (Table 10-3). The AVPU system (Table 10-4) is also used.

EXPOSURE

- Completely undress the patient to perform a thorough assessment. Take care to maintain body temperature.

RESUSCITATION

- Resuscitation occurs simultaneously with the primary survey but is presented separately for the sake of clarity.
- Ensure adequate oxygenation and ventilation of all trauma victims.
- Vascular access is the next priority. Two large-bore intravenous lines should be established. The highest success rates are obtained at the antecubital fossae or the saphenous veins. Femoral vein or intraosseous access are alternatives. Venous cutdown is an alternative if the other methods are not successful.
- Send blood for type and cross-match, complete blood count, serum electrolytes, liver transaminases, and amylase. Obtain a blood gas for patients with

significant volume loss, respiratory compromise, or toxic exposure.

- **Hypovolemic shock** occurs most commonly after major trauma and is due to blood loss. A child's blood volume compromises 8 to 9 percent of their body weight. The extent of volume depletion and shock is difficult to estimate in children and multiple parameters must be used (Table 10-5). Hypotension is a late marker for shock. Only in infants can an isolated head injury produce hypovolemic shock.
- Cardiogenic shock is rare but could occur with cardiac tamponade or direct cardiac contusion. It should be suspected in a patient with dilated neck veins who has sustained a decelerating injury, penetrating chest trauma, or sternal contusion.
- Neurogenic shock presents with hypotension without tachycardia or vasoconstriction.
- Distributive or septic shock should not be a consideration immediately after a trauma.
- Crystalloid isotonic solution is the initial resuscitative fluid in pediatric trauma patients. The initial bolus is 20 mL/kg given as rapidly as possible. Repeat fluid boluses to four times if necessary. Reassess the child's vital signs and perfusion after each bolus. If the child remains unstable, give 10 to 20 mL/kg packed red blood cells or whole blood. Approximately 300 mL of crystalloid is used to replace each 100 mL of blood lost.
- Insert a Foley catheter and use urinary output as a monitor for resuscitation. The goal for urine output is 1 mL/kg/h for children <1 year old and 2 mL/kg/h for children >1 year old.
- If there is blood at the urethral meatus or in the scrotum or if, on rectal examination, the prostate is placed abnormally, a Foley catheter should not be placed until a retrograde urethrogram (RUG) has proven that the urethra is intact. An RUG is performed by instilling contrast through a Foley catheter that has been inserted into the distal urethra with the balloon partially inflated with 0.5 to 1.0 mL of saline.
- If the initial hemoglobin is <7 mg/dL, give blood immediately since this level of hemoglobin increases cellular hypoxia.

TABLE 10-3 Pediatric Glasgow Coma Scale

EYE OPENING		
SCORE	0–1 YEAR	>1 YEAR
4	Spontaneously	Spontaneously
3	To shout	To verbal command
2	To pain	To pain
1	No response	No response

BEST MOTOR RESPONSE		
SCORE	0–1 YEAR	>1 YEAR
6		Obeys command
5	Localizes pain	Localizes pain
4	Flexion withdrawal	Flexion withdrawal
3	Decorticate	Decorticate
2	Decerebrate	Decerebrate
1	No response	No response

BEST VERBAL RESPONSE			
SCORE	0–2 YEARS	2–5 YEARS	>5 YEARS
5	Appropriate cry Smiles, coos	Appropriate words and phrases	Oriented, converses
4	Cries	Inappropriate words	Disoriented, converses
3	Inappropriate cry	Cries/screams	Inappropriate words
2	Grunts	Grunts	Incomprehensible sound
1	No response	No response	No response

NOTE: A score is given in each category. The individual scores are then added to give a total of 3–15. A score of <8 indicates severe neurologic injury.

TABLE 10-4 AVPU Method for Assessing Level of Consciousness

A	Alert
V	Vocal stimuli: responds
P	Painful stimuli: responds
U	Unresponsive

TABLE 10-5 Therapeutic Classification of Hemorrhagic Shock in the Pediatric Patient

	BLOOD LOSS PERCENT OF BLOOD VOLUME[a]			
	UP TO 15	15–30	30–40	≥40
Pulse rate	Normal	Mild tachycardia	Moderate tachycardia	Severe tachycardia
Blood pressure	Normal or increased	Decreased	Decreased	Decreased
Capillary refill	Normal	Positive	Positive	Positive
Respiratory rate	Normal	Mild tachypnea	Moderate tachypnea	Severe tachypnea
Urinary output	1–2 mL/kg/h	0.5–1.0 mL/kg/h	0.25–0.5 mL/kg/h	Negligible
Mental status	Slightly anxious	Mildly anxious	Anxious and confused	Confused and lethargic
Fluid replacement (3:1 rule)	Crystalloid	Crystalloid	Crystalloid + blood	Crystalloid + blood

[a]Assume blood volume to be 8–9% of body weight (80–90 mL/kg).

- If the child is not responding appropriately, look for continued bleeding or other causes of shock, such as tension pneumothorax or hypoxemia.
- Place an oro- or nasogastric catheter during or immediately after volume resuscitation. Nasogastric tube insertion should be avoided in a patient with extensive facial trauma.
- Monitor the patient's body temperature. Normothermia can be maintained by warming the resuscitation room and IV fluids, using radiant warmers, and covering exposed body parts.
- Obtain lateral cervical spine, chest, and pelvic radiographs. Approximately 80 percent of children with pelvic fractures also have abdominal or genitourinary injuries. Other films, including additional views of the cervical spine, are obtained during the secondary survey.
- Obtain surgical consultation in any significantly injured child as early as possible. If notified by EMS of a severely injured child coming to the facility, make early contact with the surgeon on call or referral center. See Table 10-6 for transfer criteria.
- An equipment table or Broselow tape is used to determine equipment size.

SECONDARY SURVEY AND DEFINITIVE CARE

- When the primary survey is complete and the child is stabilized, perform a directed evaluation of each body area, proceeding from head to toe. Continuously reassess vital signs and abnormal conditions identified in the primary survey.
- The components of the secondary survey are:
  ○ Complete examination
  ○ History: use an AMPLE history to determine the mechanism of injury, time, status at scene, changes in status, and complaints that the child may have.
    ▪ **A** – <u>a</u>llergies
    ▪ **M** – <u>m</u>edications
    ▪ **P** – <u>p</u>ast medical and surgical history
    ▪ **L** – time of the child's <u>l</u>ast meal
    ▪ **E** – <u>e</u>vents preceding the accident
- Laboratory and radiographic studies that were not done during the resuscitation
- Problem identification

HEAD EXAMINATION

- Reevaluate pupil size and reactivity. Perform an examination of the conjunctivae and fundi. Assess

TABLE 10-6   Reasons for Transfer of Pediatric Trauma Patients for Tertiary Care

I. **Mechanism of trauma**
   A. Falls
      1. Falls >10 feet involving patients <14 years old
      2. Falls from second floor or higher
   B. Motor vehicle–crash passenger
      1. Evidence of high-impact velocity motor vehicle accident
         a. Shattered windshield
         b. Evidence of intrusion into the passenger compartment
         c. Bent steering wheel
      2. Rollover incident with unrestrained victim
      3. Ejection of the patient from the vehicle
      4. Death of an occupant within the same passenger compartment
      5. Extraction time >20 min
   C. Auto versus pedestrian incident at >20 mph and victim <15 years old
   D. Major burns
   E. Blast injuries

II. **Physiology**
   A. Total trauma score of ≤12
   B. Pediatric Trauma Score ≤8
   C. Unstable vital signs (age appropriate)
   D. Compromise of airway, breathing, or circulation, or need for protracted ventilation
   E. Severely compromised neurologic status (Glasgow Coma Scale score of ≤8)

III. **Injuries**
   A. Penetrating injuries involving the head, neck, chest, and abdomen or groin
   B. Two or more proximal long bone fractures
   C. Traumatic amputation proximal to either the wrist or the ankle
   D. Evidence of neurologic deficit due to spinal cord injury
   E. Flail chest, major chest wall injury, or pulmonary contusion
   F. Penetrating head injury, open head injury, or CSF leak
   G. Suspicion of vascular or cardiac injury
   H. Severe maxillofacial injuries
   I. Depressed skull fracture

visual acuity by determining if the patient can read, see faces, recognize movement, and distinguish light versus dark. Check for rhinorrhea.
- Thoroughly palpate the skull and mandible.

CERVICAL SPINE

- Cervical spine (C-spine) injuries are not common in children but the presence of any of the following conditions increases the risk:
  ○ Injury above the clavicles
  ○ Injury from falling >1 floor
  ○ Motor vehicle–pedestrian crash at >30 mph
  ○ Poorly or unrestrained occupant in a motor vehicle crash
  ○ Sports injuries
- If there is a low-risk mechanism of injury and the child is awake, cooperative, and free of distracting injuries, the C-spine can be cleared in the ED with a normal lateral C-spine film and clinical examination.

The lateral film must show all seven cervical vertebrae. The child should be able to flex, extend, and rotate the neck without spasm, guarding, pain, or tenderness. Patients with an altered sensorium cannot be cleared and the cervical collar should remain in place.

- Children with high-risk mechanisms of injury should have anteroposterior (AP), odontoid, and lateral radiographic views of the cervical spine.
- Special considerations are required in four situations:
  - The child who requires immediate intubation should not have airway management delayed for a lateral C-spine film. Oral intubation should be done with in-line C-spine immobilization.
  - If an intubated child is at high risk for a neck injury, a CT scan of the cervical vertebrae should be done.
  - If a patient arrives with a helmet in place, the lateral C-spine x-ray can be done prior to removing the helmet.
  - Penetrating injuries to the neck should have entry and exit sites denoted with opaque markers on anteroposterior and lateral films of the C-spine.

CHEST

- The child should be completely exposed to inspect for wounds and respiratory effort. Sucking chest wounds require a sterile occlusive dressing. A flail chest component could be splinted, but most patients with this injury need to be intubated.
- Roll the patient, keeping in-line spine immobilization, and check the back.
- Look for pneumothorax, hemothorax, or cardiac tamponade by palpating bony parts and auscultating the thorax. Bear in mind that a child's breath sounds are easily transmitted making auscultation an insensitive test for pneumothorax. Neck vein distention is difficult to appreciate and an insensitive marker when assessing for tension pneumothorax. Therefore, an unstable child should undergo needle decompression thoracentesis if there is an injury to the thorax. After thoracentesis, tube thoracostomy(ies) should be done.
- Impaled objects protruding from the chest should be left in place until surgery.
- Aortography is indicated if the chest radiograph reveals a widened mediastinum or apical cap and there is a history of deceleration injury. First or second rib fractures increase the likelihood of vascular injury.
- Any penetrating injury to the abdomen or lower chest carries a risk of diaphragmatic injury. Radiographs showing intestinal air above the diaphragm should be considered evidence of such an injury.

ABDOMEN

- Signs suggesting abdominal injury include abdominal wall contusion, distention, abdominal or shoulder pain, and signs of peritoneal irritation and shock. Penetrating wounds to the abdomen usually need operative intervention.
- Controversies arise in diagnosing and managing blunt abdominal injuries. CT with IV, oral, and colonic contrast may be the most sensitive and useful diagnostic modality, but diagnostic peritoneal lavage provides rapid, objective evaluation of possible intraperitoneal injuries.
- DPL is more sensitive than a CT in diagnosing hollow-viscous injuries (see Table 14-3) but it is much less sensitive in diagnosing injuries to the pancreas, duodenum, genitourinary tract, aorta, vena cava, and diaphragm. Use DPL to help determine the etiology of unexplained hypovolemia and to assist in the evaluation of selected penetrating injuries to the abdomen and lower thorax. Consider performing DPL in the patient requiring urgent anesthesia and nonabdominal surgery.
- False-positive DPL tests most commonly occur with pelvic fractures. Additionally, a DPL with >100,000 RBCs may be due to a laceration of the liver or spleen. In these cases, a CT scan is more valuable for evaluating and assessing damage and determining a treatment plan in the stable patient. More than 80 percent of these patients will stop bleeding without an operative intervention.
- Ultrasound can diagnose most injuries to the liver, spleen, and kidneys, and can document intraperitoneal fluid, however, it is generally not a substitute for CT.

PELVIS

- Palpate the bony prominences of the pelvis for tenderness or instability. Examine the perineum for lacerations, hematomas or active bleeding. If not checked earlier when placing a Foley, examine the urethral meatus for blood.

RECTAL

- Perform a rectal examination to determine sphincter tone, rectal integrity, prostate position, presence of a pelvic fracture, and the presence of blood in the stool.

EXTREMITY EXAMINATION

- Examine extremities for deformity, contusions, abrasions, intact sensation, penetrating injuries, pulses, and perfusion. Palpate long bones circumferentially assessing for tenderness, crepitus, or abnormal movement.
- Straighten severe angulations of the extremities and apply splints and traction. Open fractures and wounds should be covered with sterile dressings. Inspect soft tissue injuries for foreign bodies. Irrigate wounds and debride devitalized tissues.

BACK EXAMINATION

- With the neck immobilized, roll the patient and examine the back for bruising, exit or entry wounds, and spine tenderness.

SKIN

- Examine for contusions, burns, penetration sites, petechiae, and abuse.

NEUROLOGIC EXAMINATION

- Recalculate the GCS and evaluate motor, sensory, and cranial nerves.

ADDITIONAL TREATMENT AND TESTS

- Give tetanus prophylaxis.
- Arrange for additional diagnostic tests as indicated by the primary and secondary surveys.
- Permit parents at the child's bedside as soon as the child is stabilized.

BURNS

- Burns are the second most common cause of accidental death in children < 4 years old. For the principles and procedures of burn management, see Chapter 114.

RADIOLOGIC IMAGING

- Imaging modalities used in the evaluation of the trauma patient may include CT scans, ultrasound, plain films, cystography, and pyelography.

- Indications for CT scanning of the brain include GCS < 13, deteriorating neurologic function, post-traumatic seizures, prolonged lethargy, prolonged vomiting, loss of consciousness, amnesia, and confounding medical problems, such as hemophilia (see Chap. 73).
- Indications for abdominal CT scanning include a hemodynamically stable blunt trauma victim with signs of intraabdominal injury, hematuria >20 RBCs per high-powered field or minimal hematuria with a history of deceleration injury, and a worrisome mechanism of trauma with neurologic compromise.
  ○ Double-contrast CT should be performed. Dilute gastrograffin (20 mL/kg) is instilled via a nasogastric tube 20 min prior to CT scan and intravenous contrast is infused after the initial survey is performed. Dosing for contrast media is outlined in Table 10-7.
  ○ During the CT, the Foley catheter should be clamped to evaluate the bladder and the nasogastric tube should be pulled into the esophagus to avoid artifact.
  ○ Positive findings on abdominal CT are increased if three of the following are present: gross hematuria, lap belt injury, assault or abuse as a mechanism of trauma, abdominal tenderness, trauma score >12.
  ○ The presence of positive abdominal findings, a worrisome mechanism of trauma, or significant neurologic compromise (GCS <10) independently increases the positive predictive value of abdominal CT.
- Ultrasonography may be an alternative to CT when CT is not available. If intraperitoneal fluid is found by CT or ultrasound with no apparent injury to the spleen or liver, a DPL should be performed.
- Diagnostic tests to be considered, especially in patients with a lap belt injury, include:

TABLE 10-7   Dose of Contrast Media for Radiographic Studies

AGE, YEARS	DOSE
INTRAVENOUS: 60% HYPAQUE	
0 to 9	1 mL/0.45 kg bolus
10 or more	50 mL, followed by infusion of 50 to 100 mL during scan
ORAL: 1.5% HYPAQUE (20 mL TO 1 L OF FLUID GIVEN PO OR NG)	
0–2	100 mL
3–5	150–200 mL
6–9	200–250 mL
>9	300–1000 mL
Adult	1000 mL
ORAL: GASTROGRAFIN, 20 mL/kg VIA NG TUBE 20 Min PRIOR TO SCAN	

- Thoracolumbar spine films (injuries missed by CT in 77 percent of cases)
- Abdominal films looking for free air (missed by CT in 75 percent of cases)
- If the integrity of the urethra is in doubt, a retrograde urethrogram should be performed. If the urethra is found to be intact, the catheter can be advanced to perform a cystogram.
- If there is high suspicion for a bladder injury that is not apparent on CT, a cystogram should be done to allow for optimal distention of the bladder and extravasation of contrast.
- A "1-shot" intravenous pyelogram can be performed in the ED to evaluate renovascular status if the patient is too unstable for CT. Two to 4 mL/kg of 50 percent diatrizoate sodium (Hypaque) is injected and a film of the abdomen is taken 5 min later. This will show the blood supply to the kidneys. Vascular disruption must be identified immediately because the time to irreversible injury in a devascularized kidney is only 6 h.

INJURY SEVERITY MEASURES

TRAUMA SCORES

- The Revised Trauma Score (Table 10-8) was developed for rapid assessment, triage, injury progression measurement, outcome prediction, and quality assessment

TABLE 10-8 Revised Trauma Score[a]

REVISED TRAUMA SCORE	GLASGOW COMA SCORE	SYSTOLIC BLOOD PRESSURE (mm Hg)	RESPIRATORY RATE (BREATHS/min)
4	13–15	>89	10–20
3	9–12	76–89	>29
2	6–8	50–75	6–9
1	4–5	1–49	1–5
0	3	0	0

[a]A score of 0–4 is given for each variable then added (range, 0–12). A score ≥11 indicates potentially important trauma.

TABLE 10-9 Pediatric Trauma Score[a]

VARIABLES	+2	+1	−1
Airway	Normal	Maintainable	Unmaintainable
CNS	Awake	Obtunded/LOC	Coma
Body weight	>20 kg	10–20 kg	<10 kg
Systolic BP	>90 mm Hg	90–50 mm Hg	<50 mm Hg
Open wound	None	Minor	Major
Skeletal injury	None	Closed fracture	Open/multiple fractures

[a]A score of +2, +1, or −1 is given to each variable then added (range −6 to 12). A score ≥8 indicates potentially important trauma. LOC = Loss of consciousness.

assistance. Although it is less sensitive for assessing severe injury to a single organ system, it allows for standardization of triage protocols and comparisons between groups of patients and institutions.
- The Pediatric Trauma Score (Table 10-9) was developed to reflect the unique injury pattern in children. It incorporates age into the score and can be used to triage patients and estimate prognosis but should be used with caution to predict functional outcome.

DISPOSITION AND TRANSFER

TRIAGE AND PREHOSPITAL CARE ISSUES

- Facilities that receive trauma victims must have the appropriate personnel and resources available at all times. Children should receive care at hospitals where EMS policies have established the facility as capable of receiving patients with life-threatening conditions.
- In a hospital without pediatric anesthesia or surgical consultants, early transfers to appropriately staffed facilities should be considered. Contingency plans for transfers between institutions should be established prospectively.
- Children who are clinically brain dead should be considered for continued resuscitation since they may be candidates for organ procurement. Organ donation may provide traumatized families some consolation in the face of tremendous grief.
- Psychological support is needed throughout the entire hospital course. Disposition and treatment decisions and progress reports need to be presented frequently, succinctly, and with sensitivity. Parents should be allowed to see the child as soon as is practical.

BIBLIOGRAPHY

APLS Joint Task Force: Trauma. In: Strange GR, ed: *APLS: The Pediatric Emergency Medicine Course.* Elk Grove Village, IL and Dallas, TX: American Academy of Pediatrics & American College of Emergency Physicians; 1998:59–78.

ACS Committee on Trauma: *Advanced Trauma Life Support Manual.* Chicago: American College of Surgeons, 2000.

ACS Committee on Trauma: *Trauma Systems in Resources for Optimal Care of the Injured Patient.* Chicago: American College of Surgeons, 1999.

Calkins CM, Bensard DD, Moore EE, et al: The injured child is resistant to multiple organ failure: A different inflammatory response? *J Trauma* 53:1058–1063, 2002.

Fleisher G, Ludwig S: *Textbook of Pediatric Emergency Medicine,* 4th ed. Baltimore: Lippincott, Williams & Wilkins, 2000.

Patrick DA, Bensard DD, Janik JS, Karrer FM: Is hypotension a reliable indicator of blood loss from traumatic injury in children? *Am J Surg* 184:555–559, 2002.

Schafermeyer R: Advances in trauma: Pediatric trauma. *Emerg Med Clin North Am* 11:187–205, 1993.

Sheik AA, Culbertson CB: Emergency department thoracotomy in children: Rationale for selective application. *J Trauma* 34:322, 1993.

Wright JL, Klein BL: Regionalized pediatric trauma systems. *Clin Pediatr Emerg Med* 2:3–12, 2001.

QUESTIONS

1. A 2-year-old child is injured in a motor vehicle crash that occurs in a rural area 30 to 45 min from the nearest hospital. Upon arrival at the scene, paramedics find the child unconscious with weak pulses at a rate of 180, associated with a systolic blood pressure of 80 mm Hg. Peripheral vascular access is attempted but is unsuccessful after two attempts. What is the most appropriate action in regard to vascular access at this point?
   A. Insert a femoral line.
   B. Insert an intraosseous line in an uninjured lower extremity.
   C. Transport without intravenous access.
   D. Continue to attempt to establish a peripheral line.
   E. Insert a subclavian line on the right.

2. In monitoring the response to fluid resuscitation in a shocky child, which of the following is correct?
   A. Blood pressure is the most sensitive indicator of shock.
   B. Urinary output is a straightforward, readily available monitor of fluid status.
   C. A central line should be established as part of the initial resuscitation to properly monitor fluid replacement.
   D. For children >1 year of age, urinary output should be maintained at 2 mL/kg/h and for infants <1 year of age at 1 mL/kg/h.
   E. Fluid overload is rarely a problem with pediatric trauma patients and need not be a concern if standard resuscitation guidelines of 20 mL/kg/h are not exceeded in the first several hours of the resuscitation.

3. Which of the following statements regarding diagnostic tests in the setting of abdominal trauma is correct?
   A. Diagnostic peritoneal lavage is the most sensitive and specific diagnostic modality.
   B. Noncontrast CT of the abdomen and pelvis is the most rapid, objective evaluation of possible intraperitoneal injury.
   C. Triple contrast CT is the most sensitive and useful diagnostic modality.

D. CT is more sensitive than DPL in diagnosing injury to hollow viscera.
E. DPL and CT are equally sensitive in detecting injuries to the pancreas, diaphragm, and genitourinary tract.

4. Unique aspects of trauma in the pediatric age group include which of the following?
   A. Children have a lower center of gravity and are less likely to sustain a closed head injury.
   B. Adolescents exhibit higher level of risk-taking activity than children, but less than adults.
   C. Children have more protective muscle and subcutaneous tissue and, in general, have greater protection from blunt trauma.
   D. Increased flexibility of the pediatric skeleton permits external forces to be transmitted to deeper internal structures.
   E. The diaphragm has a greater curvature allowing greater protection of the abdominal organs by the rib cage.

5. A 5-year-old child is injured in a riot and presents with signs of shock. An intravenous line is inserted and 20 mL/kg of normal saline is administered as rapidly as possible. There is no improvement in the child. What is the most appropriate subsequent action?
   A. Repeat the fluid bolus up to 4 times if necessary.
   B. Repeat the fluid bolus but at 10 mL/kg.
   C. Immediately order and administer 10 to 20 mL/kg of packed red blood cells.
   D. Initiate dopamine drip at 5 μg/kg/min and titrate to achieve blood pressure ≥100 systolic.
   E. Since hypovolemic shock appears not to be the cause, discontinue fluid resuscitation and look for other causes of shock.

ANSWERS

1. B. Intraosseous line placement should be considered early in a severely injured child, even when a blood pressure or pulse is present, if vascular access is difficult. The femoral route is the preferred route when central venous access is required, but central venous access is not preferred in the acute setting for intravenous fluid resuscitation. When transport times are brief, inordinate amounts of time should not be used up trying to establish vascular access. Attempts may continue during transport. But with prolonged transport times, vascular access becomes much more important. Subclavian lines are difficult to establish in children and are associated with significant complications.

2. B. Urinary output is a convenient and accurate method for monitoring initial fluid replacement.

Central lines are not usually required during the early management of the trauma patient. Low blood pressure is a late finding in shock and is not a sensitive monitor. Urine output for an infant <1 year of age should be maintained at 2 mL/kg/h and for an older infant or child at 1 mL/kg/h. Both inadequate fluid replacement and fluid overload are possible in the initial resuscitation of the pediatric trauma patient and close monitoring of fluid replacement is indicated.

3. C. Triple contrast CT is probably the most sensitive and useful diagnostic modality for evaluating abdominal trauma. Noncontrast CT has a very limited role. DPL may be superior for detecting injury to hollow organs, but CT is far superior for detecting injury to the pancreas, diaphragm, and genitourinary tract.

4. D. The pediatric skeleton is much more flexible than the adult skeleton, allowing for external forces to be transmitted to deeper structures without skeletal injury or external evidence of injury. This is an important factor in abdominal and thoracic injury where the markedly flexible rib cage provides much less protection than is seen in the adult. Due to the proportionately larger head of the child, the center of gravity is higher in the child and head injury is more likely. Adolescents exhibit more risk-taking activity than any other age group. Children have less protective musculature and subcutaneous tissue than adults. The diaphragm inserts at a more horizontal angle than in adults, resulting in the abdominal organs being less protected by the rib cage.

5. A. A single bolus of 20 mL/kg will frequently not be enough to replace a child's acute blood loss due to hemorrhagic shock. Repeat boluses should be given up to a maximum of 4 if needed to get a response. If the child continues to be unstable, 10 to 20 mL/kg of packed red blood cells should be given. Pressors should never be used until fluid deficits have been replaced.

11 HEAD TRAUMA

Kimberly S. Quayle
Kemedy K. McQuillen
Patricia Lee

EPIDEMIOLOGY

- Brain injury causes more death and disability in children than in any other age group and 80 percent of children who die from trauma have significant head injury.

- Falls are the most common cause of head injury. Other causes include motor vehicle accidents, bicycle accidents, and assaults, including child abuse.

PATHOPHYSIOLOGY

- Primary brain injury results from direct mechanical damage. Secondary injury results from hypoxia, ischemia, or increased intracranial pressure (ICP).

ANATOMY

- Layers of the head (from superficial to deep) (Fig. 11-1)
  ○ Scalp
  ○ **Galea:** tendinous sheath connecting the frontalis and occipitalis muscles
  ○ **Subgaleal compartment:** large subgaleal hematomas may form in this space
  ○ **Pericranium:** tightly adherent to the skull
  ○ **Outer and inner tables of the skull:** separated by the diploic space
  ○ **Dura:** thin and fibrous
    ▪ Dural attachments compartmentalize the brain. The falx cerebri divides the right and left hemispheres of the brain and the tentorium divides the anterior and middle fossa from the posterior fossa.
    ▪ Herniation across compartments causes compression of vital structures, ischemia from vascular occlusion, and infarction.
  ○ **Subdural space:** contains bridging veins that drain into dural sinuses
  ○ **Leptomeninges: Arachnoid and pia.** More vascular than dura
  ○ **Subarachnoid space:** contains CSF. An adult has approximately 1200 to 1500 mL of CSF, while 2 year olds have 70 percent and 8 year olds 90 percent of this volume.

- In infants, the open sutures and thin calvarium produce a more flexible skull capable of absorbing greater impact. This flexibility permits more severe distortion between the skull and dura, and the cerebral vessels and brain, increasing susceptibility to hemorrhage.

- Incomplete myelinization of the brain contributes to greater plasticity and increased likelihood of diffuse axonal injury.

- The disproportionately large size and weight of the head compared to the rest of the body contributes to an increased likelihood of head injury.

SPECIFIC INJURIES

- **Scalp bleeding** can lead to hemodynamically significant blood loss in infants and young children.

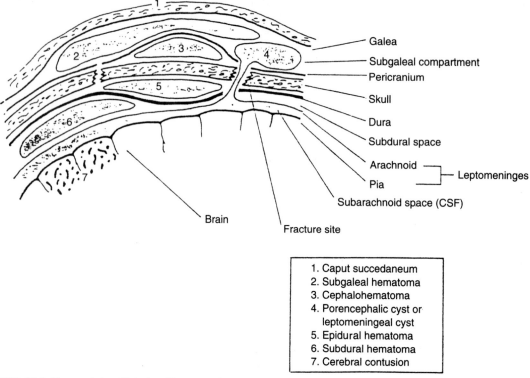

FIG. 11-1 Traumatic head injuries. [From Barkin RM, Rosen P (eds): *Emergency Pediatrics: A Guide to Ambulatory Care*, 3d ed. St. Louis: Mosby-Year Book, 1990. Reproduced with permission of Mosby-Year Book, Inc.]

Lacerations should be explored for skull integrity, depressions, or foreign bodies.

- **Subgaleal hematomas** present as an extensive soft tissue swelling hours to days after the traumatic event. They are commonly associated with a skull fracture and may persist for days to weeks.
- **Linear nondepressed skull fractures** have a high association with intracranial injury, however, intracranial injury may occur without a skull fracture.
- **"Growing fractures"** occur in children under 2 years old who sustain a skull fracture with a dural tear. Postinjury, rapid brain growth results in the development of a leptomeningeal cyst.
- **Basilar skull fractures** can occur anywhere along the base of the skull but typically occur at the petrous portion of the temporal bone. Signs include hemotympanum, CSF otorrhea or rhinorrhea, periorbital ecchymosis (raccoon eyes), and postauricular ecchymosis (Battle's sign). Diagnosis may require computed tomography (CT) imaging of the temporal bone.
- **Epidural hematomas** are as common in children as in adults but less likely to be clinically apparent. Eighty percent occur in combination with a skull fracture and meningeal artery bleeding; the remainder are venous. Signs and symptoms include headache,

vomiting, and altered mental status. Uncal herniation with pupillary changes and hemiparesis may ensue.

- Acute **subdural hematomas** are less common in children than adults. They occur after bridging veins are torn in acceleration-deceleration injuries and are often associated with diffuse brain injury. Symptoms include irritability, vomiting, and lethargy.
- **Parenchymal contusions** (bruises or tears of brain tissue) occur as the brain moves within the skull against bony irregularities of the skull. Coup injuries occur at the site of impact while contrecoup injuries occur at a site remote from the impact. Findings include altered level of consciousness, focal neurologic signs, and seizures.
- **Penetrating injuries** result from sharp-object penetration or gunshot wounds and extensive brain injury is common.
- **Concussion** is defined as a transient loss of awareness and responsiveness following head trauma. Symptoms include loss of consciousness, vomiting, headache, amnesia, or dizziness.
- **Diffuse axonal injury** is three times more common in children than in adults. It results from a shearing, acceleration-deceleration injury and can progress to coma or death.

INTRACRANIAL PRESSURE AND HERNIATION SYNDROMES

- The total volume of the intracranial vault is constant
  - Brain: 70 percent
  - CSF and interstitial fluid: 20 percent
  - Blood: 10 percent
- If one of these three components increases in volume, the other two compartments must decrease or intracranial pressure (ICP) rises. The main component of compensation is a displacement of cerebrospinal fluid into the spinal canal. Once this compensatory mechanism is maximized, any additional increases in volume cause elevation of ICP to abnormal levels (>15 to 20 mm Hg). Cerebral perfusion becomes impaired and irreversible ischemic damage to the brain ensues.
- Three types of cerebral edema are involved in brain injury:
  - **Cytotoxic:** from fluid accumulation within damaged brain and glial cells
  - **Interstitial:** from decreased absorption of fluid following brain **trauma**
  - **Vasogenic:** from the disruption of the blood–brain barrier with subsequent leakage of fluid into the perivascular brain tissue
- CSF volume may increase despite redistribution of the fluid into the spinal canal. As brain and blood volumes increase, the ventricular spaces become compressed until redistribution is no longer possible. CSF pathways can also be compressed by edematous tissue, resulting in the disruption of CSF outflow, ventricular dilation, and hydrocephalus.
- Cerebral hyperemia contributes to brain swelling in the first 24 h postinjury. As autoregulatory mechanisms attempt to maintain cerebral perfusion pressure and are ultimately lost, cerebral blood flow is increased. Hypoxia and hypercapnia also increase cerebral blood flow.
- Increased ICP may produce herniation. Cingulate herniation occurs as one cerebral hemisphere is displaced underneath the falx cerebri. A transtentorial or uncal herniation is of major clinical significance (Fig. 11-2). A mass lesion or hematoma forces the ipsilateral uncus of the temporal lobe through the space between the cerebral peduncle and the tentorium. This causes ipsilateral compression of the oculomotor nerve and an ipsilateral dilated nonreactive pupil. The cerebral peduncle is compressed causing a contralateral hemiparesis. As ICP increases and the brain stem is compressed, consciousness wanes. If herniation continues, apnea and death ensue. Uncal herniation may be bilateral if there are bilateral lesions or diffuse edema.
- Cerebellar tonsil herniation through the foramen magnum occurs infrequently and results in medullary compression, bradycardia, respiratory arrest, and death.

ASSESSMENT

- Assessment begins with a detailed history of the traumatic event. Mechanism, time, and location of injury should be ascertained as should any subsequent signs and symptoms, including loss of consciousness, seizures, vomiting, headache, visual changes, altered mental status, weakness, and amnesia.
- Child abuse should be suspected with a witnessed report of abuse, a history incompatible with the injuries, a changing or inconsistent history or a developmentally incompatible history.
- Past medical history should include prior history of seizures, neurological or bleeding abnormalities, and immunization status.

PRIMARY SURVEY

- Physical evaluation begins with the primary survey.
- Establish an **airway** by positioning, suctioning, or endotracheal intubation. Maintain cervical spine immobilization until cervical injury is excluded.
- Once the airway is established, assess **breathing/ventilation** by observing chest expansion, auscultating breath sounds, and assessing for cyanosis or respiratory distress. Treat hypoventilation with 100% oxygen, bag-valve-mask ventilation, and endotracheal intubation. Rapid sequence intubation (RSI) should be employed to minimize increases in ICP and reduce the risk of aspiration. RSI is discussed in Chapter 5, however, there are special considerations in patients with head injuries.
  - Ketamine increases ICP and is contraindicated.
  - Succinylcholine use is controversial due to concerns that it may increase ICP. Rocuronium is an alternative with a similar onset but longer duration of action.
  - When endotracheal intubation or bag-valve-mask ventilation is likely to be unsuccessful, as with major facial or laryngeal trauma, RSI is contraindicated.
- **Circulation** is assessed by evaluating the heart rate, peripheral pulses, and perfusion. Blood pressure must be maintained to ensure adequate cerebral perfusion. Hypovolemic shock is rare with isolated head injuries but can occur in infants and young children.
- Level of consciousness and pupillary response are used to determine neurologic **disability**. Level of consciousness can be assessed using the AVPU system:

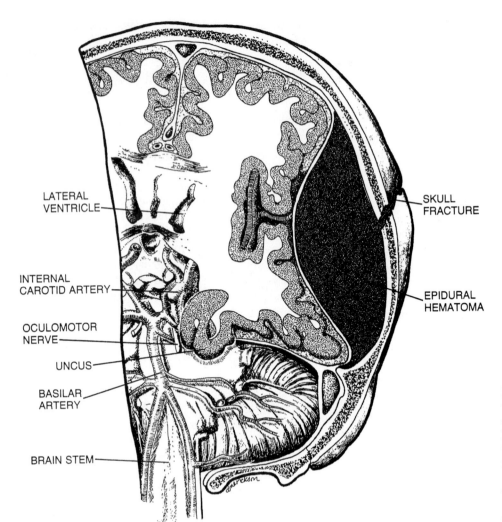

LATERAL VENTRICLE

SKULL FRACTURE

INTERNAL CAROTID ARTERY

OCULOMOTOR NERVE

EPIDURAL HEMATOMA

UNCUS

BASILAR ARTERY

BRAIN STEM

FIG. 11-2 Anterior view of transtentorial uncal herniation caused by a large epidural hematoma. (From American College of Emergency Physicians: *Emergency Medicine: A Comprehensive Study Guide*, 3d ed. New York: McGraw-Hill, 1992. Reproduced with permission of McGraw-Hill.)

Alert, responsive to **V**erbal stimulus, responsive to **P**ainful stimulus, or **U**nresponsive. The remainder of the primary survey is completed prior to returning to a more detailed secondary neurologic examination.

• During the **secondary survey**, the scalp is examined and palpated for deformity. The fontanel, if present, is palpated. Signs of basilar skull fracture are noted. Extraocular movements, muscle tone, and spontaneous movements are evaluated. The neck is palpated for tenderness or deformities. Posturing should be noted: decorticate posturing signifies damage to the cerebral cortex, white matter, or basal ganglia and decerebrate posturing suggests damage below the midbrain. In adults and older children, the Glasgow Coma Scale (GCS) is commonly used to assess and follow the level of consciousness (Table 11-1), however, it is less helpful in infants and young children due to their limited language skills. Specialized pediatric coma scales have been developed but none have been validated. During the evaluation, bear in mind that infants and children less than 2 years old may have subtle findings despite significant intracranial injury.

TABLE 11-1   Glasgow Coma Scale[a]

Eye opening (E)	Spontaneous	4
	To speech/voice	3
	To pain	2
	No response	1
Motor response (M)	Obeys commands	6
	Localizes pain	5
	Withdraws to pain	4
	Abnormal flexion-decorticate	3
	Abnormal extension-decerebrate	2
	No response	1
Verbal response (V)	Oriented	5
	Confused/disoriented	4
	Inappropriate words	3
	Incomprehensible sounds	2
	No response	1

[a]E + M + V = coma score (range: 3 to 15).

DIAGNOSTIC STUDIES

• Complete blood count, type and cross-match, electrolytes, and coagulation studies should be obtained. Blood gases, toxicology screens, and ethanol levels are obtained as needed.

- Cervical spine films should be obtained in alert patients with neck pain or neurologic deficits and in all unconscious patients.
- Computed tomography of the head is the diagnostic method of choice for identifying intracranial pathology and is indicated in children with severe injuries including altered mental status, focal neurologic deficits, known or suspected skull fractures, or penetration of the calvarium. CT is also indicated in children less than 2 years old who have seizures, irritability, loss of consciousness, or a bulging fontanel, or who vomit five or more times or for more than 6 h. CT of the head should be **considered** in children with multiple injuries, cervical spine injury, preexisting neurologic disorders, a bleeding diathesis, suspected intentional head trauma, a language barrier, or the presence of drugs or alcohol. CT should also be considered in children who vomit three to four times or have a history of resolved lethargy or irritability.
- Skull radiographs are not routinely recommended but may be useful as a screening tool in young infants with scalp hematomas, in cases of suspected unaccidental trauma, or when CT is not readily available. If skull radiographs demonstrate a skull fracture, children should be transported to a facility capable of performing head CT.

TREATMENT

- Prevention of hypoxia, ischemia, and increased intracranial pressure (ICP) is essential for children with severe head injuries to prevent secondary brain injury.
- Consult a neurosurgeon for seriously head-injured children.
- Endotracheal intubation and controlled ventilation, to prevent hypercarbia and maintain oxygenation, are frequently required for patients with severe head injury. Maintain moderate hyperventilation (P_{CO_2} 32 to 35 torr) for management of increased ICP.
- Maintain normal ICP and normal mean arterial pressure (MAP) to preserve cerebral perfusion pressure: $CPP = MAP - ICP$. Insert an arterial catheter for close monitoring of arterial pressure. Treat hypotension with isotonic fluid boluses and inotropic medications.
- Use an ICP monitor to detect acute changes in ICP and to drain CSF.
- Position the patient with the head elevated to 15° to 30° to decrease ICP.
- Consider using mannitol and loop diuretics to maintain ICP by reducing intravascular volume. Fluid restriction may also be used if the MAP is adequate.
- Syndromes of inappropriate antidiuretic hormone secretion or diabetes insipidus may occur with severe intracranial injury; follow fluid balance and electrolyte status closely.
- Treat posttraumatic seizures with phenytoin or fosphenytoin.
- Corticosteroids and hypothermia are not used routinely to treat serious brain injury.
- Monitor seriously brain-injured children in an intensive care setting.
- The care for children with less serious injuries varies. Many children are admitted for observation with serial neurologic examinations. However, in previously well children 2 to 20 years old with isolated minor head injury, or in infants at low risk who are asymptomatic and have a low-energy mechanism of trauma, observation by a reliable caregiver is sufficient. Additionally, children without a history of loss of consciousness, but with a history of seizure, headache, vomiting, or amnesia, may be observed without a head CT if they are alert and have a normal neurologic examination. Patients should return for re-evaluation if new symptoms develop or if current symptoms worsen or persist.
- The development of delayed intracranial injury is extremely rare, therefore, children with normal head CT scans, mental status, and neurologic examinations may be observed at home.
- Children with isolated nondepressed skull fractures without intracranial injury may be observed at home.

PROGNOSIS

- Although children have a greater likelihood of survival and recovery from brain injury than adults, they may be more vulnerable to long-term cognitive and behavioral dysfunction.

BIBLIOGRAPHY

Adelson PD, Kochanek PM: Head injury in children. *J Child Neurol* 13:2, 1998.

Committee on Quality Improvement, American Academy of Pediatrics: The management of minor closed head injury in children. *Pediatrics* 104:1407, 1999.

Duhaime AC, Christian CW, Rorke LB, et al: Nonaccidental head injury in infants—The shaken baby syndrome. *N Engl J Med* 338:1822, 1998.

Greenes DS, Schutzman SA: Occult intracranial injury in infants. *Ann Emerg Med* 32:680, 1998.

Klassen TP, Reed MH, Stiell IG, et al: Variation in utilization of computed tomography scanning for the investigation of minor head trauma in children: A Canadian experience. *Acad Emerg Med* 7:739–744, 2000.

Mazzola CA, Adelson PD: Critical care management of head trauma in children. *Crit Care Med* 30(11 Suppl): S393–401, 2002.

Poussaint TY, Moeller KK: Imaging of pediatric head trauma. *Neuroimaging Clin N Am* 12: 271–294, 2002.

Quayle KS: Minor head injury in the pediatric patient. *Pediatr Clin North Am* 46:1189, 1999.

Quayle KS, Jaffe DM, Kuppermann N, et al: Diagnostic testing for acute head injury in children: When are head computed tomography and skull radiographs indicated? *Pediatrics* (Online) 99:11, 1997. http://ww.pediatrics.org/cgi/content/full/99/5/e11.

Sanchez JI, Paidas CN: Childhood trauma: Now and in the new millennium. *Surg Clin North Am* 79:1503, 1999.

Schutzman SA, Barnes P, Duhaime AC, et al: Evaluation and management of children younger than two years with apparently minor head trauma: Proposed guidelines. *Pediatrics* 107: 983–993, 2001.

Zuckerman GB, Conway EE: Accidental head injury. *Pediatr Ann* 26:621, 1997.

QUESTIONS

1. An 18-month-old child is brought by parents after falling from the kitchen counter onto the concrete floor last night. The parents state that the child cried at the time of injury but seemed to act normally afterward. This morning the child has vomited three times. On examination, the child appears lethargic. A skull radiograph is obtained, which reveals a linear skull fracture: Additional concerns regarding this finding are all of the following **EXCEPT**:
   A. Epidural hematoma
   B. Subgalea hematoma
   C. "Growing fracture"
   D. Parenchymal contusion
   E. No additional concern
2. Cerebral blood flow is increased by:
   A. Decreased ventilatory rate
   B. Normal oxygenation
   C. Hypocapnia
   D. Cerebral ischemia
   E. Autoregulatory mechanisms
3. Uncal herniation is characterized by all of the following **EXCEPT**:
   A. Ipsilateral uncus moves under the falx cerebri
   B. Ipsilateral compression of the oculomotor nerve
   C. Ipsilateral dilated, nonreactive pupil
   D. Contralateral hemiparesis
   E. Brain stem compression
4. When intubation is performed on a head-injured child, which of the following is true?

   A. Succinylcholine does not increase intracerebral pressure (ICP).
   B. Ketamine does not increase ICP.
   C. Rocuronium does not increase ICP.
   D. Rapid sequence intubation increases ICP.
   E. BVM with hyperventilation increases ICP.
5. AVPU is a quick method to assess level of consciousness and represents:
   A. Appearance, Pulse, Ventilation, Unstable
   B. Apgar, Pulse, Ventilation, Unresponsive
   C. Appearance, Painful Stimulation, Verbal stimulus, Unstable
   D. Alert, Verbal stimulus, Painful stimulus, Unresponsive
   E. Alert, Purposeful, Visual, Unresponsive
6. CT scan of the brain is indicated in children less than 2 years old with all of the following **EXCEPT**:
   A. Skull fracture
   B. Fever
   C. Multiple episodes of emesis
   D. Vomiting for more than 6 h
   E. Loss of consciousness

ANSWERS

1. E. Headache, vomiting, and altered mental status are signs and symptoms of intracranial injury, such as epidural hematoma, parenchymal contusions, and concussion. Subgaleal hematomas present as an extensive soft tissue swelling hours to days after a traumatic event and are commonly associated with a skull fracture. Linear nondepressed skull fractures have a high association with intracranial injury, however, intracranial injury may occur without a skull fracture. "Growing fractures" occur in children under 2 years of age with a skull fracture and a dural tear. Postinjury, rapid brain growth results in the development of a leptomeningeal cyst.
2. A. Hypercapnia results from decreased ventilation. Cerebral hyperemia, hypoxia, and hypercapnia postinjury contribute to cerebral blood flow increase and resultant brain swelling.
3. A. Cingulate herniation occurs as one cerebral hemisphere is displaced underneath the falx cerebri.
4. C. Rocuronium does not increase ICP. BVM with hyperventilation aids in decreasing ICP as does the use of controlled RSI. Succinylcholine and ketamine may result in increased ICP
5. D. Level of consciousness can be assessed using the AVPU system: Alert, responsive to Verbal stimulus, responsive to Painful stimulus, or Unresponsive.
6. B. All of the other answers are reasons for CT brain. While fever may indicate the presence of an infection,

including meningitis, a CT is not mandatory prior to lumbar puncture for a child less than 2 years with no focal neurologic findings.

12 EVALUATION OF CHILDREN FOR CERVICAL SPINE INJURIES

David M. Jaffe
Kemedy K. McQuillen
Gary R. Strange

EPIDEMIOLOGY

- Approximately 1100 children sustain spinal injuries annually. Leading causes of injury include motor vehicle-related injuries, falls, firearms, and sports activities.

MAJOR ANATOMIC COMPONENTS OF THE CERVICAL SPINE

BONES

- Base of the skull and the first eight vertebrae, C1–7, and T1
- C1 and C2 vertebrae have unique characteristics (Figs. 12-1 and 12-2). The other vertebrae consist of a body and an arch that form a ring around the spinal canal, which contains the spinal cord and subarachnoid space (Fig. 12-3).

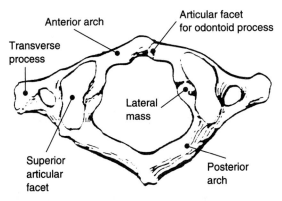

FIG. 12-1 Anatomy of C1 (atlas). (From Bonadio WA: Cervical spine trauma in children: Part I. General concepts, normal anatomy, radiographic evaluation. *Am J Emerg Med* 11:158–165, 1993. Reproduced by permission of W.B. Saunders Company, copyright 1993.)

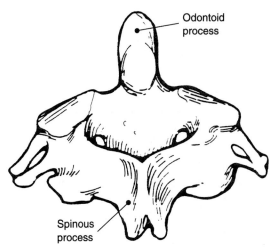

FIG. 12-2 Anatomy of C2 (axis). (From Bonadio WA: Cervical spine trauma in children: Part I. General concepts, normal anatomy, radiographic evaluation. *Am J Emerg Med* 11:158–165, 1993. Reproduced by permission of W.B. Saunders Company, copyright 1993.)

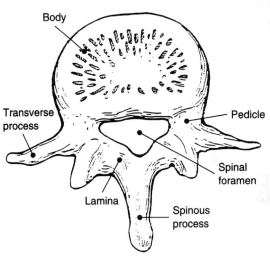

FIG. 12-3 Anatomy of a typical cervical vertebra. (From Bonadio WA: Cervical spine trauma in children: Part I. General concepts, normal anatomy, radiographic evaluation. *Am J Emerg Med* 11:158–165, 1993. Reproduced by permission of W.B. Saunders Company, copyright 1993.)

- The occiput articulates with articular facets on the lateral arches of C1. The odontoid process of C2 is articulated with the inner surface of the anterior arch of C1 and serves as a pivot point for rotation of C1 on C2.

LIGAMENTS

- Ligaments are depicted in Fig. 12-4. Additionally, the transverse ligament stabilizes the atlantoaxial joint.

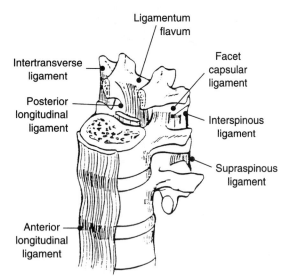

FIG. 12-4 Multilayered section of cervical spine anatomy with anterior and posterior compartments delimited by posterior longitudinal ligament. (From Bonadio WA: Cervical spine trauma in children: Part I. General concepts, normal anatomy, radiographic evaluation. *Am J Emerg Med* 11:158–165, 1993. Reproduced by permission of W.B. Saunders Company, copyright 1983.)

INTERVERTEBRAL DISKS

- The disks cushion compression forces applied to the cervical spine and support the spinal column during bending.

FACETS AND INTERFACET JOINTS

- These have synovial membranes and fibrous capsules, also absorb compression forces and limit flexion.
- Other anatomic components include muscles, nerves, and blood vessels of the neck.

UNIQUE CHARACTERISTICS OF THE PEDIATRIC CERVICAL SPINE

- Greater elasticity of ligaments, joint capsules, and cartilaginous structures
- More horizontal orientation of facet joints and uncinate processes
- Wedged anterior surfaces of vertebral bodies (Fig. 12-5)
- Underdeveloped neck musculature
- Relatively large and heavy head
- Higher center of gravity
- Anatomic fulcrum at the level of C2 and C3 (at C7/T1 in adults)
- Greater vulnerability of the vertebral arteries to ischemia

PEDIATRIC INJURY PATTERNS

- Predisposition for upper cervical spine injuries
  - 30 percent of fractures in children less than 8 years old are below the level of C3.
  - 85 percent of cervical spine fractures in adults are below the level of C3.
- Spinal cord injury without radiographic abnormality (SCIWORA) occurs in approximately 25 to 50 percent of pediatric spinal cord injuries. Injuries may be stable or unstable. Flexion-extension radiographs and computed tomography (CT) scans are normal while MRI scans reveal muscular and ligamentous disruptions, growth plate avulsions, epiphyseal separations, and subdural or epidural spinal hematomas.
- The biomechanical and anatomic features of the spine attain adult patterns between the ages of 8 and 10 years, however, adult injury patterns are not fully manifest until age 15 years.

EVALUATION AND MANAGEMENT

- Suspect spinal cord injury with severe multiple trauma; significant trauma to the head, neck, or back; or trauma associated with high-speed vehicular crashes and falls from heights.
- Evaluate the "six P's":
  - Pain: altered level of consciousness, intoxication, or an injury to another part of the body may make pain localization unreliable.
  - Position
    - Head tilt is associated with rotary subluxation of C1 on C2 or a high cervical injury.
    - Prayer position (arms folded across the chest) suggests an injury at C4 to C6.
  - Paralysis or paresis
  - Paresthesias: "pins and needles" sensation, numbness, burning or an electric shock passing down the vertebral column, especially with neck flexion.
  - Ptosis: Horner's syndrome (ptosis and a miotic pupil) suggests a cervical cord injury.
  - Priapism is present in 3 to 5 percent of spine-injured patients and indicates sympathetic nervous system involvement.
- Absence of vital signs is also associated with upper cervical cord injury.
- Test for the bulbocavernosus reflex by inserting a finger into the rectum and pulling on the glans of the penis or the head of the clitoris. A normal response is a reflex contraction of the anal sphincter. Absence of the bulbocavernosus reflex in the presence of flaccid paralysis carries a grave prognosis.

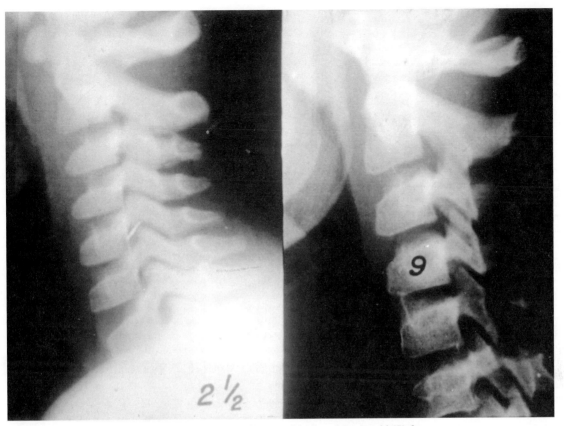

FIG. 12-5 Cross-table lateral view (CTLV) x-ray of 2 year old (*A*) and 9 year old (*B*) for comparison of cervical spine anatomy.

- Characteristic cord syndrome findings are outlined in Fig. 12-6.

ANALYSIS OF RADIOGRAPHS

- The standard screening series includes
  - Cross-table lateral view (CTLV)
    - See Fig. 12-8 for the steps in evaluating the CTLV.
    - Anteroposterior view (AP)
    - Assess the longitudinal alignment of vertebral bodies and the symmetry of the facets, pillars, and spinous processes.
  - Open-mouth view (OM)
    - Assess the alignment of the atlantooccipital and atlantoaxial joints, the margins of the lateral arches of C1 with C2, and the position of the odontoid between the lateral arches of C1. Inspect the film for any evidence of fractures.
    - In younger or uncooperative children, the Waters view can be substituted.

- Sensitivity and specificity of screening radiographs (adults)
  - CTLV alone: 82 and 70 percent, respectively

SPINAL SHOCK

- Flaccid below level of lesion
- Absent reflexes
- Decreased sympathetic tone
- Autonomic dysfunction (including hypotension)
- Sensation may be preserved; if absent = total cord transection (poor prognosis)

CENTRAL CORD

- Diminished or absent upper-extremity function
- Preservation of lower-extremity function
- Associated with extension injuries

BROWN-SÉQUARD

- Hemisection
- Ipsilateral loss of
  - Motor function
  - Proprioception
- Contralateral loss of sensation:
  - Pain
  - Temperature

ANTERIOR CORD

- Complete motor paralysis
- Loss of pain and temperature sensation
- Preservation of position and vibration
- Associated with severe flexion injuries
- See Figure 12-7

FIG. 12-6 Cord syndromes.

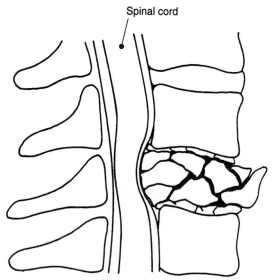

Spinal cord

FIG. 12-7 Burst fracture with anterior cord compression.

1. All seven vertebral bodies must be clearly seen, including the C7 to T1 junction.
2. Evaluate proper alignment of the posterior cervical line and the four lordotic curves: anterior longitudinal ligament line, the posterior longitudinal ligament line, the spinolaminal line, and the tips of the spinous processes.
3. Evaluate the predental space (3 mm in adults, 4–5 mm in children).
4. Evaluate each vertebra for fracture and increased or decreased density (e.g., suggestive of a compression fracture, metastatic lesion, osteoporosis).
5. Evaluate the intervertebral and interspinous spaces. (Abrupt angulation of more than 11° at a single interspace is abnormal.)
6. Evaluate if there is fanning of the spinous processes suggestive of posterior ligament disruption.
7. Evaluate prevertebral soft-tissue distance. (Less than 7 mm at C2 and less than 5 mm at C3–4 is considered normal.) Note: in children less than 2 years old, the prevertebral space may appear widened if it is not an inspiratory film.
8. Evaluate the antlantooccipital region for possible dislocation.

FIG. 12-8 Criteria for clearing the cervical spine using crosstable lateral view. (From Van Hare RS, Yaron M: The ring of C2 and evaluation of the cross-table lateral view of the cervical spine. *Ann Emerg Med* 21:734, 1992. Reproduced by permission.)

- Negative predictive value: 97 percent
  ◦ CTLV with AP and OM views: 93 and 71, respectively
  - Negative predictive value: 99 percent
- Other imaging modalities are used when the standard views are suboptimal for visualization or when clinical suspicion of a cervical spine injury is high.
  ◦ Swimmer's view to delineate the lower cervical spine
  ◦ Flexion and extension views to assess instability. These films require moving the neck out of neutral position and must be supervised. They should not be attempted in patients who have an altered sensorium or are unable to communicate.
  ◦ Supine oblique views
  ◦ Thin-section tomography
  ◦ Computed tomography is very sensitive for detecting bony injury
  ◦ MRI is highly sensitive for detecting soft tissue and spinal cord injuries and is the test of choice for diagnosing SCIWORA.
- Using the following criteria, some patients may have their cervical spine "cleared" without radiographs.
  ◦ Low risk, low energy mechanism of injury
  ◦ Verbal, awake, alert, nonintoxicated children
  ◦ No significant painful lesions elsewhere
  ◦ Normal neurologic examination
  ◦ No spine tenderness
  ◦ Normal range of motion of the neck (tested last and with care)
- Other emergency procedures (ie, endotracheal intubation or surgical intervention) should not be delayed by prolonged attempts to clear the cervical spine in the emergency department. In these cases, it should be assumed that a spine injury is present and immobilization should be maintained.

MANAGEMENT

- The pathogenesis of spinal cord injury is felt to be related to direct damage that is largely irreversible and secondary damage from ischemia, hypoxemia, and tissue toxicity.

AIRWAY

- Use the jaw-thrust maneuver to lift the mandibular block of tissue that can obstruct the airway in a supine, unconscious child. Maintain cervical spine stabilization (Fig. 12-9).
- Clear secretions with suctioning and positioning. Maintain spinal immobilization.
- In-line stabilization, rapid sequence induction and oral endotracheal intubation are the preferred techniques to achieve airway stabilization (Fig. 12-10).

BREATHING

- The spine-injured patient may hypoventilate because of diminished diaphragmatic activity, intercostal muscle paralysis, and supine positioning. Head or chest injuries and aspiration of gastric contents may further compromise ventilation.

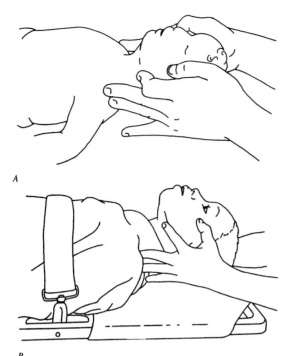

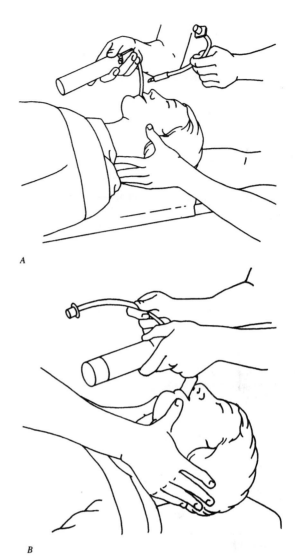

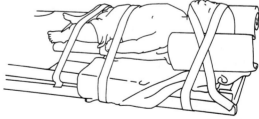

FIG. 12-9 Manual jaw-thrust and cervical spine stabilization in (*A*) an infant and (*B*) a child.

- Provide supplemental humidified oxygen and support ventilation as needed. An altered mental status or the need for prolonged ventilatory support mandates endotracheal intubation.

CIRCULATION

- Hypotension may be secondary to either hypovolemia or spinal shock. The etiology can be differentiated by the patient's pulse: in spinal shock, the pulse is slow, while hypovolemic shock is marked by a rapid pulse.
- Treat hypotension with intravenous fluids, atropine, and vasopressors.

CERVICAL SPINE IMMOBILIZATION

- Immobilization is accomplished with stiff collars (available in sizes for children as young as 1 year of age), cloth tape or straps across the forehead, and external orthoses (ie, a rigid backboard) (Fig. 12-11).
- The backboard should be modified for a child's disproportionately large head with a recess for the occiput or by elevating the chest by placing sheets or towels under the child (Fig. 12-12).
- Complications of spinal immobilization include restriction of ventilation, pain, improper spine positioning, and interference with other procedures.

FIG. 12-10 In-line stabilization for endotracheal intubation: (*A*) above and (*B*) below.

FIG. 12-11 A method for immobilization of an infant.

- A recent study has challenged the benefit of out-of-hospital immobilization among spine-injured patients and it is likely that current recommendations will change over the next decade.

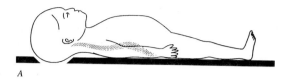

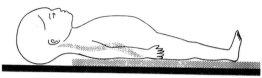

B

FIG. 12-12 Backboard modifications for children. *A.* Young child on a modified backboard that has a cutout to recess the occiput, obtaining a safe supine cervical positioning. *B.* Young child on a modified backboard that has a double-mattress pad to raise the chest, obtaining a safe supine cervical positioning. (From Herzenberg JE, Hensinger RN, Dedrick DK, et al: Emergency transport and positioning of young children who have an injury of the cervical spine. The standard backboard may be hazardous. *J Bone Joint Surg* 17:15, 1989. Reproduced by permission.)

DISABILITY

- Care should be taken to protect insensate areas of the body from hard, protruding objects, as they may cause skin necrosis.

EXPOSURE

- Patients with spinal shock may be more sensitive to temperature variations and may require supplemental warming or cooling.
- In adults with spinal cord injuries, **high-dose methylprednisolone** (30 mg/kg) followed by 5.4 mg/kg/h for 23 hours, started within 8 hours of injury, improves neurologic recovery. Although there have been no clinical trials confirming the efficacy of steroids in children, it is accepted practice to use the same regimen in pediatric patients.

BIBLIOGRAPHY

Bracken MB, Shepard MJ, Holford TR, et al: Administration of methylprednisolone for 24 or 48 hours or tirilazad mesylate for 48 hours in the treatment of acute spinal cord injury. *JAMA* 277:1597, 1997.

Hauswald M, Ong G, Tandberg D, et al: Out-of-hospital spinal immobilization: Its effect on neurologic injury. *Acad Emerg Med* 5:214, 1998.

Keiper MD, Zimmerman RA, Bilaniuk LT: MRI in the assessment of the supportive soft tissues of the cervical spine in acute trauma in children. *Neuroradiology* 40:359, 1998.

Proctor MR: Spinal cord injury. *Crit Care Med* 30(11 Suppl):S489–499, 2002.

Viccellio P, Simon H, Pressman BD, et al: A prospective multicenter study of cervical spine injury in children. *Pediatrics* 108:E20, 2001.

QUESTIONS

1. Which of the following observations is true regarding differences in cervical spine anatomy and physiology in children?
   A. The most commonly fractured vertebra in children less than 8 years of age is C6.
   B. The pediatric cervical spine is more subject to injury because there is less elasticity in the ligaments, joints, and cartilaginous structures.
   C. The facet joints are aligned in a more vertical orientation.
   D. Differences in anatomy and physiology lead to spinal cord injury without radiographic abnormality in the pediatric population.
   E. Intervertebral disks are less able to cushion compression forces applied to the cervical spine.

2. Which of the following tests is the modality of choice for assessing the supportive soft tissues of the spine and the spinal cord itself?
   A. CT
   B. Flexion and extension views
   C. MRI
   D. Three-view cervical spine series
   E. Five-view cervical spine series

3. A 3-year-old child was injured in a fall and is suspected to have a cervical spine fracture. What is the most appropriate technique for airway management?
   A. Oral endotracheal intubations with in-line stabilization and rapid sequence induction.
   B. Blind nasotracheal intubation with in-line stabilization and no pharmacologic adjuncts.
   C. Bag-valve-mask ventilation until the cervical spine is definitively immobilized.
   D. Cricothyrotomy.
   E. Oral endotracheal intubation with cervical traction and rapid sequence induction.

4. Which of the following interventions is appropriate in preventing inadvertent neck flexion when placing a child on a backboard?
   A. Padding under the occiput
   B. Padding under the shoulders and back
   C. Trendelenburg position
   D. Cloth tape across the forehead
   E. Cloth tape across the anterior mandible

ANSWERS

1. D. In the pediatric cervical spine, there is greater elasticity in the ligaments, joints, and cartilaginous structures, leading to hypermobility and greater possibility for injury to the soft tissues without bone injury. The head is relatively larger and the center of gravity higher, making injury to the upper cervical spine more likely than injury to the lower cervical spine. Facet joints are aligned more horizontally, again leading to hypermobility and less stability. Intervertebral disks function similarly in adults and children.

2. C. MRI is the modality of choice for assessing the supportive soft tissues of the spine and the spinal cord itself. MRI is useful in demonstrating cord and soft tissue injury in the presence of SCIWORA. Flexion and extension views can be used to demonstrate ligamentous injury but must be used with caution and under careful medical supervision. CT is more sensitive for bone injury. Standard cervical spine series primarily demonstrate boney injury as well.

3. A. The preferred technique for airway management in the setting of a cervical spine injury is oral intubation with in-line cervical stabilization, using rapid sequence induction. Cervical traction is not advised. Blind nasotracheal intubation is difficult and unreliable and cricothyrotomy is contraindicated in young children due to the likelihood of causing permanent tracheal damage. Prolonged bag-valve-mask ventilation increases the likelihood of gastric aspiration and it too is associated with cervical spine movement.

4. B. Padding under the shoulders and back will provide more space for the relatively large occiput and prevent the neck from being forced into flexion. Alternatively, special boards with a cutout to recess the occiput can be used.

13 THORACIC TRAUMA

Wendy Ann Lucid
Todd Brian Taylor
Kemedy K. McQuillen
Patricia Lee

EPIDEMIOLOGY

- Thoracic trauma remains the second most common cause of traumatic death after head injury. The overall mortality is about the same for blunt and penetrating trauma.

- *Isolated* chest injury is relatively infrequent, however, chest injury is a marker of injury severity and multisystem trauma mortality is 10 times higher when associated with chest injury.

- Blunt trauma accounts for approximately 83 percent of thoracic injuries. It is most commonly caused by motor vehicle crashes, falls, and bicycle accidents. Due to the compliance of the ribs and supporting structures, rib fractures and pulmonary contusions (50 percent) are more common than hemo- (10 percent) or pneumothorax (20 percent).

- Penetrating trauma accounts for approximately 15 percent of thoracic trauma. The most common causes of death are hemothorax and hemorrhagic shock with gunshot injuries and tension pneumothorax in patients who are stabbed. Cardiac injury with associated tamponade and major vascular injuries are more lethal but less common causes of death.

- Gunshot wounds to the chest are associated with abdominal injuries in 30 to 40 percent of patients. Abdominal injuries should be suspected with penetrating trauma at or below the level of the sixth rib anteriorly or below the scapula posteriorly or when stomach contents, chyme, or saliva are recovered from the chest tube.

UNIQUE ASPECTS OF PEDIATRIC THORACIC TRAUMA

- With more flexible ribs and less overlying fat and muscle, the child's chest wall is pliable and allows large forces of impact to dissipate. Although this may protect the ribs and underlying structures from injury, it allows for significant intrathoracic trauma with few or no external signs of trauma.

- The pediatric mediastinum is highly mobile and subject to extreme excursion with tension pneumothorax. This can lead to rapid ventilatory and circulatory collapse.

- Children have a proportionally larger oxygen consumption and smaller functional residual capacity, increasing their risk of hypoxia.

- A child's limited pulmonary compliance and greater chest wall compliance makes tachypnea the chief physiologic response to hypoxia.

- Children have a greater dependence on diaphragmatic breathing, which is rapidly compromised with gastric distention from aerophagia.

- Pulmonary injuries are the most common type of thoracic trauma in children. Blunt trauma tends to cause pulmonary contusion, while penetrating trauma tends to cause lacerations, and either can cause a hematoma. Pulmonary lacerations have a cavitary appearance on chest radiograph, but require surgical repair only when associated with ongoing bleeding or air leakage. Pulmonary hematoma is uncommon and is generally a self-limited injury, rarely progressing to lung abscess.

GENERAL MANAGEMENT OF THORACIC INJURY

- This section assumes that the ABCs (*a*irway, *b*reathing, *c*irculation) of trauma resuscitation have already been initiated.
- With thoracic injury, a minimal work-up includes two large-bore intravenous lines, supplemental oxygen, cardiac monitor, pulse oximetry, an arterial blood gas, hemoglobin/hematocrit, and a chest radiograph. Use of other diagnostic modalities is dictated by the clinical situation.
- With abdominal and thoracic injuries, the chest wound should be stabilized with a thoracostomy tube before the patient is placed under general anesthesia. If the clinical situation allows, the abdominal injuries are repaired first. After the abdomen is closed, a thoracotomy can then be performed for other injuries and to irrigate the chest if it is contaminated with intestinal contents.

SPECIFIC INJURIES AND MANAGEMENT

- **Traumatic pneumothorax** is often associated with significant pulmonary injury. There may be an associated hemothorax.
  - Conservative treatment includes lateral placement a large caliber, posteriorly directed chest tube. A smaller caliber, lateral or anteriorly placed chest tube may suffice if an underlying hemothorax is not suspected.
  - If there is an isolated small pneumothorax, observation with a repeat chest radiograph at 6 h may suffice. If there is no increase in size, the patient may be discharged to return in 24 h for another chest radiograph.
  - A chest tube is mandatory if the patient is to undergo mechanical ventilation or emergency transport.
- **Hemothorax** results from injury to the lung parenchyma or the intercostal or internal mammary vessels. Clinical findings include decreased breath sounds and dullness to percussion on the affected side with or without obvious respiratory distress. Visualization of a hemothorax on chest radiograph requires the presence of at least 10 mL/kg of blood.

- Place a large caliber chest tube to evacuate the hematoma and observe for ongoing bleeding. Hematoma removal prevents delayed complications of fibrosis and empyema.
- **Massive hemothorax** is rare in children and may be complicated by hypovolemic shock.
  - Initiate aggressive crystalloid fluid resuscitation and give blood as needed.
  - Place thoracostomy tubes: use a large caliber (about as wide as the intercostal space) tube and insert it laterally and in a posterior direction to allow for drainage. Consider using an autotransfusion chest tube collection system.
  - Thoracotomy may be indicated for initial evacuated blood volume exceeding 10 to 15 mL/kg, continued blood loss exceeding 2 to 4 mL/kg/h, or continued air leakage. An emergency thoracotomy and clamping of the injured area may be necessary to control bleeding until definitive treatment can be administered.
- An **open pneumothorax** (sucking chest wound) is created when the chest wall is compromised and air flows bidirectionally through the wound. The lung is unable to expand due to equal pressures between the chest cavity and atmosphere. Gas exchange is compromised and hypoxia and hypercarbia ensue. The compliant mediastinum in children complicates this condition, allowing compression of both lungs with inspiration and paradoxical breathing.
  - In the prehospital setting, place a petroleum dressing and tape three sides to create a flutter valve.
  - In the emergency department, treat breathing patients with small injuries by covering the chest wall defect with a sterile petroleum dressing and placing a thoracostomy tube through a fresh incision. In general, small chest wall defects heal spontaneously and do not require surgical repair.
  - Those patients who are not spontaneously breathing and those who have chest wall defects too large to seal will require intubation and ventilatory support. Large wounds may require urgent thoracotomy.
- **Tension pneumothorax** occurs when air flows into the pleural cavity without a means of escape. This increases the pressure against the mediastinal structures causing them to shift toward the opposite side. Cardiac decompensation ensues from mechanical impingement of blood flow and hypoxia from respiratory compromise. Signs and symptoms include severe respiratory distress, decreased breath sounds, ipsilateral hyperresonance, contralateral tracheal deviation, distended neck veins, subcutaneous emphysema, and circulatory collapse with hypotension and narrow pulse pressure.

◦ In the field, treatment is with a percutaneous needle thoracostomy attached to a flutter valve, placed just over the top of the third rib in the midclavicular line. Even if the presence or location of a tension pneumothorax is in question, and the patient is deteriorating, empiric treatment with bilateral needle thoracostomies should be initiated.

◦ Definitive treatment is accomplished using a large caliber thoracostomy tube placed laterally and directed posteriorly.

• Due to the compliance of the chest wall, children are particularly susceptible to **pulmonary contusion** with few external signs of trauma. After a blunt or high energy penetrating injury, capillary leak into the interstitial and alveolar spaces causes hypoxia and respiratory distress. Symptoms range from minimal to severe respiratory distress. The initial chest radiograph and arterial blood gas may be normal.

◦ Treatment is directed toward preventing hypoxia and respiratory failure. With an isolated pulmonary contusion, supplemental oxygen and close monitoring are often sufficient. Patients with more severe respiratory distress require intubation and ventilation with positive end-expiratory pressure (PEEP) of 5 to 10 cmH$_2$O.

◦ Acute respiratory distress syndrome (ARDS) may complicate pulmonary contusion. Excessive administration of crystalloid and aspiration of gastric contents are predisposing factors and should be avoided.

• **Traumatic asphyxia** is an injury unique to children due to their increased chest wall compliance. The pressure from a severe blow to the chest is transmitted through the superior vena cava into the capillaries of the head and neck, resulting in a deep violet color of the skin in the head and neck, bilateral subconjunctival hemorrhages, and facial edema. About one-third of these patients will experience a loss of consciousness. The condition is generally benign but serves as a marker for associated head trauma, pulmonary contusions, and intraabdominal injuries. Transient and permanent visual disturbances can occur due to retinal hemorrhages and edema.

• **Traumatic tracheal and bronchial disruptions** are rare in children, but highly lethal; half of all affected patients die within the first hour after injury. The disruption nearly always occurs adjacent to the carina. Concommitant ipsilateral tension pneumothorax and hemoptysis may be seen. Bronchoscopy is diagnostic.

◦ If necessary, establish an endotracheal or surgical airway: place a tracheostomy or cricothyrotomy below the level of the disruption.

◦ Small disruptions can be treated with a chest tube and observation, however, thoracotomy is necessary if bleeding cannot be controlled, the patient cannot be ventilated, or if tracheal obstruction occurs.

• **Traumatic esophageal rupture** is exceptionally rare in children. Clinical signs include pain and shock out of proportion to the apparent severity of injury. It may be associated with a pneumothorax that drains stomach contents or bubbles equally and continuously throughout the respiratory cycle, subcutaneous emphysema, and Hamman's sign (a mediastinal crunching sound with heartbeats). A chest radiograph, fluoroscopy with water-soluble contrast, and/or endoscopy confirms the diagnosis.

◦ Urgent surgical repair with mediastinal drainage is required unless there is extensive damage that requires a temporary esophageal diversion with delayed definitive repair.

• **Traumatic diaphragmatic hernia** is part of the "lap belt" complex, occurring predominantly on the left. It is most often caused by a blunt trauma producing a sudden increase in intraabdominal pressure and, less commonly, by penetrating trauma occurring anywhere between the nipples and umbilicus. Because many patients have no evidence of injury, up to 90 percent of these injuries are missed on initial evaluation. When present, clinical findings include external signs of trauma to the upper abdomen and lower chest wall, decreased breath sounds, bowel sounds in the chest cavity, and respiratory distress. Chest radiograph findings depend on the status of the abdominal contents and are outlined in Table 13-1. In some cases, fluoroscopy or laparotomy may be required to confirm the diagnosis.

◦ Treatment includes intubation, if there is respiratory distress, nasogastric tube placement, and surgical repair.

• **Rib fractures** are uncommon in children. If there are multiple fractures in various stages of healing or if there is no clear history of trauma, child abuse should be suspected. The posterolateral aspect of the ribs is the most susceptible to fracture. Findings include pain, point tenderness, crepitus, and deformity. Atelectasis and respiratory splinting is uncommon. Rib radiographs are of limited value.

TABLE 13-1   Chest Radiograph Findings in Traumatic Diaphragmatic Hernia

Chest radiograph with acute herniation of abdominal contents
Diagnostic with bowel or stomach presenting within the chest cavity
Presence of the nasogastric tube in the chest

Chest radiograph with diaphragmatic tear but delayed herniation of abdominal contents
Unexplained elevation of the hemidiaphragm
Unrelieved acute gastric dilation
Loculated subpulmonic hemopneumothorax
Presence of the nasogastric tube in the chest.

○ Simple rib fractures require no specific treatment other than pain management. Medication and/or intercostal nerve blocks may be necessary.

- **Flail chest** occurs when the structural integrity of the chest wall is compromised with more than two fractures to the same rib in more than two adjacent ribs. Associated pulmonary contusion is common. Signs and symptoms include tenderness, bruising, crepitus overlying the flail segments, respiratory distress, hypoxia, and paradoxical chest wall motion. Chest radiography confirms the diagnosis.
  - ○ Treatment includes supplemental oxygen, close monitoring, and pain control. Intercostal or epidural nerve blocks are preferable to narcotic analgesia due to their potential for respiratory depression. Intubated patients require ventilation with PEEP of 5 to 10 cmH$_2$O. External stabilization of the fractures is not effective.
- **Cardiac tamponade** is the most common cardiovascular injury from penetrating trauma. It is a life-threatening condition that occurs when fluid fills the pericardial space and compromises venous return. Stab wounds are the most common traumatic etiology. Clinical findings include the presence of a precordial wound, tachycardia, narrow pulse pressure, pulsus paradoxus, and Beck's triad [distant heart sounds, hypotension, and jugular venous distention (may be absent in the presence of hypovolemia)]. If untreated, hypotension progresses to pulseless electrical activity (PEA). The chest radiograph typically shows a "water bottle" cardiac silhouette. The ECG may show tachycardia with low voltage or evidence of acute myocardial infarction if a coronary artery has been lacerated. Bedside echocardiography is diagnostic but treatment should not be delayed while waiting for the echo.
  - ○ Definitive treatment requires thoracotomy, pericardiotomy, and repair of the underlying injury.
  - ○ If definitive thoracotomy is not readily available and the patient's condition is deteriorating and not responsive to aggressive fluid resuscitation, a pericardiocentesis should be done, leaving the needle or plastic angiocath in place so that repeated aspirations may be done as needed to relieve pressure. In certain circumstances, an emergency pericardial window may be necessary to open the pericardium and control the bleeding until definitive treatment can be performed. Pericardiocentesis risks include myocardial and coronary artery laceration, hemopericardium, pneumothorax, and dysrhythmia.
- **Myocardial contusion** is the most common cardiovascular injury from blunt trauma. Findings include chest wall tenderness or poorly localized chest pain. Tachycardia is the most common ECG finding. Echocardiograms rarely show abnormalities. Myocardial enzymes may be elevated. Radionuclide angiography may be useful in selected cases.
  - ○ Treatment includes cardiac monitoring and dysrhythmia management.
- **Traumatic rupture of the great vessels** is extremely rare in children. The most common site for aortic disruption is at the level of the ligamentum arteriosum. Injury may be associated with aortic dissection. Morbidity and mortality is high, with more than 50 percent of these patients dying at the scene. Blunt aortic injury is most commonly caused by rapid deceleration. Findings include anterior chest, back, or upper abdominal pain and a murmur radiating to the back. Penetrating trauma to the vena cava or pulmonary vessels is more common than penetrating injury to the aorta. Findings include an obvious wound and hypotension. Chest radiograph findings are listed in Table 13-2. CT of the chest may confirm the diagnosis but can miss small tears. Early surgical consultation with angiography is the diagnostic test of choice.
  - ○ Initial treatment includes airway management and aggressive fluid resuscitation. Associated hemopneumothorax should be treated with a thoracostomy tube unless emergency thoracotomy is indicated.
  - ○ Definitive treatment requires immediate surgical repair.
- Rare complications of blunt thoracic trauma include myocardial rupture, myocardial necrosis with subsequent aneurysm, traumatic aortic insufficiency, pericardial laceration, fatal cardiac herniation, coronary artery injury, and cardiac conduction system injury.

PROCEDURES

(*These procedures should only be performed by physicians trained in the techniques and for the appropriate indication.*)

- The technique for **thoracostomy tube placement** is identical for adults and children. Chest tube size is approximately four times endotracheal tube size. A postinsertion chest radiograph should be obtained to confirm proper placement of the tube and reexpansion of the lung.

TABLE 13-2   Chest Radiograph Findings in Aortic Injury

Widened mediastinum with obliteration of the aortic knob
Dilation of the ascending aorta
Deviation of the trachea (as evidenced by the endotracheal tube) to the right
Deviation of the esophagus (as evidenced by the nasogastric tube) to the right
Evidence of first and/or second rib fracture
Apical pleural cap (blood at the apex of the lung, seen more commonly on the left)

- The technique for **pericardiocentesis** is the same for adults and children. A 20-mL syringe attached to an 18-gauge, 3.5-inch spinal needle is required. An alligator clip with a wire can be used for cardiac monitor guidance. Atypical ventricular depolarization is seen as the needle is advanced toward the myocardium. For the subxiphoid approach, the needle is inserted at a 30° to 45° angle just left of the xiphoid process, aiming for the sternal notch.
- **Emergency department thoracotomy** is indicated in cases of cardiac tamponade or in penetrating trauma when vital signs have been lost in the emergency department or just prior to arrival. Survival after emergency thoracotomy in blunt trauma is dismal. Crossclamping of the distal thoracic aorta has been abandoned. Direct finger compression of the proximal abdominal aorta via laparotomy is as effective, with less potential for collateral injury.

LAW ENFORCEMENT

- Most states require reporting of stab wounds, gunshot wounds, assaults, and child abuse.

BIBLIOGRAPHY

Bliss D, Silen M: Pediatric thoracic trauma. *Crit Care Med* 30(11 Suppl):S409–415, 2002.

Cantor RM, Leaming JM: Evaluation and management of pediatric major trauma. *Contemp Issues Trauma* 16:229–256, 1998.

Grant WJ, Meyers RL, Jaffe RL, et al: Tracheobronchial injuries after blunt chest trauma in children—Hidden pathology. *J Pediatr Surg* 33:1707–1711, 1998.

Holmes JF, Brant WE, Bogren G, et al: Prevalence and importance of pneumothoraces visualized on abdominal computed tomographic scan in children with blunt trauma. *J Trauma* 50:516–520, 2001.

Holmes JF, Sokolove PE, Brant WE, Kupperman N: A clinical decision rule for identifying children with thoracic injuries after blunt trauma. *Ann Emerg Med* 39:492–499, 2002.

Karnak I, Senocak ME, Tanyel FC, et al: Diaphragmatic injuries in childhood. *Surg Today* 31:5–11, 2001.

Murray JA, Berne J, Asensio JA: Penetrating thoracoabdominal trauma. *Emerg Med Clin North Am* 16:107–128, 1998.

Sanchez JI, Paidas CN: Childhood trauma: Now and in the new millennium. *Surg Clin North Am* 79:1503–1535, 1999.

Tiao GM, Griffith PM, Szmuszkovicz JR, et al: Cardiac and great vessel injuries in children after blunt trauma: An institutional review. *J Pediatr Surg* 35:1656–1660, 2000.

APLS Joint Task Force: Trauma, in Strange GR (ed): *Advanced Pediatric Life Support,* 3d ed. Dallas: American Academy of Pediatrics/American College of Emergency Physicians, 1998, pp 59–78.

Schafermeyer RW: Pediatric trauma. *Emerg Med Clin North Am* 11(1):187–205, 1993.

QUESTIONS

1. All of the following are true regarding pediatric thoracic trauma **EXCEPT**:
   A. Thoracic trauma is the most common cause of traumatic death in children.
   B. Multisystem trauma mortality is 10 times higher when associated with chest injury.
   C. Blunt trauma accounts for most thoracic injury in children.
   D. Few or no external signs of trauma may be present in spite of significant underlying injury.
   E. Abdominal injuries should be suspected with penetrating thoracic trauma when the injury is below the level of the sixth rib anteriorly.

2. A 4-year-old female presents after a motor vehicle crash. Concern exists regarding the possibility of blunt chest trauma. Important differences in pediatric chest trauma from adult chest trauma are all of the following **EXCEPT**:
   A. Because the pediatric mediastinum is highly mobile, rapid ventilatory and circulatory collapse may occur with tension pneumothorax.
   B. Children have a lower oxygen consumption and larger functional, residual capacity, thereby, decreasing their risk of hypoxia.
   C. Children have a greater dependence on diaphragmatic breathing.
   D. Pulmonary injuries are the most common type of thoracic trauma.
   E. Pulmonary lacerations may have a cavitary appearance on chest radiograph.

3. A 6-year-old boy arrives as a victim of a motor vehicle collision. On arrival, he is tachypneic, hypotensive, and tachycardic. Chest radiograph reveals a pneumohemothorax. All of the following are appropriate interventions **EXCEPT**:
   A. Placement of a large caliber, posterior directed chest tube.
   B. Observation with a repeat chest radiograph at 6 h.
   C. Autotransfusion
   D. Thoracotomy may be indicated for initial evacuated blood volume exceeding 10 to 15 mL/kg.
   E. Chest tube placement is mandatory if the patient is to go to the operating room.

4. Signs of tension pneumothorax include all the following **EXCEPT**:
   A. Subcutaneous emphysema
   B. Decreased breath sounds

C. Narrow pulse pressure

D. Ipsilateral tracheal deviation

E. Distended neck veins

5. A 4-year-old girl is brought to the emergency department after being kicked in the chest by her old brother who was practicing his judo. Her parents report that initially after the injury, the child was found unconscious. On physical examination, she is found to have a deep violet color of the head and neck and bilateral subconjunctival hemorrhages. Which of the following are true characteristics of this injury?

A. This injury is not unique to children.

B. About 90 percent of all children with this condition will experience loss of consciousness.

C. Transient and permanent visual disturbances can occur.

D. The injury occurs due to a blow to the chest that interrupts the electrical activity of the heart.

E. The injury is generally chronically debilitating.

6. A 10-year-old presents as a restrained passenger in a motor vehicle collision with complaints of abdominal pain. On examination, decreased breath sounds are heard on the left chest. Chest radiograph reveals an elevated diaphragm in the left hemithorax. All of the following characteristics are true of this situation **EXCEPT**:

A. Most of these injuries are missed on initial evaluation.

B. Treatment includes intubation and surgical repair.

C. It may be associated with pneumothorax that drains stomach contents.

D. Fluoroscopy or laparotomy may be required to confirm the diagnosis.

E. It is usually caused by blunt trauma.

7. Clinical findings of cardiac tamponade may include all of the following **EXCEPT**:

A. ECG changes

B. Narrow pulse pressure

C. Pulsus paradoxus

D. Beck's triad

E. Bradycardia

ANSWERS

1. A. Thoracic trauma is the second most common cause of traumatic death in children after head injury. With more flexible ribs and less overlying fat and muscle, the child's chest wall is pliable and allows large forces of impact to dissipate. This allows significant trauma to occur to intrathoracic structures with few of no external signs of trauma.

2. B. Children have a higher oxygen consumption and lower functional residual capacity thereby, increasing their risk of hypoxia.

3. B. Conservative treatment of a pneumohemothorax includes placement of a large caliber, posteriorly directed chest tube. A smaller caliber, lateral or anteriorly placed chest tube may suffice if an underlying hemothorax is not suspected. If there is an isolated, small pneumothorax only, observation with a repeat chest radiograph at 6 h may suffice.

4. D. Signs and symptoms of tension pneumothorax include severe respiratory distress, decreased breath sounds, ipsilateral hyperresonance, contralateral tracheal deviation, distended neck veins, subcutaneous emphysema, circulatory collapse with hypotension, and narrow pulse pressure.

5. C. Traumatic asphyxia is an injury unique to children due to their increased chest wall compliance. The pressure from a severe blow to the chest is transmitted through the superior vena cava into the head capillaries. About one third of patients experience loss of consciousness. The condition is generally benign but may be a marker for associated head trauma, pulmonary contusions, and intraabdominal injuries. Transient and permanent visual disturbances may occur.

6. C. Traumatic diaphragmatic hernia is part of the "lap belt" complex, occurring predominantly on the left and occurring most often due to blunt trauma. Because most patients have no evidence of injury, up to 90 percent of these injuries are missed on initial evaluation.

7. E. Tachycardia is a common finding in cardiac tamponade. If untreated, hypotension may progress to pulseless electrical activity (PEA). The ECG typically will show tachycardia with low voltage or evidence of acute myocardial infarction if a coronary artery has been lacerated.

14   ABDOMINAL TRAUMA

Wendy Ann Lucid
Todd Brian Taylor
Kemedy K. McQuillen
Gary R. Strange

EPIDEMIOLOGY

• Serious abdominal injuries account for approximately 8 percent of admissions to pediatric trauma centers but only 15 percent of these injuries require surgery.

- Abdominal trauma is the third leading cause of traumatic death behind head and thoracic injuries, but it is the most common unrecognized cause of fatal injury in children.
- Blunt trauma accounts for 85 percent of pediatric abdominal trauma, with 9 percent of these patients dying from other injuries. Penetrating abdominal trauma accounts for 15 percent of the total cases, with 6 percent of patients dying from the penetrating wound.

PATTERNS OF INJURY

MOTOR VEHICLE CRASHES (TABLE 14-1)

- **Waddell's triad** includes head, extremity, and intra-abdominal injuries. In countries in which motorists drive on the right side of the road, the most common injuries are on the left side because children are struck when they dart into traffic; these accidents frequently result in splenic injuries.
- The **lap belt complex** (bursting injury of solid or hollow viscera and disruption of the diaphragm or lumbar spine) is characterized by ecchymosis across the abdomen and flanks (Grey–Turner sign). The injury occurs when an improperly applied restraint allows the lap belt to ride up and compress the abdomen.
- Injuries sustained in all-terrain vehicle crashes parallel motor vehicle crashes.

BICYCLE CRASHES, SPORTS INJURIES, AND FALLS

- Head trauma remains the predominant injury in bicycle crashes.
- With handlebar injuries, most children show no sign of injury for hours to days: the mean time to onset of symptoms is almost 24 h and the mean length of hospital stay exceeds 3 weeks. Traumatic pancreatitis is the most common handlebar injury, followed by injuries to the kidneys, spleen, and liver, duodenal hematoma, and bowel perforation.
- Sports-related trauma typically produces isolated organ injury due to a direct blow to the abdomen. The spleen, kidney, and gastrointestinal tract are particularly vulnerable.

- Injuries from falls include head and chest wall trauma and multiple long bone fractures. Isolated abdominal injuries are rare.

CHILD ABUSE

- Significant abdominal injury occurs in about 5 percent of child abuse cases but it represents the second most common cause of death (after head injury). The diagnosis is obscured by the delay in seeking treatment, the surreptitious nature of the visit, and the lack of external signs of trauma.

PATHOPHYSIOLOGY

- Proportionally larger solid organs, poorly muscled protuberant abdomen, and flexible, thin ribs contribute to the increased incidence of abdominal injury.
- The diagnosis of intraabdominal hemorrhage may be delayed because children are able to maintain a normal blood pressure and pulse rate with significant blood loss. Abdominal distention caused by aerophagia confounds the examination by masking or mimicking serious abdominal injury. Severe distention can also result in respiratory compromise due to interference with diaphragm motion, gastric aspiration, or vagal dampening of the normal tachycardic response. Vagal dampening can lead to precipitous circulatory collapse in the presence of hypovolemia. External signs of injury, abdominal tenderness, and absence of bowel sounds seldom give clues to the ultimate need for surgery.

MANAGEMENT

GENERAL PRINCIPLES

- A systematic approach is mandatory in evaluating the injured child. Evaluation of the abdomen is included in the primary and secondary surveys. The following interventions are particularly important:
  - A nasogastric tube to decompress the stomach and check for blood or bile

TABLE 14-1   Patterns of Injury by Mechanism

WADDELL'S TRIAD	LAP BELT COMPLEX	FALL FROM A HEIGHT
Pedestrian mechanism in child	Restrained occupant in MVC	Head injury
Midshaft femur fracture	Blowout diaphragm injury	Multiple long bone fractures
Abdominal injury	Duodenal injury	Chest wall injury
Head injury	Solid organ injury	

- A urinary catheter to check for blood and urinary retention (if there is no blood at the meatus and the prostate is normal)
- A rectal examination to check for blood, prostate position, and rectal tone
- NPO status in anticipation of surgery
- Blood sampling for type and cross-match, CBC, serum amylase, and liver transaminases
- The mechanism of injury is important and guides the secondary survey and the ordering of specific tests or procedures. External injuries such as abrasions, lacerations, bruising, and characteristic markings, such as tire tracks and seat belt marks, should be noted. All unstable patients need immediate surgical consultation.
- A traumatized child may not show signs of impending demise, history may be limited, and the child's reaction to pain may be over- or underexaggerated. Designate a team member to care for the child's emotional needs and promote their cooperation.

PENETRATING ABDOMINAL TRAUMA

- Penetrating wounds between the nipples and the groin potentially involve the peritoneal cavity.
  - The initial management does not depend on the identification of specific injury.
  - Hollow organs, due to their large volume, are most commonly injured, followed by the liver, kidney, spleen, and major vessels.
  - Location, size, and trajectory of entrance and exit wounds help identify potential underlying injuries.
  - At a minimum, place a nasogastric tube and urinary catheter; obtain an upright posteroanterior chest radiograph and supine, upright and cross-table abdominal radiographs.
  - Order a "one shot" intravenous pyelogram for deep stab wounds and gunshot wounds.
- Stab wounds enter the peritoneal cavity only one third of the time and only one third of these require a visceral repair.
- Stab wounds, though, pose the greatest threat to blood vessels, including the aorta, inferior vena cava, portal vein, and hepatic veins.
- Surgical evaluation, wound debridement, and possible exploration, along with broad spectrum intravenous antibiotics are necessary in all but the most minor of stab wounds. Conservative management, with repeated evaluations by a surgeon over 12 to 24 h, is possible if there are no:
  - Signs of shock or peritonitis
  - Blood in the stomach, rectum, or urine
  - Evidence of free air on x-ray
  - Evidence of bowel or omental evisceration
- Gunshot wounds, which injure organs directly or indirectly through kinetic energy dissipation, require immediate exploration.

BLUNT ABDOMINAL TRAUMA

- Physical examination of the pediatric trauma patient is only slightly more than 50 percent accurate. The key to management is realizing that minor mechanisms can cause major injuries, suspecting the diagnosis, and obtaining appropriate studies and consultation.
- Radiographs of the chest (supine or upright posteroanterior plus a lateral), abdomen, and pelvis can give important clues to the diagnosis of abdominal injury (Table 14-2).
- Hemoglobin and hematocrit are seldom useful early in the evaluation of a trauma patient, although an initial hematocrit <30 percent with signs of impending shock suggests significant hemorrhage and an initial hematocrit <24 percent is associated with high mortality. Subsequent hematocrit measurements are helpful for comparison to baseline.
- Immediate surgical intervention is warranted for:
  - Persistently distended abdomen after nasogastric tube placement
  - Hemodynamic instability not immediately responsive to fluid resuscitation
  - Recurrent hypotension
  - Signs of peritoneal irritation

COMPUTED TOMOGRAPHY (CT)

- CT is the procedure of choice for stable trauma patients. Indications for abdominal and pelvic CT are listed in Table 14-3. CT is useful for evaluation of liver, kidney, spleen, retroperitoneum, and, to a lesser extent, gastrointestinal injuries but has poor sensitivity

TABLE 14-2   Radiographic Clues in Abdominal Trauma

- A ground-glass appearance of the abdominal cavity may suggest intraperitoneal blood or urine
- Medial displacement of the lateral border of the stomach, as evidenced by the nasogastric tube, suggests splenic laceration or hematoma as the enlarged spleen pushes the stomach aside
- Obliteration of the psoas shadow or renal outline and fracture of the lower ribs suggest renal trauma
- Bleeding from the short gastric vessels gives the fundic mucosa a "sawtooth" appearance
- With nasogastric tube in place, the relative lack of gas in the distal small intestine suggests a duodenal or proximal jejunal hematoma
- Air injected via the nasogastric tube may increase the chance of detecting a pneumoperitoneum indicative of perforated viscus

TABLE 14-3 Comparison of Techniques for Evaluation of Abdominal Trauma

	ABDOMINAL CT	DIAGNOSTIC PERITONEAL LAVAGE	ABDOMINAL ULTRASOUND
Indication	Relatively stable patient	Relatively unstable patient	May be used as a triage tool and adjunct to the physical examination
	Multiple trauma or major thoracic, head, or orthopedic (pelvic) injury	Otherwise the same as for CT	
	Physical findings or a mechanism suggesting possible abdominal injury		Evaluation of pancreatic injury and intraabdominal fluid (presumably blood)
	Unexplained hypotension		May also be used to identify other intraabdominal injuries when CT is not readily available.
	Hematuria (gross or microscopic >20 RBC/hpf), CNS injury, spinal injury, or mental status alteration precluding serial abdominal examination.		
	Declining hematocrit <10 g/dL) or unaccountable fluid and blood requirements		
Advantage	Relatively noninvasive	May be performed on a patient who is relatively unstable or who needs to undergo urgent general anesthesia for other reasons	Available at the bedside and more readily available than CT in some locales
	High sensitivity and specificity		Can be used at the bedside for a FAST examination to evaluate for peritoneal fluid and blood
	Evaluates multiple organ systems simultaneously	Easily and rapidly performed	
Disadvantage	Generally requires intravenous with or without oral contrast	Unless grossly positive, laboratory results may delay definitive treatment	Not as sensitive as CT
	Time delay	Neither organ nor injury specific	
		Cannot asses retroperitoneal injury	
		Decision to operate is not generally based on the amount of peritoneal blood	
		Introduction of air and fluid into the abdomen may alter future diagnostic tests	
		Local peritoneal irritation may alter serial abdominal examinations	

in detecting pancreas, diaphragm, and bowel injuries. Serial abdominal examinations may be necessary to rule out occult injury. Oral and intravenous contrast media increase the sensitivity of abdominal CT, however oral contrast is difficult to administer, increases the waiting time before scanning, increases the risk of aspiration, and has limited value due to frequent lack of bowel opacification. Its role in trauma patients is being questioned.

DIAGNOSTIC PERITONEAL LAVAGE (DPL)

• In pediatric patients, close observation, serial physical examinations, and abdominal CT are utilized to

the exclusion of peritoneal lavage. DPL is useful if other modalities are unavailable or the child must undergo immediate general anesthesia for other injuries.
• The usefulness of DPL remains questionable:
  ○ It is neither organ- nor injury-specific.
  ○ It cannot reliably assess retroperitoneal injury.
  ○ It does not dictate the need for surgery with liver or splenic injuries.
  ○ It introduces air and fluid into the abdomen, making subsequent radiographic and physical examinations more difficult.
• If done, a small supraumbilical incision to avoid the bladder is preferred over the infraumbilical approach.

ABDOMINAL ULTRASOUND

- Bedside ultrasound (US) is useful in the unstable patient as an immediate triage tool and adjunct to the physical examination: it is best used for detecting intraabdominal injuries that require immediate attention rather than for making a definitive diagnosis. It is also useful when CT is not available. Its greatest utility is in detecting intraperitoneal hemorrhage and pancreatic injuries. Bedside ultrasound is often taught using the "focused abdominal sonography for trauma" (FAST) method. This examination evaluates up to six areas of the abdomen with the principal objective of identifying hemoperitoneum. However, children who are hemodynamically unstable with abdominal trauma will require laparotomy regardless of the US and those that are stable are often managed nonsurgically, even with an abdominal organ injury. As such, the role of US in pediatric abdominal trauma is still being evaluated.

NUCLEAR SCANS

- Nuclear scans are not typically used for the evaluation of acute abdominal injury, but can be useful as a follow-up for liver or splenic injuries.

SPECIFIC INJURIES AND MANAGEMENT

SOLID ORGANS

SPLEEN

- The spleen is the most commonly injured abdominal organ in blunt trauma. It is second only to the liver in lethal injury. It is most commonly injured in motor vehicle accidents, although, for patients with mononucleosis, splenic swelling may occur and seemingly inconsequential injuries can result in rupture.
- Findings with splenic injury include left upper quadrant pain radiating to the left shoulder (Kehr's sign), left upper quadrant tenderness, splenic enlargement, or diffuse abdominal pain. Splenic rupture may lead to shock and posttraumatic cardiac arrest. Persistent unexplained leukocytosis or hyperamylasemia also suggests splenic injury.
- Although abdominal radiographs may reveal a medially displaced gastric bubble secondary to the enlarged spleen, abdominal CT is the study of choice to identify splenic injury.
- The thick, elastic splenic capsule and the orientation of lacerations parallel to the vessels commonly results

in spontaneous cessation of bleeding and allows nonsurgical management in 90 percent of splenic injuries. Conservative management includes hospitalization for 7 to 10 days of bed rest, followed by a regimen of limited activity. Delayed rupture can occur at any time and is most common on the third to fifth day. Children who develop hypotension and do not respond to volume resuscitation require surgery: splenorrhaphy or partial splenectomy may be done to preserve some splenic function.
- Postsplenectomy, there is an increase risk of infection and lethal sepsis, particularly with encapsulated organisms. Pneumococcal and *H. influenzae* vaccines should be given to patients undergoing partial or complete splenectomy.

LIVER

- The liver is the second most commonly injured abdominal organ in blunt trauma but is the most common source of *lethal* hemorrhage. Fortunately, most liver injuries are minor and discovered incidentally by abnormal liver enzymes or CT scan.
- Mechanisms of injury are similar to those in splenic trauma. Symptoms depend on the extent of injury and range from nonspecific diffuse abdominal pain to right upper abdomen tenderness and liver enlargement to posttraumatic cardiac arrest.
- Children with liver injuries who are not in shock or who respond to volume resuscitation rarely require surgery to control bleeding. However, nonsurgical management is not without complications.
  - With late laparotomy, transfusion requirements may be greater than 50 percent of total blood volume (TBV) and there may be bleeding into the biliary tract (hematobilia).
- Conservative management includes careful monitoring of vital signs, serial abdominal examinations, and hematocrit measurements.
- Large, stellate lacerations and hematomas that have eroded through Glisson's capsule tend to require surgery: in most cases, direct suturing and drainage are sufficient.
- Circulating blood volume should be restored in anticipation of surgery.

PANCREAS

- The pancreas is rarely seriously injured in blunt trauma due to its deep position in the upper abdomen; however, its fixed position anterior to the vertebral column makes it vulnerable to a direct blow to the upper abdomen as is seen with bicycle handlebar injuries.

- Pancreatic injuries are difficult to diagnose.
- Traumatic pancreatitis without major injury is most common, followed by pancreatic hematomas, and transection of the body or duct.
- Pancreatic transections often lead to pancreatic pseudocyst formation within 3 to 5 days and result in chronic intermittent attacks of abdominal pain, nausea, vomiting, and weight loss.
- Acutely, the leakage of pancreatic fluid into the lesser peritoneal sac causes a chemical peritonitis and pancreatic ascites.
- The classic triad of epigastric pain radiating to the back, a palpable abdominal mass with or without acute peritonitis or ascites, and hyperamylasemia is rarely present in children.
- CT or ultrasound may help identify pancreatic injury or show evidence of edema. There may be an elevated serum amylase, but normal levels do not preclude a pancreatic injury.
- Simple traumatic pancreatitis is treated with bowel rest, nasogastric suction, intravenous fluids, and pain medication. Severe pancreatic injury typically requires surgical drainage with repair or partial resection of the pancreas. Pancreatic pseudocyst treatment involves 6 to 8 weeks of total parenteral nutrition followed by surgical drainage.

ABDOMINAL WALL

- Hematomas of the abdominal wall muscles and injury to the spine and other skeletal structures may occur in abdominal trauma. The psoas muscle is particularly susceptible to hematoma in patients with hemophilia or on warfarin.
- Tenderness, bruising, swelling, or a mass of the abdominal wall may indicate hematoma or contusion; however, certain types of ecchymoses, that may occur hours after the injury, are indicative of intraabdominal injury:
  - **Grey-Turner sign,** or *ecchymosis* in the abdominal or flank area, may represent a retroperitoneal hematoma
  - **Cullen's sign,** a bluish discoloration around the umbilicus, may represent an intraperitoneal hemorrhage.
- Most abdominal wall injuries are self-limited. Differentiation between abdominal wall and deeper injury can be difficult, so a low threshold for abdominal CT is warranted.
- At discharge, instruct patients and caregivers to return for vomiting, increasing pain, abdominal distention, hematuria, and fever. Arrange for follow-up and reexamination within 24 h.

HOLLOW ORGANS

- Hollow visceral organ injuries rarely occur in blunt abdominal trauma. Perforations of the duodenum and proximal jejunum are the most common and are usually associated with a lap belt or handlebar injury. The diagnosis of a perforated viscus is difficult: tenderness may not develop until 6 to 12 h after injury when peritonitis or obstruction occur. Abdominal CT is not sensitive for these injuries, and repeated physical examinations remain the most reliable diagnostic tool. A perforated viscus requires surgical repair.
- Intramural hematomas of the duodenum or jejunum can cause symptoms of intestinal obstruction with pain, bilious vomiting, and gastric distention.
  - The diagnosis is made with ultrasound or an upper GI series, which reveals a "coiled spring" sign.
  - An intramural hematoma rarely requires surgery.
  - If it causes a traumatic pancreatitis, treatment is supportive with nasogastric suction and parenteral nutrition for up to 3 weeks.
- If there is a large abdominal wall defect that allows evisceration, keep the bowel moist with saline-soaked gauze and do not allow the patient to assume a dependent position that would increase edema of the bowel wall.

Bibliography

APLS Joint Task Force: Trauma. In: Strange GR, ed. *Advanced Pediatric Life Support,* 3d ed. Dallas: American Academy of Pediatrics/American College of Emergency Physicians, 59–78, 1997.

Brown CK, Dunn KA, Wilson K: Diagnostic evaluation of patients with blunt abdominal trauma: A decision analysis. *Acad Emerg Med* 7:385–396, 2000.

Cantor RM, Leaming JM: Evaluation and management of pediatric major trauma. *Contemp Issues Trauma* 16:229–256, 1998.

Gaines BA, Ford HR: Abdominal and pelvic trauma in children. *Crit Care Med* 30(11 Suppl):S416–423, 2002.

Melanson SW, Heller M: The emerging role of bedside ultrasonography in trauma care. *Emerg Med Clin North Am* 16: 165–189, 1998.

Patel JC, Tepas JJ: The efficacy of focused abdominal sonography for trauma (FAST) as a screening tool in the assessment of injured children. *J Pediatr Surg* 34:44–47, 1999.

Rothrock SG, Green SM, Morgan R: Abdominal trauma in infants and children: Prompt identification and early management of serious and life-threatening injuries. Part I: Injury patterns and initial assessment. *Pediatr Emerg Care* 16:106–115, 2000. Part II: Specific injuries and ED management. *Pediatr Emerg Care* 16:189–195, 2000.

Sanchez JI, Paidas CN: Childhood trauma: Now and in the new millennium. *Surg Clin North Am* 79:1503–1535, 1999.

Schafermeyer RW: Pediatric trauma. *Emerg Med Clin North Am* 11:187–205, 1993.

QUESTIONS

1. The principal objective of the focused abdominal sonographic scan for trauma (FAST scan) is:
   A. Establishing a specific organ diagnosis
   B. Identifying hemoperitoneum
   C. Assessment for retroperitoneal injury
   D. Assessment of hollow visceral organs
   E. Differentiation of abdominal wall from intraabdominal injuries

2. A 10-year-old boy is brought to the ED by his parents 24 h after a bike crash. He reports vague upper abdominal soreness where he was struck by the handlebar of the bike. He shows no other signs of significant trauma. What is the most common injury associated with this mechanism?
   A. Small bowel rupture
   B. Duodenal hematoma
   C. Subcapsular hematoma of the spleen
   D. Renal contusion
   E. Traumatic pancreatitis

3. A 5-year-old girl is injured in a motor vehicle crash and presents with stable vital signs but significant abdominal tenderness. CT scan reveals splenic laceration with subcapsular hematoma. Appropriate management includes:
   A. Immediate splenectomy
   B. Exploration and partial splenectomy
   C. Hospitalization for observation and frequent examination for 3 to 5 days
   D. Hospitalization for observation and frequent examination for 7 to 10 days
   E. Bedrest at home with daily rechecks for 3 days

ANSWERS

1. **B.** The principal objective of the FAST scan is identifying hemoperitoneum. It is best used for detecting intraabdominal injuries that require immediate attention rather than for a definitive diagnosis.

2. **E.** All of these injuries are associated with handlebar injury but traumatic pancreatitis is the most common result.

3. **D.** Conservative management with hospitalization for 7 to 10 days of bedrest, followed by a regimen of limited activity is the preferred management. This preserves the spleen and prevents the increased susceptibility to infection associated with splenectomy.

Partial splenectomy also is superior to total splenectomy in preserving splenic function. Delayed spontaneous rupture can occur at any time but is most common on days 3 to 5. Conservative management **MUST** include close observation and frequent examination.

15 GENITOURINARY AND RECTAL TRAUMA

Wendy Ann Lucid
Todd Brian Taylor
Kemedy K. McQuillen
Patricia Lee

EPIDEMIOLOGY

- The incidence of urinary tract injury in children with multiple trauma is second only to injury of the central nervous system. Most GU injuries involve the kidneys.

- Hematuria heralds the possibility of injury to the kidneys, ureter, bladder, or urethra. The kidneys and renal pedicle may be sources for major bleeding and should be considered for patients with hypovolemic shock.

- A dipstick urine analysis is the initial screening test for hematuria in the emergency department. It is highly sensitive for blood but cannot quantify the amount of hematuria or differentiate among myoglobinuria, hemoglobinuria, and true hematuria. In the early postinjury period, not all GU trauma will present with hematuria.

- The GU system can often be evaluated simultaneously with diagnostic tests being done to evaluate the abdomen. The GU system should be evaluated before surgery in appropriate cases of penetrating trauma and for patients with significant hematuria.

GENERAL MANAGEMENT PRINCIPLES

- Children are more likely than adults to sustain GU injuries. **Blunt abdominal trauma** accounts for more than 90 percent of GU injuries and more than 10 percent of children with blunt abdominal injuries also have GU injuries.

- Physical examination clues can be found in the abdomen, flank, pelvis, and genitalia. The genital and rectal examinations should precede the insertion of a urinary catheter. Signs of urethral injury include blood at the meatus or a high-riding prostate.

- Radiographic clues to GU injury include the loss of the psoas shadow on the abdominal radiograph (indicating retroperitoneal blood), scoliosis with concavity to the side of injury, or lower rib or transverse process fractures.

- Monitor urine output and perform a urinalysis on all trauma patients. If a urine dipstick is positive for blood, perform a microscopic examination. Hematuria may be present with GU trauma or an underlying renal malformation and may be *absent* with renal vascular (pedicle) or ureteral injuries. Indications for further GU evaluation are listed in Table 15-1.

- Consider sexual and physical abuse when evaluating perineal injuries: burns to the perineum, inconsistent mechanism of injury, evidence of previous injury, or the child reporting abuse need further evaluation and a child protective services referral.

- Complications of GU trauma include hemorrhage, urinary extravasation, renal parenchymal damage, infection, delayed hypertension, and renal dysfunction.

- **Penetrating trauma** between the nipples and perineum requires at least a one-shot intravenous pyelogram (IVP) before surgery to rule out GU injuries (see Table 15-1).

DIAGNOSTIC STUDIES

- A **computed tomography** (CT) scan of the abdomen with intravenous contrast is 98 percent accurate in evaluating the kidneys. It provides information about structure and function and may be more valuable than arteriography when vascular injuries are suspected. Nonionic contrast media should be considered if the patient is younger than 1 year old, had a previous reaction to contrast, is unstable, or has significant medical conditions including renal, heart or lung

TABLE 15-1 Indications for Diagnostic Evaluation of the Genitourinary (GU) Tract in Pediatric Trauma

Blunt trauma
    Multiple trauma
    Gross or microscopic hematuria (>20 RBCs/hpf) or shock
    Palpable flank mass, hematoma, ecchymosis, or tenderness
    Lower rib or thoracic or lumbar spine fractures
    Deceleration injuries (motor vehicle accident or fall from height) with
        crush injuries to the abdomen or pelvis with or without other signs
        Pelvic fracture
Penetrating trauma
    Any injury that can reasonably be expected to injure the GU tract
    Anticipated surgery for lower chest, abdomen, or pelvis for gunshot
      or deep stab wound

disease, diabetes, sickle cell anemia, or dehydration. Nonionic studies may overestimate the amount of urinary extravasation and should not be used as absolute criteria for surgery.

- **Intravenous pyelography** (IVP) has an accuracy of more than 90 percent and may be used for isolated renal injuries without shock or significant physical findings (Fig. 15-1, Tables 15-1 and 15-2). An emergency IVP includes a "scout KUB" followed by injection of contrast media (1 to 2 mL/kg) and films at 1, 5, and 10 min. A one-shot IVP at 5 min can be substituted in unstable patients. Prompt bilateral function, well-defined anatomy, and no extravasation exclude major renal injury. In a stable patient, a formal IVP or CT is recommended to accurately delineate the injury prior to surgery.

- **Renal ultrasound** (US) may be useful for following perirenal hematomas or urinomas or to limit radiation exposure in pregnancy. Bedside US and the focused abdominal sonography for trauma (FAST) have limited value for GU injuries.

- **Retrograde pyelography** is useful for delineating ureteropelvic disruption if the IVP is indeterminate.

- **CT cystography** can be done in conjunction with an abdominal CT to evaluate for bladder rupture.

- **CT and digital subtraction angiography** has replaced renal angiography.

- **Radioisotope renal scanning** can be used as an alternative for patients allergic to ionic contrast media for evaluating renovascular injuries.

SPECIFIC INJURIES AND MANAGEMENT

- The **kidneys** are the second most commonly injured solid organ in blunt trauma. Less perirenal fat, weaker abdominal muscles, more compliant ribs, proportionally larger kidneys, and frequent congenital abnormalities are all contributory. Only 20 percent of trauma patients have *isolated* renal injuries.

- Due to their relatively fixed position within Gerota's fascia, the kidney parenchyma and vascular pedicle are susceptible to injury with rapid deceleration. Renal pedicle injuries often present with vascular thrombosis and absent hematuria, and the kidney is nearly always lost despite early surgical intervention.

- Penetrating trauma is often associated with adjacent visceral injuries.

- Due to the high incidence of anomalous kidneys with pediatric renal trauma (15 percent), evaluation by IVP for microscopic hematuria is recommended.

- Delayed complications of renal trauma include acute tubular necrosis with renal failure, delayed bleeding,

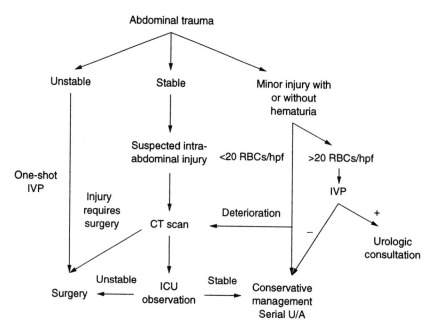

FIG. 15-1 Renal evaluation after trauma.

TABLE 15-2 Diagnostic Evaluation of Pediatric Genitourinary (GU) Injury: Patients Meeting Criteria for GU Evaluation

Abdominal CT
  Stable patient
  Multiple trauma
  IVP equivocal or severe injury requiring better definition
IVP
  Unstable patient (one-shot IVP)
  Isolated GU trauma
  Penetrating wounds
  Suspected ureteral injury

CT, computed tomography; IVP, intravenous pyelography.

infection, abscess formation, arteriovenous fistula, chronic pyelonephritis, hydronephrosis, chronic calculi, pseudocyst, and renin-mediated hypertension.

○ Blunt trauma patients without other injuries, who present with isolated microscopic hematuria of greater than 20 RBCs/hpf require only a follow-up urinalysis in 48 to 72 h to ensure resolution of the hematuria. If bleeding persists, a formal evaluation should be performed. More significant bleeding requires urgent investigation. Significant renal injuries or suspicious mechanisms of injury require hospital observation (Table 15-3 and Fig. 15-1).

○ Patients with direct communication between the renal arterioles and calyx, injury to the renal pedicle, expanding retroperitoneal hematoma, severe kidney laceration causing extensive extravasation, and frank transsection of a portion of the main collecting system require immediate surgery. Less serious injuries that may require delayed surgical

intervention include retroperitoneal extravasation secondary to communication between the renal calyx and the perinephric space and persistent or infected urinoma resulting from a small urinary leak. Management of grade IV and V injuries (see Table 15-3) is controversial.

• **Ureteral injuries** occur in less than 5 percent of GU trauma. Penetrating trauma is the most common mechanism.

○ Traumatic avulsion of the ureter occurs most commonly at the right ureteropelvic junction or in the proximal 4 cm of the ureter. Symptoms include fever, ileus, hematuria, and flank or abdominal pain. The diagnosis is often delayed since hematuria can be absent or transient. IVP shows extravasation of contrast at the level of the kidney without filling of the ureter. Retrograde pyelography may be necessary to delineate the extent of the injury. Delays in diagnosis can cause fistulas, ureteral strictures, and abscesses. Nephrectomy is frequently necessary.

○ Ureteral transection is treated with prompt ureteropyelostomy. The kidney salvage rate is higher than 95 percent.

• **Bladder injury** represents about 25 percent of urologic traumas and is generally due to motor vehicle accidents. It is often associated with multisystem trauma: pelvic fracture is associated with GU injury 75 percent of the time, and 10 percent of pelvic fractures result in bladder injury.

○ **Bladder contusions** are self-limited and account for about two thirds of bladder injuries. Patients may be asymptomatic or have microscopic hematuria and pain.

TABLE 15-3   Classification of Renal Injury

GRADE	MINOR RENAL INJURY	OBSERVATION (85%)
I	Contusion	Parenchymal injury without fracture of the parenchyma or capsule as evidenced by delayed or underfilling of the renal calyces on IVP
II	Shallow cortical laceration	Intact capsule with superficial parenchymal laceration without extension into the collecting system; no urinary extravasation on IVP
III	Deep cortical lacerations	Lacerated capsule with superficial parenchymal laceration without extension into the collecting system; no urinary extravasation on IVP
IV	Forniceal laceration	Disruption of the collecting system and parenchymal junction without injury to the parenchyma and capsule
	MAJOR RENAL INJURY	**CONSIDER SURGERY (15%)**
IV	Deep parenchymal laceration	Extension of the laceration into the collecting system with intact or disrupted capsule
V	Shattered kidney	Parenchyma is ruptured in multiple fragments with distortion of the intrarenal collecting structures with intact or disrupted capsule
V	Renal pedicle injury	Laceration or thrombus at the pedicle involving the renal artery or vein as evidenced by lack of contrast in the affected kidney on IVP

IVP, intravenous pyelography.

○ In young children the bladder is an intraabdominal organ, especially when full, placing it at greater risk for rupture.

○ **Bladder rupture** is divided into extraperitoneal, intraperitoneal; and combined: extraperitoneal ruptures are most common.

○ It has a mortality rate of 11 to 44 percent, which increases when the diagnosis is delayed, a not uncommon occurrence because many patients are initially asymptomatic.

○ Acute findings include gross hematuria, blood at the urethral meatus, inability to void, or little urine upon urinary catheter placement (Table 15-4).

○ Delayed symptoms include persistent hematuria, peritonitis, sepsis, and renal failure.

○ Intraperitoneal absorption of urine leads to elevated blood urea nitrogen (BUN) levels.

○ Bladder rupture is diagnosed by cystography that includes maximally full, post drainage, and oblique films (Table 15-5). To avoid obscuration of findings by extravasated dye, an IVP or abdominal/ pelvic CT should be done prior to the cystogram.

○ In males, a retrograde urethrogram should precede attempts to pass a urinary catheter due to the high incidence of associated urethral injuries.

○ Small, uncomplicated extraperitoneal bladder tears can be managed conservatively with suprapubic or urinary catheter drainage for 7 to 14 days.

○ Extraperitoneal tears with an associated pelvic fracture require surgical exploration and repair.

○ Intraperitoneal bladder rupture requires surgical exploration, repair, debridement, and bladder drainage.

• A more flexible pelvis makes **urethral** injuries uncommon in children. Most result from blunt trauma (80 percent motor vehicle accidents) and can result in

TABLE 15-4   Indications for Cystogram in Pediatric Trauma Patients

Penetrating injury to lower abdomen and pelvis
Blunt lower abdominal or perineal trauma with significant microscopic hematuria (>20 RBCs/hpf), gross hematuria,[a] or blood at the meatus[a]
Significant pelvic fracture[a]
Unable to void[a] or little urine with urinary catheterization

[a]A retrograde urethrogram should be considered before attempting urethral catheterization in these instances.

TABLE 15-5   Findings with Bladder Injury

CRYSTOGRAM FINDINGS	RADIOGRAPHIC FINDING
Bladder contusion	Teardrop shape or elevation of the bladder due to a perivesical hematoma without extravasation of contrast. Lateral deviation and obliteration of the soft tissue planes by pelvic hematoma may also be present.
Extraperitoneal bladder rupture	Postvoid films with significant rupture reveal a typical "sunburst" pattern as the contrast extravasates outside the peritoneal cavity. However, there may only be small streaks of contrast with minor bladder ruptures.
Intraperitoneal bladder rupture	Extravasation into the peritoneal cavity around the bowel and intraabdominal organs and or in the pericolic gutters, giving a typical hourglass appearance.

strictures, incontinence, impotence, diverticulae, fistulas, and chordee.

○ The proximal (posterior) urethra extends from the neck of the bladder to the urogenital diaphragm and the distal (anterior) urethra extends from the urogenital diaphragm to the meatus. The urethra is relatively fixed at the urogenital diaphragm, the symphysis pubis, and the bladder neck.

○ Ninety percent of proximal urethral injuries are associated with pelvic fractures and symptoms include difficulty voiding, blood at the urethral meatus (90 percent), abdominal pain, and, in males, a high-riding, floating, or boggy prostate. Distal urethral injuries are less common and may only present long after the injury when urethral strictures become symptomatic. Acute symptoms include difficulty voiding and discoloration and edema of the scrotum, perineum, abdominal wall, or along the shaft of the penis due to extravasation of blood or urine.

○ Early urologic consultation is recommended. Care should be taken to avoid converting partial tears of the urethra into transsections by attempting to pass urethral catheters. Indications for retrograde urethrogram before catheter placement are listed in Table 15-6. Extravasation of contrast media with some contrast also in the bladder indicates partial urethral tear. Extravasation alone indicates a complete transsection.

• **Scrotal and testicular injuries** result from the testis being forced against the pubic ramus. Injuries occur with straddle injuries, birth trauma, sports injuries, dog bites, and arthropod envenomations. Significant straddle injuries should be screened with a radiograph of the pelvis to rule out a fracture of the pubic ramus. Doppler ultrasound is often used in the evaluation of scrotal or testicular trauma. Equivocal findings may require a ^{99m}technetium radionucleotide scan. Diagnostic studies must be done promptly as a delay of 4 to 6 h may result in the loss of the testis. Surgical exploration remains the most rapid and definitive method for evaluation of significant scrotal trauma, and other modalities should be reserved for less obvious cases.

○ **Testicular or epididymal rupture** results in tearing of the inelastic tunica albuginea with extrusion of the seminiferous tissue. Rupture should be suspected when there is a recurrence of pain with delayed onset of scrotal swelling from several hours to 3 days after the injury. Complications include epididymoorchitis characterized by localized red-

ness, warmth, swelling, and fever. Management is early surgical exploration. Delayed diagnosis frequently results in orchiectomy

○ **Testicular dislocation** occurs when the testis is forcibly displaced from the scrotum into the inguinal, acetabular, crural, perineal, penile, or abdominal region, or extruded from the scrotum through a laceration. Findings include scrotal pain, nausea, vomiting, and an empty hemiscrotum after trauma. Closed relocation of the testis may be possible. Immediate urologic consultation should be obtained.

  ▪ Once testicular torsion, rupture, dislocation, and large expanding hematoma have been excluded, the patient may be discharged with urologic follow-up. The use of a scrotal support and cold packs may be beneficial.

• **Penile injuries** occur from complications of circumcision, direct blows, zipper entrapment of the foreskin, and tourniquet injuries. Urinalysis should be performed with significant injury.

○ Superficial lacerations of the penis can be repaired similarly to any other laceration, but damage to deeper structures should be considered if there is marked swelling, ecchymosis, or blood at the meatus.

○ Fracture of the penis occurs when the erect penis is forced against a solid object, such as the pubis, during sexual intercourse. The patient hears a "cracking" sound followed by pain, swelling, and deformity of the penis. Most can be treated conservatively unless there is severe penile deformity or urethral involvement. Management decisions should be made with urologic consultation.

○ Zipper injuries to the foreskin occur most commonly in boys 3 to 6 years of age. Bone cutters are used to break the bridge of the sliding piece of the zipper, allowing it to fall apart and release the entrapped foreskin. Local anesthesia is not usually required.

○ Tourniquet injuries occur when a band of hair surrounds the coronal groove and cuts into the shaft of the penis. Only rarely are the urethra and corpora involved. Removal of the band and treatment of infection is usually all that is required. Urology follow-up is necessary if deeper injury is suspected.

• **Vulvar and vaginal injuries**, including vulvar hematomas, vaginal tears and lacerations, and urethral, rectal, or bladder injuries, often result from blunt trauma. Complications include urinary retention, secondary infection, and urinary tract infection.

○ Vulvar injuries are usually minor and are treated with rest and cold packs. Patients with significant straddle injuries should have a pelvis radiograph to rule out a fracture of the ramus. Large hematomas

---

TABEL 15-6 Indications for Retrograde Urethrogram in Pediatric Trauma Patients

Penetrating injury to lower abdomen and pelvis suspected of involving the lower genitourinary tract

Blunt lower abdominal or perineal trauma with significant microscopic hematuria (>20 RBCs/hpf), gross hematuria, or blood at the meatus

Significant pelvic fracture

Inability to void

High-riding, floating, or boggy prostate in males

Discoloration or edema due to extravasation of blood or urine into the scrotum, perineum, or abdominal wall or along the shaft of the penis

Laceration of the vagina secondary to significant trauma

may require surgical drainage and are susceptible to secondary infection. Urethrogram or cystoscopy may be needed to rule out urethral injury; a suprapubic catheter may be necessary.

- ○ Most vaginal injuries are minor, but complete vaginal examination is warranted to exclude significant injury. Large lacerations can cause significant bleeding.
- ○ **Sexual abuse** is estimated to occur in one of five girls during childhood. Abuse should be considered with all perineal injuries.
- **Rectal injuries** are uncommon in children and are primarily the result of impalement. The injuries are often significant and may have minimal signs of external trauma. There may be associated vaginal injury. Sedation or general anesthesia is often required to facilitate examination and anoscopy.
- **Retroperitoneal blood vessels** are rarely injured in blunt trauma except with rapid deceleration or severe physical abuse. Penetrating trauma is much more likely to cause significant vascular injury. Upper retroperitoneal injury typically results in a retroperitoneal hematoma that is confined to the retroperitoneal space. If the peritoneal membrane is disrupted, though, there can be massive intraperitoneal hemorrhage. Lower retroperitoneal injury is often associated with pelvic fracture and involves the iliac vessels, with venous injuries being more common than arterial. Retroperitoneal vascular injuries should be suspected when hypovolemia cannot be otherwise explained.

Bibliography

Advanced Pediatric Life Support Joint Task Force: Trauma. In: Strange G, ed. *Advanced Pediatric Life Support: The Pediatric Emergency Medicine Course,* 3d ed. Dallas: American Academy of Pediatrics/American College of Emergency Physicians, 59–78, 1998.

Christopher NCD: Genitourinary tract trauma in the pediatric patient. *Emerg Med Rep* 5:113–120, 2000.

Rothrock SG, Green SM, Morgan R: Abdominal trauma in infants and children: Prompt identification and early management of serious and life-threatening injuries. Part I: Injury patterns and initial assessment. *Pediatr Emerg Care* 16:106–115, 2000.

Rothrock SG, Green SM, Morgan R: Abdominal trauma in infants and children: Prompt identification and early management of serious and life-threatening injuries. Part II: Specific injuries and ED management. *Pediatr Emerg Care* 16:189–195, 2000.

Schafermeyer RW: Pediatric trauma. *Emerg Med Clin North Am* 11:187, 1993.

Tarman GJ, Kaplan GW, Lerman SL: Lower genitourinary injury and pelvic fractures in pediatric patients. *Urology* 59:123–126, 2002.

QUESTIONS

1. Which of the following is true regarding GU trauma in children:
   A. Adults are more likely than children to sustain GU injury.
   B. The absence of hematuria rules out GU trauma.
   C. Most GU injuries involve the bladder.
   D. Penetrating trauma between the nipples and perineum requires at least a one-shot IVP before surgery to rule out GU trauma.
   E. A CT scan of the abdomen with IV contrast is inadequate for evaluating most renal trauma.

2. A 6-year-old girl presents as a restrained passenger in a high-speed motor vehicle collision. Urinalysis reveals hematuria. Which of the following is **NOT** correct regarding work-up for hematuria following traumatic injury?
   A. Follow-up urinalysis in 48 to 72 h if only isolated microscopic hematuria of <20 rbcs/hpf in the absence of other injury.
   B. Utilization of the dipstick urine analysis as a sensitive screening test.
   C. IVP or CT to accurately delineate injury prior to surgery.
   D. Absence of hematuria rules out significant injury.
   E. Retrograde pyelography may be used to evaluate ureteral injuries.

3. Findings associated with traumatic rupture of the ureter include all of the following **EXCEPT**:
   A. Fever
   B. Ileus
   C. Hematuria
   D. Abdominal pain
   E. Contrast filled bladder

ANSWERS

1. D. Children are more likely than adults to sustain GU injury. Most GU injuries involve the kidneys. In the early postinjury period, not all GU trauma will present with hematuria. A CT scan of the abdomen with IV contrast is 98 percent accurate in evaluate the kidneys. Nonionic contrast media should be considered if the patient is younger than 1 year old.

2. D. Hematuria may be present with GU trauma or an underlying renal malformation and may be absent with renal vascular (pedicle) or ureteral injuries.

3. E. Ureteral injuries occur in less than 5 percent of GU trauma. Penetrating trauma is the most common mechanism. Traumatic avulsion of the ureter occurs most commonly at the right ureteropelvic junction or in the proximal 4 cm of the ureter. The diagnosis is often delayed since hematuria can be absent or transient. IVP shows extravasation of contrast at the level of the kidney without filling of the ureter or bladder. Symptoms include fever, ileus, hematuria, and flank or abdominal pain.

16   MAXILLOFACIAL TRAUMA

Alan E. Jones
Stephen A. Colucciello
Kemedy K. McQuillen
Patricia Lee

EPIDEMIOLOGY

- The highest incidence of facial fractures is between 8 and 10 years of age and the most frequently fractured bones are the nose (45 percent), mandible (32 percent), orbit (17 percent), and zygoma/maxilla (5 percent). The most common facial fractures in children requiring hospitalization are mandibular fractures.
- Causes include motor vehicle crashes, including auto/pedestrian incidents, falls, sporting injuries, altercations, child abuse, and gunshot wounds.
- Associated injuries include skull fractures, intracranial injuries, intraocular injuries, and cervical spine fractures. Skull fractures are particularly common in child abuse.

UNIQUE ASPECTS OF PEDIATRIC MAXILLOFACIAL TRAUMA

- Large fat pads cushion impact and lessen forces transmitted to the facial bones.
- A high ratio of cancellous to cortical bone provides greater resilience and results in a higher incidence of incomplete and greenstick fractures.
- Because of their prominent skull and small face and mandible, younger children tend to fracture the upper face, while older children tend to fracture the lower face.

- LeForte fractures are uncommon under 5 years of age, prior to pneumatization of paranasal sinuses. For this reason, orbital and frontal skull fractures predominate in children under 5. Maxillary and mandibular fractures predominate in older children.

EMERGENCY MANAGEMENT

- The most urgent complication of facial trauma is airway compromise resulting from loss of tongue support, hematoma formation, or uncontrolled bleeding. Simple maneuvers, such as chin-lift-jaw thrust, pulling the tongue forward (manually or with a large suture or towel clip), and oropharyngeal suctioning, provide immediate benefit. If cervical spine injury is not a consideration, the child should be allowed to sit up and lean forward.
- If simple airway maneuvers do not suffice or if there is uncontrolled bleeding into the pharynx, orotracheal intubation with in-line immobilization should be done. Nasotracheal intubation should not be attempted.
  ○ When uncuffed endotracheal tubes are used and oropharyngeal bleeding persists, pack the pharynx with absorbent gauze to prevent aspiration.
- If the child cannot be intubated, a surgical airway must be established. In children younger than 12 years of age, this can be accomplished with percutaneous transtracheal jet ventilation or emergency tracheostomy. Cricothyroidotomy can be used in older children.
- Infants under the age of 3 months are obligate nose breathers, and nasal or midface trauma can lead to complete airway obstruction.
- Severe nasal hemorrhage should be controlled with external pressure. If bleeding continues, a foley catheter and nasal packing can be used. Insert the catheter along the floor of the nose, inflate the balloon in the nasopharynx, pull it anteriorly, and then place an anterior pack.

HISTORY

- Historical evaluation should include determination of timing and mechanism of injury, loss of consciousness, visual problems, facial anesthesia, or pain with jaw movement.

PHYSICAL EXAMINATION

- Physical examination includes face-to-face and tangential (from the child's head looking down or from the chin looking up) inspection for swelling, ecchymosis, and deformity; palpation for bony deformity and crepitus; and gross observation of function (posttraumatic Bell's palsy can suggest a temporal bone fracture).

- Evaluate the **eyes** for the presence of the pupillary light reflex, hyphema, subconjunctival hemorrhage, and extraocular movements. Note the presence of proptosis or enophthalmos (unequal pupil height may indicate orbital floor fracture). Retract the lids for adequate visualization of the globe. Document visual acuity. Look for periorbital ecchymosis: ecchymosis present immediately after injury reflects direct trauma. Raccoon's eyes secondary to basilar skull fracture occur 4 to 6 h after injury. Bilateral periorbital ecchymosis also occurs with LeFort II and III fractures. Carefully palpate the *entire* orbital rim for tenderness or deformity. Anesthesia above or below the eye may be secondary to supraorbital or infraorbital nerve injury. Subcutaneous emphysema about the eyes and maxillae indicates a communication with a sinus or nasal antrum. This may not be present until the child blows his or her nose. Telecanthus, an increased width between the medial canthi of the eyelids, with flattening of the medial canthus, is associated with nasal ethmoid injury.

- Examine the **ear** canal for lacerations and cerebrospinal fluid (CSF) leak and the tympanic membrane (TM) for hemotympanum or rupture. Hemotympanum occurs with a basilar skull fracture and is present several hours before ecchymosis appears over the mastoid area (Battle's sign). TM rupture may occur with mandibular condyle fractures. Check the pinna for sub perichondral hematoma.

- **Midface** evaluation includes simultaneous palpation of the zygomatic arches to detect flattening. Intraoral palpation of the arch is helpful in detecting minimally displaced fractures. LeFort fractures may be identified by elongation of the midface or by manipulation of the central maxillary arch.

- Palpate the **nose** for crepitus and deformity. Examine the inside of the nose for septal hematoma; pressure with a cotton swab will confirm its soft, doughy swelling. Look for CSF rhinorrhea by placing a drop of bloody nasal secretions on a sheet and assessing for a double ring: this sign may also occur with normal nasal secretions.

- Do a careful **intraoral and mandibular examination**. Check for anesthesia of the upper or lower lip to assess for injury to the inferior orbital nerve or inferior alveolar/mental nerve, respectively. Anesthesia may be secondary to fracture of the bony canal or direct nerve contusion. Observe movement of the patient's jaw and palpate the condyles through a full range of motion. Deviation to one side indicates ipsilateral subcondylar fracture. Trismus, malocclusion, and difficulty in jaw movement may be secondary to mandibular fracture, temporomandibular joint (TMJ) injury, or a depressed zygoma impinging on the mandible or muscles of mastication. Apply a distracting pressure upon the dental arches to assess for traumatic diastasis of the hard palate. Grasp and manipulate each tooth to assess for laxity and remove teeth that are in danger of falling out. Save permanent teeth in saline moistened gauze. To test for bony disruption, stress the mandible with lateral and medial pressures on the dental arches and up and down manual pressure. Ask the patient to bite down upon a tongue blade while torque is applied. In the presence of a mandibular fracture, there will be pain and reflex opening of the mouth.

- **Facial lacerations** may involve underlying vital structures. Involvement of the medial third of the upper or lower eyelids may result in lacrimal apparatus disruption; while the parotid duct and the buccal branch of the facial nerve can be injured if a deep wound crosses a line drawn from the tragus to the mid portion of the upper lip. Suspect laceration of the parotid duct if saliva enters the wound or if blood is expressed at Stensen's duct when the parotid gland is massaged. Facial nerve injuries are surgically repaired if they are posterior to a vertical line drawn through the lateral canthus. More anterior injuries are usually not repaired.

RADIOGRAPHY

- Radiography of the face should never delay evaluation and treatment of serious, life-threatening injuries.

- Three radiographic views of the face [Waters, posteroanterior (PA), and lateral films] can detect the vast majority of facial bone fractures. These plain films provide an excellent screening tool for maxillofacial trauma. Additional radiographic views include the panoramic (Panorex) radiograph, to define the anatomy of the mandible, the Towne's view, to image the condyles and ramus of the mandible, and the submental vertex view (jug-handle or zygomatic arch view), to demonstrate the zygomatic arches and the base of the skull. Radiographs of the nose are of limited usefulness.

- The **computed tomography** scan is the definitive test for delineation of maxillofacial fractures. CT is particularly helpful in the presence of orbital fractures.

SPECIFIC INJURIES

- **Nasal fractures** are the most common pediatric facial fracture. Control of hemorrhage is obtained with external digital pressure and, if that is ineffective, nasal packing. An "open book" nasal fracture is especially severe, with nasal bones separation along the midline suture.
  - Referrals can be made based on physical examination, reports of difficulty breathing through the nose, or radiographs showing a nasal fracture. For optimal repair of displaced nasal fractures, consultation should take place within 5 to 6 days postinjury, after which time, fractures begin to unite and manipulation becomes increasingly difficult.
- **Septal hematomas** must be recognized and treated. If untreated, they can result in infection, septal perforation, and collapse of the septum with a "saddle" deformity of the nose.
  - To drain the hematoma, a #11 blade is used to make an L-shaped incision through the mucoperiosteum along the floor of the nose and extended vertically. The nasal antrum is then packed to prevent re accumulation. The child needs to follow up with an appropriate specialist.
- **Nasal-ethmoidal-orbital (NEO)** fractures occur when the bony structures of the nose are driven backward into the intraorbital space. They present with telecanthus and increased mobility on the bimanual test. To perform the bimanual test, a clamp is inserted into the nose and the tip is pressed against the medial orbital rim opposite the canthal ligament. Counter pressure is then applied with a finger against the external surface of the canthal ligament. With a fracture, there will be movement between the clamp and index finger. A CT scan of the face, including coronal views, should be done. Associated injuries include lacrimal system disruption as well as orbital and optic nerve problems.
- The most common **orbital fracture** is a blowout fracture, which occurs when a blunt object strikes the globe, suddenly increasing the intraorbital pressure and decompressing the contents through the orbit, most commonly the floor. Blowout fractures also occur through the medial wall, the roof, and the greater wing of the sphenoid bone. With an orbital floor fracture, the inferior ocular muscles may be trapped causing diplopia on upward gaze. The Waters view may reveal a soft tissue mass projecting into the sinus cavity **(teardrop sign)** or depression of the bony fragments into the **sinus (open bomb bay door sign)**. CT scans are diagnostic.
  - Patients with NEO or orbital fractures should be instructed not to blow their nose. Antibiotics have not been proven to reduce complications. Urgent consultation is required in the presence of exophthalmus or extraocular muscle entrapment.
- **Supraorbital fractures** involve the superior orbital rim or orbital roof and may present with exophthalmus, ptosis, and impairment of upward gaze. The **superior orbital fissure syndrome** results in paralysis of extraocular muscles, ptosis, and anesthesia in the ophthalmic division of the trigeminal nerve. The **orbital apex syndrome** is a combination of the superior orbital fissure syndrome plus optic nerve damage and results in blindness.
  - These syndromes represent surgical emergencies and require immediate consultation and decompression.
- Linear, nondisplaced fractures of the anterior wall of the **frontal sinus** may be treated with observation and antibiotics. If the posterior wall is involved, a CT scan should be done to evaluate for depression and underlying brain injury and neurosurgical and maxillofacial consultation should be obtained.
- The incidence of **maxillary fractures** increases with age, as the paranasal sinuses develop. Associated intracranial injuries must be suspected.
- The **malar complex** is often broken in a tripod fashion, with fractures at the infraorbital rim, across the zygomatic–frontal suture and along the zygomatic–temporal junction. Inward displacement of this fragment results in mandible impingement and trismus. The zygomatic arch itself is frequently fractured in isolation.
- **LeFort fractures** of the midface are classified based on the horizontal level of the fracture. They may result in lengthening of the midface, occlusal abnormalities, and orbital ecchymosis. They can have concomitant basilar skull fractures. CT scans are diagnostic.
  - LeFort I: transverse fracture that separates the hard palate from the lower portion of the pterygoid plate and nasal septum. Traction on the upper incisors produces movement of the hard palate and dental arch.
  - LeFort II (pyramidal fracture): separates the central maxilla and palate from the rest of the craniofacial skeleton. Traction on the upper incisors will move the central pyramid of the face, including the nose.
  - LeFort III (craniofacial dysjunction): separates the face from the cranium. The entire face, including inferior and lateral portions of the orbital rim, move as a unit.
    - Children with LeFort fractures must be admitted with a maxillofacial specialist consultation.
- **Mandible fractures** are the second most common pediatric facial fracture and are often multiple. The most frequently injured areas are the condyle (70 percent), followed by the body, angle, and symphysis. Physical

examination is key in diagnosing these injuries, as radiographs may be non diagnostic. Crush injuries to the condyle prior to the age of 5 years have the greatest potential for developmental arrest. Complications include severe facial deformity, micrognathia, and ankylosis of the temporomandibular joint (TMJ).

- ◦ Treatment is based on age, state of dentition, fracture location, bony integrity, and the presence of associated injuries.
- **Soft tissue injuries** should be cleaned, irrigated, and conservatively debrided. Foreign bodies should be removed. Landmarks should be aligned for good cosmetic closure. Repair of lacerations to the salivary duct or to the lacrimal drainage system should be performed by a specialist. Eyebrows should not be shaved. Hematomas of the pinna should be drained with needle aspiration or incision and a pressure dressing applied.
- **Penetrating wounds to the posterior pharynx** endanger the carotid artery, jugular vein, and cranial nerves. Color flow Doppler, angiography, or magnetic resonance imaging may be indicated after specialist consultation.

PAIN MANAGEMENT AND ANESTHESIA

- Acute maxillofacial injuries are extremely painful. Local anesthesia with wound infiltration or nerve block is the primary method of achieving immediate pain control. The most useful maxillofacial nerve blocks are mental, inferior alveolar, infraorbital, and supraorbital. Systemic analgesia is often necessary. Conscious sedation may be needed for patients who are unable to cooperate.

BIBLIOGRAPHY

Antonyshyn O: Principles in management of facial injuries. In: Georgiade GS, Riefkohl R, Levin LS, eds. *Plastic, Maxillofacial, and Reconstructive Surgery.* Baltimore: Williams & Wilkins, 1997.

Chase DC: Maxillofacial injuries. In: Buntain WL, ed. *Management of Pediatric Trauma.* Philadelphia: WB Saunders, 200–218, 1995.

Dodson TB, Kaban LB: Special considerations for the pediatric emergency patient. *Emerg Med Clin North Am* 18:539–547, 2000.

Druelinger L, Guenther M, Marchand EG: Radiographic evaluation of the facial complex. *Emerg Med Clin North Am* 18:393–410, 2000.

Ellis E, Scott K: Assessment of patients with facial fractures. *Emerg Med Clin North Am* 18:411–448, 2000.

Koltai PJ, Rabkin D: Management of facial trauma in children. *Pediatr Clin North Am* 43:1253–1275, 1996.

LeFort R: Etude experimentale sur les fractures de le machoire superieure. *Rev Chir* 23:208,360,479, 1901.

Rhea JT, Rao PM, Novelline RA: Helical CT and three-dimensional CT of facial and orbital injury. *Radiol Clin North Am* 37:489–513, 1999.

Schultz RC: Facial fractures in children and adolescents. In: Cohen M, ed. *Mastery of Plastic and Reconstructive Surgery.* Boston: Little, Brown, 1188–1198, 1995.

Yagiela JA: Anesthesia and pain management. *Emerg Med Clin North Am* 18:449–470, 2000.

QUESTIONS

1. The most frequently fractured pediatric facial bone is the:
   A. Mandible
   B. Orbit
   C. Zygoma
   D. Maxilla
   E. Nose

2. The most common pediatric facial fracture requiring hospitalization is the:
   A. Mandible
   B. Orbit
   C. Zygoma
   D. Maxilla
   E. Nose

3. A 3-year-old boy presents with facial trauma after a motor vehicle crash. Unique aspects of pediatric maxillofacial trauma may include all of the following **EXCEPT**:
   A. Greater resilience of bone due to high ratio of cancellous to cortical bone
   B. Greater incidence of incomplete and greenstick fractures
   C. Younger children tend to fracture the lower face, whereas older children will tend to fracture the upper face.
   D. LeForte fractures are uncommon in children under 5 years of age prior to pneumatization of paranasal sinuses.
   E. Increased incidence of orbital and frontal skull fractures in children under 5 years of age

4. Airway control is paramount in patients with maxillofacial trauma. Appropriate interventions in controlling the airway to be considered are all of the following **EXCEPT**:
   A. Nasotracheal intubation
   B. Endotracheal intubation
   C. Jaw-thrust maneuver

D. Percutaneous transtracheal jet ventilation
E. Forward pull on tongue with towel clip

5. A temporal bone fracture is suggested by which of the following findings:
   A. Subcutaneous emphysema
   B. Dental pain
   C. Enophthalmos
   D. Bell's palsy
   E. Decreased hearing

6. Basilar skull fracture is suggested by all of the following findings except:
   A. Raccoon's eyes
   B. Hemotympanum
   C. Battle's sign
   D. Periorbital ecchymoses
   E. Subcutaneous emphysema

7. Telecanthus may occur with which of the following injuries:
   A. Basilar skull fracture
   B. Nasoethmoidal orbital fracture
   C. Blowout fracture
   D. Supraorbital fracture
   E. Frontal sinus fracture

8. The most frequently injured area of the mandible is the:
   A. Body
   B. Angle
   C. Symphysis
   D. Condyle
   E. Ramus

ANSWERS

1. E. The highest incidence of facial fractures is between 8 and 10 years of age and the most frequently fractured bones are the nose (45 percent), mandible (32 percent), orbit (17 percent), and zygoma/maxilla (5 percent)

2. A. Mandible fracture is the most common pediatric facial fracture requiring hospitalization.

3. C. Because of their prominent skull and small face and mandible, younger children tend to fracture the upper face. Older children tend to fracture the lower face. Pneumatization of the paranasal sinuses occurs after the age of 5 years. Therefore, orbital and frontal skull fractures predominate in children under 5 years of age. Maxillary and mandibular fractures predominate in older children.

4. A. The most urgent complication of facial trauma is airway compromise. Nasotracheal intubation should not be attempted.

5. D. Posttraumatic Bell's palsy can suggest a temporal bone fracture.

6. D. Periorbital ecchymosis that occurs immediately after injury reflects direct trauma. Raccoon's eyes secondary to basilar skull fracture occurs 4 to 6 h after injury. Hemotympanum occurs with a basilar skull fracture and is present several hours before ecchymosis appears over the mastoid area (Battle's sign). Subcutaneous emphysema about the eyes and maxilla indicates a communication with a sinus or nasal antrum.

7. B. Nasoethmoidal orbital fractures occur when the bony structures of the nose are driven backward into the intraorbital space, creating telecanthus, or widening of the space between the eyes. Blowout fractures are orbital fractures that occur when a blunt object strikes the globe causing sudden increase in intraorbital pressure and decompressing the contents through the orbit, most commonly the floor. With an orbital floor fracture, the inferior ocular muscles may be trapped, causing diplopia on an upward gaze. Supraorbital fractures involve the superior orbital rim or orbital roof and may present with exophthalmus, ptosis, and impairment of upward gaze.

8. D. The most frequently injured areas are the condyle (70 percent) followed by the body, angle, and symphysis.

17 EYE TRAUMA

D. Mark Courtney
Stephen A. Colucciello
Kemedy K. McQuillen
Patricia Lee

EPIDEMIOLOGY

• Ocular trauma is the leading cause of noncongenital blindness in people under 20 years old. Ocular trauma results from falls, motor vehicle collisions, accidental blows to the eye during recreational or sporting activities, fireworks, BB guns, and child abuse.

HISTORY

• The history should include the circumstances surrounding the injury, preexisting eye abnormalities or use of prescription lenses, exposure to power tools or metal striking metal, and the presence of double vision. If present, double vision should be clarified as monocular or binocular: monocular diplopia implies a problem with the lens or retina, whereas binocular diplopia is associated with extraocular muscle injuries or entrapment. Assess past medical issues including sickle cell disease and coagulopathy.

PHYSICAL EXAMINATION

- The examination of the eye should be performed after life-threatening injuries have been addressed.
  - Inspect the eyes and assess extraocular movements.
  - In trauma, initial **visual acuity** is the best predictor of ultimate visual outcome. It is the vital sign of the eye and should be documented in every child with an ocular injury or visual complaint. If the child wears glasses, measure acuity with the glasses on. If the glasses have been lost, correct refractive error by having the child look through a pinhole in a piece of paper. Lack of correction with pinhole testing suggests pathology in the retina or optic nerve. If the child is unable to read an eye chart, ask him or her to finger count at 3 feet; if that fails, assess for light perception.
  - Begin with the lids and periorbital structures and work centrally. Examine for swelling, subcutaneous emphysema, penetrating injury, and ecchymosis. Retract swollen lids with fingers, lid retractors, or bent paper clips. Examine the eye for abnormal tear drainage; **epiphora** may be secondary to injury of the canalicular system.
  - Examine the conjunctiva for injection, perilimbal injection, and chemosis. Check sclera carefully for disruption or penetration. Document subconjunctival hemorrhage.
  - Evaluate the pupils for asymmetry or irregularity. Pupillary dilatation occurs with direct blows to the eye (posttraumatic mydriasis), anticholinergic medication, or with a third nerve palsy. Pilocarpine drops will constrict a pupil that is dilated secondary to a third nerve lesion but will have no effect on pharmacologic mydriasis. Never overlook the possibility of a glass eye.
  - The lens should be transparent and the margins should not be visible. Examine the anterior chamber for abnormal depth. To assess optic nerve function, perform the swinging flashlight test. A pupil that initially dilates when illuminated by light has a sensory (afferent) defect (Marcus Gunn pupil).
  - On funduscopic examination, the vitreous should be clear and the optic disk sharp.
  - Check **intraocular pressure** if globe rupture or penetrating injury is not a concern. Normal intraocular pressure is between 15 and 20 mm Hg.

MEDICATIONS

- **Topical anesthetics** (EG, tetracaine) have an onset of action within 1 min and last for 15 to 20 min. They should never be prescribed for home use because they impede corneal healing and result in the loss of normal protective reflexes.
- **Cycloplegics** (ie, homatropine and cyclopentolate hydrochloride) dilate the eye and decrease pain by preventing ciliary spasm. Atropine has a long duration of action and should not be used in the emergency setting.
- **Ocular steroids** should not be used without first consulting an ophthalmologist.
- Ensure adequacy of **tetanus prophylaxis** in all patients with ocular injuries.

SPECIFIC INJURIES

- Simple, superficial **lid lacerations** may be repaired by the emergency physician.
- The following lacerations required specialized repair:
  - Lacerations of the medial third of either lid: lacrimal system may be involved. Check for lacrimal system involvement by instilling fluorescein into the eye and checking for wound fluorescence with a Wood's lamp or cobalt blue light.
  - Lacerations with fat in the wound: underlying globe injury may be present.
  - Lacerations of lid margins: risk for lid deformity and abnormal lid movement.
  - Levator palpebrae muscle involvement: posttraumatic ptosis may develop.
  - Lacerations of the tarsal plate (dense band of fibrous tissue in the upper lid).
- **Subconjunctival hemorrhage** may herald more serious injury. Clues to an underlying globe injury include decreased visual acuity, severe pain, photophobia, and extension of hemorrhage beyond the limbus. Lateral subconjunctival hemorrhages are associated with zygomatic fractures (tripod fractures). Uncomplicated subconjunctival hemorrhages usually resolve within 2 weeks.
- Children with **corneal abrasions** complain of a foreign body sensation, pain, and photophobia and present with blepharospasm and a red eye. Infants may present with only crying. Corneal abrasions will fluoresce with fluorescein and a cobalt blue or Wood's light. Multiple vertical striations (ice-rink sign) suggest an upper lid foreign body that can be detected with lid eversion and inspection. Topical anesthetics prior to examination decrease blepharospasm and pain. Corneal abrasions in the absence of trauma may

represent herpetic dendrites. These can be differentiated from a corneal abrasion by the presence of a decreased corneal reflex. In the case of herpes keratitis, ophthalmologic consultation is required.

○ Treat corneal abrasions with ophthalmic antibiotics to prevent infection and topical mydriatic agents to decrease ciliary spasm and provide comfort. Eye patching is not indicated unless there is a Bell's palsy and incomplete lid closure. Abrasions should be rechecked in 48 h if patients are still symptomatic.

• Patients with **posttraumatic iritis** present 1 to 2 days after a blunt eye injury with photophobia, pain, and tearing. They often have marked blepharospasm, perilimbal injection (ciliary flush), and pain on accommodation. Pain on accommodation is tested by having the patient look at a distant object and then quickly focusing on an object inches away. Slit lamp examination reveals cells in the anterior chamber, the hallmark of iritis.

○ Treat the pain with a topical cycloplegic, oral anti-inflammatory medication, and dark sunglasses. Symptoms usually resolve within a week. Ocular steroids may be used but only after consultation with an ophthalmologist.

• **Hyphemas** are defined by blood in the anterior chamber and are almost always secondary to blunt trauma. They may present with a diffuse red haze or as a layer of blood and are described by the percentage of the anterior chamber that is filled. A 100 percent hyphema, known as an "eight ball," may cause complete loss of light perception. Untreated, hyphemas may result in permanent corneal staining with loss of visual acuity and deprivational amblyopia. Rebleeding is a poor prognostic factor that occurs in up to 25 percent of patients. It can obstruct aqueous outflow causing increased intraocular pressure. Hemoglobinopathies and coagulopathies predispose to rebleeding.

○ Treatment includes shielding the eye and bed rest with 30 degrees of head elevation. An ophthalmology consultation should always be obtained and the use of mydriatics, ocular steroids, osmotic agents, acetazolamide, or antifibrinolytics should be left to the ophthalmologist. Patients should avoid platelet-active medications (ie, aspirin).

• Blunt ocular trauma can result in **lens subluxation** or **dislocation**. Subluxation causes monocular diplopia, whereas dislocation results in profoundly blurred vision. The lens may sublux either posteriorly or anteriorly, resulting in a deep or shallow anterior chamber and a visible lens margin. **Iridodonesis**, or shimmering of the iris provoked by rapidly changing gaze, is associated with posterior dislocation. If the capsule of

the lens is disrupted a cataract can develop. Lens injuries should be referred to an ophthalmologist.

• Children with **retinal injuries** complain of light flashes or a "curtain" over the visual field. Central vision will be spared if the macula remains unaffected. Funduscopy may reveal boat-shaped, preretinal hemorrhages, flame-shaped, superficial hemorrhages, round, purple-gray deep hemorrhages, or linear, exudative hemorrhages associated with shaken baby syndrome. Retinal injuries require ophthalmology consultation.

• **Retrobulbar hemorrhage**, bleeding behind the globe, may result in extraocular motion deficits, proptosis, and compromise of the optic nerve producing an afferent pupillary defect (Marcus Gunn pupil). Surgical decompression may be necessary. In rare instances, a lateral canthotomy is required in the ED.

• Perform a slit lamp examination to assess for **conjunctival and scleral lacerations**. Clues to scleral disruption include decreased visual acuity, an abnormal anterior chamber, low intraocular pressure (less than 6), and a positive **Sidle test**. To perform the Sidle test, place fluorescein on the cornea and observe for an aqueous leak under the cobalt blue light of the slit lamp. Tonometry is contraindicated if a scleral laceration is seen.

○ Treat small conjunctival lacerations with topical antibiotic drops. If the patient has a scleral laceration, place an eye shield, administer intravenous antibiotics, provide sedation, and obtain an ophthalmology consultation.

• Patients with **corneal foreign bodies** present with redness, tearing, and a foreign body sensation. To look for the foreign body, anesthetize the cornea and evert the lid by folding the lid upward over a cotton swab placed on the middle of the upper lid. Remove the foreign body with a cotton applicator soaked in topical anesthetic. If this is unsuccessful, attempt removal with a slit lamp and an eye spud or a 25-gauge needle on a tuberculin syringe. Iron-containing foreign bodies may leave rust rings that can be referred to a specialist for removal or removed in the ED with an ophthalmic burr.

○ After the foreign body is removed, instill a mydriatic agent and a topical antibiotic and recheck the child in 24 h. Prescribe appropriate analgesia.

○ If there is a **scleral foreign body**, consult an ophthalmologist for evaluation in the ED.

• **Intraocular foreign bodies** are vision-threatening injuries. Exposure to power tools and metal striking metal predisposes to an occult intraocular foreign body. Iron (siderosis) and copper (chalcosis) are particularly toxic to the eye, whereas glass and plastic are less inflammatory. Organic foreign bodies pose a high risk for intraocular infection. Findings include decreased visual acuity, pupillary distortion, and relatively little pain. Metallic objects may be seen by routine radiography or a computed tomography scan of the orbit. Ocular ultrasound is sensitive for both metallic and nonmetallic penetrations. Magnetic resonance imaging (MRI) accurately detects organic, plastic, and glass particles but may cause further injury if the foreign body is metal.

- ○ Cover the eye with a metal shield, keep the child at rest, and administer broad spectrum intravenous antibiotics, usually a first-generation cephalosporin and an aminoglycoside. Do not use topical antibiotics.
- ○ If the child requires intubation, succinylcholine and ketamine should be avoided as they may increase intraocular pressure and cause extrusion of orbital contents.
- ○ Foreign bodies that protrude from the eye must be removed in the operating room.
- • **Chemical injuries to the eye** (acid or alkali) require immediate irrigation with normal saline prior to examination and visual acuity testing. Irrigation takes precedence over all but life-saving interventions. The extent of caustic injury is dependent on the quantity, the pH, and the duration of the exposure. Alkalis result in liquefaction necrosis with saponification and deep penetration, and cause a more serious injury than do acids that produce a coagulation necrosis with limited penetration. Complications of caustic injuries include blindness, perforation, corneal neovascularization, secondary glaucoma, cataract formation, and retinal damage.
- ○ Begin irrigation in the prehospital setting and, in the ED, perform double lid eversion to expose the fornices and continue irrigation. A Morgan lens is useful. An alternative to the Morgan lens is a nasal oxygen cannula connected to intravenous bags of NS and placed on the bridge of the nose. This allows bilateral irrigation of the eyes through the nasal prongs. Check the pH in the conjunctival sac after 20 min and 2 L of NS irrigation, and continue irrigation until the pH is between 7.4 and 7.6. Recheck the pH 10 min after irrigation is stopped to ensure a stable level. Confirm that all particulate matter is removed. In cases of a bad alkali exposure, continuously irrigate the eyes until stopped by the ophthalmologist.
- ○ Hydrofluoric acid exposure may require irrigation with a magnesium oxide solution. Consult a poison center for the latest recommendations.
- • **Ultraviolet keratitis** occurs with prolonged glare from the snow or unprotected eye exposure when staring at an eclipse or using a tanning booth or welder's torch. Unprotected vision of an eclipse can also cause severe retinal damage and blindness. Eight to 12 h after exposure, patients present with bilateral photophobia, eye pain, tearing, blepharospasm, and scleral and perilimbal injection. Slit lamp examination using fluorescein shows thousands of punctate, shallow lesions on the cornea (keratitis).
- ○ Treat with cycloplegia and oral analgesia. Recovery usually takes 24 to 48 h.
- • Lids are more often damaged from thermal injury than is the globe. Use the slit lamp and fluorescein to evaluate for corneal injury and apply topical antibiotics to burned lids. Third degree burns require admission.

BIBLIOGRAPHY

Brunette DD, Ghezzi K, Renner GS: Ophthalmologic disorders. In: Rosen P, Barkin R, eds. *Emergency Medicine: Concepts and Clinical Practice.* St. Louis: CV Mosby, 2698–2719, 1998.

Ferrari LR: The injured eye. *Anesth Clin North Am* 14:125–150, 1996.

Marshall DH, Brownstein S, Addison DJ, et al: Air guns: The main cause of enucleation secondary to trauma in children and young adults in the greater Ottawa area in 1974–93. *Can J Ophthalmol* 30:187–192, 1995.

Napier SM, Baker RS, Sanford DG, et al: Eye injuries in athletics and recreation. *Surv Ophthalmol* 41:229–244, 1996.

Rubin SE, Catalano RA: Ocular trauma and its prevention. In: Nelson LB, ed. *Harley's Pediatric Ophthalmology.* Philadelphia, Saunders; 482–498, 1998.

Smith GA, Knapp JF, Barnett TM, et al: The rockets' red glare, the bombs bursting in air: Fireworks-related injuries to children. *Pediatrics* 98:1–9, 1996.

Tingley DH: Consultation with the specialist: Eye trauma: Corneal abrasions. *Pediatr Rev* 20:320–322, 1999.

QUESTIONS

1. Pupillary dilatation may occur as a result of all of the following **EXCEPT**:
   - A. Posttraumatic mydriasis
   - B. Anticholinergic medication
   - C. Third nerve palsy
   - D. Pilocarpine drops
   - E. Cycloplegics
2. All of the following lacerations require specialized repair **EXCEPT**:
   - A. Lacerations with fat in the wound
   - B. Lacerations of the lid margins
   - C. Lacerations of the supraorbital rim

D. Lacerations of the tarsal plate

E. Laceration with levator palpebrae muscle involvement

3. Characteristics of posttraumatic iritis are all of the following **EXCEPT**:

A. Presents 1 week after a blunt eye injury

B. Photophobia

C. Blepharospasm

D. Perilimbal injection

E. Pain with accommodation

4. Monocular diplopia may be caused by:

A. Lens subluxation

B. Retinal injury

C. Increased intraocular pressure

D. Hyphema

E. Posttraumatic iritis

5. Signs of a scleral laceration include all of the following **EXCEPT**:

A. Decreased visual acuity

B. Abnormal anterior chamber

C. Positive Sidle test

D. Low intraocular pressure by tonometry

E. Vitreous hemorrhage

6. Management of intraocular foreign bodies includes all of the following **EXCEPT**:

A. CT scan of orbit

B. MRI of orbit

C. Ocular ultrasound

D. Avoidance of succinylcholine and ketamine

E. Topical antibiotics

ANSWERS

1. D. Pilocarpine drops will cause papillary constriction. Cycloplegics, such as homatropine and cyclopentolate hydrochloride, dilate the eye.

2. C. All of the other lacerations require specialized repair by ophthalmologist due to concern about underlying injury to the eye and its surrounding structures. Lacerations with fat in the wound may indicate an underlying globe injury. Lacerations of the lid margins are at risk for lid deformity and abnormal lid movement. Lacerations involving the levator palpebrae muscle may result in posttraumatic ptosis.

3. A. Posttraumatic iritis generally presents within 1 to 2 days following blunt eye injury.

4. A. Blunt ocular trauma can result in lens subluxation. Subluxation causes monocular diplopia. The lens may sublux either posteriorly or anteriorly, resulting in a deep or shallow anterior chamber and a visible lens margin. Iridodonesis, or shimmering of the iris provoked by rapidly changing gaze, is associated with posterior dislocation.

5. D. Tonometry is contraindicated if a scleral laceration is seen.

6. E. The orbit can be imaged for an intraocular foreign body by several methods including the CT scan of the orbit (metallic objects), MRI (organic, plastic, and glass), ocular ultrasound (metallic and nonmetallic). If the child requires intubation, succinylcholine and ketamine should be avoided as they may increase intraocular pressure and cause extrusion of orbital contents. The eye should be covered with a metal shield and broad spectrum intravenous antibiotics should be given. Topical antibiotics should be avoided.

18 ORTHOPEDIC INJURIES

Valerie A. Dobiesz
Russell H. Greenfield
Kemedy K. McQuillen
Patricia Lee

EPIDEMIOLOGY

- Fractures account for 10 to 15 percent of all childhood injuries.

UNIQUE ASPECTS OF THE PEDIATRIC SKELETON

- Growing bone is more porous with fewer lamellar components than adult bone. This makes it less dense, more malleable, and able to withstand greater force before breaking.

- Pediatric bone allows less propagation of the fracture, making comminution less likely.

- Incomplete (greenstick) and torus (buckle) fractures, plastic deformation, and bowing injuries are more common in children than in adults.

- With metaphyseal fractures, the active growth of children's bones facilitates remodeling, corrects longitudinal malalignment, and allows for the acceptance of greater degrees of angulation. Remodeling will occur if a fracture is adjacent to a hinged joint and has an angulation of <30 degrees in the plane of motion, and if the child has 2 or more years of bone growth remaining.

- The pediatric periosteum is extremely strong, thick, and resistant to tearing. It minimizes the frequency of open fractures, decreases the amount of fracture displacement, and aids in fracture reduction. It also possesses increased osteogenic capability, allowing for more rapid healing and minimizing the risk of nonunion.

- The physis (epiphyseal plate or growth plate) is the weakest structure in the pediatric skeleton and is injured more frequently than the surrounding ligaments. This makes pediatric sprains uncommon. The physis is also the place where anatomic alignment of fracture fragments is most critical to avoid growth imbalance.
- Following an injury, there is increased blood flow to the growth plate resulting in accelerated longitudinal bone growth. This makes overriding fracture fragments desirable in certain instances, especially with diaphyseal femur fractures.

TERMINOLOGY

- Table 18-1 outlines terms commonly used to describe fractures and Fig. 18-1 is a diagram demonstrating anatomic terms related to the immature bone.

- An open fracture is one in which there is a break in the skin and communication with the underlying fracture. Antibiotics, operative wound debridement, and fracture reduction are required with open fractures.

PHYSEAL INJURIES

- Up to 18 percent of fractures involve the physis. They are classified using the Salter–Harris classification system (with or without the Ogden modification) as it describes the relationship of the fracture to the growth plate, epiphysis, metaphysis, and joint. The Salter–Harris classification has prognostic and therapeutic implications (Table 18-2, Fig. 18-2).
- Most Salter–Harris type I or II fractures are at low risk for growth disturbance and are treated with closed reduction. The risk of growth disturbance is greater with fracture types III to V and these injuries often require operative intervention.

TABLE 18-1   Fracture Terminology

Anatomic location
  Epiphysis: present at the end of each long bone; completely cartilaginous at birth except at distal femur; secondary ossification centers develop
    that replace cartilage over time
  Apophysis: traction epiphysis; nonarticular site of ligament and tendon attachment (example: distal humeral condyles); not directly involved in
    longitudinal growth but contribute to bony contour
  Physis (growth plate) or epiphyseal plate: cartilaginous structure between epiphysis and metaphysis responsible for longitudinal bone growth;
    injury may result in growth disturbance or arrest
  Metaphysis: flared end of diaphysis adjacent to physes representing new bone; structurally weak area; diaphyseal: central shaft of long bone
Diaphyseal: central shaft of long bone
  Articular: involves portion of epiphysis comprising joint surface
  Epicondylar: distal humeral site of muscle attachments
  Supracondylar: part of metaphysis located cephalad to condyles and epicondyles
  Transcondylar: across the condyles of humerus or distal femur
  Intercondylar: intraepiphyseal; fracture disrupts articular surface and separates condyles from one another
  Subcapital: metaphyseal area of proximal femur and radius
Fracture pattern
  Avulsion: bone fragment pulled off by action of tendon or ligament
  Longitudinal: fracture line follows long axis of bone
  Transverse: fracture line at right angle to long axis of bone
  Oblique: fracture line angled at 30–60 degrees from long axis of bone
  Spiral: encircling oblique fracture (has torsional component)
  Impacted: fracture ends compressed together
  Comminuted: any fracture with more than two fracture fragments
  Bowing: (plastic deformation) significant bend in bone without fracture; commonly seen in ulna and fibula in association with fracture of
    respective paired bone
  Torus: "buckle fracture," metaphyseal compaction of trabecular bone and buckling of cortical bone
  Greenstick: incomplete fracture of cortex on convex (tension, elastic phase) side of bone with only a bend in cortex of concave side (compression,
    plastic phase); most common fracture pattern in children
  Pathologic: fracture through abnormal, weakened bone (examples: tumors, osteomyelitis, cysts, inherited metabolic disorders)
Fracture fragment positions
  Alignment: refers to longitudinal relationship of one fragment to another
  Displacement: deviation of fracture fragments from anatomic position (displacement of distal fragment described in relation to proximal one;
    varus displacement: toward midline of body; valgus displacement: away from midline of body)
  Angulation: direction of apex of angle formed by fracture fragments (will be opposite to direction of displacement of distal fragment)
  Distraction: degree to which fracture surfaces are separated
  Bayonet deformity: overlapping fracture surfaces with resultant shortening
  Butterfly fragment: wedge-shaped fragment arising at apex of force applied to shaft of long bone

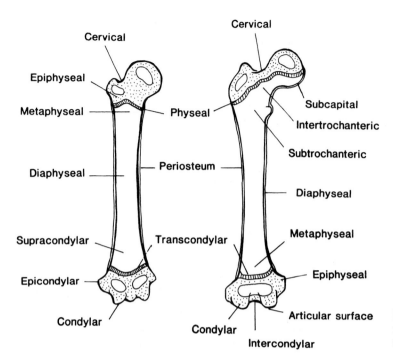

FIG. 18-1 Illustration of a pediatric humerus and femur depicting specific anatomic sites and descriptive terminology.

TABLE 18-2 Classification of Epiphyseal Injuries

TYPE	DESCRIPTION
	SALTER–HARRIS SYSTEM
I	Complete separation of the epiphysis and most of the physis from metaphysis. Prognosis for normal growth is good. Commonly results from shearing force in newborns and young infants. May be seen in victims of abuse. Diagnosis may be difficult; if radiographic studies are normal but patient is tender over the growth plate immobilization and orthopedic referral are recommended.
II	Fracture line propagates along physis and extends into metaphysis; result is displaced metaphyseal fragment, often with epiphyseal displacement. Most common epiphyseal injury; associated with low risk of growth disturbance. Usually occurs in children over 10 years of age.
III	Fracture line extends from physis through epiphysis to articular surface of the joint. Anatomic reduction necessary to restore normal joint mechanics and prevent growth disturbance, bony bridging, and posttraumatic arthritis.
IV	Fracture line begins at articular surface, crosses the epiphysis and growth plate, and extends into the metaphysis, splitting off a metaphyseal fragment (example: humeral lateral condyle fractures). Open reduction and internal fixation usually required to ensure anatomic reduction and avoid angular deformity and loss of joint function. Significant incidence of growth disturbance.
V	Results from longitudinal compression of the growth plate. Rare injury associated with apparently normal x-rays. Diagnosis usually made in retrospect when premature closure of the physis and growth abnormalities develop.
	ADDITIONAL TYPES FROM THE OGDEN SYSTEM
VI	Peripheral shear injury to borders of growth plate. Angular deformity may develop due to formation of osseous bridge between metaphysis and epiphysis.
VII	Intraarticular intraepiphyseal injury where ligament pulls off distal portion of epiphysis rather than tearing.
VIII	Fracture through region of metaphysis with temporary disruption of circulation.
IX	Fracture involving significant damage to or loss of periosteum.

• Salter II fractures are the most common physeal injury (75 percent).

BIRTH TRAUMA

• Fractures of the clavicle, humerus, hip, and femur can occur during difficult deliveries (Fig. 18-3).

CHILD ABUSE

• Most child abuse occurs in children less than 2 years old and up to 50 percent of fractures in children younger than 1 year old are the result of non-accidental trauma. Clues to the presence of non-accidental trauma include a delay in seeking medical attention, a mechanism that is inconsistent with the injury, and an

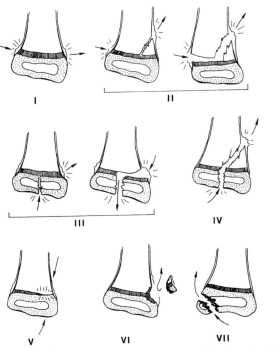

FIG. 18-2 Classification of growth plate injuries described by Salter and Harris (I to V) and Ogden (VI to VII).

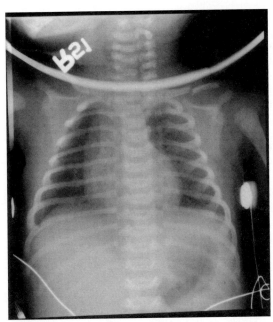

FIG. 18-3 Fracture of the middle third of the clavicle secondary to shoulder dystocia in a newborn.

injury that is developmentally unlikely. Long bone fractures in a young child, femur fractures in the non-ambulatory child, and non-supracondylar fractures of the humerus are highly suggestive of abuse. Spiral fractures are common in both accidental and un-accidental trauma. Radiographic findings suggestive

TABLE 18-3   Radiographic Findings Suggestive of Child Abuse

High Risk for Abuse
  Metaphyseal lesions
  Posterior rib fractures
  Scapular fractures
  Spinous process fractures
  Sternal fractures
Moderate Risk for Abuse
  Multiple fractures, especially bilateral
  Fractures of different ages
  Epiphyseal separation
  Vertebral body fractures and subluxations
  Digit fractures
  Complex skull fractures
Low Risk for Abuse
  Clavicular fractures
  Long bone shaft fractures
  Linear skull fractures

of unaccidental trauma are listed in Table 18-3. Metaphyseal-epiphyseal junction fractures are pathognomonic for child abuse. They are frequently bilateral and result from periosteal avulsion of bone and cartilage when there is a twisting motion or downward pull on an extremity. The radiographic findings of a chip of bone or a larger "bucket handle" fracture may not be visible until 7 to 10 days after the injury when new subperiosteal bone formation is seen (Fig. 18-4).

- A skeletal survey should be performed on any child younger than 2 years old when abuse is suspected. The survey includes anteroposterior (AP), lateral, and oblique views of the chest; AP views of the pelvis; AP views of all extremities; lateral views of the lumbar and cervical spine; and AP and lateral views of the skull. If abuse is strongly suspected and the initial skeletal survey is not diagnostic, a follow-up survey is recommended 2 weeks after the initial study.

CLINICAL EVALUATION

- Resuscitative efforts and attention to life-threatening injuries take precedence over orthopedic injuries.
- Ascertain historical information including the time and mechanism of injury, direction and degree of force involved, and history of previous injury.
- Observe and palpate the limb for deformity, swelling, pain, or abnormal motion. Examine the joints above and below the injury. Carefully inspect the surrounding soft tissue for any breaks that may signify an open fracture. Perform serial neurovascular assessments of the limb to monitor for compartment syndrome and recheck the neurovascular status before and after any manipulations.
- Splint the injured extremity before moving the patient to prevent further injury.

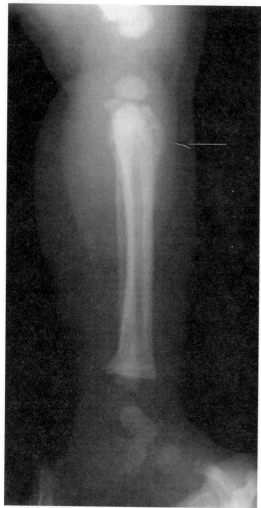

FIG. 18-4 Periosteal reaction with metaphyseal irregularity in a 3-month-old child (*arrow*). This metaphyseal corner fracture is highly suggestive of unaccidental trauma.

• Obtain at least AP and lateral views of the injury. The films should include the joints above and below the injury since dislocations can occur with diaphyseal fractures (eg, Monteggia fractures). Comparison views of the uninjured extremity may be helpful.

THERAPEUTIC CONSIDERATIONS

• Treat pain with enteral or parenteral medication, local or regional blocks, and immobilization of the injured extremity. Fractures that are open, significantly malaligned, associated with neurovascular compromise, or involve a growth plate or a joint require immediate orthopedic consultation. Other fractures can be splinted by the primary care physician and referred for definitive care within 3 days.

• Discharge instructions should include the proper use of ice, elevation, and analgesia. Patients should be instructed to return immediately for severe pain, swelling, or discoloration of the limb.

BIBLIOGRAPHY

Bachman D, Santora S: Orthopedic trauma. In: Fleisher GR, Ludwig S, eds. *Textbook of Pediatric Emergency Medicine.* Baltimore: Williams & Wilkins, 1236–1244, 2000.

Bright RW: Physeal injuries. In: Rockwood CA, Wilkins KE, King RE, eds. *Fractures in Children.* Philadelphia: JB Lippincott, 87–186, 1996.

Canale, ST: Physeal injuries. In: Green NE, Swiotkowski MF, eds. *Skeletal Trauma in Children*, vol 3. Philadelphia: WB Saunders, 17–58, 1998.

DiScala, C, Sege R, et al: Child abuse and unintentional injuries: A 10-year retrospective. *Arch Pediatr Adolesc Med* 54:16–22, 2000.

Hennrikus WL, Shaw BA, Gerardi JA: Injuries when children reportedly fall from a bed or couch. *Clin Orthop* (407): 148–151, 2003.

Jones E: Skeletal growth and development as related to traumas. In: Green NE, Swiontkowski MF, eds. *Skeletal Trauma in Children.* Philadelphia: WB Saunders, 1–16, 1998.

Leventhal JM, Thomas SA, Rosenfield NS, et al: Fractures in young children: Distinguishing child abuse from unintentional injuries. *Am J Dis Child* 147:87, 1993.

Ogden JA, Ogden DA, Ganey TM: Biological aspects of children's fractures. In: Rockwood CA, Wilkins KE, Beaty JH, eds. *Fractures in Children.* Philadelphia: JB Lippincott, 19–52, 1996.

Peterson HA: Physeal and apophyseal injuries. In: Rockwood CA, Wilkins KE, Beaty JH, eds. *Fractures in Children.* Philadelphia: JB Lippincott, 103–166, 1996.

Salter RB, Harris WR: Injuries involving the epiphyseal plate. *J Bone Surg [Am]* 45A:587, 1963.

Section on Radiology: Diagnostic imaging of child abuse. *Pediatrics* 105:1345–1348, 2000.

QUESTIONS

1. Unique aspects of the pediatric skeleton include all of the following except:
   A. Pediatric periosteum is extremely strong, thick, and resistant to tearing.
   B. Pediatric bones are less likely to have comminuted fractures.
   C. Remodeling occurs if a fracture is adjacent to a hinged joint and has an angulation of <30 degrees in the plane of motion, and if the child has 2 or more years of bone growth remodeling.
   D. The epiphysis is the strongest structure and is injured less frequently than the surrounding ligaments.

E. Following an injury, there is accelerated longitudinal bone growth.

2. A 7-year-old boy presents with a fracture of the distal radius. The radiograph shows a fracture line that extends through the epiphysis and into the metaphysis. The mother is concerned about problems with future growth of the forearm following the fracture. You advise her that in her son's situation:

A. Salter–Harris II type fractures are at low risk for growth disturbance and can be treated with closed reduction.

B. Salter–Harris I type fractures are at low risk for growth disturbance and can be treated with closed reduction.

C. Salter–Harris III type fractures have a higher risk for growth disturbance.

D. Salter–Harris V type fractures have the highest risk for growth disturbance.

E. Her son does not have a Salter–Harris fracture.

3. Radiographic findings suggestive of child abuse include all of the following **EXCEPT**:

A. Metaphyseal-epiphyseal junction fracture

B. Salter–Harris II fracture

C. Bucket handle type fracture

D. Bone chip type fracture

E. Femur fracture in non-ambulatory child

ANSWERS

1. D. The physis (epiphyseal plate or growth plate) is the weakest structure in the pediatric skeleton and is injured more frequently than the surrounding ligaments

2. A. According to the Salter–Harris classification, the boy has a Salter–Harris II type fracture, which has a low risk for growth disturbance.

3. B. Salter–Harris II fractures are frequently seen in children in accidental trauma. Clues to the presence of child abuse (unaccidental trauma) include a delay in seeking medical attention, a mechanism that is inconsistent with injury, and an injury that is developmentally unlikely. Long bone fractures in a young child, femur fractures in the non-ambulatory child, and non-supracondylar fractures of the humerus are highly suggestive of abuse. Spiral fractures are common in both accidental and unaccidental trauma. Metaphyseal-epiphyseal junction fractures are pathognomonic for child abuse, with findings of a chip of bone or a larger "bucket handle" fracture.

19 INJURIES OF THE UPPER EXTREMITIES

Timothy J. Rittenberry
Russell H. Greenfield
Kemedy K. McQuillen
Patricia Lee

CLAVICLE AND ACROMIOCLAVICULAR JOINT

- **Clavicle fractures** are the most common fracture in childhood and most commonly result from a fall onto the shoulder. Greater than 90 percent involve the distal third of the clavicle. The medial clavicular epiphysis is the last growth plate to close, making patients up to age 25 years more susceptible to Salter–Harris type I or II fractures of the clavicle than to sternoclavicular joint dislocations. Clavicle fractures that occur during delivery may be present acutely as a pseudoparalysis (normal hand and forearm movement without movement of the arm) or weeks after delivery when callus formation causes a clavicle deformity. Older children present with pain with or without a deformity. With displaced fractures, vascular injuries must be considered: pulse abnormalities and swelling suggests laceration or compression of the subclavian vessels. Lung injuries occur infrequently. An anterior-posterior (AP) radiograph of the clavicle confirms the diagnosis. If clinical suspicion is high and the AP view does not reveal a fracture, a 30-degree cephalic view can be helpful. Specialized imaging studies are rarely needed.
  - Most clavicle fractures heal well without complication and reduction is rarely necessary. Injuries due to birth trauma require only careful handling of the infant. In other children, a sling, sling and swath, or shoulder strap provides immobilization and pain relief. Patients with significantly overriding fracture fragments, an open fracture, or a vascular complication require operative intervention.
- **Acromioclavicular joint** separations are rare in children: trauma to the distal clavicle produces metaphyseal fractures rather than ligamentous tearing. Diagnosis is by non-weighted radiographs. These fractures heal well with a sling and swathe.

SHOULDER DISLOCATIONS

- **Shoulder dislocations** are rare in children: the forces that cause shoulder dislocation in adults usually cause displaced Salter–Harris type II proximal humerus fractures in young children.

- Anterior dislocations are more common than posterior or inferior dislocations. With an anterior dislocation, patients present with the arm held in slight abduction and external rotation. There is loss of the normal contour of the shoulder and the humeral head may be palpated anterior to the glenoid fossa.
- Posterior dislocations occur following seizures or electrical injuries and patients present with the arm held in adduction and internal rotation. The anterior shoulder appears flat and the humeral head may be palpated posteriorly.
- The axillary nerve can be injured with shoulder dislocations and its function should be assessed by checking sensation over the deltoid muscle.
- Anteroposterior and true scapular lateral or transaxillary radiographs are diagnostic and also delineate associated greater tuberosity fractures, damage to the glenoid labrum, and compression fractures of the posterolateral humeral head (Hill–Sachs deformity). Complications include fractures, rotator cuff injuries, and recurrent dislocations.
  ○ Reduction of anterior dislocations is accomplished with traction-countertraction, scapular manipulation, or external rotation techniques after the administration of adequate analgesia and relaxation. Orthopedic consultation is recommended in all cases of posterior shoulder dislocation.

HUMERUS FRACTURES

- Salter–Harris type I **proximal humerus fractures** occur most commonly between the ages of 5 and 11 years; while type II proximal humerus fractures tend to occur between 11 to 15 years of age. Most are not displaced. Radiographs should include two perpendicular views of the humerus that include the distal clavicle and acromion.
- In most cases, sling and swathe immobilization is adequate. Pinning or internal fixation may be required if the proximal epiphysis is displaced more than 50 percent, angulation is greater than 40 degrees, or there is significant malrotation.
- Most **humeral shaft fractures** are the result of a direct blow, however, unaccidental trauma should be suspected in a child less than 3 years of age with a spiral humerus fracture. Mid-shaft fractures heal well, even with angulations of up to 20° and as much as 2 cm of overlap. Radial nerve injury can complicate fractures of the middle to distal humerus and its function should be assessed before and after any

manipulation. Acute radial nerve palsy has an excellent long-term prognosis.
- Immobilize young children in a sling and swathe and adolescents in a sugar tong splint.

ELBOW

- The diagnosis of elbow injuries by radiography is complicated by the presence of numerous epiphyses and ossification centers. At a minimum, radiographic evaluation of the elbow consists of an AP view with the joint in extension and a true lateral view with the elbow flexed at a right angle. In some cases, comparison views of the unaffected elbow are helpful.
- The anterior humeral line and the radiocapitellar line are two reference lines useful in detecting occult elbow injuries. On a true lateral view of the elbow, the anterior humeral line is drawn along the anterior cortex of the distal humerus and intersects the middle third of the capitellum. Posterior displacement of the capitellum relative to the anterior humeral line suggests a supracondylar fracture. Also on a lateral view of the elbow, and regardless of the degree of flexion or extension, the radiocapitellar line, drawn down the axis of the proximal radius, should bisect the capitellum. Failure to do so suggests a radial neck fracture or radial head dislocation.
- Fat pads are also helpful in detecting occult fractures. On a lateral film of a normal elbow flexed at 90 degrees, the anterior fat pad sits in the coronoid fossa and appears as a small lucency, while the posterior fat pad sits deep down in the olecranon fossa and is not visible. The presence of *any* posterior fat pad or an exaggerated anterior fat pad (sail sign) is always abnormal and suggests blood within the joint capsule and an occult fracture of the distal humerus, proximal ulna, or radius (Fig. 19-1).

SUPRACONDYLAR HUMERUS FRACTURES

- Supracondylar humerus fractures result from a fall onto an outstretched hand causing hyperextension of the elbow. The olecranon process is thrust into the olecranon fossa, resulting in fracture with posterior displacement of the distal fragment (Fig. 19-2). Supracondylar fractures most commonly occur in children 3 to 10 years of age and have a high risk for neurovascular complications. Brachial artery disruption, compression, contusion, or vasospasm may present with pallor and cyanosis of the fingers, prolonged capillary refill, or absence of the radial pulse. These

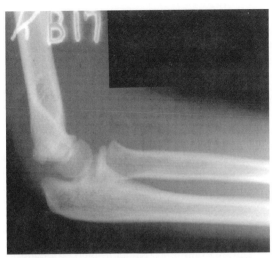

FIG. 19-1 Fracture through the medial epicondyle extending into the olecranon fossa. Note the posterior fat pad sign, signifying the presence of blood within the joint space.

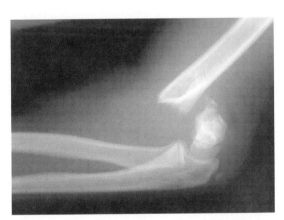

FIG. 19-2 Comminuted supracondylar fracture with large joint effusion. The patient required fasciotomy and skin grafting due to neurovascular compromise.

injuries need prompt reduction and, if the vascular status is not improved, surgical exploration. These patients are at risk for developing a forearm compartment syndrome, Volkmann's ischemic contracture, and a nonfunctional hand and wrist. Radial, median, and ulnar nerve injuries occur in 10 to 20% of children with supracondylar fractures and have a good prognosis for recovery. Cubitus varus is a late complication of supracondylar humerus fractures.

- Supracondylar fractures are treated with closed reduction and immobilization, transcutaneous pinning, and open reduction-internal fixation depending on the degree of displacement and rotational and angular deformities. Urgent orthopedic consultation is critical and some children require admission for 24 to 48 hours of observation.

MEDIAL AND LATERAL CONDYLES

- **Lateral condyle (capitellum) fractures** occur when there is a fall on the outstretched arm with forearm supination or elbow flexion. The peak in incidence is at 6 years old and children present with swelling and tenderness most pronounced at the lateral elbow. On radiographs, the capitellum is displaced from the trochlea or radiocapitellar line. Complications include nonunion, loss of elbow mobility, and growth arrest leading to eventual cubitus valgus and tardy ulnar palsy.
- Management is usually operative in all but nondisplaced fractures.
- **Medial condyle (trochlea) fractures** rarely occur, but when present, require precise anatomic reduction due to the intraarticular nature of the injury (Fig. 19-3). The most frequent complications are nonunion and ulnar nerve injury.

MEDIAL EPICONDYLAR FRACTURES

- Medial epicondylar fractures occur most commonly in children between 7 and 15 years of age. They can occur acutely, as is seen when they accompany an elbow dislocation (Fig. 19-4), or more insidiously with repetitive motion (Little Leaguer's elbow).
- Treatment is nonoperative unless there is severe displacement or an ulnar nerve injury.

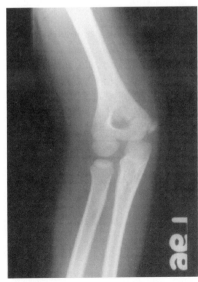

FIG. 19-3 Nondisplaced fracture of the medial condyle in a 5-year-old.

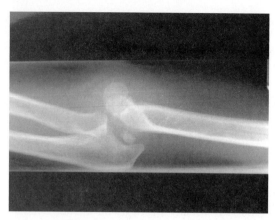

FIG. 19-4 Posterior elbow dislocation with avulsion of the medial epicondyle.

FRACTURE-SEPARATION OF THE DISTAL HUMERAL PHYSIS

- When this injury is present in children less than 3 years of age, physical abuse should be suspected. The fracture can also occur following birth trauma. Differentiation from elbow dislocation is difficult due to the lack of capitellar ossification. Treatment is with closed reduction and orthopedic consultation is warranted

ELBOW DISLOCATIONS

- Elbow dislocations occur infrequently. They are usually the result of a fall onto the slightly flexed, outstretched arm in an adolescent. Most dislocations are posterior. Associated fractures of the medial epicondyle, coronoid process, radial head, or olecranon are common (see Fig. 19-4). Ulnar and median nerve injuries are more common than brachial artery injuries.
- Reduce the dislocation after providing analgesia and muscle relaxation. Flex the elbow to 60 degrees, supinate the forearm, and, while an assistant stabilizes the proximal humerus, apply longitudinal traction at the wrist. After reduction, gently flex and immobilize the elbow and recheck the neurovascular status of the arm. On a postreduction radiograph, verify that the medial epicondyle is extraarticular.

RADIAL HEAD SUBLUXATION

- Nursemaid's elbow is the most common pediatric elbow injury. It occurs when abrupt axial traction is applied to the extended, pronated forearm, causing entrapment of the annular ligament between the radial head and capitellum. The child presents with the forearm held in pronation with the elbow in slight flexion. There is minimal swelling and only mild tenderness over the radial head. The diagnosis is based on clinical features and radiographs are not necessary.
- Reduction is accomplished with either supination or pronation. Using the supination method, the thumb is held over the radial head while the forearm is supinated and flexed at the elbow. Radial traction prior to supination and flexion may be helpful. With the pronation method, the thumb is held over the radial head while the forearm is hyperpronated. With both methods, a palpable or audible "pop" signals successful reduction and the patient should start using the arm within 15 minutes. No additional treatment is necessary.
- If normal use does not follow reduction attempts, x-rays should be obtained. If the radiographs are normal, splint the arm and arrange for orthopedic follow-up within 3 days. The recurrence rate for nursemaid's elbow approaches 30 percent.

FRACTURES OF THE RADIUS AND ULNA

- These fractures are very common during childhood. Although an isolated fracture of one bone can occur, concomitant fractures or dislocations are not uncommon. For this reason, forearm x-rays should always include the wrist and elbow. Complications are uncommon and include vascular compromise and compartment syndrome.
- Most proximal radius fractures in children less than 5 years old involve the metaphyseal neck: Salter–Harris type I and type II fractures are most common. These fractures are associated with elbow dislocations and are often seen with injury to the medial epicondyle, olecranon, and coronoid process. An abnormal fat pad sign or radiocapitellar line on x-ray suggests an occult radial head or radial neck fracture. Minimally displaced or nondisplaced fractures can be treated in a posterior splint with the elbow flexed at 90 degrees. Complications include restriction of pronation and supination and myositis ossificans.
- Olecranon fractures tend to occur with other elbow injuries, such as radial head dislocations, radial neck fractures, and fractures of the medial epicondyle. Isolated olecranon epiphyseal fractures are rare and usually due to a direct blow to the posterior elbow. Nondisplaced injuries may be treated in a posterior splint. Nonunion and ulnar nerve neuropraxia are infrequent complications.

- Most forearm diaphyseal fractures are either greenstick or bowing injuries (Fig. 19-5). The potential for remodeling of a bowing injury is minimal in children older than 4 years. Bowing may restrict pronation and supination and result in permanent deformity.

- Overriding of fracture fragments in the presence of an isolated fracture of one of the forearm bones suggests a Monteggia (proximal ulna fracture with radial head dislocation; Fig. 19-6) or Galeazzi fracture (fracture of the middle to distal radius with distal radioulnar joint dislocation; Fig. 19-7). Closed reduction is usually successful.

- Fractures of the distal third of the radius and ulna are common in children 6 to 12 years of age. Torus fractures are immobilized in a long arm splint (Fig. 19-8). Tenderness over the physis of the distal radius with a normal radiograph suggests a nondisplaced Salter–Harris type I injury. Splinting with orthopedic

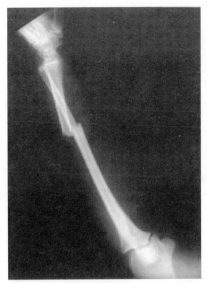

FIG. 19-7 Galeazzi fracture in a 16-year-old.

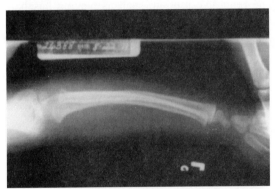

FIG. 19-5 Illustration depicting a greenstick fracture of the radium with associated plastic deformity of the ulna. Radiographic appearance of mid-shaft bowing injury of both the radius and ulna.

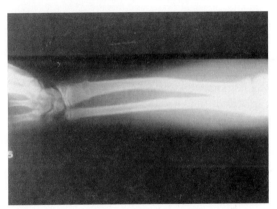

Fig. 19-8 Torus fracture of the distal radius.

follow-up is appropriate. When reducing forearm fractures, it is important to correct rotational abnormalities. Complications are uncommon, but vascular compromise or compartment syndrome can develop with any forearm fracture.

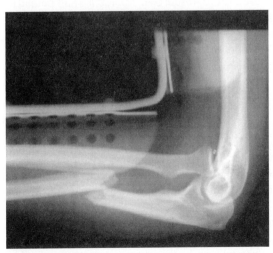

FIG. 19-6 Fracture of the proximal ulna with radial head dislocation (Monteggia fracture). A line bisecting the proximal radius completely misses the capitellum.

BIBLIOGRAPHY

Green NE: Fractures and dislocations about the elbow. In: Green NE, Swiontkowski MF, eds. *Skeletal Trauma in Children.* Vol 3. Philadelphia: WB Saunders, 259–317, 1998.

Kaplan RE, Lillis KA: Recurrent nursemaid's elbow (annular ligament displacement) treatment via telephone. *Pediatrics* 110(1 Pt 1):171–174, 2002.

Macias CG, Bothrer J, Wiebe R: A comparison of supination/ flexion to hyperpronation in the reduction of radial head subluxation, *Pediatrics* 102:e10, 1998.

Rittenberry TJ, Townes DA: Pediatric orthopedics: The upper extremity. In: Hart RG, Rittenberry TJ, Uehara DT, eds: *Handbook of Orthopaedic Emergencies.* Philadelphia: Lippincott-Raven, 420–437, 1999.

Villalba K, Kroger KJ: Upper extremity injuries. In: Reisdorff EJ, Roberts MR, Weigenstein JG, eds. *Pediatric Emergency Medicine.* Philadelphia, WB Saunders, 948–960, 1993.

Wilkens KE: Fractures and dislocations of the elbow region. In: Rockwood CA, Wikins KE, Beaty JH, eds. *Fractures in Children.* Philadelphia: Lippincott-Raven, Vol 3, 420–437, 1996.

Wu J, Perron AD, Miller MD, et al: Orthopedic pitfalls in the ED: Pediatric supracondylar humerus fracture. *Am J Emerg Med* 20:544–550, 2002.

QUESTIONS

1. The most common fracture in childhood is the:
   A. Distal radius
   B. Distal humerus
   C. Clavicle
   D. Nasal bone
   E. Distal fibula
2. The most common pediatric elbow injury is:
   A. Posterior elbow dislocation
   B. Medial epicondyle fracture
   C. Capitellum fracture
   D. Radial head subluxation
   E. Medial condyle fracture
3. A 15-year-old boy presents following a fall from his bicycle with complaints of pain to his right shoulder. Physical examination reveals his arm held in slight abduction and external rotation with associated loss of the normal contour of the shoulder. The humeral head may be palpated anterior to the glenoid fossa. Associated problems with this injury may include all of the following except:
   A. Axillary nerve injury
   B. Rotator cuff injury
   C. Hill–Sachs deformity
   D. Greater tuberosity fracture
   E. Posterior shoulder dislocation
4. An elbow fracture is suggested by which of the following findings?
   A. Anterior fat pad
   B. Posterior fat pad
   C. Anterior humeral line intersects the middle third of the capitellum.
   D. Radiocapitellar line bisects the capitellum
   E. Epiphyseal growth plate
5. Complications of a supracondylar fracture include all of the following except:
   A. Volkmann's ischemic contraction
   B. Brachial artery disruption
   C. Forearm compartment syndrome
   D. Cubitus varus
   E. Little Leaguer's elbow

ANSWERS

1. C. Clavicle fractures are the most common fracture in childhood and most commonly result from a fall onto the shoulder. Greater than 90% involve the distal third of the clavicle.
2. D. Radial head subluxation (nursemaid's elbow) is the most common pediatric elbow injury.
3. E. The above injury represents an anterior shoulder dislocation.
4. B. The presence of **ANY** posterior fat pad or an exaggerated anterior fat pad (sail sign) is always abnormal and suggests blood within the joint capsule and an occult fracture of the distal humerus, proximal ulna, or radius.
5. E. The repetitive motion, such as playing baseball (Little League), can result in a medial epicondylar fracture.

20 INJURIES OF THE HAND AND WRIST

Dennis T. Uehara
Kemedy K. McQuillen
Patricia Lee

EPIDEMIOLOGY

- Hand fractures represent 5 to 7 percent of all pediatric fractures.
- Isolated crush injuries are common in younger children while injuries related to athletic competition are more prevalent in older children.

PHYSICAL EXAMINATION

- **OBSERVE** for lacerations, puncture wounds, soft tissue swelling, deformity, color, and position. The resting hand should demonstrate increasing flexion from the index through little finger and increasing flexion of the joints, from the DIP through MCP joints. Abnormalities imply a tendon laceration. Check alignment with the fingers in extension and flexion. Check for malrotation by having the patient alternately flex the fingers to the palm. Each finger should converge to the tubercle of the scaphoid. Alternatively, with the fingers in flexion, compare the planes of the fingernails. The nail plates should be roughly parallel and symmetric to the opposite hand. Any abnormal tilting is evidence of a rotational deformity.

- Gently **PALPATE** the patient's hand while it is resting on a flat surface. Tenderness over the radial or ulnar aspect of an interphalangeal (IP) joint indicates a collateral ligament tear, over the volar aspect of an IP joint indicates a volar plate injury, and over the ulnar aspect of the thumb MCP joint indicates a gamekeeper's thumb (torn ulnar collateral ligament of the thumb). Pain over the anatomic snuff box is presumptive for a scaphoid fracture. A felon is diagnosed with the presence of erythema, warmth, swelling, and tenderness over the distal finger pad.
- Assess **CIRCULATION** using color, capillary refill and skin temperature. A cyanotic edematous hand indicates venous insufficiency while a pale cool hand with poor capillary filling indicates arterial insufficiency. Control arterial bleeding with pressure. Because the digital nerve runs superficial to the artery, arterial bleeding from a volar laceration implies a concomitant digital nerve laceration.
- Test **SENATION** with two point discrimination: normal two-point discrimination is 3 to 5 mm. In uncooperative patients, skin wrinkling and sweating can be assessed. Following digital nerve injury, the ability to sweat is lost, and the skin takes on a smooth, silky texture. Skin wrinkling is also lost after a digital nerve injury: soaking the hand in warm water will not result in the normal wrinkling of the skin distal to the nerve injury.
- Test **MOTOR** function of the ulnar, median, and radial nerves (test against resistance):
  ○ Ulnar nerve: have the patient abduct the index finger while the examiner palpates the first dorsal interosseus muscle
  ○ Median nerve: have the patient palmar abduct the thumb while the examiner palpates the belly of the abductor pollicis brevis muscle
  ○ Radial nerve: have the patient extend the fingers and wrist
- Examine for **TENDON** injury (do all maneuvers against resistance).
  ○ Flexor digitorum profundus: immobilize the PIP and MCP joints and have the patient flex the DIP joint
  ○ Flexor pollicis longus: immobilize the thumb's MCP joint and have the patient flex the interphalangeal (IP) joint
  ○ Flexor digitorum superficialis: immobilize the MCP joint and have the patient flex the PIP joint. (Note: this test does not work for the index finger)
  ○ Flexor digitorum superficialis (index finger): have the patient hyperextend the DIP joint against the

thumb (thumb index pinch). Patients with a superficialis laceration will not be able to hyperextend the DIP joint but can accomplish pinch by DIP joint flexion.
  ○ Flexor carpi radialis: have the patient flex and radially deviate the wrist
  ○ Flexor carpi ulnaris: have the patient flex and ulnarly deviate the wrist
  ○ Alternative testing may be needed in uncooperative patients.
    ▪ With the elbow resting on the table, allow the wrist to fall naturally into flexion: fingers with an intact tendon system will fall into extension. The opposite will occur when the wrist is relaxed in extension.
    ▪ To assess the flexor tendons passively, squeeze the ulnar-volar surface of forearm at the junction of the middle and distal thirds. This will cause flexion of the fingers, especially the three ulnar fingers. Similarly, to test the flexor pollicis longus, press the mid-volar aspect of the distal forearm and assess flexion of the interphalangeal joint of the thumb.
  ○ Table 20-1 describes the tests for extensor tendon function.

FRACTURES OF THE PHALANGES

- **DISTAL PHALANX FRACTURES** tend to be crush or hyperextension injuries. With crush injuries, the soft tissue damage is more significant than the orthopedic injury. Treatment includes wound care, nail bed approximation with absorbable suture, nail plate replacement in the eponychial fold, and finger splinting. Hyperflexion injuries include an open Salter–Harris type I or II fracture with a mallet deformity in the preadolescent and an open displaced Salter–Harris type III fracture in the adolescent (Fig. 20-1). Fractures may not be seen on x-ray until the epiphysis is ossified. Clinical clues include a mallet deformity and an inability to extend the DIP joint. Treatment consists of wound care, replacement of the nail plate if needed, and splinting of the DIP joint in slight hyperextension. Open reduction and Kirschner-wire fixation is done if closed reduction is not successful
- **MIDDLE AND PROXIMAL PHALANGEAL FRACTURES** are usually Salter–Harris type II fractures (Fig. 20-2). After reducing them with flexion and adduction, place an ulnar gutter splint and refer the patient to an orthopedist. Salter–Harris type III fractures are ligament or tendon avulsion injuries and, when displaced, require Kirschner-wire fixation. Shaft fractures tend to have no or minimal displacement.

TABLE 20-1   Extensor Tendons of the Hand

COMPARTMENT	TENDON	INSERTION	TEST OF FUNCTION
First	Abductor pollicis longus	Dorsum of the base of the thumb metacarpal	Extension and abduction of the thumb
	Extensor pollicis brevis	Dorsum of the base of the thumb proximal phalanx	Extension and abduction of the thumb
Second	Extensor carpi radialis longus and extensor carpi radialis brevis	Dorsum of the base of the index metacarpal Dorsum of the base of the long metacarpal	Making first while extending the wrist
Third	Extensor pollicis longus	Dorsum of the base of the thumb distal phalanx	Lifting the thumb off the surface of the table while the palm is flat on the table
Fourth	Extensor digitorum communis	Dorsum of the bases of the proximal phalanges	Extension of the fingers at the MCP joints
	Extensor indicis proprius	Dorsum of the base of the index finger proximal phalanx	Extension of the index finger at the MCP joint with the hand in a fist
Fifth	Extensor digiti minimi	Dorsum of the extensor hood of the little finger	Extension of the little finger while making a fist
Sixth	Extensor carpi ulnaris	Dorsum of the base of the little finger metacarpal	Extension and ulnar deviation of the wrist

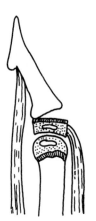 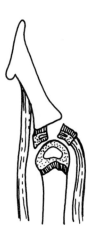

Child   Adolescent

FIG. 20-1 Mallet injuries are caused by avulsion of the extensor tendon from the distal phalanx or from a fracture of the dorsal base of the distal phalanx. An extension lag at the distal interphalangeal (DIP) joint is present, and the patient is unable to actively extend the DIP joint. In children a Salter–Harris type I or II fracture is seen. In the adolescent, a Salter–Harris type III fracture occurs. These fractures may be difficult to detect radiographically since the epiphysis is not fully ossified in children. Inability to actively extend the DIP joint and a mallet deformity reveal the extent of injury. *Source:* Uehara DT: Injuries of the hand and wrist, in Strange, Ahrens, Lelyveld, Schafermeyer (eds): *Pediatric Emergency Medicine: A Comprehensive Guide.*

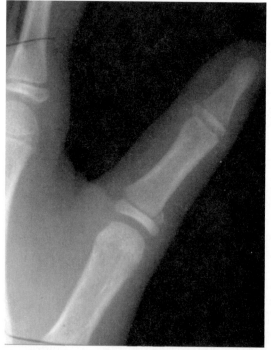

FIG. 20-2 Salter–Harris type II fracture of the proximal phalanx of the thumb.

Splinting and referral is sufficient for displaced and nondisplaced fractures.

- **METACARPAL FRACTURES** most commonly occur in the neck. They rarely require reduction and can be treated with an ulnar gutter splint with orthopedic referral. Although rare, a displaced intraarticular fracture of the base of the thumb metacarpal is an unstable Salter–Harris type III fracture that is treated by open reduction and Kirschner-wire fixation. Most other metacarpal fractures are undisplaced or minimally displaced. Displaced or undisplaced metacarpal fractures can be splinted and referred. Occasionally, displaced fractures require Kirschner-wire fixation.

- **CARPAL FRACTURES** are rare in children due to the elasticity imparted by the cartilage surrounding the carpal bones. The most commonly fractured carpal bone is the scaphoid. Patients present after a fall on the outstretched hand with tenderness in the "anatomic snuff box" and limited range of motion from pain and swelling. Initial x-rays often appear normal. Treatment is a thumb spica splint and orthopedic referral. Most injuries are avulsions or nondisplaced fractures through the distal third of the bone so nonunion and avascular necrosis are rare. Other carpal bone fractures are very rare in children and are treated with splinting and orthopedic referral.

- **WRIST FRACTURES** are common in children, with the distal radial metaphysis being most com-

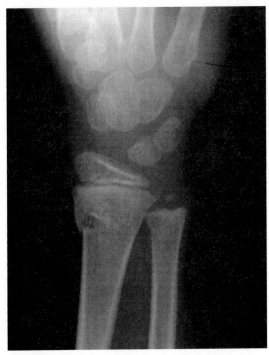

FIG. 20-3 Undisplaced distal radius fracture.

monly involved (Fig. 20-3). With a displaced fracture, patients present after a fall on an outstretched hand with swelling, deformity, and tenderness. Undisplaced fractures have minimal or no swelling and deformity. Radiographs commonly show Salter–Harris type I and II fractures. Undisplaced and minimally displaced fractures are splinted and referred. Displaced fractures require reduction, immobilization in a long arm cast and referral.

DISLOCATIONS

- A **DISTAL INTERPHALANGEAL JOINT** (DIP) dislocation results from a hyperextension force, generally displaces dorsally and is often open. Reduction consists of traction-countertraction followed by flexion. After reduction, test active motion to ensure that the extensor and flexor tendons are functioning and that the volar plate is not interposed in the joint.

- **PROXIMAL INTERPHALANGEAL JOINT** (PIP) dislocations most commonly occur dorsally as a result of an axial load with concomitant hyperextension. Reduce it by applying longitudinal traction to the middle phalanx, slightly hyperextending the finger, correcting any ulnar or radial deformity, and then gently flexing the finger into position. After reduction, test active range of motion and stress test of the collateral ligaments and volar plate. Place the finger in a splint immobilizing the PIP (20° to 30° of flexion) and MCP joints (60° to 70° of flexion) and refer the patient to an orthopedic surgeon. Volar dislocations are rare and may be irreducible. These dislocations can result in a late boutonnière deformity and orthopedic referral is required.

- **METACARPOPHALANGEAL JOINT** (MCP) joint dislocations most commonly involve the thumb (Fig. 20-4) and are a result of hyperextension. In the simple reducible dislocation, the proximal phalanx assumes a dorsal point at a 90° angle to the metacarpal. It is reduced with gentle traction-countertraction. After joint stability is assessed, the finger is splinted and the patient referred. With a complex irreducible dislocation, the proximal phalanx assumes a bayonet position parallel to the metacarpal. The volar plate is interposed in the joint and the metacarpal head may be trapped in the intrinsic muscles. This dislocation is treated with open reduction.

- **CARPOMETACARPAL DISLOCATIONS** are rare in pediatrics. They require prompt orthopedic consultation for surgical intervention.

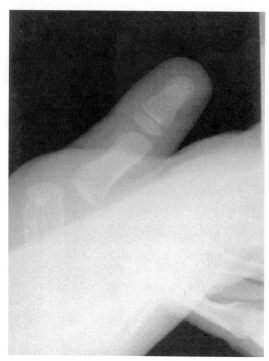

FIG. 20-4 Carpometacarpal dislocation of the thumb.

BIBLIOGRAPHY

Doraiswamy NV: Childhood finger injuries and safeguards. *Injury Prev* 5:298–300, 1999.

Doraiswamy NV, Baig H: Isolated finger injuries in children—incidence and etiology. *Injury* 31:571–573, 2000.

Garcia-Mata S: Carpal scaphoid fracture nonunion in children. *J Pediatr Orthop* 22(4):448–451, 2002.

Huurman WW: Injuries to the hand and wrist. *Adolesc Med* 9:611–625, 1998.

Kocher MS, Waters PM, Micheli LJ: Upper extremity injuries in the pediatric athlete. *Sports Med* 30:117–135, 2000.

MacGregor DM, Hiscox JA: Fingertip trauma in children from doors. *Scot Med J* 44:114–115, 1999.

Mahabir RC, Kazemi AR, Cannon WG, et al: Pediatric hand fractures: A review. *Pediatr Emerg Care* 17:153–156, 2001.

Mastey RD, Weiss AP, Akelman E: Primary care of hand and wrist athletic injuries. *Clin Sports Med* 16:705–724, 1997.

Pershad JM, Monroe K, Kinh W, et al: Pediatric wrist injuries. *Acad Emerg Med* 7:1152–1155, 2000.

Rettig A: Epidemiology of hand and wrist injuries in sports. *Clin Sports Med* 17:1152–1155, 1998.

Rockwood CA, Wilkins KE, King RE: *Fractures in Children,* 3d ed. Philadelphia: JB Lippincott, 1991.

QUESTIONS

1. 1-year-old boy presents with a laceration to the index finger of his hand. When the hand is immersed in warm, no wrinkling of the skin distal to the injury is seen. All of the following is true of this injury EXCEPT:
   A. The ability to sweat distal to the injury is absent
   B. No further treatment is necessary
   C. Normal two point discrimination is 3–5 mm
   D. The digital nerve runs superficial to the digital artery
   E. The skin will have smooth silky texture

2. Examination of the normal hand will reveal all the following EXCEPT:
   A. Normal ulnar nerve function: the patient abducts the index finger while the examiner palpates the first dorsal interosseus muscle
   B. Flexor digitorum profundus: immobilize the PIP and MCP joints and have the patient flex the DIP joint
   C. Squeezing the ulnar-volar surface of the forearm at the junction of the middle and distal thirds will cause flexion of the fingers.
   D. When the elbow rests on a table and the wrist is allowed to fall naturally into flexion, the finger will fall into extension
   E. Flexor carpi radialis: flex and ulnarly deviate the wrist

3. An 18-month-old girl is brought by her parents after she got her fingers caught in the car door. On examination, she is unable to extend her right 3rd distal phalanx and has an obvious partial nail avulsion with crushed tissue. Which of the following is true regarding this injury?
   A. The bony defect is more significant than the soft tissue injury
   B. Treatment includes nail bed approximation with absorbable suture followed by nail plate replacement and finger splinting.
   C. The absence of a fracture by radiograph rules out fracture
   D. A mallet finger is diagnosed by an inability to flex the DIP joint
   E. Treatment of mallet finger is by splinting the DIP in slight hyperflexion

4. A 7-year-old boy presents with a right wrist injury after he fell on his outstretched hand while rollerblading. Which of the following is true about wrist injuries in children?
   A. Carpal fractures are common in children
   B. The scaphoid is the most commonly fractured bone in the pediatric wrist
   C. The distal radial epiphysis is commonly fractured in falls on outstretched hand
   D. Nonunion and avascular necrosis of the scaphoid is common
   E. Most wrist injuries require operative repair

5. Which of the following is true regarding finger dislocations?
   A. PIP dislocations most commonly occur dorsally as a result of an axial load with concomitant hyperextension
   B. After reduction of a PIP dislocation, immobilize finger in hyperextension
   C. Volar dislocations are common and are treated with simple reduction
   D. MCP dislocations are the result of hyperflexion
   E. After reduction, splint immediately and do not allow the finger to move through range of motion

ANSWERS

1. B. Normal two point discrimination is 3–5 mm. In uncooperative patients, skin wrinkling and sweating can be assessed. Following digital nerve injury, the ability to sweat is lost and the skin takes on a smooth, silky texture. Sin wrinkling is also lost. Operative repair is necessary to restore digital nerve function.
2. E. Flexor carpi radialis is tested by flexion and radial deviation of the wrist.
3. B. Distal phalanx fractures tend to be crush or hyperextension injuries. With crush injuries, the soft tissue damage is more significant than the orthopedic injury. Treatment includes wound care, nail bed approximation with absorbable suture, nail plate replacement in the eponychial fold, and finger splinting. Fractures may not be seen until the epiphysis is ossified. A mallet finger is diagnosed by an inability to extend the DIP joint. Treatment consists of splinting the DIP joint in slight hyperextension.
4. B. Carpal fractures are rare in children due to the elasticity of cartilage surrounding the carpal bones. The scaphoid is the most commonly fractured bone in the wrist of children. Initial x-rays often appear normal. Most injuries are avulsions or nondisplaced fractures through the distal third of the scaphoid so nonunion and avascular necrosis are rare. The distal radial metaphysis is most commonly involved in wrist fractures. Most injuries are treated with splinting and orthopedic referral.
5. A. PIP dislocations most commonly occur dorsally as a result of an axial load with concomitant hyperextension. After reduction, test active range of motion to ensure that the extensor and flexor tendons are functioning and that the volar plate is not interposed in the joint. After reduction of a PIP dislocation, splint the finger in 20–30 degrees of flexion. MCP dislocations most commonly involve the thumb and are the result of hyperextension.

21 INJURIES OF THE PELVIS AND HIP

Edward P. Sloan
Russell H. Greenfield
Kemedy K. McQuillen
Patricia Lee

PELVIC FRACTURES

- The pediatric pelvis is elastic and pliable, allowing for significant displacement without a fracture.
- Isolated or single breaks in the pelvic ring are considered stable pelvic fractures. Multiple disruptions in the pelvic ring render the pelvis unstable. Examples of an unstable pelvis include the free-floating pubis seen with bilateral pubic rami fractures (Fig. 21-1) and a Malgaigne fracture, or disruption of the pubis anteriorly and the sacroiliac joint posteriorly.
- Compression injuries cause acetabular fractures or triradiate cartilage injuries. They are often associated with hip dislocations. Growth arrest can occur with these injuries, causing the formation of a shallow, dysplastic acetabulum (Fig. 21-2).
- Avulsion fractures occur as a result of muscle traction stress in adolescents. They are usually caused by the strong contraction of the sartorius and hamstring muscles, resulting in damage to the anterior superior and inferior iliac spines or ischial tuberosity. They are stable injuries that are managed conservatively.

PHYSICAL EXAMINATION

- The examination of a child with a possible pelvic fracture includes observation for ecchymosis and swelling and palpation for point tenderness. The pelvis should be stressed by pressing posteriorly on the iliac crests and by applying direct pressure on the symphysis pubis. Suspect a fracture if these maneuvers produce pain, crepitus, or movement of the pelvic ring. If a fracture is present, evaluate for underlying visceral injuries with a careful examination of the abdomen, rectum, and vagina.
- An anteroposterior pelvis radiograph and pelvic CT scan are diagnostic.

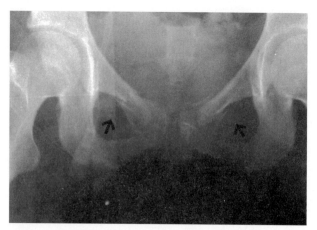

FIG. 21-1 Bilateral superior pubic rami fractures. Associated injury to the bladder and urethra should be suspected.

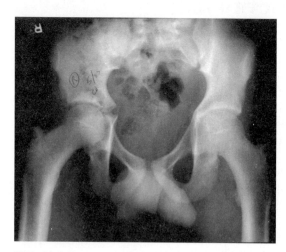

FIG. 21-2 Fracture through the triradiate cartilage of the right acetabulum. Growth arrest is a common complication of this type of injury.

HIP DISLOCATIONS AND FRACTURES

HIP DISLOCATIONS

- Posterior hip dislocations are most common and patients with this injury present with the leg held flexed and internally rotated. Patients with anterior hip dislocations present with the leg flexed and externally rotated and those with central hip dislocations, with the femoral head protruding through the acetabulum into the pelvis, present without a rotational deformity. Other findings include pain and limited range of motion. Hip dislocations can be complicated by acetabular fractures and sciatic nerve injuries. An anteroposterior pelvis radiograph and pelvic CT scan are diagnostic. Complications include recurrent dislocations, avascular necrosis of the femoral head, degenerative arthritis, and sciatic nerve injury.

- Treatment is with prompt closed reduction; if it is delayed by more than 12 hours, there is an increased risk of avascular necrosis. Operative intervention is required if the acetabulum is disrupted or if there are bony fragments in the joint postreduction.

HIP FRACTURES

- Hip fractures involve the epiphysis (transepiphyseal) or the femoral neck and trochanters (cervico-trochanteric). Transepiphyseal fractures often occur in patients with preexisting slipped capital femoral epiphysis (SCFE). Complications include avascular necrosis of the femoral head, premature closure of the physis, and shortening and angulation of the lower extremity.
- Depending on the location of the fracture and the degree of displacement, open reduction and internal fixation is often required.

SLIPPED CAPITAL FEMORAL EPIPHYSIS

- SCFE is a disruption of the capital femoral physis with slippage of the femur superiorly and in the anterolateral direction away from the epiphysis.
- SCFE is most common in overweight adolescent males but can also occur in rapidly growing adolescents who are tall and thin.
- It is classified as acute (symptoms for less than 3 weeks), chronic, stable, and unstable.
- Findings include a limp; hip pain that radiates to the groin, thigh, or knee; hip tenderness; limited internal rotation and flexion; and shortening of the leg.
- Diagnostic radiographs include a lateral hip view and AP and frog-leg views of the pelvis.
  - On the AP or frog-leg view of the pelvis, a line drawn along the superior edge of the femoral neck should transect at least 20 percent of the epiphysis. With a SCFE, this line will no longer pass through the epiphysis (Fig. 21-3).
  - SCFE is considered to be severe if the amount of slippage is >50 percent of the metaphyseal width.
  - Other x-ray findings include asymmetry between the affected and normal hip and irregular widening of the epiphyseal line.
  - Most patients can be treated as outpatients with crutches, instructions to be non–weight-bearing and close orthopedic follow-up.
  - If the slip is acute and unstable and the patient has intractable pain, hospital admission and operative intervention may be warranted.

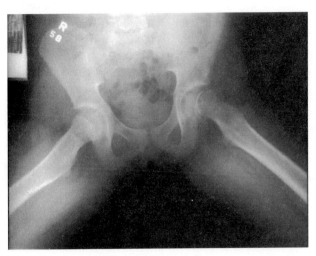

Fig. 21-3 Frog-leg view of the pelvis revealing a slipped left femoral capital epiphysis.

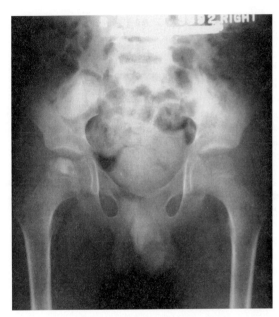

FIG. 21-4 Legg–Calvé–Perthes disease of the left femoral head.

LEGG–CALVÉ–PERTHES DISEASE (LCPD)

- LCPD is an idiopathic avascular necrosis of the femoral head.
- LCPD is more common in Caucasians and boys, with a peak incidence between the ages of 4 and 9 years.
- Patients with LCPD may present with a limp, pain in the hip or knee that may be worsened with exercise, and limited internal rotation and abduction of the hip.
- Radiographic studies include AP and frog-leg views of the pelvis and a lateral hip view. They may show a small femoral head, widened medial joint space, and evidence of epiphyseal collapse. If LCPD is suspected and radiographs are normal, a bone scan or MRI should be obtained (Fig. 21-4).
- There is bilateral involvement in up to 15 percent of children.
- Treatment includes no weight bearing, crutches, NSAIDs, and close orthopedic follow-up.

FEMUR FRACTURES

- Pediatric fractures of the femur are common, peaking at 3 years old.
  - They result from birth trauma, underlying bone pathology, or child abuse, with a spiral femur fracture in a nonambulatory child highly suggestive of abuse.
  - Midshaft fractures are most common, however, fractures of the distal epiphysis also occur, usually in older children. There may be an ipsilateral hip dislocation.
  - Patients with femur fractures should be admitted for pain control.
  - Femur fractures are treated with casting, skeletal traction, or surgery; plates and/or intermedullary rods are sometimes needed for shaft fractures.
- Complications of distal femur epiphyseal injuries include growth arrest, vascular compromise, peroneal nerve palsy, and recurrent displacement.
- Long-term orthopedic follow-up is required for these patients.

BIBLIOGRAPHY

Bachman D, Santora S: Orthopedic trauma, in Fleisher GR, Ludwig S, Henretig FM, et al (eds): *Textbook of Pediatric Emergency Medicine*, 4th ed. Philadelphia: Lippincott Williams & Wilkins, 2000, pp 1435–1478.

Della-Giustina K, Della-Giustina DA: Emergency department evaluation and treatment of pediatric orthopedic injuries. *Emerg Med Clin North Am* 1999;895–922.

Grisoni N, Connor S, Marsh E, et al: Pelvic fractures in a pediatric level I trauma center. *J Orthop Trauma* 16(7):458–463, 2002.

Kehl DK: Slipped capital femoral epiphysis, in Morrisey RT, Weinstein SL (eds): *Lovell and Winter's Pediatric Orthopedics*, 5th ed. Philadelphia: Lippincott Williams & Wilkins, 2001, pp 999–1034.

Kutty S, Thornes B, Curtin WA, Gilmore MF: Traumatic posterior dislocation of hip in children. *Pediatr Emerg Care* 17(1):32–35, 2001.

Loder RT, et al: Acute slipped capital femoral epiphysis: the importance of physeal stability, J Bone Joint Surg Am 75(8): 1134–1140, 1993.

Loder RT, Aronson DD, Greenfield ML: The epidemiology of bilateral slipped capital femoral epiphysis. *J Bone Joint Surg* 1993;1141–1147.

Perron AD, Miller MD, Brady WJ: Orthopedic pitfalls in the ED: slipped capital femoral epiphysis. *Am J Emerg Med* 20(5):484–487, 2002.

Quintana EC, Friedman M, Selbst SM: Pitfall in pediatric emergency medicine. *Foresight: Risk Management for Emergency Physicians* 2001;1–3.

Rockwood CA, Wilkins KE, Beaty JH (eds): *Fractures in Children*, 5th ed. Philadelphia: Lippincott Williams & Wilkins, 2001.

Weinstein SL: Legg–Calvé–Perthes syndrome, in Morrisey RT, Weinstein SL (eds): *Lovell and Winter's Pediatric Orthopedics*, 5th ed. Philadelphia: Lippincott Williams & Wilkins, 2001, pp 957–998.

QUESTIONS

1. A 6-year-old boy presents with a complaint of right knee pain for 4 days that is made worse by exercise. Radiographs of the hip and pelvis reveal a small femoral head, widened medial joint space, and moderate epiphyseal collapse. Which of the following is true regarding this condition?
   A. Treatment includes NSAIDS and moderate weight bearing.
   B. It is more common in children between the ages of 9 and 15 years.
   C. It is more common in females.
   D. On examination, the child walks with a limp and internal rotation and abduction of the hip is limited.
   E. Bilateral involvement is present in more than 80% of cases.

2. A 14-year-old boy presents with a complaint of left groin pain for 4 days. The pain is described as dull and radiates to the anteromedial thigh. No antecedent trauma is known. A radiograph is obtained which reveals asymmetry between the affected and normal hip and irregular widening of the epiphyseal line. Which of the following are true about this condition?
   A. It is characterized by slippage of the femur inferiorly and in the anteromedial direction toward the epiphysis.
   B. When reading the radiograph, a line drawn along the superior edge of the femoral neck will transect at least 20 percent of the epiphysis.
   C. Bilateral involvement is found in less than 15% of cases.
   D. It is seen more commonly in females.

   E. Most patients can be treated as outpatients with no weight bearing, NSAIDs, and close orthopedic follow-up.

3. A 7-year-old female presents as a restrained passenger involved in a motor vehicle collision. Radiographs determine that she has sustained a pelvic fracture. Which of the following is true about pediatric pelvic fractures?
   A. The pediatric pelvis is elastic and pliable and, therefore, significant internal injuries may occur without a fracture.
   B. Avulsion injuries of the ischial tuberosity are unstable and should be treated by operative repair.
   C. Growth arrest is an infrequent complication of a hip dislocation with associated acetabular fracture
   D. Triradiate cartilage injuries are generally caused by direct blow.
   E. A single break in the pediatric pelvic ring is considered unstable.

4. Pediatric femur fractures have all the following characteristics **EXCEPT**:
   A. A spiral fracture in a nonambulatory child may be the result of child abuse.
   B. They may be the result of underlying bone pathology.
   C. They may occur with a contralateral hip dislocation.
   D. The peak incidence is at 3 years of age.
   E. Midshaft fractures are the most common.

5. The following characteristics of hip dislocation are true **EXCEPT**:
   A. Posterior hip dislocations are the most common.
   B. May be complicated by acetabular fractures
   C. May be associated with sciatic nerve injury
   D. Operative intervention for reduction is the method of choice to prevent avascular necrosis.
   E. Recurrent dislocations are a frequent complication.

ANSWERS

1. D. Legg–Calvé Perthes disease is an idiopathic avascular necrosis of the femoral head. It is more common in Caucasians and boys, with a peak incidence between the ages of 4 and 9 years. Patients with LCPD may present with a limp, pain in the hip or knee that may be worsened with exercise, and limited internal rotation and abduction of the hip. There is bilateral involvement in up to 15% of children. Treatment includes no weight bearing, NSAIDs, and close orthopedic follow-up.

2. E. Slipped capital femoral epiphysis is a disruption of the capital femoral physis with slippage of the

femur superiorly and in the anterolateral direction away from the epiphysis. It is most common in overweight adolescent males. It presents with a limp; hip pain that radiates to the groin, thigh or knee; hip tenderness; limited internal rotation and flexion; and shortening of the leg. With a SCFE, a line drawn along the superior edge of the femoral neck will no longer pass through the epiphysis. SCFE is bilateral in up to one third of children.

3. A. The pediatric pelvis is elastic and pliable, allowing for significant displacement without a fracture. Avulsion injuries are generally stable injuries and are managed conservatively. Hip dislocation is a frequent complication of acetabular fractures. These injuries frequently result in growth arrest. Triradiate cartilage injuries occur due to compression injury. An isolated or single break in the pelvic ring is considered a stable fracture.

4. C. Pediatric femur fractures are common and peak at 3 years of age. They result from birth trauma, underlying bone pathology, or child abuse with a spiral fracture in a nonambulatory child. Midshaft fractures are the most common. There may be ipsilateral hip dislocation.

5. D. Posterior hip dislocations are the most common type and patients will present with the leg held flexed and internally rotated. Hip dislocations can be complicated by acetabular fractures and sciatic nerve injury. Complications include recurrent dislocations, avascular necrosis of the femoral head, degenerative arthritis, and sciatic nerve injury. Treatment is with prompt closed reduction; if it is delayed by more than 12 hours, avascular necrosis may occur. Operative intervention is required if the acetabulum is disrupted or if there are bony fragments in the joint postreduction.

22 INJURIES OF THE LOWER EXTREMITIES

Edward P. Sloan
Russell H. Greenfield
Kemedy K. McQuillen
Valerie A. Dobiesz

KNEE AND PATELLAR FRACTURES

- In children, the knee ligaments are stronger than the adjacent growth plates and cartilage, making fractures more common than ligamentous sprains. Sprains can occur with fractures of adjacent bones.

- Thick cartilage surrounding the osseous center of the patella makes childhood patellar fractures uncommon. Bipartite patellae, however, are not uncommon and can be mistaken for a fracture. They can be differentiated from a fracture by their smooth, contoured bony segments in the superior-lateral portion of the patella.
- Avulsion fractures of the knee occur and may disrupt the knee's extensor mechanism.
- Knee dislocations are associated with extremity fractures and neurovascular disruption.
- Fractures of both the distal femur and proximal tibiafibula result in a floating knee.
- The physical examination of the knee should include inspection for effusion, alignment, and ecchymosis; palpation for tenderness; and assessment of neurovascular function, range of motion, ligamentous laxity, and competence of the extensor mechanism.

OSGOOD–SCHLATTER DISEASE

- Also known as traumatic tibial apophysitis, Osgood–Schlatter disease is caused by avulsion of the chondral portion of the tibial tuberosity and is usually seen in physically active teenagers involved in activities that involve repetitive use of quadriceps. It is bilateral in up to 25 percent of patients and usually self-limited.
- Findings may include pain below the knee exacerbated by physical activity and kneeling, tenderness, and swelling over the tibial tuberosity.
- Knee radiographs may reveal irregularity or prominence of the tibial tuberosity.
  ○ Treatment includes temporary restriction of activity and NSAIDs.

PROXIMAL TIBIA AND TIBIAL SHAFT FRACTURES

- Proximal tibial injuries are less common than distal femur fractures and result from forceful twisting in younger children and car bumper injuries in older children (Fig. 22-1). Complications include vascular compromise, growth abnormalities, and compartment syndrome.
- Tibial diaphysis (shaft) fractures occur commonly: a spiral fracture of the tibial shaft in young children is termed a toddler's fracture.
- Stress fractures of the tibial shaft also occur, causing pain in the proximal tibial shaft. Radiographs may reveal a radiolucent line and periosteal reaction of the tibial shaft. Orthopedic consultation is advised to exclude other diagnoses, such as osteogenic sarcoma and osteomyelitis.

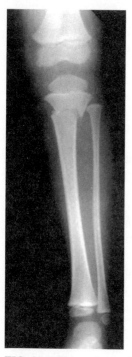

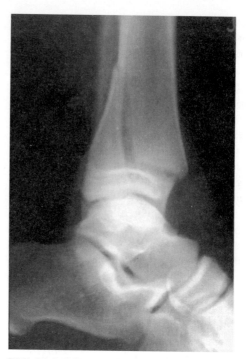

FIG. 22-1 This patient suffered a fracture of the proximal tibial metaphysis after being struck by a car. Complications associated with this injury include damage to the posterior tibial artery and the development of a valgus deformity.

FIG. 22-2 Salter–Harris type II fracture of the distal tibia. An associated greenstick fracture of the fibula commonly occurs with this injury.

FIBULAR FRACTURES

- Fibular fractures occur in younger children due to twisting injuries and, in older children, due to motor vehicle trauma.
- The peroneal nerve may be injured with fibular head fractures and is manifest by the loss of dorsiflexion (foot drop).
- Similar to a Maisonneuve fracture in adults, a fibular shaft fracture can also occur as a result of disruption of the distal tibial epiphys. For this reason, children with a significant ankle injury should be examined for proximal fibula tenderness.

ANKLE FRACTURES

- The ankle joint is formed by the tibia, fibula, and talus.
- In children, the strength of the ankle ligaments makes distal tibial and fibular epiphysis injuries more likely than ligamentous injuries.
- The physical examination should include palpation of the base of the fifth metatarsal, the calcaneus, and the proximal fibula.
- Diagnostic radiographs include the anteroposterior (AP), lateral, and mortise views. The lateral view should

include the posterior malleolus, the talus, calcaneus, and the base of the fifth metatarsal. On the mortise view, a uniform 3- to 4-mm space between the tibia, talus, and fibula should be visualized.

- Medial ankle injuries occur as a result of foot pronation, eversion, and external rotation: Salter–Harris type II fractures of the distal tibia are common (Fig. 22-2). Salter–Harris type III and IV distal tibial epiphysis fractures are often complicated by growth arrest, and the triplane fracture, a type IV fracture that has multiple tibial epiphysis and metaphysis fragments, requires operative intervention.
- Lateral ankle injuries occur as a result of supination with foot inversion and external rotation: Salter–Harris type I and II distal fibular fractures can occur. Type III and IV fractures are uncommon. Infrequently, the talofibular ligament can cause a fracture of the distal fibular epiphysis, an injury that can be treated as an ankle sprain when seen in isolation. If the physis is tender to palpation, it is best to assume there is a Salter–Harris type I or V injury.
- Salter–Harris type II to IV injuries, especially those that cause ankle mortise disruption, should be managed aggressively with orthopedic consultation.
- In ankle fractures with dislocation, the ankle mortise remains intact and the tibial epiphyseal plate is displaced: forced reduction can cause the growth plate

germinal layer to be damaged. As such, provide an anatomic reduction with gentle traction only if there is vascular compromise or an inability to stabilize the ankle. Otherwise, the reduction can take place after admission.

FOOT FRACTURES

- Most pediatric foot fractures involve the forefoot and occur due to falls, crush injuries, or lawnmower injuries. Hindfoot fractures are rare.
- The talus is most commonly fractured in its neck due to forced dorsiflexion (Fig. 22-3).
  - Talar fractures are rare in children and may be complicated by avascular necrosis. Treatment includes splinting the ankle in plantar flexion and orthopedic consultation.
  - Transchondral fractures, which occur at the cartilaginous surface of the talar dome, occur in older children: chronic pain and arthritis can result.
- The calcaneus is the most commonly fractured tarsal. A fall with a direct load is the most common mechanism (Fig. 22-4).
- There are three significant differences in pediatric calcaneal injuries as compared with adults:
  - Bohler's angle is unreliable in detecting injury because the angle is normally found in nonadolescent children.
  - Nonoperative therapy is more successful because comminution occurs less commonly.
  - Concomitant injury of the lumbar spine, renal pedicle, and contralateral calcaneus are less common.
- Fractures of the cuboid, navicular, and cuneiforms usually result from direct trauma to the midfoot. Irregularities of these bones during growth make fracture exclusion difficult, but conservative management is usually effective.
- Midfoot fractures are rare due to the strong fibrous tissues that surround these bones. They are difficult to detect because of the irregularities of these bones.
  - Lisfranc's fracture occurs at the base of the second metatarsal, where the stability of the midfoot is maintained. They occur as a result of forced abduction and plantar flexion, as is seen with jumping from the tiptoe position (Fig. 22-5). Vascular compromise is the major complication and orthopedic consultation is prudent.
  - The Jones' fracture is a metatarsal neck fracture at the base of the fifth metatarsal (Fig. 22-6).
  - Crush injuries that cause multiple metatarsal fractures are managed conservatively because a compartment syndrome of the foot can occur.

TALAR FRACTURES

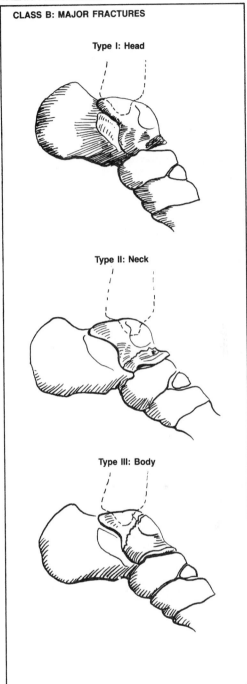

CLASS B: MAJOR FRACTURES

Type I: Head

Type II: Neck

Type III: Body

FIG. 22-3 Talus neck fracture in a child. (Used with permission from King RE, Powell DF: Injury to the talus. In: Jahss MH (ed): *Disorders of the Foot and Ankle,* 2d ed, Philadelphia: Saunders, 1991, p 2308.)

- Phalangeal injuries due to direct trauma can be buddy taped once a rotational deformity has been excluded.
- Phalangeal fractures that occur as a result of the foot being stuck in the spokes of a bicycle wheel can result in neurovascular compromise.

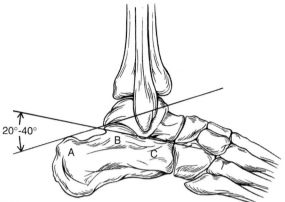

FIG. 22-4 Angles used to assess the calcaneus. *A.* Bohler's angle *B.* Calcaneus pitch. (Used with permission from Shereff MT: Radiographic analysis of the foot and ankle. In: Jahss MH (ed): *Disorders of the Foot and Ankle,* 2d ed, Philadelphia: Saunders, 1991, p 104.)

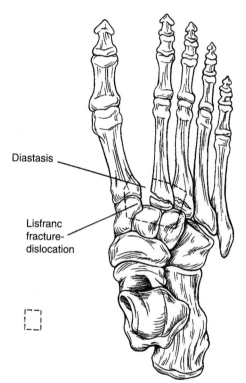

FIG. 22-5 Lisfranc's dislocation of the second metatarsal. (Used with permission from Ogden JA: *Skeletal Injury in the Child,* 2d ed, Philadelphia: Saunders, 1990, p 887.)

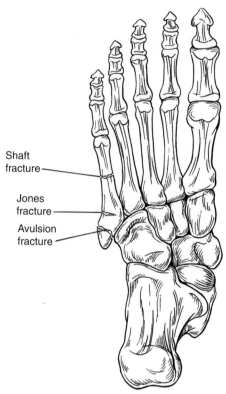

FIG. 22-6 Displaced fracture of the base of the fifth metatarsal in an adolescent. Note that the apophysis is not united. Also, note that the fracture is perpendicular to the metatarsal shaft, and that the apophysis is parallel to the long axis of the metatarsal shaft. (Used with permission from Harris JH, Harris WH, Novelline RA: *The Radiology of Emergency Medicine,* 3d ed, Baltimore: Williams & Wilkins, 1993, p 1032.)

BIBLIOGRAPHY

Adirim TA, Cheng TL: Overview of injuries in the young athlete. *Sports Med* 33:75–81, 2003.

Bachman D, Santora S: Orthopedic trauma. In: Fleisher GR, Ludwig S, Henretig FM, et al, eds. *Textbook of Pediatric Emergency Medicine,* 4th. ed. Philadelphia: Lippincott Williams & Wilkins, 1435–1478, 2000.

Della-Giustina K, Della-Giustina DA: Emergency department evaluation and treatment of pediatric orthopedic injuries. *Emerg Med Clin North Am* 1999;17:895–922.

Rockwood CA, Wilkins KE, Beaty JH (eds): *Fractures in Children,* 5th ed. Philadelphia: Lippincott Williams & Wilkins, 2001.

Sloan EP, Rittenberry TJ: Ankle and foot injuries. In: Reisdorff EJ, Roberts MR, Weigenstein JG, eds. *Pediatric Emergency Medicine.* Philadelphia: Saunders, 974–982, 1993.

QUESTIONS

1. A 12-year-old male presents with the complaint of right knee pain after playing basketball. He is noted to have tenderness and swelling to the proximal tibia. He is afebrile and there are no skin changes surrounding the area. A knee radiograph reveals an irregularity of the tibial tuberosity. The optimal management of this patient would be:

   A. A cortisone injection to the knee joint

B. Long leg posterior mold, crutches, and urgent orthopedic follow up

C. Orthopedic consultation in the ED for possible surgical intervention

D. Arthrocentesis to rule out infection

E. Temporary restriction of activity and NSAIDs

2. Which of the following is true regarding injuries to the knee in children?

A. Ligamentous injuries are more common than fractures.

B. Bipartite patellae is the most common fracture of the patella.

C. Knee dislocations are benign injuries and typically spontaneously reduce.

D. Avulsion fractures of the knee may disrupt the knee's extensor mechanism.

E. Range of motion should be avoided in evaluation of traumatic knee injuries.

3. A spiral fracture of the lower third of the tibial shaft in young children is referred to as a:

A. Jones' fracture

B. Toddler's fracture

C. Maissonneuve fracture

D. Triplane fracture

E. Torus fracture

4. Which of the following is true regarding ankle injuries in children?

A. Medial ankle injuries result from foot inversion.

B. Standard radiographs of the ankle are the anteroposterior (AP) and lateral views.

C. The tibia, fibula, and the calcaneus form the ankle joint.

D. Sprains are more common than fractures.

E. If the physis is tender to palpation and the radiographs are negative, assume there is a Salter–Harris type I or V injury.

5. A 10-year-old girl presents complaining of bilateral heel pain after falling off the roof of a garage. On physical examination, the only finding is tenderness and ecchymosis to the calcaneous bilaterally. Which of the following is true regarding this injury?

A. Pediatric calcaneal injuries are identical to those in adults.

B. Bohler's angle is unreliable in children.

C. Operative management is generally needed.

D. Concomitant injury to the lumbar spine, renal pedicle are more common than in adults.

E. The calcaneus is the least commonly fractured tarsal bone.

ANSWERS

1. E. This patient has Osgood–Schlatter disease, which is caused by avulsion of the chondral portion of the tibial tuberosity. This is typically seen in physically active teenagers in activities that involve repetitive use of quadriceps. Treatment includes temporary restriction of activity, NSAIDs, and it is usually self-limited.

2. D. Fractures are more common than ligamentous injuries in children as the knee ligaments are stronger. A bipartite patella is a normal variation in the patella usually in the superior-lateral portion and is not a fracture. Knee dislocations are severe injuries typically associated with extremity fractures and NV injuries. An avulsion fracture of the knee may disrupt the knee's extensor mechanism. A complete examination of the knee should include a range of motion assessment.

3. B. A spiral fracture of the tibial shaft in young children is termed a toddler's fracture.

4. E. Medial ankle injuries occur with foot eversion. Standard radiographs should include the AP, lateral, and a mortise view. The tibia, fibula, and the talus form the ankle joint. In children, the strength of the ankle ligaments makes distal tibia and fibular epiphysis injuries more likely than ligamentous injuries. In general, if the physis is tender to palpation, it is best to assume there is a Salter–Harris type I or V injury and to treat this conservatively.

5. B. Pediatric calcaneal injuries are different than adults in the following ways: Bohler's angle is unreliable in detecting injuries, nonoperative therapy is more successful, and concomitant injuries are less common. The calcaneus is the most commonly fractured tarsal bone.

23   SOFT TISSUE INJURY AND WOUND REPAIR

Jordan D. Lipton
Kemedy K. McQuillen
Valerie A. Dobiesz

SKIN AND SOFT TISSUE ANATOMY AND BIOMECHANICS

- The skin is composed of the dermis, which provides most of the skin's tensile strength, and the epidermis, which protects the dermis from infection and desiccation. Dermal capillaries are fed by the nutrient vessels of the skin, and the epidermis, which has no blood supply, is fed by diffusion of nutrients from the dermis. The subcutaneous tissue beneath the dermis is composed of loose connective and adipose tissue, large vessels, and nerves.

- The most cosmetically pleasing scar results when the long axis of the wound is along "Langer's lines" (Fig. 23-1). Greater scarring is also more likely when there is marked retraction of wound edges (>5 mm) or a when a wound intersects the transverse axis of the joint. When a wound intersects the transverse axis of a joint, post repair function can also be compromised.

CLASSIFICATION OF MINOR INJURIES

- **Lacerations** are cuts through the skin. Those that involve the dermal capillaries bleed and those through the subcutaneous fat produce gaping wounds. Lacerations can be associated with occult injuries and require thorough exploration to detect deeper injuries.
- The three main classes of lacerations are:
  ○ **Shear injuries** are caused by sharp objects with little damage to adjacent tissues but can cause nerve, tendon, and vascular damage. Shear injuries heal the fastest and have the lowest incidence of infection.
  ○ **Tension lacerations** occur when stresses cause the skin to tear in irregular shapes. There is associated damage to the surrounding tissues.
  ○ **Compression lacerations** occur during a crush injury and have irregular, often stellate, wound edges. There is significant injury to the adjacent skin, they heal most poorly, and have a higher incidence of wound infection.
- With **abrasions**, skin layers are scraped or sheared away. Superficial abrasions involve only the cornified epidermis, have little or no bleeding, and heal rapidly. Deeper abrasions involving the dermis bleed more and are more susceptible to infection, tattooing, and foreign body retention.
- **Contusions** result from crush injuries and manifest as swelling and pain from localized bleeding and edema. Secondary ischemic injuries occur infrequently. Treatment includes elevation, ice, and monitoring of circulation and neurologic function.
- **Hematomas** are confined collections of extravasated blood. They are associated with most types of wounds and must be monitored for signs of infection.

PREHOSPITAL CARE

- Prehospital care of minor wounds includes initial attention to the ABCs (airway, breathing, and circulation). Bleeding can be controlled with direct manual pressure or a pressure dressing. Inflation of a sphygmomanometer proximal to the bleeding site can also be used to control bleeding, even for prolonged transport times. Always check neurovascular status distal to the injury and assess for associated injuries prior to nonemergent interventions.

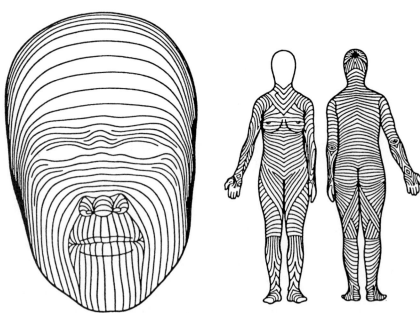

A   *B*

FIG. 23-1 Lines of skin tension.

HISTORY AND PHYSICAL EXAMINATION

- Prior to assessing a minor wound, exclude more serious injuries that take precedence.
- Include in the history the type of force (blunt or sharp), time and mechanism of the injury, whether there are other injuries, the potential for wound contamination or foreign bodies, and prehospital wound care. Additional history includes tetanus immunization status, past medical history, allergies, and medications. Consider unaccidental trauma when the history is inconsistent with the injury.
- Physical examination should assess the length and depth of the wound, the neurovascular status, the presence of foreign bodies and contaminants, and involvement of underlying structures (nerves, tendons, muscles, ligaments, vessels, bones, joints, and ducts). With the exception of the neurologic examination, the examination can be done after anesthesia is administered. Test sensation by measuring two-point discrimination: for children younger than 5 years, use a pinprick to provide a sensory and a partial motor assessment. Use an ophthalmoscope to look for beads of sweat, as loss of sweating also provides a clue to denervation. Check peripheral pulses, skin temperature and color, and capillary refill to evaluate circulation. Test tendons, muscles, and ligaments distal to an injury. Have the child manipulate a toy or light pen to help evaluate motor function.

MANAGEMENT

INSTRUMENTS, SUTURES, STAPLES, TAPE, AND TISSUE ADHESIVES

- The selection of the closure technique will depend on the location and nature of the laceration: sutures, staples, surgical tape, or tissue adhesives may be used (Tables 23-1 and 23-2).
  - The most common type of needle used for wound repair is the cutting needle. They come in two grades: cuticular and plastic. Plastic needles, identified by the letter P next to the needle size, are recommended for ED wound repair.
  - Lacerations can also be closed using **staples**, which induce a minimal inflammatory reaction and produce similar cosmetic results to suturing. Do not use staples to repair hand or face lacerations and avoid their use in areas that will undergo computed tomography (CT) or magnetic resonance imaging (MRI).

TABLE 23-1 Advantages and Disadvantages of Common Wound Closure Techniques

TECHNIQUE	ADVANTAGES	DISADVANTAGES
Suture	Time honored	Requires removal
	Meticulous closure	Requires anesthesia
	Greatest tensile strength	Greatest tissue reactivity
	Lowest dehiscence rate	Highest cost
		Slowest application
		Highest risk of needle stick
Staples	Rapid application	Less meticulous closure
	Low tissue reactivity	May interfere with imaging techniques
	Low cost	
	Low risk of needle stick	
Tissue adhesive	Rapid application	Lower tensile strength than sutures
	Patient comfort	Dehiscence over high-tension areas
	Resistant to bacterial growth	Not useful on hands
	No need for removal	Cannot bathe or swim
	Low cost	
	Low or no risk of needle stick	
Surgical tape	Least reactive	Frequently falls off
	Lowest infection rates	Lower tensile strength than sutures
	Rapid application	Highest rate of dehiscence
	Patient comfort	Requires use of toxic adjuncts
	Low cost	Cannot be used in areas with hair
	No risk of needle stick	Cannot get wet

- **Steri-strips** applied with an adhesive, such as tincture of benzoin, are effective in closing small linear lacerations that are under minimal tension (Fig. 23-2). Taped wounds are more resistant to infection than sutured wounds and do not require another visit for removal. Tape can also be used for skin closure of partial thickness wounds and of wounds that are closed in a layered fashion with well-approximated wound edges.
- **Tissue adhesive** is another option for closing superficial wounds that are under minimal tension. It should not be used on mucous membranes or around the eyes.

ANALGESIA, LOCAL ANESTHESIA, NERVE BLOCKS, AND SEDATION

- Analgesia, anesthesia, nerve blocks, and sedation are discussed in more detail in Chapter 24. Most wounds are adequately anesthetized using local infiltration of 1 to 2 percent lidocaine, with or without epinephrine. It has a rapid onset of action and lasts approximately

TABLE 23-2   Suture Types and Characteristics

TYPE AND MATERIAL	PROPERTIES
Nonabsorbable	
Silk	Easy to handle Lies flat when tied Forms secure knot due to presence of braid Induces more tissue reaction and has higher infection potential than other nonabsorbables
Cotton	Similar to the properties of silk
Nylon	Synthetic Less tissue reactivity and infection potential Does not tend to lie flat More difficult to handle than silk/cotton Decreased knot security due to lack of braid requires more throws per knot
Polypropylene	Similar to the properties of nylon sutures, although slightly easier to handle
Polyester	Infection potential greater than nylon and polypropylene, but less than silk and cotton Easier to handle and better knot security than nylon and polypropylene
Metal	Low tissue reactivity and infection potential Difficult to handle Uncomfortable for patient during healing
Polybutester	Equivalent to nylon and polypropylene in tensile strength and low infection potential Stretches easily, thus advantageous for wounds that tend to swell
Absorbable	
Plain gut	Phagocytosed by macrophages Maintains tensile strength for ~7 days High tissue reactivity and infection potential
Chromic gut	Similar to the properties of plain gut sutures, but maintains tensile strength for ~2–3 weeks
Fast-absorbing	Similar to the properties of plain gut sutures, but breaks down gut within 5–7 days, thus does not require removal with scissors
Polyglycolic acid and polyglactin	Synthetic Cause less tissue reactivity and have lower infection potential than gut sutures Absorbed by enzymatic hydrolysis Braided, thus hold knots well, but have lots of drag through tissues if not coated with materials that reduce friction Gradually loses tensile strength over ~4 weeks
Polydioxanone, polyglyconate, and glycoside	Synthetic monofilament (pass more smoothly through tissues) Cause less tissue reactivity than gut sutures Absorbed by enzymatic hydrolysis
Trimethylene carbonate	Retain ~60% of tensile strength at 28 days

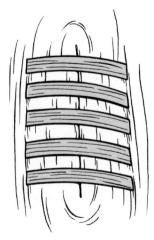

FIG. 23-2 Skin-closure tapes should be applied perpendicular to the wound edges and spaced so that the edges do not gape.

one-half to 2 h. Epinephrine should not be used in regions supplied by end arteries (fingers, nose, lip, ears, genitalia, and toes). The maximum doses of lidocaine and lidocaine with epinephrine are 4.5 mg/kg and 7 mg/kg, respectively. A longer-acting agent, such as bupivacaine, can be used for prolonged closure times. Bupivacaine's onset of action is moderate and it lasts 2 to 6 h.

• Decrease the pain of injection by adding bicarbonate to the lidocaine (1:10 dilution), using a 25- to 27-gauge needle, and injecting slowly into the wound margins. When possible, perform infiltration prior to irrigation.

• Topical lidocaine-adrenaline-tetracaine (LAT) also provides effective anesthesia for facial and scalp lacerations. It should not be used on mucous membranes or in regions supplied by end arteries due to the vasoconstrictive effect of the adrenaline.

  ○ The mixture should be applied to the wound using a saturated cotton ball that is held in place by a caregiver wearing gloves.

- Transient anesthesia can also be obtained by applying 4 percent lidocaine to an abrasion that requires mechanical scrubbing.

- Use regional nerve blocks for large lacerations and for lacerations in areas where the anatomy will be distorted if local infiltration is performed.

- Physical restraint is generally required for younger children. Papoose boards or a folded sheet can be used. Conscious sedation may be needed in children who are uncooperative.

WOUND CLEANING AND PREPARATION

- Universal precautions, including gloves, mask, and eye protection, should be worn during wound preparation.

- **Hemostasis** can be achieved with direct pressure, wound elevation, dilute epinephrine (1:100,000) application, lidocaine with epinephrine infiltration, absorbable gelatin powder or sponge packing, tourniquets, or blood pressure cuff placement and inflation proximal to the wound. Limit tourniquet time to 45 min. Electrocautery can also be used on small, oozing vessels. Do not suture or clamp vessels blindly because of the risk of injuring adjacent structures. Persistently bleeding small arteries require ligation, however, this should not be done in the wrists or hands without consulting a hand surgeon.

- After anesthesia, perform **wound exploration** and remove foreign material.

  ○ Radiographs with a radiopaque marker are occasionally required for precise localization of a foreign body. Other studies that can help localize foreign bodies include CT, MRI, xeroradiography, and ultrasonography.

  ○ If an inert foreign body is small and cannot easily be removed, it may be left in place and the patient or parent informed of its presence. Organic foreign bodies require removal to prevent inflammatory reactions and infection.

- **Hair removal**: Since infection rates are higher in wounds that are shaved, clip hair if it interferes with the procedure. Preferably, moisten the hair with lubricating jelly to keep it out of the way. Never shave or clip the eyebrows. They serve as landmarks for alignment during wound repair and, if removed, can take 6 to 12 months to grow back.

- **Irrigate** with 5 to 8 psi of normal saline or tap water to remove bacteria and debris. An 18- to 20-gauge plastic catheter attached to a 30-mL syringe delivers 6 to 8 psi. Irrigate with the tip of the catheter within 5 cm of the intact skin and use 200 to 300 mL of fluid for an average-sized low-risk wound. For increasing size or contamination, use more fluid. Normal saline or tap water is the standard fluid, however, dilute (1%) povidone-iodine solution may be considered in moderate- or high-risk wounds. Nonionic surfactant agents (Shur-Clens, Pharma Clens) should be reserved for scrubbing rather than irrigating. Hydrogen peroxide has no role in wound irrigation. During irrigation, splatter can be minimized by irrigating through the middle web space of the irrigator's hand while cupping the hand above the wound, attaching a 4 × 4 inch gauze to the irrigation catheter, or by using a plastic shield. An alternative to commercially available plastic shields is formed by puncturing the base of a sterile plastic medication cup with the irrigation needle.

- **Antisepsis and scrubbing**: Prior to wound irrigation and repair, and after a gauze sponge is folded and placed in the wound, clean the skin surrounding the wound. Various antiseptic skin cleansers can be used, including povidone-iodine (Betadine scrub) and chlorhexidine gluconate (Hibiclens). Nonionic surfactants, such as Shur-Clens and Pharma Clens, mechanically lift bacteria from the skin but possess no bactericidal activity. Avoid mechanical scrubbing of the wound unless there is gross contamination. If the wound needs to be scrubbed, use a fine-pore sponge (eg, Optipore) to minimize tissue abrasion and a nonionic surfactant to minimize tissue toxicity and inflammation.

- **Debride** contaminated wounds or wounds with nonviable tissue. Debridement increases a wound's ability to resist infection, shortens the period of inflammation, and creates a sharp, trimmed wound edge that is easier to repair and more cosmetically acceptable. If a wound is debrided, it can be undermined to avoid a wide scar.

- **Primary wound closure** is performed on new lacerations (<24 h on the face and <12 h on other areas of the body) that are relatively clean with minimal tissue devitalization. Use 3-0 suture for tissues with strong tension, such as fascia in an extremity, and 6-0 suture for tissues with light tension, such as the subcutaneous tissue of the face.

- **Deep (buried) sutures** minimize skin tension, improving the cosmetic result, provide 2 to 3 weeks of additional support after skin sutures are removed, preserve the normal muscle function if the muscular fascia is sutured, reduce the likelihood of hematoma or abscess formation by minimizing dead space, and prevent the development of pitting caused by inadequate healing of deep tissues. Deep sutures can increase the risk of infection and damage nerves, arteries, and tendons. In hands and feet, especially, placement of deep sutures increases the risk of infection and should be avoided.

- The most common deep suture is the **buried knot stitch**; it begins and ends at the base of the wound and buries the knot below the dermis (Fig. 23-3).
- With the **buried horizontal mattress stitch**, the suture is passed at the dermal-epidermal junction and the knot is placed subcuticularly.
- The **subcuticular stitch** is a running buried suture at the dermal-epidermal junction that is used for skin closure (Fig. 23-4). The suture enters the skin approximately 1 cm from one end of the laceration, emerges at the subcuticular plane at the wound apex, and passes through the subcuticular tissue on alternate sides of the laceration. The point of entry of each stitch is directly across from or slightly behind the exit point of the previous stitch. At the other end of the laceration, the needle is burrowed into the dermis and exits the skin 1 cm from the end. After ensuring that there is no skin puckering, tape the free suture ends in place. If absorbable suture is used, this stitch can be left in place or, if nonabsorbable suture is used, it can be removed in 2 to 3 weeks.

- **Skin closure** is accomplished with nonabsorbable synthetic sutures. Place sutures the same depth and width on both sides of the incision. A key to closure is edge eversion, which is obtained by entering the skin at a 90-degree angle, and, in some cases, by using a skin hook. For wounds with edges that tend to invert despite proper technique, vertical mattress stitches can be used (see below).

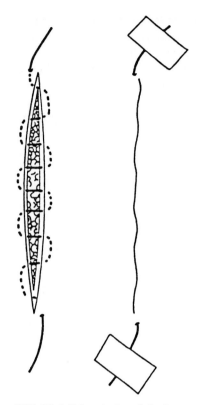

FIG. 23-4 Subcuticular stitch. See text for discussion.

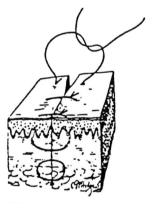

FIG. 23-5 Simple interrupted stitch (with buried subcutaneous stitch). See text for discussion.

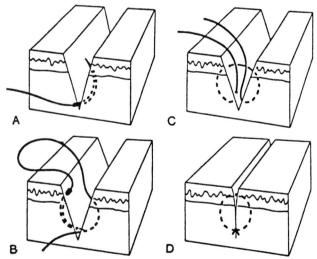

FIG. 23-3 Buried subcutaneous stitch. This is particularly useful when approximating the subcutaneous tissue just beneath the skin edge, because it prevents irritation of the skin edge by the knot.

- The **simple interrupted stitch** is used most frequently for skin closure (Fig. 23-5). It involves placing, tying, and cutting separate loops of suture. If one stitch in the closure fails, the remaining stitches will hold the wound together. It is useful for stellate lacerations, wounds with multiple components, lacerations that change direction, and for approximating landmarks.

○ The **running or continuous stitch** is rapid, easily removed, stronger than interrupted sutures, more effective for hemostasis, and distributes tension more evenly along its length (Fig. 23-6). It should not be used over joints since, if one point were to break, the entire stitch would unravel. To begin a simple continuous stitch, place an interrupted stitch

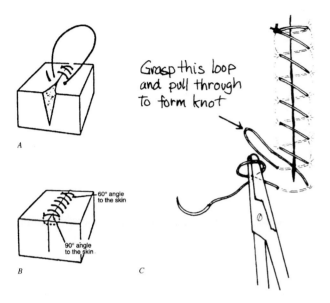

FIG. 23-6 The simple continuous stitch. *A/B.* This continuous suture is begun with a single suture that is tied to anchor the rest of the suture. The needle should be passed perpendicular to the skin edge and the suture threads should lie perpendicular to the wound margin, as with the simple interrupted suture. *C.* To finish and tie off this continuous suture, grab the loop formed at the free end after insertion of the needle through the skin at its midpoint with the needle holder and pull on this loop. It will come together as if it were a single thread. Tie the needle end of the suture material and this "looped" free end as a simple interrupted suture would be tied. To complete the simple continuous stitch, a series of square knots is tied, with the loop as one of the ties.

at one end of the wound and cut only the free end of the suture. Continue suturing in a coil pattern, ensuring that the needle passes perpendicularly across the laceration with each pass. After each pass, tighten the loop slightly so that tension is equally distributed. To complete the stitch, place the final loop just beyond the end of the laceration and tie the suture with the last loop used as the tail. An interlocking continuous stitch can be used to reduce slippage of loops and for more irregular lacerations (Fig. 23-7). It is performed by pulling the needle through the previous loop each time it exits the skin. It can, however, increase the degree of scarring if the loops are tied too tightly.

○ The **horizontal mattress stitch** is used for single-layer closure of lacerations under tension (Fig. 23-8). It approximates skin edges, provides eversion, and decreases the time needed to suture because 50 percent of knots are tied.

○ A **running horizontal mattress suture** can be used in areas of the body where loose skin could overlap or invert easily, such as the upper eyelids (Fig. 23-9).

○ The **half-buried horizontal mattress stitch (corner stitch)** is used for closure of complex wounds with angulated (V-shaped) flaps (Fig. 23-10). Enter and exit the skin directly across from the flap and course the suture loop within the subcuticular tissue of the flap.

○ The **vertical mattress stitch** causes more ischemia and necrosis within its loop than other stitches (Fig. 23-11). It is useful in areas with little subcutaneous tissue. The stitch begins in the same way as a simple interrupted stitch, but after the loop is made, reenter and reexit the skin approximately 1 to 2 mm from the wound edge and tie.

○ The knot used most commonly is the surgeon's knot followed by one to four half-knots, usually formed

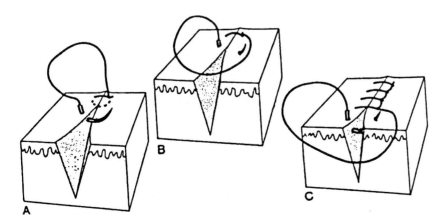

FIG. 23-7 Continuous single lock stitch. See text for discussion.

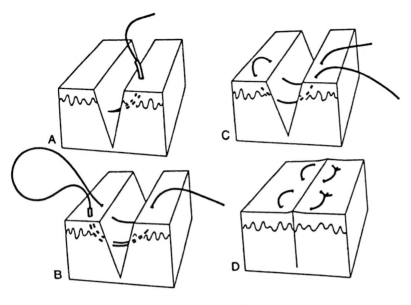

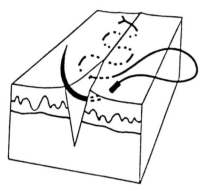

FIG. 23-8 Horizontal mattress stitch. *A.* The needle is passed 0.5–1 cm away from the wound edge deeply into the wound. *B.* The needle is then passed through the opposite side and reenters the wound parallel to the initial suture. *C.* One must enter the skin perpendicularly to provide some eversion of the wound edges and must enter and exit both the wound and skin at the same depth, otherwise "buckling" and irregularities occur in the wound margin. *D.* The suture loop is then tied as shown.

FIG. 23-9 Continuous mattress stitch. See text for discussion.

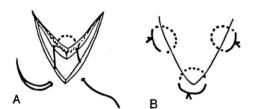

FIG. 23-10 A, B. Half-buried horizontal mattress stitch. This minimizes the vascular compromise at a corner flap. See text for discussion.

as instrument ties. The single surgeon's knot allows for some give if tissue edema develops.

○ **Correction of dog ears** is required when wound edges are not precisely aligned and there is an excess of skin on one or both ends. To repair a dog ear, elevate the excess skin with a skin hook and make an oblique incision from the apex of the wound toward the side of the dog ear, undermine

the flap, lay it flat, excise the excess triangle of skin, and complete the closure (Fig. 23-12).

○ **Tissue adhesives** are rapidly and painlessly applied (Fig. 23-13). Clean, debride, and dry the wound before applying the adhesive. Use it topically and avoid placing adhesive between the wound margins, within the wound, or in the eyes. Tissue adhesives should be used only if lacerations can be well approximated manually and without excessive tension. At least three coats of adhesive should be applied to provide adequate strength to the wound. It sloughs off within 7 to 10 days and acts as its own waterproof dressing and antimicrobial barrier. Petroleum-based ointments break down the adhesive and should not be used.

• **Secondary wound closure** allows wounds to heal by granulation and reepithelialization. It is used to manage ulcerations, drained abscess cavities, deep puncture wounds, older or infected lacerations, and many animal bites. Daily packing is performed with saline-soaked gauze or iodoform gauze strips until granulation tissue closes the potential space.

• **Delayed primary (tertiary) closure** is used on wounds 3 to 5 days after they have been initially cleansed, debrided, and packed with saline-soaked gauze. It is used on wounds that are too contaminated for primary closure but not associated with significant tissue loss or devitalization.

WOUND DRESSING, DRAINS, AND IMMOBILIZATION

• After laceration repair with sutures or staples, cleanse the skin of blood and povidone-iodine, and apply

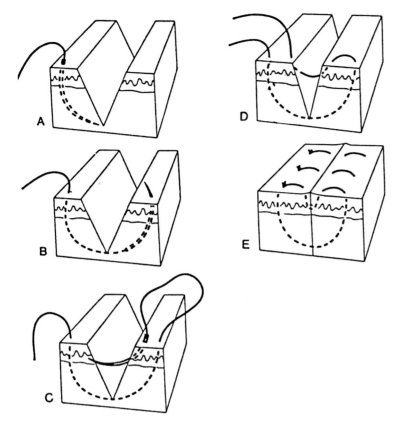

FIG. 23-11 A–E. Vertical mattress stitch. See text for discussion.

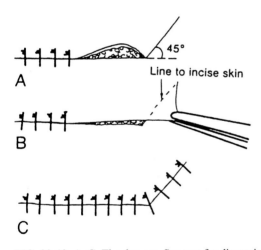

FIG. 23-12 A–C. The dog ear. See text for discussion.

antibiotic ointment or a semiporous nonadherent dressing (Adaptic, Telpha, Xeroform, or Vaseline gauze). Cover the wound with sterile gauze, an adhesive bandage (Band-Aid) or an occlusive or semiocclusive dressing (Op-Site, Tegaderm, DuoDerm, or Biobrane). If hematoma formation is a concern, apply a pressure dressing.

- **Drains** act as foreign bodies and should not be used in sutured wounds.

- If a wound is overlying a joint, **splint** it in the position of function for 7 to 10 days. In small children, a bulky dressing can act as a splint.
- **Prophylactic antibiotics** are indicated for patients who are prone to infective endocarditis, have orthopedic prostheses, wounds that are more than 12 to 24 hours old, or have a wound infection due to inappropriate care at home. Other indications include wounds that are heavily contaminated with feces or saliva, extensive intraoral lacerations, mammalian bites, wounds in immunocompromised hosts, contaminated or devitalized wounds, or wounds involving cartilage, joint spaces, tendons, or bones. If used, antibiotics should be given in the ED within 3 h of the injury.
  ○ The choice of antibiotics depends on the type of wound and contamination.
    ▪ Provide coverage for staphylococci and streptococci species with penicillinase-resistant penicillins, middle-generation cephalosporins, or erythromycin.
    ▪ Wounds contaminated with saliva can be treated with the same agents.
    ▪ Feces contamination requires coverage against facultative organisms, coliforms, and obligate anaerobes. Agents include second- and third-generation cephalosporins, or clindamycin and an aminoglycoside.

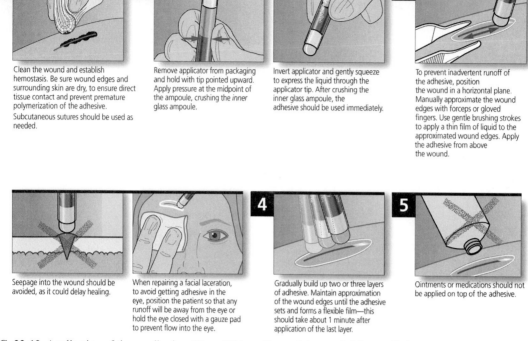

FIG. 23-13 Application of tissue adhesive. (From Ethicon, Inc., a Johnson & Johnson Co.)

- ▪ Trimethoprim-sulfamethoxazole and parenteral third-generation cephalosporins are effective for wounds that are contaminated with fresh water.
  - ○ Despite the fact that no definitive studies have examined the appropriate duration of prophylaxis, most practitioners provide 3 to 5 days of oral antibiotics.
- • **Tetanus prophylaxis** begins with appropriate wound care. If the wound is tetanus prone, determine the child's immunization status (Fig. 23-14). If the child has a tetanus-prone wound and was not immunized, partially immunized, or has an unknown immunization status, treat them as if they have no protection: give human tetanus immune globulin (HTIG) 250 U IM and complete or initiate primary immunization.

POSTOPERATIVE WOUND CARE AND SUTURE REMOVAL

- • Patients and parents should be informed that all wounds heal with scars, regardless of the quality of care, and the final appearance of the scar cannot be predicted until 6 to 12 months after the repair.
- • They should be educated regarding signs of infection and counseled that there is always the possibility of a residual foreign body in the wound.

- • Instruct the family to keep the wound dry for 24 to 48 h; changing the dressing only if it becomes soiled or soaked by exudate. After the initial 1 to 2 days, the dressing should be removed to check for signs of infection. After 2 days, lacerations are bridged by epithelial cells, making the wound impermeable to the entry of bacteria.
- • If parental reliability is questionable, the patient should have the wound examined in the ED in 2 to 3 days.
  - ○ If there are no signs of infection, instruct the patient or parents to gently wash the wound daily with soap and water.
  - ○ The wound should be protected with a dressing during the middle week, with daily dressing changes.
  - ○ Once the dressing is removed, patients and parents should be instructed that sunscreen (SPF 15 or greater) should be applied to the scar for at least 6 months to prevent hyperpigmentation of the scar.
  - ○ Table 23-3 outlines appropriate times for suture removal.
    - ▪ Skin tape should be applied after suture removal to ameliorate wound contraction and scar widening.

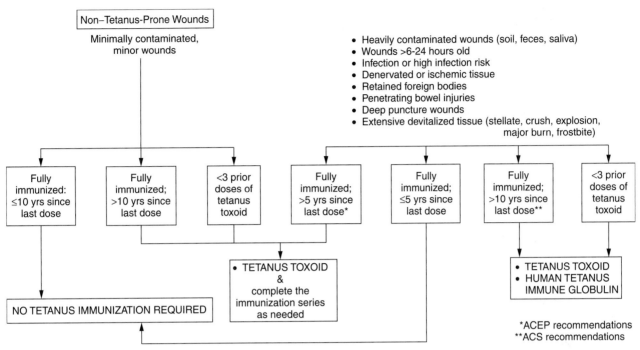

FIG. 23-14 Tetanus immunization guidelines.

MANAGEMENT OF SELECTED INJURIES

- **Abrasions** should be cleaned and dressed with a non-adherent dressing or antibiotic ointment and a dressing that can be changed daily after cleaning. Deeper abrasions are treated with cleansing and a fine-mesh gauze dressing. Foreign bodies need to be removed to avoid infection and tattooing of the wound. Large abrasions may require general anesthesia or conscious sedation to permit adequate debridement. Topical anesthesia with 2 or 4 percent lidocaine or LAT solution, infiltration of local anesthetic, or nerve blocks can be used for smaller abrasions. Large or deep abrasions should be reexamined in 2 to 3 days.
- **Scalp lacerations** can involve any or all of the five anatomic layers in the scalp.
  - Skin
  - Superficial fascia
  - Galea aponeurotica
  - Subaponeurotic areolar connective tissue
  - Periosteum
  - A rich vascular supply and vessels that tend to remain patent when cut are responsible for the profuse bleeding associated with scalp injuries. Usually, the bleeding is halted by rapid suturing. Hemostasis can also be controlled with direct pressure, placement of a wide, tight rubber band around the scalp, infiltration of local anesthetic with epinephrine into the wound, Raney scalp clips, or large vessel ligation.
  - In scalp wounds that penetrate the galea, bacteria can be carried by "emissary veins," and a wound infection can result in osteomyelitis, meningitis, or an intracranial abscess. Approximation of galeal lacerations will help control bleeding and safeguard against the spread of infection.
  - Scalp wounds are best closed with a single layer of sutures that incorporates the skin, the subcutaneous fascia, and the galea.
  - Superficial scalp lacerations are amenable to staple closure.
- **Forehead lacerations** that are limited to the area above the supraorbital rim can be anesthetized with supraorbital and supratrochlear nerve blocks, avoiding tissue distortion associated with local infiltration. Close the forehead in layers taking care to align landmarks.
- Patients with **eyelid lacerations** need a thorough eye examination to exclude concomitant eye injury. Simple, superficial lid lacerations may be repaired by the emergency physician using 6-0 nonabsorbable suture or fast absorbing gut. The following lacerations, however, require specialized repair:
  - Lacerations of the medial third of either lid: lacrimal system may be involved. Check for lacrimal system involvement by instilling fluorescein into

TABLE 23-3 Repair of Soft Tissue Injuries by Body Location

LOCATION	ANESTHETIC	REPAIR/MATERIAL	TYPE OF CLOSURE	SUTURE REMOVAL (DAYS)
Scalp	Lidocaine 1% with epinephrine	3-0 or 4-0 nylon[a]; ± 3-0 polyglycolic acid[b] (galea) Staples if galea intact	Single tight layer with simple interrupted, vertical mattress, or horizontal mattress for hemostasis; galea requires close approximation, but preferably with single-layer closure	7–10
Pinna (ear)	Lidocaine 1% (field block)	5-0 polyglycolic acid[b] (perichondrium); 6-0 nylon[a] (skin)	Simple interrupted; stent dressing	4–6
Eyebrow	Lidocaine 1% with epinephrine	4-0 or 5-0 polyglycolic acid[b] (and 6-0 nylon)[a]	Layered closure	4–5
Eyelid	Lidocaine 1%	6-0 nylon[a] 2-OCA	Horizontal mattress	3–5
Lip	Lidocaine 1% with epinephrine or mental node block	4-0 or 5-0 polyglycolic acid[b] or (chromic) gut (mucosa); 5-0 polyglycolic acid[b] (SQ, muscle); 6-0 nylon[a] (skin)	Three layers (mucosa, muscle, skin) if through and through, otherwise two layers	3–5
Oral cavity	Lidocaine 1% with epinephrine or field block Sedation may be necessary	4-0 or 5-0 polyglycolic acid[b] or (chromic) gut	Simple interrupted or horizontal mattress	7–8 or allow to dissolve
Face	Lidocaine 1% with epinephrine or field block	4-0 or 5-0 polyglycolic acid[b] (SQ); 6-0 nylon[a] (skin) 2-OCA (skin)	If full-thickness, layered closure	3–5
Neck	Lidocaine 1% with epinephrine	4-0 polyglycolic acid[b] (SQ); 5-0 nylon[a] (skin)	Two-layered closure	4–6
Trunk	Lidocaine 1% with epinephrine	4-0 polyglycolic acid[b] (SQ fat); 4-0 or 5-0 nylon[a] (skin)	Single or layered closure	7–12
Extremity	Lidocaine 1% with epinephrine	3-0 or 4-0 polyglycolic acid[b] (SQ, fat muscle) 4-0 or 5-0 nylon[a] (skin)	Single or layered; splint if over joint	10–14 (joint) 7–10 (other)
Hands and feet	Lidocaine 1% (lidocaine 2% or bupivacaine 0.25% for field block)	4-0 or 5-0 nylon[a]	Single-layer closure with simple interrupted or horizontal mattress; splint if over joint	10–14 (joint) 7–10 (other)
Nailbeds	Digital nerve block with lidocaine 2% or bupivacaine 0.25%	5-0 polyglycolic acid[b]		Allow to dissolve

[a]Nylon or polypropylene.

[b]Polyglycolic and (Dexon) or polyglactin (Vicryl).

the eye and watching for wound fluorescence with a Wood's lamp or cobalt blue light.
  ○ Lacerations with fat in the wound: underlying globe injury may be present.
  ○ Lacerations of lid margins: risk for lid deformity and abnormal lid movement.
  ○ Levator palpebrae muscle involvement: posttraumatic ptosis may develop.
  ○ Lacerations of the tarsal plate (dense band of fibrous tissue in the upper lid).
• **Ear lacerations** require cleaning, debridement of devitalized tissue, and coverage of exposed cartilage to avoid chondritis.

  ○ Anesthesia of the external ear is performed by infiltrating the base of the auricle to block the auriculotemporal, greater auricular, and occipital nerves.
  ○ Cartilage should be approximated with 5-0 absorbable suture placed through the posterior and anterior perichondrium. Keep tension to a minimum to prevent tearing of the cartilage.
  ○ The skin should then be approximated with 5-0 nonabsorbable suture ensuring that all cartilage is covered.
  ○ After repair, dress the ear with a mastoid compression dressing to prevent a perichondral hematoma,

which can lead to necrosis of cartilage and "cauliflower ear."

- **Lip lacerations** require careful attention to ensure a good cosmetic result (Fig. 23-15). Prior to repair, inspect the oral mucosa and teeth for lacerations and trauma. Consider performing a mental nerve block for lower lip lacerations or an infraorbital nerve block for upper lip lacerations to prevent obscuration of landmarks by local infiltration of anesthetic. If local anesthetic is used, prior to infiltration paint a thin line of methylene blue along the vermilion border on each side of the laceration. This will be used as a landmark during repair. After anesthesia, cleanse and irrigate the wound and place the middle stitch at the vermilion border. If deep sutures are required, leave the initial stitch untied and proceed with deep closure. Through-and-through lip lacerations require three-layer closure: approximate the orbicularis oris muscle with 4-0 or 5-0 absorbable suture, the mucosa with 5-0 absorbable suture and, after irrigation of the outside surface, the skin with 6-0 nonabsorbable suture. Through-and-through lip lacerations are prone to infection and prophylaxis with penicillin or erythromycin is recommended.

- **Distal fingertip injuries** heal remarkably well in children. Treatment consists of a digital block or local infiltration, cleansing and dressing of the wound with antibiotic ointment or non-adherent gauze, and a splint or bulky dressing for protection. Frequent wound checks should be scheduled to watch for infection.
  - More proximal amputations require a hand surgeon.
  - Close nailbed lacerations with 6-0 absorbable sutures: avoid tying the sutures too tightly and tearing through tissue. Keep debridement to a min-

imum. Use the nail or foil from the suture pack to stent open the space between the paronychium and eponychium to prevent the formation of adhesions with the nailbed. If there is an underlying fracture, splint the finger and prescribe prophylactic antibiotics (cephalosporin or dicloxacillin).

- A **paronychium** is a cutaneous abscess at the lateral aspect of fingernails or toenails. They are painful, swollen, erythematous, and tender. For fingers, the cuticle can be incised with a number 11 blade, and the abscess drained and irrigated with a normal saline-povidone- iodine solution. Prescribe systemic antibiotics only when there is a cellulitis or lymphangitis. Paronychia of the toes are often caused by ingrown toenails and the ingrown portion of the nail should be removed to avoid a recurrence. A digital nerve block is mandatory for this procedure.

- A **subungual hematoma** is a collection of blood under a nail. If the nail is intact, pressure from the hematoma causes substantial pain. As long as the nail and surrounding nail fold are intact the hematoma can be drained by trephinating the nail with electrocautery. Prior to trephination, cleanse the nail using povidone-iodine, and once blood escapes through the nail, remove the cautery to avoid nail bed damage. Dress the digit with dry sterile gauze and splint for protection.

- **Puncture wounds to the foot** have the potential to result in cellulitis, plantar space infections, abscesses, retained foreign bodies, and osteomyelitis. To start, obtain a radiograph to exclude bony involvement, air in the joint spaces, and radiopaque foreign bodies. Anesthetize the wound locally or with a posterior

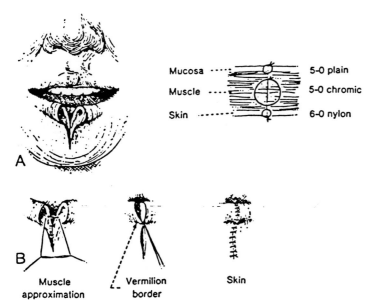

FIG. 23-15 Repair of through-and-through lip laceration.

tibial or sural nerve block, unroof the puncture site, cleanse and debride the wound, and remove any foreign bodies. If jet irrigation is performed, be aware of irrigation fluid that is not returned: this fluid can carry bacteria and debris deeper into the wound and increase swelling. Prophylactic antibiotic use is controversial, but should include *Pseudomonas* coverage, especially if the puncture wound occurs through the sole of a sneaker.

- Specialty consultation should be considered for:
  ○ complex or extensive wounds
  ○ wounds with large tissue defects
  ○ wounds in which there is tendon, nerve, joint, or critical vessel involvement
  ○ lacerations involving the parotid or lacrimal ducts
  ○ lacerations of the eyelid tarsal plates
  ○ lacerations over fractures
  ○ facial lacerations in which cosmetic results are a concern
  ○ wounds about which there is physician uncertainty.

BIBLIOGRAPHY

Bruns TB, Robinson BS, Smith RJ, et al: A new tissue adhesive for laceration repair in children. *J Pediatr* 132:1067–1070, 1998.

Christoph RA, Buchanan L, Begalla K, et al: Pain reduction in local anesthetic administration through pH buffering. *Ann Emerg Med* 17:117, 1998.

Hollander JE, Singer AJ: Laceration management. *Ann Emerg Med* 34:356–367, 1999.

Jankauskas S, Cohen IK, Grabb WC: Basic technique of plastic surgery. In: Aston SJ, Beasley RW, Thorne CHM, eds. *Grabb and Smith's Plastic Surgery,* 5th ed. Philadelphia: Lippincott-Raven, 1997.

Knapp JF: Updates in wound management for the pediatrician. *Pediatr Clin North Am* 46:1202–1213, 1999.

Quinn JV, Wells GA, Sutcliffe T, et al: Tissue adhesive versus suture wound repair at one year: Randomized clinical trial correlating early, three-month, and one year cosmetic outcome. *Ann Emerg Med* 32:645–649, 1998.

Roberts JR, Hedges JR, eds: *Clinical Procedures in Emergency Medicine,* 3d ed. Philadelphia: WB Saunders, 1998.

Schilling CG, Bank DE, Borchert BA, et al: Tetracaine, epinephrine (adrenaline), and cocaine (TAC) versus lidocaine, epinephrine, and tetracaine (LAT) for anesthesia of lacerations in children. *Ann Emerg Med* 25:203–208, 1995.

Trott A: *Wounds and Lacerations: Emergency Care and Closure,* 2d edition. St. Louis: Mosby, 1997.

Valente JH, Forti RJ, Freundlich LF, et al: Wound irrigation in children: saline solution or tap water? *Ann Emerg Med* 41:609–616, 2003.

QUESTIONS

1. Which of the following is the most effective way to control bleeding in a pediatric patient with a laceration?
   A. Application of a tourniquet
   B. Direct pressure
   C. Clamping of vessels with a hemostat
   D. Injection of lidocaine with epinephrine (1:10,000)
   E. Inflation of a blood pressure cuff proximal to the injury

2. Which of the following is true regarding wound closure techniques?
   A. Staples are effective on hand and face lacerations.
   B. Tissue adhesives are effective on joint lacerations.
   C. Steri-strips are effective for large gaping wounds.
   D. Staples produce similar cosmetic results to suturing.
   E. Steri-strips must be removed in 3 to 5 days.

3. Which of the following is true regarding the use of lidocaine for wound anesthesia?
   A. The maximum dose is 4.5 mg/kg
   B. Epinephrine can be added to use on nose lacerations.
   C. The pain of injection may be decreased by injecting rapidly.
   D. Topical lidocaine-adrenaline-tetracaine may be used on lip lacerations.
   E. Bupivacaine is a shorter acting agent that may be used.

4. A 10-year-old boy presents with a 2-cm linear laceration to his eyebrow. Which of the following is optimal in the management of this patient?
   A. The eyebrow should be shaved.
   B. The wound should be irrigated with hydrogen peroxide.
   C. The wound may be sutured if <48 h old.
   D. A 6-0 suture should be used.
   E. Tissue adhesives are very effective in this area.

5. Which of the following is true regarding deep (buried) sutures in wound repairs?
   A. Are useful in laceration repairs of the hands and feet
   B. May improve the cosmetic result
   C. Decrease the risk of infection
   D. Nonabsorbable synthetic sutures should be used
   E. Increases the likelihood of hematoma formation

6. Which of the following is an indication for prophylactic antibiotic use?
   A. A facial laceration that is 6 h old
   B. Any laceration using tissue adhesive
   C. A wound heavily contaminated with saliva

D. Any wound where hair is shaved

E. When deep (buried) sutures are used

7. Which of the following wound care instructions are appropriate to tell the parents after repairing a laceration?

A. If proper technique is used no scar will form.

B. Instructions to apply sunscreen to the scar for at least 6 months once dressings are removed.

C. All sutures should be removed at 5 days to prevent scarring.

D. The wound should be kept dry and not be washed until sutures removed.

E. The child should be seen urgently by a plastic surgeon for scar revision.

8. A 5-year-old female presents with an eyelid laceration. Which of the following does not require specialized repair and may be safely done in the ED?

A. Lacerations with fat exposed in the wound

B. Lacerations of the lid margins

C. Lacerations with muscle involvement

D. Lacerations of the tarsal plate

E. Lacerations of the lateral third of the upper lid

9. A 10-year-old male presents with a through-and-through upper lip laceration that crosses the vermilion border. Which of the following is true regarding repair of this injury?

A. Anesthesia of the upper lip may be accomplished with an infraorbital nerve block.

B. The initial suture should be placed at the most superior aspect of the laceration to the most distal.

C. The skin should be closed first then the oral mucosa.

D. A 4-0 non-absorbable suture is used on the oral mucosa.

E. No prophylactic antibiotics are recommended.

10. A 15-year-old female presents with a painful right thumb nail injury after hitting it with a hammer. On examination, the skin and nail are intact and there is a dark bluish discoloration of the nail. Which of the following is the most appropriate treatment of this injury?

A. Ice, elevation, and analgesics

B. Digital block and removal of the nail

C. Trephination of the nail with electrocautery

D. Aluminum splint to the thumb, ice, analgesics

E. Analgesics

ANSWERS

1. B. The most effective way to control bleeding is with direct manual pressure or a pressure dressing. Clamping of vessels with a hemostat should never be done. Inflation of a blood pressure cuff proximal

to the injury may be used if direct pressure is unsuccessful.

2. D. Staples induce minimal inflammatory reaction and produce similar cosmetic results to suturing. Tissue adhesives and steri-strips should not be applied to areas of tension. Steri-strips do not require removal.

3. A. The maximum dose of lidocaine is 4.5 mg/kg. Epinephrine and lidocaine-adrenaline-tetracaine should not be used in regions supplied by end arteries (fingers, nose, lip, ear, genitalia, and toes). The pain of injection is decreased by adding bicarbonate to the lidocaine, using a 25- to 27-gauge needle, and injecting slowly into the wound margins. Bupivacaine is a longer acting agent.

4. D. The eyebrows should never be shaved or clipped as they serve as landmarks for alignment during wound repair and may take 6 to 12 months to grow back. Hydrogen peroxide has no role in wound irrigation. Lacerations on the face may be repaired up to 24 h. A 6-0 suture is used on tissues with light tension, such as the face. Tissue adhesives should be used with caution around the eye.

5. B. Deep (buried) sutures minimize skin tension improving the cosmetic result and reduce the likelihood of hematoma or abscess formation by minimizing dead space. They should not be used on the hands and feet as it increases the risk of infection. Absorbable sutures should be used. Deep sutures can increase the risk of infection and damage nerves, arteries, and tendons.

6. C. Prophylactic antibiotics are indicated for wounds heavily contaminated with feces or saliva.

7. B. All wounds heal with scars, regardless of the quality of care. Sunscreen should be applied to the scar for at least 6 months to prevent hyperpigmentation of the scar. The location of the wound determines the time frame for suture removal. The wound should be kept dry for 24 to 48 h and then may be gently washed with soap and water. Final appearance of the scar cannot be predicted until 6 to 12 months and referral to plastic surgery for wound revision is not done urgently.

8. E. Lacerations of the medial third of either lid are at risk for involvement of lacrimal system. Superficial lacerations of the lateral lid, if not involving the lid margin, no fat in the wound, or no muscle or tarsal plate involvement, may be safely sutured.

9. A. To not distort the landmarks, an infraorbital nerve block may be used for upper lip lacerations. The initial suture should be placed at the vermilion border. A three-layer closure should be used; initially repair of the orbicularis oris muscle, then mucosa with 5-0 absorbable suture, and, finally, the

outer skin. Prophylactic antibiotics are recommended in through-and-through lip lacerations.

10. C. This patient has a subungual hematoma, which is a collection of blood under the nail. The hematoma can be drained by trephinating the nail with electrocautery.

24   EMERGENCY DEPARTMENT PROCEDURAL SEDATION AND ANALGESIA

Alfred Sacchetti
Michael J. Gerardi
Kemedy K. McQuillen
Gary R. Strange

TERMINOLOGY

- **Procedural sedation**, to paraphrase the American College of Emergency Physicians, is a technique of administering sedatives or dissociative agents with or without analgesics to induce a state that allows the patient to tolerate unpleasant procedures while maintaining cardiorespiratory function. It is intended to result in a depressed level of consciousness that allows the patient to maintain his or her airway. The degree of sedation needed is determined by the treating physician and the procedure to be performed.

PATIENT ASSESSMENT

- The procedural sedation and analgesic (PSA) needs of any patient are determined by the nature of the patient complaint, the status of the child, the child's response to the problem, and the preferences of the treating clinician.
- Children being considered for sedation or analgesia should undergo a focused history that includes past medical problems, prior sedation or analgesia, allergies, upper respiratory infections, and recent meals. Although the timing of the last oral intake is questioned, all children in the emergency department (ED) setting should be assumed to have a full stomach.
- The physical examination should address the patient's immediate problem plus assess respiratory rate, temperature, heart rate, pulse oximetry, the oropharynx, posterior pharynx, and chest.
- Childhood sedation is complicated by a larger tongue, more reactive tonsils and adenoids, and frequent upper respiratory infections (URIs), adding nasal or respiratory tract congestion as a potential source of airway obstruction.
- An **American Society of Anesthesiologists (ASA) Score** should be assigned to any child undergoing PSA. The ASA scoring system is summarized in Table 24-1. ASA 1 or 2 patients are good candidates for PSA in the emergency department. ASA 3 patients may be managed in either area depending on the nature of the problem and the capabilities of the treating physician. ASA 4 or 5 patients are generally better treated in a formal procedural unit.
- **Levels of pain** can be quantitated using a number of scoring systems. Figure 24-1 contains examples of visual analog or observational pain scoring systems.

PATIENT MONITORING

- Patients receiving analgesia for pain or anxiety generally do not require additional monitoring unless unusually high doses are required. In that case, respiratory or blood pressure monitoring may be warranted.
- Patients undergoing PSA require additional monitoring. Electronic monitoring should be in place prior to the initiation of sedation. These patients also require an additional health care provider to monitor the patient from a PSA standpoint. The medical provider should understand monitoring equipment, recognize the signs and symptoms of respiratory depression, and be able to manage acute respiratory problems.
- Monitoring should assess the patient's ventilation and oxygenation.
  - Continuous pulse oximetry will provide assessment of oxygenation, heart rate, and, in some newer equipment, respiratory rate. However, pulse oximetry only reports oxygen status and does not reflect the patient's ventilatory status: if supplemental oxygen is provided, hypoventilation may be present without a change in oxygenation.

TABLE 24-1 American Society of Anesthesiologists Physical Status Classification

CLASS	CHARACTERISTICS
I	A normal healthy patient
II	A patient with mild systemic disease
III	A patient with severe systemic disease
IV	A patient with severe systemic disease that is a constant life threat
V	A moribund patient who is not expected to survive without the procedure
E	Emergency procedure

Neonatal or Infant Observational Scale

Observation	Score		
	0	1	2
Face	Normal or relaxed	Occasional grimace, frown, withdrawn	Constant frown, grimace, clenched jaw
Cry	No cry	Moans or whimpers	Crying steadily, screams or sobs
Consolability	Content	Reassured by occasional touching, hugging, or talking	Difficult to control or comfort
Legs	Normal relaxed	Uneasy, restless, tense	Kicking or legs drawn up

Visual Pictorial Type Scale

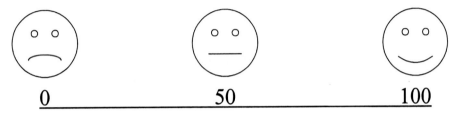

Numeric Visual Analog Scale

0		25		50		75		100

FIG. 24-1 Pediatric pain scales.

○ For those in whom it is important to maintain normal arterial CO_2 tensions, a continuous end-tidal capnometer can be added.

○ Cardiac monitoring is generally not needed unless hypovolemia or cardiac abnormalities are an issue.

○ Blood pressure measurements should be obtained in children in whom hypovolemia or hypertension is a concern.

○ Monitoring should be continued until the clinical effects of the drug therapy have worn off and the child's respiratory and mental status have returned to baseline.

• A flow sheet that includes ASA class, relevant medical history, baseline airway, respiratory and neurologic status, doses and timing of medications, vital signs (including pulse oximetry), and discharge findings should be used for all children undergoing PSA.

• Prior to discharge, children should be able to tolerate sips of fluids and ambulate without assistance unless there is an unavoidable barrier to ambulation, such as lower extremity injury. Discharge instructions should include the need for close supervision and modified activities (eg, no climbing) in the short term as well as reasons to seek medical attention.

ROUTES OF ADMINISTRATION

• **Intravenous (IV)** administration offers the greatest flexibility for titrating medications to patient response. An additional advantage to the IV route is the potential for initiating patient controlled analgesia (PCA). PCA permits the patient to control the dose of analgesia and is effective in children as young as 5 years old.

• **Intramuscular (IM)** and **subcutaneous (SQ)** injections provide reliable delivery but are not easily titrated.

- **Oral (PO)** administration should be reserved for drugs with predictable actions. The timing of repeat doses is difficult to determine due to delays in absorption.
- **Transmucosal (TM)** drug administration is quicker in onset than PO administrations, but slow enough to make titration difficult.
  ○ Delivery can be through the oral, buccal, nasal, and rectal routes.
  ○ Transmucosal medications include midazolam, fentanil, sufentanil, ketamine, thiopental, methohexital, and diazepam.
- **Transdermal (TD)** delivery of analgesics can be used to prepare patients for procedures involving percutaneous punctures.
- **Inhalation** sedative analgesics are well tolerated, painless, and easy to administer, however, they require specialized equipment and patient cooperation.

SEDATIVE AND ANALGESIC AGENTS

- Medications most commonly used for PSA are listed in Table 24-2. PSA drugs are divided into four general classes: pure analgesics, sedative analgesics, pure sedatives, and others. There is no single agent that is ideal in all situations, so physicians using these agents must be familiar with their indications, all of their actions, relative contraindications, and potential alternatives.
  ○ **Pure analgesic agents** include aspirin, acetaminophen, and nonsteroidal antiinflammatory drugs (NSAIDs). These agents are used for antipyresis and mild pain. Keterolac, the only parenteral NSAID available in the United States, is especially effective in prostaglandin-mediated conditions, such as biliary or renal colic, although its use in other painful conditions generally requires supplementation with

Table 24-2   Common Pediatric Procedural Sedation and Analgesic Agents

MEDICATION	ROUTE	DOSE (mg/kg)	TYPICAL MAXIMUM (mg/kg)[a]	DURATION	COMMENTS
Sedative Analgesics					
Meperidine	IV, IM	1.0–2.0	100	3–4 h	Chronic accumulation risk
Morphine	IV, IM, SQ	0.1–2.0	10	2–4 h	
Fentanyl	IV	0.001–0.002	0.05	20 min	Rigidity, apnea, lower dose <6 mo
	TM	0.005–0.010			
Remifentanil	IV	0.001	0.05	4–6 min	Rigidity, apnea
Hydromorphone	IV	0.01–0.02	2		
Hydrocodone	PO	0.2	10	4–6 h	
Codeine	PO	1–1.5	60	4–6h	
Sedatives					
Diazepam	IV	0.05–0.2	10	2–4 h	
Lorazepam	IV, IM	0.02–0.05	2	6–8 h	
Midazolam	IV, IM	0.01–0.1	2	1–3 h	
Pentobarbital	IV, IM	2.0–5.0	200	2–4 h	
Thiopental	IV	3.0–5.0	500	20 min	Intubation doses
	PR	15–25		1–2 h	
Methohexital	IV	1–1.5	100	20 min	Intubation doses
	PR	18.0–25.0		1–2 h	
Chloral Hydrate	PO	50–75	1,000	10–24 h	Caution post procedure
Propofol	IV	0.25–1.0	75	20 min	Apnea
	Infusion	1–3 mg/kg/h		20 min	
Etomidate	IV	0.1–0.3	30	20 min	
Other Agents					
Ketamine	IV	1.0–1.5	100	30–90 min	
	IM	4.0–5.0		2–4 h	
	PO	5.0–6.0		6 h	
Nitrous oxide	Inhalation	30–50%		1–2 min	
Diphenhydramine	PO	1.0–1.5	50		
Droperidol	IV, IM	0.01–0.05	5	4–6 h	Possible dystonic reaction
Dexmedetomidine	IV	0.2–0.7 µg/kg/h		5–6 min	Hypotension and bradycardia
Reversal Agents					
Naloxone	IV, IM	0.1	2 mg	20 min	
Flumazenil	IV	0.01	0.2 mg	30 min	

[a]Typical maximum dose represents dose that is effective in most patients. Since all patients respond differently, it is possible that for some patients, a dose in excess of this dose may be required. If such a higher dose is utilized, precautions in monitoring the patient should be taken.

a narcotic. When combined, pure analgesics and narcotics are synergistic: there are many oral combination therapies that take advantage of this effect.

○ **Sedative analgesic agents** include synthetic and naturally occurring narcotics, which work through stimulation of opioid receptors in the central nervous system. Differences in the effects of the various agents result from differential receptor binding preferences. Narcotic analgesics provide dose-dependent pain relief with mild sedation and can be administered PO, IV, IM, SQ, TM, and intrathecally. Adverse effects include nausea, transient itching or urticaria from histamine release, and cardiovascular and respiratory depression. Narcotics can be reversed through administration of competitive antagonists such as naloxone or nalmephine.

- *Morphine* is the classic narcotic analgesic and is used to treat moderate to severe pain. Although it is frequently administered with a phenothiazine or hydroxazine, there is no evidence that that addition of these agents potentiates the analgesic effects or decreases the incidence of emesis.

- *Meperidine* is another analgesic that is very similar to morphine. Unlike morphine, meperidine is metabolized to an active metabolite, normeperidine, which has a longer serum half-life than that of its parent compound. It produces a dysphoric reaction and seizures if allowed to accumulate. For this reason, meperidine should not be used if multiple doses will be required.

- *Hydromorphone* is a more potent semisynthetic narcotic that is frequently used in sickle cell anemia patients and PCA pumps.

- *Fentanyl citrate* is a synthetic short-acting narcotic approximately 100 times more potent than morphine. It has a rapid onset and a 20-min duration of action. Unlike other narcotics, fentanyl has few cardiovascular effects, making it appropriate for hypovolemic and cardiac patients. A side effect of fentanyl, chest wall rigidity, can occur if the drug is administered too rapidly. This can be reversed with naloxone or skeletal muscle paralysis. Fentanyl is the only narcotic that can be administered through the PO transmucosal route. Provided as a "lollipop," the child sucks on the fentanyl-containing hard candy until he or she becomes drowsy. Unfortunately, transmucosal fentanyl causes vomiting in up to 30 percent of children. A cogeniter of fentanyl, *sufentanil* can be administered intranasally. Respiratory monitoring is required if using either of these drugs. Reduced doses should be used in very young infants, as they are more sensitive to the respiratory depressant effects. Fentanil can also be given transdermally in patients with chronic pain.

- *Remifentanil* is a synthetic narcotic with an onset of 15 to 30 s and a 4- to 6-min duration. Its potency and cardiovascular effects are similar to those of fentanyl but up to 80 percent of nongeneral anesthesia patients experience hypoxia and apnea. It is used for PSA, anesthesia, and RSI.

- *Codeine*, *hydrocodone*, and *oxycodone* are less potent narcotics generally administered orally and in combination with a pure analgesic.

• **Pure sedatives** are also referred to as sedative hypnotic agents. Most of these agents exert their effect through gamma-aminobutyric acid (GABA) receptors, an essential part of the central nervous system's negative feedback loop. Side effects include dose-related cardiovascular and respiratory depression. Subtherapeutic doses of these agents will cause disinhibition with agitated, uncontrolled behavior. Treatment with additional doses will take the child through disinhibition to somnolence.

○ *Barbiturates* are the classic sedative agents and include pentobarbital, thiopental, and methohexital. Thiopental and methohexital are both extremely fast acting with profound sedation within 30 s of IV administration. Apnea should be anticipated when these medications are used. Respiratory depression may be ameliorated with lower, slowly administered doses. Rectal administration of either of these agents is also effective with an extremely rapid onset of action. Pentobarbital is a rapid-acting, less-potent sedative hypnotic used primarily in sedation for diagnostic studies. It can be administered IV or IM. After vascular access is obtained, 2.5 mg/kg is given over 30 s. If not effective after 1 to 2 min, half the dose can be repeated twice for a total dose of 5 mg/kg.

○ *Benzodiazepines*, unlike the barbiturates, can be reversed with the competitive antagonist flumazenil. Diazepam and lorazepam are moderate to long-acting anxiolytics with good sedative hypnotic properties. They are more commonly used for seizure control, agitation, and skeletal muscle relaxation for joint reduction than for PSA. Midazolam is a shorter-acting, more potent benzodiazepine commonly used for PSA. It can be given PO, PR, IV, IM, and intranasally.

○ *Propofol* is an ultra–short-acting sedative hypnotic used for RSI and PSA. Propofol has a very fast onset of action with a duration of 6 to 8 min. For short procedures, such as the reduction of a large joint dislocation, a 0.5 mg/kg bolus is given and then titrated with 0.1 mg/kg boluses as needed.

With prolonged sedation, the bolus is generally followed by a continuous infusion. Propofol will induce apnea and hypotension if pushed rapidly.

○ *Etomidate* is another sedative hypnotic agent that is used for RSI and as a sedative for short, painful procedures. It has minimal effect on the cardiovascular system and is cerebral protective. It can cause significant myoclonic jerks that may interfere with joint relocation.

○ *Chloral hydrate*, although effective, has fallen out of favor because of its long duration of action. Given in the range of 50 to 75 mg/kg, chloral hydrate's actions are seen in 30 min, but residual effects may last for 3 days.

○ *Diphenhydramine* is an antihistamine with prominent sedative side effects that can be used in children undergoing painless diagnostic studies. Its use in young children can cause paradoxical irritability.

○ *Dexmedetomidine*, related to clonidine, is a central acting β2-agonist with potent sedative, analgesic, and anxiolytic actions. It does not produce respiratory depression but can cause hypotension and bradycardia. Pediatric clinical trials are limited, and this drug should be used only for older adolescents.

• Other agents include ketamine, droperidol, and nitrous oxide.

○ *Ketamine* is a dissociative agent that produces a trance-like cataleptic state through disruption of communications between the cortical and limbic systems. Ketamine produces rapid sedation, analgesia, and amnesia. Through mild sympathomimetic effects, it can decrease bronchospasm, increase heart rate, and maintain and even slightly raise systemic blood pressure. Generally, it does not cause respiratory depression but transient apnea has been reported when the drug was given rapidly to extremely young infants. Complications of ketamine include emesis, increased intracranial pressure, laryngospasm, increased salivation, which can be limited by pretreatment with atropine or glycopyrrolate, and emergence reactions. Emergence reactions appear to be related to the child's level of anxiety prior to the procedure, age younger than 5 years, and the existence of underlying medical conditions. Limiting stimuli during recovery may help to lessen these reactions. Prophylactic midazolam given with the initial dose of ketamine does not decrease the incidence of emergence reactions. Because of the increased salivation, care should be taken when using ketamine in children with active URIs.

○ *Droperidol* is a butyrophenone that has fallen out of favor since its association with significant cardiac dysrhythmias. Its use is no longer recommended.

○ *Nitrous oxide* is a sedative analgesic that does not function through opioid receptor stimulation. It is administered as an oxygen and nitrous oxide mixture, it has an onset of 2 to 3 min and a similar duration of action. This drug is not metabolized and is excreted only through exhalation by the lungs. The sedation and analgesia produced by this drug is dose dependent: at a minimum, a 30 percent nitrous oxide to 70 percent oxygen mixture is necessary for brief anxiolysis and short, painful procedures. Most nitrous oxide systems are designed for self-administration although modifications have been designed to provide continuous flow systems for children as young as 4 years old. Specialized equipment and staff training is the limiting factor in the widespread use of this modality. Because it diffuses freely into gas-filled cavities, nitrous oxide should not be used in patients with pneumothorax or bowel obstruction.

• Nonpharmacologic sedation and analgesia may be effective in children who are susceptible to suggestion.

○ Conversation, story telling, or visual or tactile stimuli are helpful in diverting a child's attention from brief, painful procedures.

○ Music via earphones or videos may be used for a more prolonged procedure.

○ In newborns, a highly concentrated sugar solution has been shown to decrease observational scores during painful procedures.

The **selection of PSA agents** is dictated by the intended effect on the child, the child's age and baseline behavior.

• A sedative hypnotic agent is ideal for painless diagnostic procedures. A narcotic analgesic should be used for painful procedures.

• Combinations may be used to take advantage of the desired properties of each. The most frequent combinations pair short-acting sedatives with short-acting narcotics such as fentanyl/midazolam or fentanyl/propofol. Extra care should be taken with such combinations because adverse effects may be increased.

○ Doses lower than those of either agent alone should be used initially when combining agents.

• Combining a local anesthetic with a sedative can also produce effective patient control.

• Potential agents for different scenarios are listed in Table 24-3.

• For very painful conditions, a parenteral narcotic should be used. Less severe pain can be managed with an oral narcotic/pure analgesic combination.

TABLE 24-3   Clinical Scenarios and Possible Sedation Analgesia Options[a]

| | OPTIONS | | |
SCENARIO	1	2	3
Moderate systemic pain	Morphine	Meperidine	Hydromorphone
Severe systemic pain	Morphine PCA	Fentanyl PCA	Hydromorphone
Fracture care	Regional anesthesia	Ketamine	Fentanyl/midazolam
Urgent diagnostics	Propofol	Pentobarbital	Midazolam
Dislocation	Propofol	Morphine and diazepam	Etomidate
Lumbar puncture[b]	Ketamine	Midazolam	Morphine
Sexual abuse examination	Midazolam	Ketamine and midazolam	Propofol
RSI adjunct	Propofol	Etomidate	Ketamine
Burn care	Nitrous oxide	Ketamine	Morphine
Abscess I&D	Ketamine	Morphine	Remifentanil[c]
Laceration repair	Ketamine	Distraction	Fentanyl/midazolam
Acute agitation control	Droperidol	Lorazepam	Diazepam
Anxiolysis	Lorazepam	Diazepam	Pentobarbital
Nonurgent diagnostics	Sleep deprivation	Diphenhydramine	Midazolam
Scheduled outpatient diagnostic study	Sleep deprivation	Return to ED or sedation unit	Chloral hydrate

[a] This table contains potential sedation or analgesia regimens. Other medications are also applicable for these scenarios, and selection of agents depends on a combination of patient characteristics and individual physician preference. PCA, patient-controlled analgesia; RSI, rapid sequence intubation; I&D, incision and drainage.
[b] Risk of hypoxia with lateral positioning.
[c] Theoretical application at present.

- Localized extremity pain can be managed with regional anesthesia.
- PCA is an excellent option for any child old enough to use a delivery pump and is particularly useful for constant painful conditions that may take time to resolve, such as sickle cell crisis or pancreatitis.
- Sedation options for painless diagnostic studies are as much based on route of delivery as pharmacologic profile. For departments adept at obtaining vascular access, an intravenous route will allow titration of an agent and a shorter clinical duration of action. Infants and small toddlers may be candidates for intramuscular, oral, or transmucosal drugs.

The approach to PSA in **children with special health care needs** (CSHCN) is the same as for any other child except that selection of the PSA agent must take into account the child's acute problem and preexisting conditions.

- Coordination of sedation with a child's medication schedule should be attempted: neuropsychiatric or seizure medications may cause somnolence following routine dosing and a painless diagnostic study can be done during this time.
- Children with cardiovascular problems should be managed with agents such as fentanyl, which have little blood pressure or heart rate effects.
- Children with respiratory pathology or anatomic upper airway difficulties may best be served with regional anesthesia or a drug with minimal ventilatory effects, such as ketamine.
- Children with hepatic or renal failure may be more sensitive to drugs and titrated with smaller doses and more prolonged postprocedure observation.
- Emergency physicians should also not hesitate to involve anesthesiology colleagues to help with CSHCN patients, particularly those who are ASA class 3 or above.

BIBLIOGRAPHY

American College of Emergency Physicians: Clinical policy for procedural sedation and analgesia in the emergency department. *Ann Emerg Med* 31:663–677, 1998.

Berde CB, Sethna NF: Analgesics for the treatment of pain in children. *N Engl J Med* 347:1094–103, 2002.

Coté CJ, Notterman DA, Karl HW, et al: Adverse sedation events in pediatrics: A critical incident analysis of contributing factors. *Pediatrics* 105:805–814, 2000.

D'Agostino J, Terndrup TE: Chloral hydrate versus midazolam for sedation of children for neuroimaging: A randomized clinical trial. *Pediatr Emerg Care* 16:1–4, 2000.

Dickinson R, Singer A, Carrion W: Etomidate for pediatric sedation prior to fracture reduction. *Acad Emerg Med* 8: 74–77, 2001.

Green SM, Kupperman N, Rothrock SG, et al: Predictors of adverse events with intramuscular ketamine sedation in children. *Ann Emerg Med* 35:35–42, 2000.

Luhmann JD, Kennedy RM, Porter FL, et al: A randomized clinical trial of continuous flow nitrous oxide and midazolam for sedation of young children during laceration repair. *Ann Emerg Med* 37:1, 2001.

McQuillen KK, Steele DW: Capnography during sedation/analgesia in a pediatric emergency department. *Pediatr Emerg Care* 16:401–404, 2000.

Pomeranz ES, Chudnofsky CR, Deegan TJ, et al: Rectal methohexital sedation for computed tomography imaging of stable pediatric emergency department patients. *Pediatrics* 105:1110–1114, 2000.

Rodriguez E, Jordan R: Contemporary trends in pediatric sedation and analgesia. *Emerg Med Clin North Am* 20:199–222, 2002.

Sacchetti AD, Schafermeyer R, Gerardi M, et al: Pediatric analgesia and sedation. *Ann Emerg Med* 23:237–250, 1994.

Sherwin TS, Green SM, Khan A, et al: Does adjunctive midazolam reduce recovery agitation after ketamine sedation for pediatric procedures? A randomized double-blind placebo controlled trial. *Ann Emerg Med* 35:229–238, 2000.

QUESTIONS

1. A 5-year-old child with congenital heart disease presents to the ED with an angulated forearm fracture. The child is on multiple cardiac medications. You need to use PSA for the reduction but are concerned about the child's cardiovascular status and potential adverse interactions with the cardiac medications. Which of the following would be a good choice for PSA in this patient?
   A. Ketorolac
   B. Morphine
   C. Fentanyl
   D. Midazolam
   E. Propofol

2. A 16-year-old male is brought to the ED with a severe asthma attack. He is on albuterol and prednisone at home and has received albuterol by inhalation while en route to the hospital. He had been intubated twice in the past. On presentation, he is in severe respiratory distress, incoherent, and thrashing about on the cart. Which of the following would be the best choice for sedating this patient as you prepare to intubate him?
   A. Etomidate
   B. Propofol
   C. Chloral hydrate
   D. Ketamine
   E. Midazolam

3. A 40-kg child has been given midazolam, 0.4 mg IV (0.01 mg/kg) to sedate him for a complex laceration repair. A few minutes after administration of the medication, the child becomes agitated and tries to run away from his parents and you. What is the best course of action?

   A. Use physical restraints and proceed with the laceration repair.
   B. Defer the laceration repair until after psychiatric evaluation.
   C. The child is intolerant of benzodiazepines. Administer chloral hydrate, 2 g PO.
   D. A subtherapeutic dose of midazolam has been administered. Administer an additional dose of midazolam, 1.6 mg IV (0.05 mg/kg).
   E. Administer DPT, 40 mg/20 mg/20 mg IM; wait 5 min and proceed with the repair.

4. Which of the following statements is true regarding monitoring during procedural sedation and analgesia?
   A. Cardiac monitoring is generally not needed.
   B. Continuous blood pressure monitoring is required for all patients.
   C. Monitoring must be continued until the procedure is fully completed.
   D. Pulse oximetry will provide assessment of oxygenation, ventilation, and heart rate.
   E. In addition to performing the procedure, the physician should be vigilant in assessing the monitors throughout the procedure.

ANSWERS

1. C. Unlike other narcotics, fentanyl has few cardiovascular effects, making it appropriate for hypovolemic and cardiac patients. Ketorolac is a pure analgesic and would provide no sedation. Morphine, midazolam, and propofol all have the potential to produce hypotension.

2. D. Ketamine produces rapid sedation, analgesia, and amnesia. It can decrease bronchospasm, making it an excellent choice for use with an asthmatic patient.

3. D. Subtherapeutic doses of many sedatives will result in disinhibition and agitated, uncontrolled behavior. This is especially true of midazolam. It has been described as paradoxical hyperexcitability but is really just under-dosing of the medication. Treatment with additional doses will take the child through disinhibition to somnolence. Use of physical restraints during a procedure without sedation is barbaric and unnecessary. A psychiatric consult is not indicated. The child is not intolerant of benzodiazepines and chloral hydrate is a poor substitute for midazolam. It is slow acting and its side effects can persist for days. DPT is an illogical combination of drugs that works in an unpredictable and slow fashion. Proceeding with the procedure 5 min after administration would

be equivalent to doing the procedure without sedation or analgesia.

4. A. Cardiac monitoring is generally not needed unless the patient is hypovolemic or has cardiac problems. Blood pressures are assessed prior to the procedure and periodically monitored, especially if the child is hypovolemic or hypertensive. Monitoring must be continued until the effects of the drugs have worn off, not just until the procedure is done. Pulse oximetry allows you to monitor oxygenation and heart rate but does not monitor ventilation. A patient can be hypoventilating for some time before he or she begins to desaturate and become hypoxic. The person performing the procedure will not be able to pay adequate attention to the monitors. An additional healthcare provider is required to monitor the patient during the procedure.

25 UPPER AIRWAY EMERGENCIES

Richard M. Cantor
Kemedy K. McQuillen
Valerie A. Dobiesz

PATHOPHYSIOLOGY

AIRWAY CONSIDERATIONS

- The small caliber of the airway makes it vulnerable to occlusion, results in greater baseline airway resistance, causes an augmented degree of turbulence with any increase in respiratory effort, and causes an exponential rise in airway resistance and a secondary increase in the work of breathing with any process that narrows the airway
- The infant is primarily a nasal breather so any obstruction of the nasopharynx results in a significant increase in work of breathing.
- The young child's large tongue can occlude the oropharynx. Mental status depression can cause upper airway obstruction secondary to loss of muscle tone of the tongue. Tilting the head or lifting the chin can correct this blockage.
- Enlarged tonsils and adenoids are vulnerable to trauma during clinical interventions such as insertion of an oral or nasal airway.
- The pediatric trachea is distensible due to incomplete closure of semiformed cartilaginous rings. Overextension of the neck contributes to compression and secondary upper airway obstruction.
- The cricoid ring is the narrowest portion of the upper airway and is often the site of occlusion in foreign body aspiration.

- Immaturity of the musculoskeletal and central nervous systems can contribute to the development of respiratory failure.
- In infancy, the diaphragm is the primary respiratory muscle. Abdominal distention interferes with diaphragmatic function and causes secondary ventilatory insufficiency. Also, the infant's diaphragm possesses muscle fibers that are more prone to fatigue.
- The chest wall of the pediatric patient is very compliant, preventing adequate stabilization with increased respiratory distress.
- Infants are less sensitive to hypoxemia secondary to poor development of central respiratory control, and they may have an insufficient response to disease states.

SIGNS OF DISTRESS

- The work of breathing and respiratory rate increase to meet oxygen and ventilation requirements; respiratory failure ensues when respiratory efforts cannot maintain adequate respiratory function. Tachypnea (Table 10-3) is the most common response to increased respiratory needs. Although most commonly due to hypoxia and hypercarbia, tachypnea may also be secondary to metabolic acidosis, pain, or a central nervous system insult. Infants and children use accessory muscles as a compensatory mechanism to support the increased work of breathing. Nasal flaring, intercostal, subcostal, sub- and suprasternal, and supraclavicular retractions are commonly seen. Grunting, or the closure of the glottis at the end of expiration, generates additional positive end-expiratory pressure to prevent alveoli collapse and is an ominous sign.
- Children with upper airway compromise will assume a "position of comfort" to optimally maintain the

airway. Children with stridor will often assume an upright position, lean forward, and generate their own jaw thrust to facilitate opening of the upper airway. They may also prefer to breathe through an open mouth. Patients with lower airway disease will assume a "tripod position," consisting of upright posture, leaning forward, and support of the upper thorax by the use of extended arms. This allows for use of the thoraco abdominal axis for the work of breathing.

- With excessive negative intrathoracic pressure, venous return to the heart increases and left ventricular volume is compromised. This results in a pulsus paradoxus greater than 20 mm Hg (normal 0 to 10 mm Hg). An elevated pulsus paradox correlates with severe respiratory distress.
- Cyanosis is an ominous sign. It represents inadequate oxygenation or oxygen delivery. Respiratory cyanosis tends to be central and can improve with crying.

GENERAL MANAGEMENT PRINCIPLES

- Children with respiratory distress require supplemental oxygen. It can be delivered by mask with or without a rebreather apparatus, nasal prongs, face tent, oxygen hood, or oxygen tubing.
- Children in distress should be allowed to assume a position of comfort in a comfortable, nonthreatening environment. Avoid unnecessary procedures and maintain normothermia and hydration.
- Frequently assess the degree of respiratory distress. Consider obtaining an arterial blood gas: the Pa_{CO_2} provides an estimate of ventilatory sufficiency and the pH represents the balance between metabolic demand and respiratory expenditure. A normal or high level of Pa_{CO_2} suggests respiratory fatigue and may herald the rapid development of respiratory failure. Tachypnea does not guarantee adequate ventilation, since many patients cannot generate adequate tidal volumes and are effectively hypoventilating.
- Percutaneous oximetry only reflects oxygenation and may falsely represent the adequacy of ventilation. Using the pH, assess the degree of acidosis. The respiratory system is the primary compensatory mechanism for overall balance: in patients with excessive work of breathing, generation of lactate from respiratory musculature may remain uncompensated by hyperventilation, resulting in profound acidemia.
- Look for signs and symptoms of respiratory distress and failure including agitation, irritability, inability to feed, ineffective respiratory effort, and somnolence. There may be an increased work of breathing and respiratory rate or hypoventilation and apnea.

- Diaphoresis, retractions, grunting, and flaring may be present. Auscultation of the chest may reveal decreased air entry, poor breath sounds, and, ultimately, bradypnea: bradycardia results. Acidosis, hypercapnea, and hypoxemia may be seen on arterial blood gas.

ASSESSMENT AND MANAGEMENT OF SPECIFIC CLINICAL SCENARIOS

- Stridor, the hallmark of upper airway compromise, results from inspiratory turbulence through a narrow lumen. It may originate anywhere from the anterior nares to the subglottic region. In the infant, stridor is often the result of a congenital anomaly involving the tongue (macroglossia), larynx (laryngomalacia), and trachea (tracheomalacia). Congenital forms of stridor are often chronic in their presentation. The most common causes of **acute** upper airway obstruction are listed in Tables 25-1 and 25-2.

EPIGLOTTITIS (SUPRAGLOTTITIS)

- Epiglottitis is a true upper airway emergency that is potentially life-threatening. It occurs at any time of the year and in all age groups. Up to 25 percent of pediatric cases will be in infants less than 2 years of age.
- It can present acutely with fever, sore throat, dysphagia, a muffled voice or stridor, respiratory distress, and signs of toxicity. In severe cases, there may be profound drooling.
- The child often assumes a position of comfort by sitting upright, with the mouth open, and the head, neck, and jaw extended. Other children may present less acutely with a severe sore throat, dysphagia, and no respiratory distress. Croup-like presentations in patients who fail to respond to traditional therapies may also herald epiglottitis. Adults may only complain of a sore throat.
- Most cases of epiglottitis are caused by *H. influenzae* type b with accompanying bacteremia. Other agents include *Streptococcus pneumoniae*, *Staphylococcus aureus*, and group A beta-hemolytic streptococci. Blood cultures will be positive in 80 to 90 percent of affected individuals.
- If unrecognized, epiglottitis will be complicated by airway obstruction and respiratory arrest. Factors contributing to deterioration include patient fatigue, aspiration of secretions, and sudden laryngospasm.
- All maneuvers that agitate the child should be avoided, including separation from parents, alteration

TABLE 25-1   Features of Upper Airway Disorders

DISEASE PROCESS	AGE GROUP	MODE OF ONSET OF RESPIRATORY DISTRESS
Severe tonsillitis	Late preschool or school age	Gradual
Peritonsillar abscess	Usually >8 yr	Sudden increase in temperature, toxicity, and distress, with unilateral throat pain, "hot potato speech"
Retropharyngeal abscess	Infancy–3 yr	Fever, toxicity, and distress after URI or pharyngitis
Epiglottitis	2–7 yr	Acute onset of hyperpyrexia, with distress, dysphagia, and drooling
Croup	3 mo–3 yr	Gradual onset of stridor and barking cough, after mild URI
Foreign body aspiration	Late infancy–4 yr	Choking episode resulting in immediate or delayed respiratory distress

URI, upper respiratory infection.

TABLE 25-2   Clinical Features of Acute Upper Airway Disorders

	SUPRAGLOTTIC DISORDERS (EPIGLOTTITIS)	SUBGLOTTIC DISORDERS (CROUP)
Stridor	Quiet	Wet and loud
Voice alteration	Muffled	Hoarse
Dysphagia	+	−
Postural preference	+	−
Barky cough	−	+
Fever	+ +	+
Toxicity	+ +	−
Trismus	+	−

of optimal airway posture (lying down), fearful events (rectal temperatures, blood work, and radiographs), and gagging (forcible tongue blade examination of the oral cavity, suctioning).

- Diagnostic radiographs include anteroposterior and lateral views of the soft tissues of the neck. These radiographs should not be done if they cause agitation and airway compromise. Direct visualization, culture of the epiglottis, and intubation should be done in the operating suite by an expert in intubation. If the child decompensates prior to going to the operating suite, the ED physician should be prepared to manage the airway; bag-valve-mask (BVM), endotracheal intubation, needle cricothyrotomy, cricothyrotomy, and tracheostomy supplies should be immediately available. Attempt BVM ventilation first and, if unsuccessful, attempt intubation. If unable to intubate, perform a needle or surgical cricothyroidotomy.
- Give intravenous antibiotics (cefotaxime 50 mg/kg every 6 h) and transfer the patient to an intensive care unit.

CROUP (VIRAL LARYNGOTRACHEOBRONCHITIS)

- Croup is an infection that affects the upper respiratory tract and accounts for 90 percent of stridor with fever. The subglottic region is most commonly affected, resulting in edematous, inflamed mucosa with a fibrinous exudate.
- Infecting agents include parainfluenza types 1, 2, and 3 (most common); adenovirus; respiratory syncytial virus (RSV); and influenza.
- Winter is the peak season and it most commonly occurs in children between 1 and 3 years of age. They often present with several days of nonspecific upper respiratory infection (URI) symptoms followed by a characteristic brassy or barking cough, inspiratory stridor, and fever. Temperatures above 102°F or the presence of a toxic appearance are atypical but may indicate atypical epiglottitis or bacterial tracheitis. Symptoms tend to be exaggerated at night, worsen over 3 to 5 days, and resolve within the week.
- Uneventful recovery is the norm; however, a small percentage may develop complete upper airway obstruction.
- Scores that quantify the severity of croup are listed in Table 25-3.
  - Mild croup is treated on an outpatient basis if the child is able to take oral liquids, is well hydrated, and has reliable parents. Home therapy includes sitting in a steam-filled bathroom or going out into the cool night air. Discharge instructions should include follow up within 24 h and instructions to return if symptoms worsen.
  - Patients with mild to moderate croup can be discharged if the child improves with cool, humidified oxygen therapy, the parents are reliable, and the child is older than 6 months of age.

TABLE 25-3   Clinical Croup Score[a]

	SCORE
Inspiratory Breath Sounds	
Normal	0
Harsh with ronchi	1
Delayed	2
Stridor	
None	0
Inspiratory	1
Inspiratory and expiratory	2
Cough	
None	0
Hoarse cry	1
Bark	2
Retractions and Flaring	
None	0
Flaring, suprasternal retractions	1
As under 1, plus subcostal and intercostal retractions	2
Cyanosis	
None	0
In air	1
In 40% O_2	2

[a]A score of 4 or more indicates moderately severe airway obstruction. A score of 7 or more, particularly when associated with Pa_{CO_2} >45 and Pa_{O_2} <70 (in room air), indicates impending respiratory failure.

○ Patients with moderate croup (stridor at rest) tend to be treated as inpatients. Oxygen, cool mist, and racemic epinephrine (0.5 mL of a 0.25 percent solution dissolved in 2.5 mL of normal saline) delivered by nebulizer usually result in symptomatic improvement. The peak effect of racemic epinephrine is seen at 10 to 30 min, and it lasts up to 2 h. If stable, discharge of racemic epinephrine recipients after 2 to 3 h of ED observation is safe.

○ Children with severe croup may be treated with racemic epinephrine as often as every 20 min (as an inpatient) to avoid intubation. Corticosteroids (dexamethasone, 0.6 mg/kg/dose IM, PO, or nebulized) are helpful in preventing the progression of croup to complete obstruction and may shorten the duration of illness. With severe croup (score >10 or a 3 in any category), admit the child to an intensive care setting and treat with oxygen, mist, racemic epinephrine, and corticosteroids. Heliox may be useful with severe obstruction. If a child develops respiratory failure and requires intubation, an endotracheal (ET) tube 1 mm smaller than expected for age should be used. As with epiglottitis, in all cases of croup, allow the patient to assume a position of comfort. Obtain soft tissue radiographs of the neck if the diagnosis is in question.

BACTERIAL TRACHEITIS

• Bacterial tracheitis, also referred to as membranous tracheitis, is an infection of the subglottic region. It occurs in the same age group as croup; however, these children usually look toxic and have a high fever. Pus may be produced during spasms of brassy or barking cough and inspiratory and expiratory stridor may be present.

• Bacterial tracheitis can progress to full airway obstruction and, as with epiglottitis, airway management is best achieved in the operating room. Upon intubation, a normal epiglottis with subglottic pus, inflammation, and in some cases, a pseudomembrane, confirms the diagnosis.

• Infecting organisms include *S. aureus, Streptococcus* spp, *H. influenzae,* and *Pneumococcus.*

• Broad spectrum antibiotics, such as ceftriaxone or another third-generation cephalosporin, are required.

RETROPHARYNGEAL ABSCESSES

• Retropharyngeal abscesses are seen in children younger than 3 years old secondary to suppurative cervical lymphadenopathy and in older children, following penetrating trauma to the posterior oropharynx.

• Organisms include group A beta hemolytic *Streptococcus, S. aureus*, and anaerobes.

• Findings may include a stiff neck, high fever, muffled voice, difficulty swallowing, drooling, and, less frequently, inspiratory stridor. A swelling of the posterior pharynx wall is diagnostic. Visualizing the oral cavity and posterior pharynx is acceptable in an older cooperative child as long as it does not cause agitation.

• A lateral neck film will demonstrate swelling of the prevertebral soft tissue at the level of the pharynx and a normal epiglottis and aryepiglottic folds. Usually, a CT scan of the neck is not necessary but, if done, will identify soft tissue swelling and, in selected cases, the presence of air.

• Definitive therapy involves operative drainage of the abscess. Children with cellulitis without a collection of pus are treated with antibiotics. Antibiotics should cover the common organisms. Clindamycin is a good empiric choice. Treat severe airway obstruction with intubation under direct visualization to avoid abscess rupture. Observe children with partial airway obstruction in a PICU setting.

PERITONSILLAR ABSCESSES

- Peritonsillar abscesses tend to affect children over the age of 8 years. They are the most common deep infections of the head and neck, usually representing complications of bacterial tonsillitis or a superinfection of an Epstein-Barr infection.
- Most are polymicrobial in origin, including group A *Streptococcus* (predominant), *Peptostreptococcus, Fusobacterium,* and other mouth flora, including anaerobes.
- Patients present with drooling, dysphagia, a "hot potato" voice, and ipsilateral ear pain, with progression to trismus, dysarthria, and toxicity. The pharynx is erythematous, with unilateral tonsillar swelling that may displace the uvula and soft palate. Fluctuance may be present and cervical adenopathy is common.
- Complications include sternocleidomastoid spasm and torticollis, fascitis, mediastinitis, and airway obstruction.
- Laboratory evaluation includes a white blood cell count (elevated), throat culture, and testing for Epstein-Barr virus.
- An experienced otolaryngologist should perform direct tonsillar needle aspiration.
- Most patients require admission for drainage, intravenous hydration, and antibiotics (nafcillin or a third-generation cephalosporin).

FOREIGN BODY ASPIRATIONS

- Most foreign body aspirations occur in children younger than 5 years, with 65 percent of deaths affecting infants younger than 1 year.
- Common agents are foods (eg, peanuts, hard candies, and frankfurters) and items commonly found in the home (eg, disk batteries, coins, and marbles).
- Symptoms range from a mild cough to complete upper airway obstruction. Fifty percent of children will not have a history of foreign body ingestion or choking.
- Diagnostic radiographs include anteroposterior and lateral views of the upper airway from the nasopharynx to the carina. Inspiratory and expiratory chest radiographs and bilateral decubital views may be obtained to demonstrate the failure of the affected hemithorax to lose volume.
- Esophageal foreign bodies at the thoracic inlet or carina can impede the upper airway and mimic airway obstruction.
- If a child younger than 1 year has an acute airway obstruction, give four back blows followed by chest thrusts.
- If the child is older than 1 year, use repetitive abdominal thrusts. If unsuccessful, use direct laryngoscopy and Magill forceps to remove the foreign body. If still unsuccessful, attempt vigorous BVM ventilation in preparation for bronchoscopy.
- With an incomplete obstruction, provide supplemental oxygen, allow a position of comfort, avoid noxious stimuli, and arrange for controlled airway evaluation in the operating room.

BIBLIOGRAPHY

Bernstein T, Brilli R, Jacobs B: Is bacterial tracheitis changing? A 14-month experience in a pediatric intensive care unit. *Clin Infect Dis* 27:458–462, 1998.

Blotter JW, Yin L, Glynn M, et al: Otolaryngology consultation for peritonsillar abscess in the pediatric population. *Laryngoscope* 110:1698–1701, 2000.

Damm M, Eckel HE, Jungehulsing M, Roth B: Management of acute inflammatory childhood stridor. *Otolaryngol Head Neck Surg* 121:633–638, 1999.

Hvizdos KM, Jarvis B: Budesonide inhalation suspension: A review of its use in infants, children and adults with inflammatory respiratory disorders. *Drugs* 60:1141–1178, 2000.

Kumar RK, Mashell K: Acute epiglottitis. *J Pediatr Child Health* 34:594, 1998.

Malhotra A, Krilov LR: Viral croup. *Pediatr Rev* 22:5–12, 2001.

Perkin RM, Swift JD: Infectious causes of upper airway obstruction in children. *Pediatr Emerg Med Reports* 7:117–128, 2002.

Rittichier KK, Ledwith CA: Outpatient treatment of moderate croup with dexamethasone: Intravenous versus oral dosing. *Pediatrics* 106:1344–1348, 2000.

Rosekrans JA: Viral croup: Current diagnosis and treatment. *Mayo Clin Proc* 73:1102–1106, 1998.

White CB, Foshee WS: Upper respiratory tract infections in adolescents. *Adolesc Med* 11:225–249, 2000.

Wright RB, Pomerantz WJ, Luria JW: New approaches to respiratory infections in children: bronchiolitis and croup. *Emerg Med Clin North Am* 20:93–112, 2002.

QUESTIONS

1. Which of the following is **FALSE** regarding the pediatric airway?
   A. A child's tongue can occlude the oropharynx.
   B. The cricoid ring is the narrowest portion of the upper airway.
   C. Infants are less sensitive to hypoxemia.
   D. Enlarged tonsils and adenoids are vulnerable to trauma during airway interventions.
   E. Overextension of the neck is helpful in maintaining a patent airway.

2. A 2-year-old male arrives in the ED in moderate respiratory distress. He is noted to be grunting. Which of the following is true regarding this patient?
   A. Grunting is from accessory muscle use.
   B. Grunting is a good clinical indicator.
   C. Grunting generates additional positive end-expiratory pressure.
   D. This patient can be triaged as non urgent.
   E. There is no clinical significance to grunting.

3. A 10-year-old male asthmatic presents with a history of cough and wheezing for 2 days. On arrival, he is retracting and is tachypneic. He is sitting upright, leaning forward, and supporting himself with extended arms. Which of the following is most accurate regarding this patient?
   A. Pulse oximetry adequately reflects the ventilatory status,
   B. This patient does not require supplemental oxygen,
   C. A decreased Pa_{CO_2} level on his ABG would indicate respiratory failure.
   D. His tachypnea will provide adequate ventilation.
   E. Somnolence is an ominous finding in this patient.

4. A 5-year-old girl presents with a 1-day history of high fever, sore throat, stridor, and dysphagia. She appears toxic and has been drooling. She was previously healthy. Which of the following is true regarding her condition?
   A. The most common cause is *H. influenzae* type B.
   B. An immediate IV should be placed and antibiotics given.
   C. A tongue blade examination should be done.
   D. AP radiographs of the neck would reveal narrowing of the subglottic structures.
   E. This is a benign self-limited disease.

5. Which of the following is true regarding viral laryngotracheobronchitis?
   A. The most common etiology is respiratory syncytial virus.
   B. Summer is the peak season.
   C. The age range is typically 5 to 10 years.
   D. They have a characteristic brassy or barking cough.
   E. Treatment consists of broad spectrum antibiotics.

6. What is the most common organism causing bacterial tracheitis (membranous laryngotracheobronchitis)?
   A. *Mycoplasma*
   B. *Staphylococcus aureus*
   C. *H. influenzae*
   D. *Pneumococcus*
   E. *Pseudomonas*

7. A 2-year-old male presents to the ED with a high fever, muffled voice, and difficulty swallowing. He is noted to have swelling of the prevertebral soft tissue at the level of the pharynx on lateral neck radiographs. Which of the following is true regarding this condition?
   A. The condition typically occurs in children between 3 and 7 years of age.
   B. A swelling or mass in the posterior pharynx wall is diagnostic.
   C. Typically, the etiology is viral.
   D. Definitive treatment is tonsillectomy.
   E. CT scans are contraindicated in these patients.

8. A 15-year-old female presents with the complaint of a sore throat for 1 week, fever, trismus, muffled voice, and drooling. She has a displaced uvula on examination. Which of the following is true regarding this condition?
   A. The most common organism is viral.
   B. Cervical adenopathy is rare.
   C. Emergent tonsillectomy is indicated.
   D. Antibiotics are not indicated.
   E. Treatment includes hydration, antibiotics, and drainage of the infection by needle aspiration or I & D.

ANSWERS

1. E. Overextension of the neck contributes to compression and secondary upper airway obstruction and should be avoided in young children.

2. C. Grunting, or the closure of the glottis at the end of expiration, generates additional positive end-expiratory pressure to prevent alveoli collapse and is an ominous sign.

3. E. This patient is in respiratory distress and children with respiratory distress require supplemental oxygen. Pulse oximetry only reflects oxygenation and not the ventilatory status. A normal or high level of Pa_{CO_2} suggests respiratory fatigue or impending respiratory failure. Tachypnea does not guarantee adequate ventilation since many patients cannot generate adequate tidal volumes and are effectively hypoventilating. Signs and symptoms of respiratory distress and failure include agitation, irritability, inability to feed, and somnolence.

4. A. This patient has the classic presentation for acute epiglottitis and is most commonly caused by *H. influenzae* type B. All maneuvers that agitate the child such as blood draws, IV insertion, or insertion of a tongue blade should be avoided. Lateral neck x-rays reveal a swollen epiglottis similar to a thumbprint. This is a true upper airway emergency that is potentially life-threatening.

5. D. The most common cause of croup is parainfluenza virus. Winter is the peak season and it most commonly occurs in children between 1 and 3 years of age. Children often present with several days of nonspecific URI symptoms followed by a characteristic brassy or barking cough, inspiratory stridor, and fever. Treatment options consist of cool mist, oxygen, racemic epinephrine, and dexamethasone. Antibiotics are not needed.

6. B. The most common cause is *Staphylococcus aureus*. These patients present similar to croup but generally look toxic and have a high fever.

7. B. This patient has a retropharyngeal abscess, which is seen in children younger than 3 years old. A swelling or mass of the posterior pharynx wall is diagnostic. The etiology is bacterial and includes group A beta hemolytic *Streptococcus, S. aureus*, and anaerobes. Definitive treatment involves operative drainage of the abscess. A CT scan is not always necessary but can be helpful in establishing the diagnosis.

8. E. This patient has a peritonsillar abscess. Most are polymicrobial in origin, including group A *Streptococcus, Peptostreptococcus, Fusobacterium*, and anaerobes. Cervical adenopathy is common. Antibiotics, such as nafcillin or a third-generation cephalosporin, are indicated. Most patients require hydration, antibiotics, and drainage of the infection with either needle aspiration or incision and drainage. The patient may require admission.

26 ASTHMA

Kathleen Brown
Kemedy K. McQuillen
Patricia Lee

EPIDEMIOLOGY

- Asthma is the most common chronic disease of childhood and affects at least 5 percent of the population of the United States.
- Asthma was traditionally defined as an intermittent, reversible obstructive airway disease but it is now known to be a chronic inflammatory disorder of the airways. It manifests as recurrent episodes of wheezing, dyspnea, chest tightness, and cough. Episodes are associated with variable airflow obstruction that is usually reversible.

PATHOPHYSIOLOGY

- Asthma symptoms result from the synergistic effects of increased airway responsiveness, inflammation, mucus production, and submucosal edema.
  - Airway responsiveness, or the ease with which airways narrow in response to various nonallergic stimuli, is influenced by inhaled pharmacologic agents and physical stimuli. The level of airway responsiveness correlates with the severity of asthma symptoms and medication requirements.
  - Airway inflammation contributes to the development of obstruction and airway hyper-responsiveness, while increased mucus production and submucosal edema exacerbate obstruction.
  - The early bronchospastic response is an antigen-antibody reaction that causes mediators such as histamine, leukotrienes, and chemotactic factors to be released, attracting inflammatory cells to the area (Fig. 26-1).
- It is the convergence of these inflammatory cells that correlates with the late asthmatic response.
  - Eosinophils play a large role in this process by releasing substances that cause inflammation in the bronchial wall.
  - Histamine, which is released from mast cells, causes smooth muscle constriction and bronchospasm and increases mucosal edema and mucus secretion.
  - Leukotrienes cause smooth muscle contraction and mucosal edema.
  - These products also cause a sloughing of mucosal cells, which results in a loss of epithelium and exposure of nerve fibers to irritants.
  - An alteration of the sensory nerve endings may contribute to bronchial hyperreactivity. Once bronchial hyperactivity is present, nonspecific triggers may produce acute bronchospasm. Triggers include:
    - Upper respiratory infection (most common)
    - Inhaled allergens
    - Exercise
    - Cold air
    - Anxiety
- The chronic stage of asthma is caused by continuous or repeated exposure to allergens resulting in the development of fibrosis, remodeling of the bronchioles, and irreversible airway disease. Parasympathetic activity maintains airway tone and causes bronchoconstriction by stimulation of cholinergic receptors resulting in smooth muscle contraction and secretions from the submucosal glands. The sympathetic β2-adrenergic receptors in the bronchial tree do

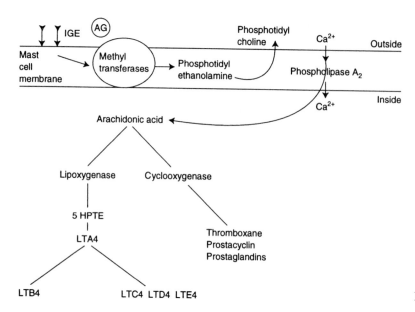

FIG. 26-1 Pathophysiology of asthma.

not play a role in maintaining airway tone, but are vital in reversing airway constriction.

- For the following reasons, children are more prone to obstruction and more vulnerable to respiratory failure than are adults:
  ○ The peripheral airways are smaller and offer greater resistance to airflow.
  ○ Infants do not possess the collateral ventilation channels that are present in older children and adults.
  ○ In infancy, the diaphragm is the primary muscle of respiration. Its fibers are more prone to fatigue and its excursion is easily compromised by abdominal distention.
  ○ The chest wall is very compliant, preventing adequate stabilization during periods of respiratory distress.

CLINICAL PRESENTATION

- Include in the history the patient's or parents' perception of the severity of the attack, precipitating factors, history of past attacks, medications (last doses, recent changes), and duration of symptoms. Ascertain if there is a family history of asthma, atopy, or allergic disease.
- Begin the physical examination with a general assessment of the patient's degree of distress by evaluating alertness, anxiety, fluid status, general health, positioning, ability to speak, and presence of cyanosis. Measure vital signs: tachycardia may be related to hypoxemia or previously administered medications;

increased respiratory rates are usually seen in asthmatic exacerbations, but the respiratory rate may decrease with fatigue in severe asthma. Listen to the lungs for wheezing that results from turbulent airflow. Initially present only on exhalation, wheezing progresses to involve inhalation as the obstruction worsens. The wheezing may be localized and may shift in location. If airway obstruction is severe, there will be little airflow and wheezing may not be present. Bronchospasm can also present as a persistent cough with clear lungs. In addition to wheezing, evaluate for diffuse or localized rales, asymmetric breath sound, tracheal deviation, or subcutaneous emphysema. Observe for the use of accessory muscles.

LABORATORY AND RADIOGRAPHIC FINDINGS

- Chest radiograph findings include hyperinflation, peribronchial cuffing, and subsegmental atelectasis. Chest radiographs should be done in a child who presents with first-time wheezing to exclude other etiologies (Table 26-1). They should also be done if there is suspicion of consolidation, effusion, pneumothorax, or impending respiratory failure.
- In children older than 5 years, spirometry should be used to assess the degree of respiratory compromise. The peak expiratory flow rate (PEFR), the simplest spirometry test, is employed most commonly. A PEFR less than 30 to 50 percent of predicted, or the patient's personal best, indicates severe airway obstruction.

TABLE 26-1   Differential Diagnosis in a Wheezing Infant

Anaphylaxis
Aspiration
Bronchiolitis
Bronchopulmonary dysplasia
Congestive heart failure
Cystic fibrosis
Extrinsic airway compression
Foreign body aspiration
Immotile cilia
Immune deficiency
Mediastinal masses
Pneumonia
Vascular rings

- Oximetry is another tool that may help assess severity. It correlates with ventilation perfusion mismatching and, therefore, the degree of obstruction.
- Blood gases are not necessary for most asthma flares but may be helpful with severe exacerbations. Early on, hypoxia will be present because of ventilation perfusion mismatching. P_{CO_2} will be decreased early in the disease secondary to compensatory hyperventilation. As the obstruction progresses, the number of alveoli being adequately ventilated and perfused decreases and CO_2 retention occurs. Thus a "normal" or slightly elevated P_{CO_2} in a patient with an asthma exacerbation may be a sign of muscle fatigue and impending respiratory failure. Eventually, the hypoxia and hypercapnia lead to acidosis.

DIFFERENTIAL DIAGNOSIS

- The diagnosis of asthma or reactive airways disease should be considered in all children with *recurrent* wheezing or episodic coughing and symptom-free intervals, especially if there is a family history of asthma, atopy, or allergies. A personal history of atopy or allergies is also suggestive of the diagnosis.
- The diagnosis of asthma depends on documentation of reversible airway disease with pulmonary function tests (PFTS). In general, children less than 6 years old are unable to perform these tests and are considered to have reactive airways disease based on presenting signs and symptoms.
- Table 26-1 lists other etiologies for wheezing in an infant or child: all that wheezes is not asthma.
  - A history of prematurity or ventilatory support will help in identifying the infant with bronchopulmonary dysplasia (BPD).
  - Cardiac examination may reveal other signs of cardiac failure in an infant with congenital heart disease.

- An association of signs and symptoms with feeding may suggest a tracheoesophageal fistula, gastroesophageal reflux, or recurrent aspiration.
- Clues to identifying the presence of a lower airway foreign body may come from the history (sudden onset, observed aspiration), chest examination (asymmetry), or radiographic studies (localized air trapping).
- A patient with cystic fibrosis may have clubbing of the digits, poor weight gain, or symptoms of malabsorption.

TREATMENT

- Every patient with an acute asthma exacerbation needs rapid cardiopulmonary assessment. The choice and intensity of therapy depend on the severity of the exacerbation and the patient's response to initial treatment. Recommended doses are summarized in Table 26-2.
  - **Oxygen** should be considered in all patients with acute asthma exacerbations. Hypoxia can lead to hypoventilation and acidosis causing pulmonary vasoconstriction, pulmonary hypertension, and right heart failure.
  - Asthmatic patients are often dehydrated due to vomiting or decreased intake and may require **intravenous fluids**. Closely monitor fluid administration, though, because acute asthma is associated with increased secretion of antidiuretic hormone, increased capillary permeability, and increased interstitial fluid; overhydration may result in pulmonary edema. Antibiotics should be used only if there is evidence of concurrent infection.
  - **β-Adrenergic agonists** remain the first line treatment in emergent asthma therapy. Bronchodilation is produced by stimulation of β2-adrenoreceptors, which mediate an increase in cyclic AMP via adenyl cyclase. Cyclic AMP stimulates binding of calcium ions to the cell membrane, reducing the mycoplasmal calcium concentration with resultant bronchodilation (smooth muscle relaxation) and stabilization of mast cells (Fig. 26-2). Stabilization of mast cells retards the release of histamine and other inflammatory products. β-agonists also improve mucociliary clearance.
  - **Aerosolized albuterol** is the most commonly used adrenergic agent in this country because it combines a long duration of action with β2 selectivity. It can be delivered by a metered dose inhaler (with an aerochamber or spacer) or a jet nebulizer. Only 10 percent of the output from an MDI and 1 to 5 percent of the output from a jet nebulizer produce particles in the 1- to 5-μm range that are deposited

TABLE 26-2   Medications for an Acute Asthma Exacerbation

MEDICATION	ROUTE	DOSE
β-Adrenergic agents		
Albuterol (5 mg/mL)	Nebulizer	0.15 mg/kg q15–20 min × 3; then q1–4h prn (minimum 2.5 mg, maximum 5 mg)
	Continuous nebulization	0.3–0.5 mg/kg/hr to 20 mg/hr
90 μg/puff	MDI	4–8 puffs q20 min × 3; then q1–4h prn
Epinephrine (1:1,000 solution)	SC	0.01 mg/kg (maximum 0.3 mg)
Terbutaline (0.1%)	SC	0.01 mg/kg (maximum 0.3 mg)
	IV	Loading dose 10 μg/kg Infusion 0.4 μg/kg/min; may titrate up to 6 μg/kg/min
Corticosteroids		
Methylprednisolone	IV	2 mg/kg (maximum 125 mg)
Prednisone/prednisolone	PO	ED dose: 2 mg/kg Discharge: 1–2 mg/kg/day × 5 days (maximum 60 mg)
Anticholinergics		
Ipratropium bromide (500 μg/2 mL)	Nebulizer	250–500 μg q20 min × 2–3 doses (usually with albuterol); then q2–4h prn
18 μg/puff	MDI	4–8 puffs as needed
Magnesium sulfate	IV	50–75 mg/kg over 20 min (maximum 2.5 g)
Ketamine	IV	Induction: 1–2 mg/kg

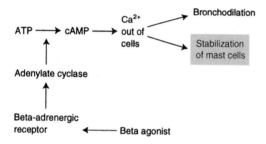

FIG. 26-2 Mechanism of action of β-adrenergic agonists.

in the lower airways. The rest of the particles escape into the room or are dissolved in mucus membranes and swallowed. Low flow rates (6 to 7 L/min) and greater breath-holding periods optimize drug deposition in the lower airways. Dosing is 0.15 mg/kg every 20 min or 0.3 mg/kg/h via continuous nebulization. Since so much of the drug escapes into the atmosphere, many physicians administer "unit doses" (usually 2.5 or 5 mg albuterol/3 mL NS) to all patients regardless of size. Repeat dosing should be guided by ongoing reassessment of the patient's clinical status. Other adrenergic medications are sometimes used in the treatment of acute asthmatic exacerbations.

○ Parenteral administration of **epinephrine** (0.01 mL/kg up to 0.3 mL of the 1:1000 solution subcutaneously) should be reserved for patients who are unable to generate adequate tidal volume to deliver aerosolized drug to the bronchial tree. It is more toxic and no more effective than albuterol.

○ **Subcutaneous terbutaline** (0.01 mg/kg up to 0.25 mg), which is more β2 specific, may be used as an alternative to subcutaneous epinephrine. It is preferred to subcutaneous epinephrine in the pregnant patient, because subcutaneous epinephrine has been associated with fetal malformations from decreased uterine blood flow.

○ **Intravenous terbutaline** is also safe and effective in pediatric patients with severe asthma exacerbations. Intravenous isoproterenol, previously used in severe asthmatics, causes significant cardiac toxicity, especially in hypoxic patients, and should be avoided.

○ **Older inhaled β-adrenergic agents** (isoetharine, metaproterenol) stimulate β1 and β2 receptors and have more undesirable side effects than albuterol.

○ **Inhaled epinephrine,** which is available without a prescription, is shorter acting than other inhaled β-agonists.

○ **Salmeterol,** a longer acting β2-agonist, has a slower onset than albuterol and is not intended for frequent repetitive administration.

○ **Levalbuterol** (Xiopenex) is the pure R-isomer of albuterol that was designed to provide bronchodilation with fewer side effects. Research results are mixed as to its efficacy.

○ β-adrenergic agonist side effects are largely due to sympathomimetic effects and include tremors, anxiety, nausea, headache, vomiting, tachycardia, arrhythmia, hypertension, and hypotension.

- Non-sympathomimetic side effects include decreased oxygen saturation (secondary to V/Q mismatching), which is common, and paradoxical bronchospasm, which is rare.
- Metabolic side effects, often related to dose and route of administration, include hypokalemia, hypophosphatemia, hyperglycemia, and lactic acidosis.

- When **corticosteroids** are used in the treatment of asthma, they decrease the duration and severity of symptoms, hospitalization rates, relapse rates, and the need for β-agonists. Corticosteroids reverse inflammation and restore responsiveness to β-adrenergics by increasing receptor numbers and lowering their threshold. Oral and parenteral corticosteroids are known to be equally efficacious with a benefit that occurs promptly enough to influence the patient's disposition from the ED. In the ED, 2 mg/kg of prednisone or its equivalent should be given as an initial bolus; it can be given orally or intravenously. Inhaled steroids in the acute setting may also be used. Corticosteroid toxicity is chiefly related to duration of use and not to dose: after a short course of therapy, adrenal suppression is minimal and clinically insignificant, immune suppression is clinically insignificant in patients with normal baseline immune function, growth suppression does not occur, and the incidence of adverse psychiatric effects is low.

- **Anticholinergics,** such as ipratropium bromide, act through interruption of parasympathetic transmission to the bronchial tree by decreasing the intracellular cyclic GMP (Fig. 26-3). This decreases bronchial tone and dilates the airways. The addition of nebulized ipratropium to the first three albuterol doses is associated with decreased hospitalization rates in children with moderate to severe asthma exacerbations. Side effects include dry mouth and a metallic taste.

- Currently, **methylxanthines** are rarely used in the treatment of acute asthma and do not contribute to bronchodilation with maximal β-agonist use. They have a narrow therapeutic-toxic window, with side effects including tachycardia, arrhythmias, nausea, vomiting, headaches, dizziness, and nervousness.

- **Magnesium** (50–75 mk/kg with a maximum dose of 2.5 g) produces bronchodilation via counteraction of calcium-mediated smooth muscle constriction. Its use in severe asthma exacerbations improves pulmonary function tests and decreases admission rates.

- **Heliox** ameliorates airway resistance and turbulence in the bronchi; may decrease work of breathing, delay fatigue, and respiratory failure; and facilitates medication delivery. Research on its benefit is inconclusive.

- Indications for **intubation and mechanical ventilation** of an asthmatic patient include decreased level of consciousness, apnea, exhaustion, a rising Pa_{CO_2} after treatment, $Pa_{O_2} > 60$ mm Hg, or a pH <7.2. Intubation does nothing to change lower airway obstruction and may not result in immediate improvement. It also puts the patient at risk for serious complications. When intubating an asthmatic patient, use the largest diameter tube appropriate for the patient's size to avoid increasing resistance. Although sedation is normally contraindicated in patients with asthma, sedation and paralysis may be accomplished with a modified rapid sequence induction using ketamine, known to have bronchodilatory properties, and succinylcholine. Pancuronium is thought to have bronchodilatory properties; however, its long duration of action outweighs this benefit. Vecuronium or rocuronium are recommended by most investigators when muscle paralysis is indicated for prolonged mechanical ventilation in a severe asthma exacerbation. Once intubated, patients with asthma will require sedation and paralysis to maintain effective ventilation. They should be allowed a long expiratory time to avoid air trapping and breath stacking. Watch for hypotension as intrinsic positive endexpiratory pressure (PEEP) can cause increased intrathoracic pressure with decreased venous return to the heart. Monitor intubated asthmatic patients carefully for the development of pneumothorax or pneumomediastinum. Ventilator settings should be adjusted to provide for adequate oxygenation with as low a peak pressure and PEEP as possible. The use of permissive hypercapnea with P_{CO_2} levels as high as 70 to 90 mm Hg is associated with decreased morbidity and mortality.

DISPOSITION AND OUTCOME

- Objective criteria are not helpful in determining disposition, however, the following risk factors are associated with increased mortality: previous intubation (greatest predictor of subsequent death), two or more

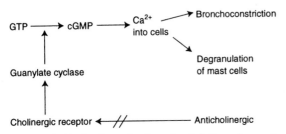

FIG. 26-3 Mechanism of action of anticholinergic agents.

hospitalizations in the last year, three or more ED visits in the last year, use of systemic steroids, rapid progression of attacks, hypoxic seizures, severe night-time wheezing, barotrauma, self-weaning from medications, lack of perception of the severity of the disease, poor medical management, poor access to medical care, and smoke exposure.

- Patients discharged from the ED should be started on a short course of corticosteroids and instructed to continue β-agonists. Steroid bursts for less than 5 days, if done no more than four times a year, do not require tapering. The most commonly used regimen is 1 to 2 mg/kg/day (maximum of 60 mg) of prednisone for 5 days. It can be given as a single daily dose at 7 to 8 AM to coincide with the surge in endogenous cortisol production or it can be given in divided doses to minimize gastrointestinal upset.

- Other drugs may be considered. Cromolyn sodium stabilizes mast cells and prevents histamine release. It is used for prophylaxis and has almost no toxicity. Monteleukast, a leukotriene receptor antagonist, is safe and effective in children as young as 4 years of age. The use of inhaled steroids is encouraged for chronic treatment in moderately severe asthmatics and the addition of inhaled steroids to oral steroids in patients discharged from the ED decreases the rate of relapse.

- Despite the mortality and morbidity associated with this disease, the prognosis for most children with asthma is good. At least half of all children with asthma will be symptom free by adulthood.

BIBLIOGRAPHY

Afilalo M, Guttman A, Colacone A, et al: Efficacy of inhaled steroids (beclomethasone dipropionate) for treatment of mild to moderately severe asthma in the emergency department: A randomized clinical trial. *Ann Emerg Med* 33:304–309, 1999.

Baren JM, Zorc JJ: Contemporary approach to the emergency department management of pediatric asthma. *Emerg Med Clin North Am* 20:115–138, 2002.

Chiang VW, Burns JP, Rifai N, et al: Cardiac toxicity of intravenous terbutaline for the treatment of severe asthma in children: A prospective assessment. *J Pediatr* 137:73–77, 2000.

Ciarallo L, Brousseau D, Reinert S. Higher-dose intravenous magnesium therapy for children with moderate to severe acute asthma. *Arch Pediatr Adolesc Med* Oct;154:979–983, 2000.

Gawchik SM, Saccar CL, Noonan M, et al: The safety and efficacy of nebulized levalbuterol compared with racemic albuterol and placebo in the treatment of asthma in pediatric patients. *J Allergy Clin Immunol* 103:615–621, 1999.

Laviolette M, Malmstrom K, Lu S, et al: Montelukast added to inhaled beclomethasone in treatment of asthma. *Am J Respir Crit Care Med* 160:1862–1868, 1999.

Parameswaran K, Belda J, Rowe BH: Addition of intravenous aminophylline to β-2 agonists in adults with acute asthma. *Cochrane Database of Systematic Reviews.* Issue 4, 2000.

Qureshi F: Management of children with acute asthma in the emergency department. *Pediatr Emerg Care* 15:206–214, 1999.

Rowe BH, Bota GW, Fabris L, et al: Inhaled budesonide in addition to oral corticosteroids to prevent asthma relapse following discharge from the emergency department: A randomized controlled trial. *JAMA* 281:2119–2126, 1999.

Rowe BH, Travers AH, Holroyd BR, et al: Nebulized ipratropium bromide in acute pediatric asthma: Does it reduce hospital admissions among children presenting to the emergency department? *Ann Emerg Med* 34:75–85, 1999.

Schuh S, Reisman J, Alshehri M, et al. A comparison of inhaled fluticasone and oral prednisone for children with severe acute asthma. *N Engl J Med* 343:689–694, 2000.

Stephanopoulos DE, Monge R, Schell KH, et al: Continuous intravenous terbutaline for pediatric status asthmaticus. *Crit Care Med* 26:1744–1748, 1998.

QUESTIONS

1. Children with asthma are more prone to respiratory failure than adults because of all of the following **EXCEPT**:
   A. Smaller peripheral airways
   B. Lower resistance to flow
   C. Lack of collateral ventilation channels
   D. Diaphragm is primary muscle of respiration
   E. Chest wall has increased compliance

2. A 2-year-old presents with sudden onset wheezing. Physical examination reveals decreased breath sounds on the right lung fields with minimal response after albuterol. Chest radiography shows hyperinflation of right lung. Appropriate management should be:
   A. Admission for bronchoscopy
   B. Continuous nebulizer therapy
   C. Antibiotic therapy
   D. Chest tube
   E. Corticosteroid

3. Asthma may be suggested by all of the following chest radiographic findings except:
   A. Pleural effusion
   B. Hyperinflation
   C. Peribronchial cuffing
   D. Subsegmental atelectasis
   E. Small cardiac silhouette

4. Severe airway obstruction is indicated with what value for the peak expiratory flow rate?
   A. 10%

B. 10 to 20%
C. 20 to 25%
D. 25 to 30%
E. 30 to 50%

5. Which of the following statements is **FALSE** regarding the interpretation of arterial blood gas in an asthmatic patient?
   A. The P_{CO_2} level will be low early in the disease.
   B. The P_{CO_2} level will be high early in the disease.
   C. Hypoxia will be present because of ventilation perfusion mismatching.
   D. A normal blood gas can be found in a patient with severe asthma exacerbation.
   E. Hypoxia and hypercapnia can lead to acidosis.

ANSWERS

1. B. Children's airways are smaller and thus have an increased resistance to flow.
2. A. The sudden onset of wheezing in a child without previous asthma accompanied by the findings in a single lung with hyperinflation suggests the presence of an inhaled foreign body. The child should be evaluated by bronchoscopy if no improvement with β-agonist agents.
3. A. Chest radiographs should be done in a child who presents with first-time wheezing. Typical findings are hyperinflation, peribronchial cuffing, subsegmental atelectasis, and a small cardiac silhouette.
4. E. A peak expiratory flow rate (PEFR), is employed commonly to evaluate the amount of respiratory compromise. A PEFR less than 30 to 50% of predicted or the patient's personal best, indicates severe airway obstruction.
5. B. Early in the disease, the P_{CO_2} will decrease due to compensatory hyperventilation. Early on, hypoxia will be present because of ventilation perfusion mismatching. As the obstruction progresses, the number of alveoli being adequately ventilated and perfused decreases and CO_2 retention occurs. Thus a "normal" or slightly elevated P_{CO_2} in a patient with an asthma exacerbation may be the sign of muscle fatigue and impending respiratory failure. Eventually, the hypoxia and hypercapnia lead to acidosis.

27 BRONCHIOLITIS

Kathleen Brown
Kemedy K. McQuillen
Patricia Lee

EPIDEMIOLOGY

- Bronchiolitis occurs almost exclusively in children younger than 2 years old.
- It is most common between the ages of 2 and 6 months, accounts for approximately 17 percent of all infant hospitalizations, and is most common in winter and spring.
- The most common etiologic agent is respiratory syncytial virus (RSV). Other pathogens include parainfluenza, influenza, mumps, adenovirus, echovirus, rhinovirus *Mycoplasma pneumoniae* (in school aged children) and, *Chlamydia trachomatis*. Adenovirus is associated with a particularly severe form of bronchiolitis that can lead to bronchiolitis obliterans.

PATHOPHYSIOLOGY

- Infection produces inflammation of the bronchiolar epithelium, which leads to necrosis, sloughing, and luminal obstruction. As ciliated epithelium sloughs, it is replaced by cuboidal cells that cannot mobilize secretions and debris. Edema also contributes to airway obstruction. The obstruction of the bronchioles and small bronchi is not uniform throughout the lungs and this causes ventilation/perfusion mismatching and hypoxia. The hypoxia leads to compensatory hyperventilation, air trapping, and atelectasis. If the obstruction is severe, hypercapnia may occur. The epithelium usually regenerates within 3 to 4 days, however, functional regeneration of ciliated epithelium takes about 2 weeks.
- In bronchiolitis obliterans, the destruction of the normal ciliated epithelium is extensive and the normal cells are replaced by stratified undifferentiated epithelium with an intense inflammatory response that extends to the alveoli. During the reparative phase, fibrosis and scarring lead to small airway obliteration.

CLINICAL PRESENTATION

- Typically, a child with bronchiolitis will have a runny nose, low-grade fever, and decreased appetite for 1 to 2 days prior to the development of tachypnea and increased work of breathing. In some children, lower tract symptoms may develop over hours. Hyperventilation with respiratory rates of 70 to 90 breaths/min is not uncommon. There may be nasal flaring and intercostal retractions. The chest is often hyperexpanded and hyperresonant and respirations may be shallow due to the air trapping. Wheezing, prolonged expiration, and musical rales are common. The liver and spleen may be displaced downward because of hyperinflation and flattening of the diaphragm. Respiratory thoracoabdominal asynchrony correlates with the degree of obstruction. Fever is often present. Despite these findings, the patient usually appears nontoxic. Respiratory fatigue can occur and apnea is not uncommon, especially in very young and premature infants. It generally occurs early in the illness, often prior to the onset of other respiratory symptoms.

LABORATORY AND RADIOGRAPHIC FINDINGS

- A chest radiograph is useful in ruling out the other disease processes. It may reveal hyperinflation, peribronchial cuffing (thickening of the bronchiole walls), and subsegmental atelectasis.
- A leukocyte count is usually within the normal range. Viral cultures or rapid tests (complement fixation or indirect immunofluorescent antibody testing) may be useful in confirming the diagnosis.
- Hypoxia is common, and oxygen saturation should be assessed with a pulse oximeter.
- Respiratory rates higher than 60 breaths/min correlate well with hypercarbia.

DIFFERENTIAL DIAGNOSIS

- The differential diagnosis for bronchiolitis is the same as for asthma (see Table 26-1). Response to bronchodilators does not exclude bronchiolitis, since some children with bronchiolitis may have some degree of bronchospasm. Congenital heart disease, cystic fibrosis, vascular rings, other congenital anomalies, and foreign body aspirations may mimic bronchiolitis.

TREATMENT

- Monitor patients with oximetry and provide **oxygen** as needed.
- Administer **intravenous hydration** judiciously if children have difficulty drinking secondary to their

increased work of breathing. Avoid overhydration as it may cause pulmonary edema.
- Administer a broad spectrum **antibiotic**, such as cefuroxime, if a bacterial superinfection is suspected.
- The role of **corticosteroids** in the treatment of bronchiolitis is controversial. Most studies suggest they are of no benefit, however, newer research is challenging this belief.
- The use of **bronchodilators** is also controversial. Most investigators recommend that patients with bronchiolitis, especially those with a history of wheezing, should be given a trial of a β-adrenergic agent. If there is no response to the trial dose, then therapy should be discontinued. Nebulized epinephrine has also been shown to be beneficial in the treatment of bronchiolitis.
- **Ribavirin** is an antiviral drug that may reduce the duration of mechanical ventilation in children with a lower respiratory infection due to RSV. The current recommendation suggests that its use should be based on clinical circumstances and the experience of the physician.
- **RSV immunoglobulin** can be used to prevent or attenuate RSV infection in high-risk neonates.
- Two to five percent of infants hospitalized for bronchiolitis will require **mechanical ventilation**. Suggested indications include P_{CO_2} of 60 to 65 mm Hg, recurrent apneic spells, decreasing mental status, and hypoxia despite O_2 therapy. Complications of intubation and mechanical ventilation include air trapping and the development of air leaks.
- Nasal or endotracheal **continuous positive airway pressure** may circumvent the need for mechanical ventilation.
- For patients unresponsive to conventional therapy, **extracorporeal membrane oxygenation** may be helpful.

DISPOSITION AND OUTCOME

- Bronchiolitis is a short-lived, self-limited disease that lasts a few days and most patients do not require admission. Follow-up within 24 hours is recommended for those who are discharged.
- Suggested criteria for admission include age (adjusted for prematurity) younger than 6 weeks, hypoxemia, persistent respiratory distress, and dehydration. Children with a history of prematurity, congenital heart disease, bronchopulmonary dysplasia, underlying lung disease, or compromised immune function are at the highest risk for morbidity and mortality and should also be admitted. The mortality rate for infants with RSV bronchiolitis is 1 to 3 percent; however, the

mortality rate for infants with congenital heart disease and RSV bronchiolitis is 37 percent. Fifteen to 30 percent of infants hospitalized for bronchiolitis require admission to an intensive care unit for ventilatory support.

- Up to 50 percent of infants with RSV bronchiolitis will go on to have recurrent wheezing. The only factor shown to increase the likelihood of subsequent wheezing is a family history of asthma or atopy. Patients with bronchiolitis obliterans have a much poorer prognosis and usually develop debilitating chronic lung disease.

BIBLIOGRAPHY

Cade A, Brownlee KG, Conway SP, et al: Randomized placebo controlled trial of nebulized corticosteroids in acute respiratory syncytial viral bronchiolitis. *Arch Pediatr Adolesc Med* 82:126–130, 2000.

Dobson JV, Stephens-Groff SM, McMahon SR, et al: The use of albuterol in hospitalized infants with bronchiolitis. *Pediatrics* 101:361–368, 1998.

Flores G, Horwitz RI: Efficacy of β_2-agonists in bronchiolitis: A reappraisal and metaanalysis. *Pediatrics* 100:233–239, 1997.

Garrison MM, Christakis DA, Harvey E, et al: Systemic corticosteroids in infant bronchiolitis: A meta-analysis. *Pediatrics* 105:44, 2000.

Hall CB: Respiratory syncytial virus a: A continuing culprit and conundrum. *J Pediatr* 135:S2–S7, 1999.

Kellner JD, Ohlsson A, Gadomoski AM, et al: Bronchodilators for bronchiolitis. *Cochrane Database of Systematic Reviews* Issue 4, 2000.

Linzer JF, Guthrie CC: Managing a winter season risk: bronchiolitis in children. *Pediatr Emerg Med Reports* 8:13–24, 2003.

Randolph AG, Wang EL: Ribavirin for respiratory syncytial virus infection of the lower respiratory tract. *Cochrane Database of Systematic Reviews* Issue 4, 2000.

Richter H, Seddon P: Early nebulized budesonide in the treatment of bronchiolitis and the prevention of postbronchiolitic wheezing. *J Pediatr* 132:849–853, 1998.

Rodriguez WJ: Management strategies for respiratory syncytial virus infections in infants. *J Pediatr* 135:S45–S50, 1999.

Schuh S, Coates AL, Binnie R, et al. Efficacy of oral dexamethasone in outpatients with acute bronchiolitis. *J Pediatr* 140:27–32, 2002

Wright RB, Pomerantz WJ, Luria JW: New approaches to respiratory infections in children: bronchiolitis and croup. *Emerg Med Clin North Am* 20:93–112, 2002.

QUESTIONS

1. Bronchiolitis obliterans is most commonly caused by:
   A. Adenovirus
   B. *Chlamydia trachomatis*
   C. Respiratory syncytial virus
   D. Parainfluenza virus
   E. Influenza virus

2. A 4-month-old female presents to the emergency department with a runny nose, fever of 100.8°F, decreased appetite, and increased respiratory rate. On examination, the child is found to be tachypneic with diffuse wheezing. Chest radiograph reveals hyperinflation and peribronchial cuffing. An RSV aspirate is positive. If the child should require mechanical ventilation, what medication has been found to reduce the duration of mechanical ventilation?
   A. Cephalosporin
   B. Ribavirin
   C. Corticosteroid
   D. Albuterol
   E. Nebulized epinephrine

3. All of the following are risk factors for increased morbidity or mortality in children with bronchiolitis **EXCEPT**:
   A. Bronchopulmonary dysplasia
   B. Previous pneumonia
   C. Congenital heart disease
   D. Prematurity
   E. Immunocompromise

4. What percentage of infants with RSV bronchiolitis will go on to have recurrent wheezing?
   A. 20%
   B. 33%
   C. 50%
   D. 70%
   E. 80%

ANSWERS

1. A. Adenovirus is associated with a particularly severe form of bronchiolitis that can lead to bronchiolitis obliterans.

2. B. Ribavirin is an antiviral drug that may reduce the duration of mechanical ventilation in children with a lower respiratory infection due to RSV.

3. B. Suggested criteria for admission include age (adjusted for prematurity) <6 weeks, hypoxemia, persistent respiratory distress, and dehydration. Children with a history of prematurity, congenital heart disease, bronchopulmonary dysplasia, underlying lung disease,

or immunocompromise are at the highest risk for morbidity and mortality and should be admitted.

4. C. Up to 50% of infants with RSV bronchiolitis will go on to have recurrent wheezing.

28 PNEUMONIA

Kathleen Brown
Kemedy K. McQuillen
Patricia Lee

EPIDEMIOLOGY

- Pneumonia is an inflammation of the lung tissue, most commonly caused by infection, and is defined by pulmonary infiltrates on a chest radiograph. It is more frequent in childhood than any other age and the incidence varies inversely with age.
- Seasonal variations occur, especially among viral etiologies: parainfluenza occurs most commonly in the fall, respiratory syncytial virus (RSV) in the winter, and influenza in the spring. Bacterial pneumonia occurs throughout the year but is more common in the colder months when crowding promotes transmission of infectious agents. *Mycoplasma pneumoniae* and *Chlamydia trachomatis* disease is endemic, although *M. pneumoniae* may cause epidemic outbreaks, particularly in the fall.

ETIOLOGY

- The predominant pathogens that cause pneumonia in infants and children are dependent on age of the patient, vaccination status, presence of underlying disease, daycare attendance, and exposure history. Table 28-1 summarizes the most common etiologic agents by age group. The immediate newborn period is the only time when pneumonia is most frequently bacterial. Most infections in this age group are caused by aspiration of the organisms that colonize the mother's genital tract. Beyond the neonatal period, most (60 to 90 percent) pneumonias are nonbacterial. Infrequent viral agents, not listed in the table, include rhinoviruses, measles, and varicella.
- Infants between 3 weeks and 3 months old may develop afebrile pneumonia (pneumonitis syndrome) typified by cough, tachypnea, and sometimes respiratory distress in the absence of fever. It is most commonly

TABLE 28-1   Common Etiologies of Pneumonia

AGE	VIRAL AGENTS	BACTERIAL AGENTS
Birth–2 weeks	CMV, HSV, Rubella	Group B *Streptococcus* *Escherichia coli* and other coliforms *Listeria monocytogenes*
2 weeks–2 mo	RSV Adenovirus Influenza EBV Parainfluenza	*Staphylococcus aureus* *Haemophilus influenzae* *Streptococcus pneumoniae* *Chlamydia trachomatis*
2 mo–3 yr	RSV Parainfluenza Adenovirus Influenza EBV	*S. pneumoniae* *Mycoplasma pneumoniae* *S. aureus* *H. influenzae*
3–12 yr	Influenza Adenovirus Parainfluenza EBV	*M. pneumoniae* *S. pneumoniae*
13–19 yr	Influenza Adenovirus Parainfluenza EBV	*M. pneumoniae* *S. pneumoniae*

CMV, cytomegalovirus; HSV, herpes simplex virus; RSV, respiratory syncytial virus; EBV, Epstein–Barr virus.

caused by viral infections but may also be caused by *C. trachomatis, Mycoplasma hominis,* and *Ureaplasma urealyticum.*
- Once children reach school age, *M. pneumoniae* is the most frequent bacterial cause of pneumonia however *S. pneumoniae* remains a common pathogen.
- Gram-negative bacilli, including *Pseudomonas,* should be considered in patients who have recently been hospitalized and anaerobic infections should be considered in children at risk for aspiration. Immunocompromised hosts are susceptible to all the infectious agents previously listed, as well as opportunistic organisms such as *Pneumocystis carinii,* CMV, and fungal disease.
- Unusual causes of bacterial pneumonia include *Mycobacterium tuberculosis, Legionella pneumophila, Chlamydia psittaci, Francisella tularensis,* and rickettsial infections. There has also been a resurgence of virulent group *A. Streptococcus* pneumonia.

PATHOPHYSIOLOGY

- There are a number of mechanisms that protect the lung from infection. Normally, infectious particles are filtered in the nose, entrapped and cleared by the mucus and ciliated epithelium in the respiratory tract, or eliminated by alveolar macrophages or systemic, humoral, and cell-mediated immune mechanisms.

Additionally, infants have maternal antibodies that protect them from several infectious agents. Alterations in any of these mechanisms may predispose a child to pneumonia.

- In a child without predisposing abnormalities, the infectious agent most commonly gains access to the lung secondary to a viral upper respiratory tract infection. The virus may spread contiguously to the lower respiratory tract or it may damage the normal defense mechanisms, allowing bacteria to infect the lower respiratory tract. The bacteria may normally colonize the child's upper airway or be transmitted person to person by airborne droplet spread. Less commonly, infecting agents (e.g., varicella, measles, rubella, CMV, EBV, and HSV) may be acquired through hematogenous spread.

- Once bacteria enter the lung, an acute inflammatory response ensues and causes fluid exudation, fibrin deposition, and infiltration of alveoli with polymorphonuclear leukocytes followed by macrophages. The fluid in the alveoli creates the lobar consolidation seen on chest radiograph. Viral agents, *Mycoplasma*, and *Chlamydia* cause inflammation with a predominantly mononuclear infiltrate of submucosal and interstitial structures. This leads to sloughing of epithelial cells into the airways.

CLINICAL PRESENTATION

- Presentation varies with patient age, causative agent, and disease severity.
  - Older children tend to present with fever, pleuritic chest pain, dyspnea, increased sputum production, and tachypnea. In the newborn, pneumonia tends to present as part of a sepsis syndrome, whereas in the infant, the symptoms may be nonspecific and include fever, apnea, poor feeding, abdominal pain, vomiting or diarrhea, hypothermia, grunting, bradycardia, lethargy, or shock.
- The history may also suggest the etiologic agent.
  - Viral pneumonia tends to have a gradual onset, is often preceded by upper respiratory symptoms, and may be associated with a rash.
  - Bacterial pneumonia may also be preceded by a viral upper respiratory infection but has a more sudden onset with fever, chills, lethargy, and poor intake with or without pleuritic chest pain.
    - *S. aureus* pneumonia is notorious for having a particularly rapid symptom progression.
    - A history of a maternal chlamydial infection during pregnancy or neonatal conjunctivitis (present in 50 percent of cases) suggests *C. trachomatis* pneumonia.

- *M. pneumoniae* pneumonia presents insidiously with malaise, fever, headache, and sore throat. Cough usually begins 3 to 5 days after the onset of illness. Patients with underlying disorders may manifest an increased severity of disease.
  - Physical examination findings vary with patient age, microbial etiology, and infection severity. Tachypnea is the most frequent sign; however, tachypnea is nonspecific and may occur with fever, anxiety, metabolic disease, cardiac disease, or other respiratory problems. Conversely, the best physical examination finding for excluding pneumonia is the absence of tachypnea. Normal respiratory rates are listed in Table 10-4. Auscultatory findings are less reliable in children but may include localized rales, wheezing, and decreased air entry. In younger children, decreased breath sounds rather than rales are often noted. Infants may have grunting respirations. Abdominal distention and pain may be present. Severe pneumonia may be associated with altered mental status, accessory muscle use, retractions, nasal flaring, splinting, and cyanosis. Infants may demonstrate paradoxical breathing.
  - Physical findings give clues as to the etiologic agent. Viral pneumonia causes diffuse findings on chest examination and will often cause wheezing, prolonged expiration, and hyperinflation. Bacterial pneumonia tends to produce more localized findings, fever, and signs of toxicity. An infant with chlamydial pneumonia is usually afebrile and nontoxic appearing with a distinct staccato cough (ie, short, abrupt onset) and diffuse rales on auscultation. Patients with *Mycoplasma* pneumonia have pharyngitis and rales. Ten percent of these patients will also have a rash, which may be papular, vesicular, urticarial, or erythema multiforme–like.

LABORATORY AND RADIOGRAPHIC FINDINGS

- Chest radiographs may show diffuse interstitial infiltrates, hyperinflation, peribronchial thickening, and atelectasis with viral pneumonia and segmental or lobar consolidation with bacterial infection. However, these findings are not an absolute and cannot be used to determine treatment.

- Blood cultures should be obtained in infants who have high fever, appear ill, or require hospitalization. They are positive in approximately 10 percent of patients with pneumococcal disease and more frequently with *S. aureus*, HIB, and group A streptococcal pneumonias.

- Sputum cultures may isolate the causative organism but are difficult to obtain in children younger than 8 years old.
- Nasopharyngeal cultures and rapid tests may isolate viruses, *Chlamydia*, pertussis, and *Mycoplasma*.
- Bacterial antigen testing is available but is not very sensitive or specific. Serologic testing can also be done for viruses, *Mycoplasma*, parasites, and fungi.
- Skin testing for tuberculosis should be considered in patients with apical, cavitary pneumonias or those not responding to traditional therapy.
- More invasive diagnostic procedures, such as endotracheal cultures, percutaneous lung puncture, bronchoalveolar lavage, or open lung biopsy, may be necessary in immunocompromised patients or in those with severe disease that is unresponsive to empiric therapy.
- In bacterial pneumonia, the white blood count is usually elevated with a left shift. Lymphocytosis is common with viral, chlamydial, and pertussis pneumonias although, initially, viral pneumonia provokes a significant polymorphonuclear cell response.
  ○ Children with hemoglobinopathies, such as sickle cell disease, may develop a leukemoid reaction (ie, extreme leukocytosis) with a viral pneumonia.
  ○ Patients with mycoplasmal pneumonia tend to have normal white blood cell and differential counts and an elevated erythrocyte sedimentation rate.
  ○ Chlamydial and parasitic infections often produce an eosinophilia.
- Cold agglutinins have been demonstrated to be positive in up to 92 percent of patients with *M. pneumoniae* but may also be positive in viral infections. They are less consistently positive in young children. To perform the bedside test for cold agglutinins, place several drops of blood in a coagulation profile tube and place in ice water for 15 to 30 s. The presence of floccular agglutination is considered a positive test: the agglutination should disappear upon rewarming.

DIFFERENTIAL DIAGNOSIS

The differential diagnosis of pneumonia includes congestive heart failure, atelectasis, primary and metastatic tumors, and congenital abnormalities, such as pulmonary hypoplasia or congenital lobar emphysema. Conditions that may simulate pneumonia on x-ray include radiologic imaging problems (ie, poor inspiration, prominent thymus), recurrent or acute aspiration, atelectasis, tumors, collagen vascular disorders, allergic alveolitis, chronic pulmonary diseases (eg, cystic fibrosis, asthma), and congenital abnormalities (eg, pulmonary sequestration).

TREATMENT

- Assess the patient for hypoxia and provide oxygen if needed. Provide additional respiratory support as dictated by the patient's condition. Assess the patient's fluid status and, if necessary, provide hydration.
- Most children with pneumonia can be managed as outpatients. If a bacterial etiology is suspected, start the child on an appropriate antibiotic based on the most likely etiologic organism (Table 28-2). Arrange 24-h follow up for all children who are discharged.
- Indications for admission include:
  ○ Hypoxia
  ○ Respiratory distress
  ○ Toxic appearance
  ○ Dehydration
  ○ Age less than 3 months
  ○ Impaired immune function
  ○ Infections unresponsive to oral therapy
  ○ The presence of underlying disease and the ability of the caregivers to provide care should also be considered.
  ○ Age younger than 1 year or the finding of a pleural effusion or pneumatocele on chest x-ray suggests a pathogen other than *S. pneumoniae* (particularly HIB or *S. aureus*). These infections can be rapidly progressive: consider hospitalizing these patients.
- Provide empiric intravenous antibiotic therapy for those who require admission. Empiric coverage should be guided by the age of the patient.
  ○ In the newborn, ampicillin in combination with an aminoglycoside or a third-generation cephalosporin is preferred. The ampicillin provides coverage against *Listeria* and *Enterococcus* species.

TABLE 28-2   Empiric Parenteral Antibiotic Therapy for Inpatient Treatment of Pneumonia in Immunocompetent Patients

AGE	THERAPEUTIC AGENT(S)
0–1 mo	Ampicillin + aminoglycoside or ampicillin + cefotaxime
1–3 mo	Ampicillin + cefotaxime (consider erythromycin or clarithromycin if *Chlamydia* pneumonitis is suspected)
3 mo–5 yr	Cefuroxime, cefotaxime, or ceftriaxone (consider the addition of a macrolide if the patient's course is suspicious for *Mycoplasma pneumoniae*)
>5 yr	Macrolide (consider adding cefuroxime in severely ill patients)
All ages	Add vancomycin, if resistant *Streptococcus pneumoniae* is suspected. If the patient's course is suspicious for *Staphylococcus aureus* infection, consider addition of an antistaphylococcal agent.

- In children with afebrile pneumonia or pneumonitis syndrome, treatment should consist of erythromycin or clarithromycin.
- In children older than 3 months, a cephalosporin alone (cefuroxime, cefotaxime, or ceftriaxone) is sufficient. In children who are unresponsive to this therapy or with a suggestive clinical presentation, a macrolide antibiotic should be used to treat presumptive *Mycoplasma* and chlamydial infections.
  - If staphylococcal disease is suspected, nafcillin should be added.
  - Ceftazidime or ceftriaxone should be used for a nosocomial pneumonia and ceftazidime for pneumonia caused by *Pseudomonas aeruginosa.*
  - Children with cystic fibrosis often develop acute infectious exacerbations secondary to *S. aureus* and *Pseudomonas,* often with resistance to standard antibiotics. The duration of therapy varies with the clinical response, predisposing host factors, and suppurative complications: 7 to 10 days is sufficient for most uncomplicated cases.
  - Parenteral therapy, if initiated, should be continued until clinical improvement occurs.
  - Whenever the case of pneumonia is complicated or prolonged, roentgenographic follow-up at 4 to 6 weeks is recommended to ensure complete resolution.
- If viral pneumonia is suspected, antibiotic therapy is not warranted.
  - In RSV pneumonia, ribavirin therapy should be considered utilizing the guidelines discussed for bronchiolitis in Chapter 27.
  - Children with fulminant viral pneumonias, such as varicella in the immunocompromised host, may require treatment with acyclovir.
  - Lymphocytic interstitial pneumonia in HIV positive children should include a combination of prednisone and zidovudine.
  - Bone marrow and solid organ transplant patients with CMV pneumonia may require ganciclovir and gammaglobulin.
- If the patient has a reactive airway disease component, bronchodilator therapy should be considered.

OUTCOME

- Childhood pneumonia has a mortality rate of less than 1 percent in industrialized nations but it accounts for 5 million deaths annually in children younger than 5 years old in developing countries.
- Most viral pneumonias will resolve spontaneously without specific therapy. Complications include dehydration, bronchiolitis obliterans, and apnea.

Apnea is seen most commonly in very young infants with RSV, chlamydia, or pertussis infections. Pleural effusions may occur with viral pneumonias but are not common. Indications for admitting patients with RSV pneumonia are the same as for RSV bronchiolitis (see Chap. 27).

- Uncomplicated bacterial pneumonia usually responds rapidly to antibiotic therapy. Delay in improvement or deterioration after therapy has begun should prompt an evaluation for complications including pleural effusions, empyemas, pneumothorax, pneumatoceles, dehydration, and development of additional infectious foci.
  - Pleural effusions complicate approximately 10 percent of pneumococcal pneumonias and 25 to 75 percent of HIB pneumonias.
  - Other foci of infection are frequently seen with HIB and include meningitis, septic arthritis, epiglottitis, soft tissue infections, and otitis media.
  - *S. aureus* pneumonias have a high rate of complications including empyema (80 percent) and pneumatocele (40 percent).
  - Mycoplasma pneumonia is occasionally complicated by pleural effusions, meningitis, encephalitis, arthritis, and hemolytic anemia.

BIBLIOGRAPHY

Davies HD, Matlow A, Petric M, et al: Prospective comparative study of viral bacterial and atypical organisms identified in pneumonia and bronchiolitis in hospitalized infants. *Pediatr Infect Dis J* 15:371–376, 1996.

Davies HD, Wang EE, Manso D, et al: Reliability of the chest radiograph in the diagnosis of lower tract respiratory infections in young children. *Pediatr Infect Dis J* 15:600–660, 1996.

DeMuri GP: Afebrile pneumonia in infants. *Prim Care Clin Office Pract* 23:849–860, 1996.

Klig JE, Chem L: Lower respiratory infections in children. *Curr Opin Pediatr* 15:121–126, 2003.

Margolis P, Gadomski A: Does this infant have pneumonia? *JAMA* 279:308–313, 1998.

McCracken GH: Etiology and treatment of pneumonia. *Pediatr Infect Dis J* 19:373–377, 2000.

Nelson JD: Community-acquired pneumonia in children: Guidelines for treatment. *Pediatr Infect Dis J* 19:251–253, 2000.

Schaad UB: Antibiotic therapy of childhood pneumonia. *Pediatr Pulmonol* 18S:146–149, 1999.

Sinanaiotis CA: Community-acquired pneumonia in children: Diagnosis and treatment. *Pediatr Pulmonol* 18S:144–145, 1999.

QUESTIONS

1. The most frequent age group that may sustain a bacterial pneumonia is:
   A. Newborn
   B. Toddler
   C. Adolescent
   D. Adult
   E. Elderly
2. The most frequent bacterial cause of pneumonia in school age children is:
   A. *Streptococcus pneumoniae*
   B. *Haemophilis influenzae*
   C. *Chlamydia trachomatis*
   D. *Mycoplasma pneumoniae*
   E. *Mycoplasma hominis*
3. The most frequent sign of pneumonia is:
   A. Fever
   B. Tachycardia
   C. Tachypnea
   D. Low pulse oximetry
   E. Rales
4. A 2-week-old male presents with a fever of 102°F. Chest radiography reveals bilateral infiltrates. Appropriate choice for antibiotic selection would be:
   A. Ceftriaxone
   B. Ampicillin and gentamycin
   C. Amoxicillin and cefotaxime
   D. Trimethoprim/sulfamethoxazole
   E. Levafloxin and ampicillin
5. An 8-year-old male with a history of cystic fibrosis presents with a progressive productive cough and a fever of 101°F. Chest radiography reveals bilateral infiltrates. Appropriate antibiotic therapy should be:
   A. Ceftazidime
   B. Erythromycin
   C. Amoxicillin
   D. Ceftriaxone
   E. Levafloxin
6. Pleural effusions are frequently associated with which of the following bacterial pneumonias?
   A. *Staphylococcus aureus*
   B. *Pseudomonas aeruginosa*
   C. *Mycoplasma pneumoniae*
   D. *Haemophilus influenzae* type b
   E. *Chlamydia trachomatis*

ANSWERS

1. A. The immediate newborn period is the only time when pneumonia is most frequently bacterial. Most infections in this age group are caused by aspiration of the organisms that colonize the mother's genital tract. Beyond the neonatal period, most pneumonias are nonbacterial.
2. D. Once children reach school age, *Mycoplasma pneumoniae* is the most common bacterial cause of pneumonia although, *S. pneumoniae* remains a frequent cause.
3. C. Tachypnea is the most frequent sign of pneumonia.
4. B. In the newborn, ampicillin in combination with an aminoglycoside or a third-generation cephalosporin is preferred. The ampicillin provides coverage against *Listeria* and *Enterococcus* species.
5. A. Children with cystic fibrosis may develop pneumonia due to *S. aureus* or *Pseudomonas* and appropriate antibiotic therapy is ceftazidime.
6. D. Pleural effusions are found in approximately 10% of pneumococcal pneumonias and 25 to 75% of HIB pneumonia.

29 PERTUSSIS

Kathleen Brown
Kemedy K. McQuillen
Patricia Lee

EPIDEMIOLOGY

• Pertussis is a respiratory infection seen in any age group but most commonly in infants younger than 6 months.
• Over the past three decades, there has been a fourfold increase in the incidence of pertussis in this country. In 1993, it became the most commonly reported vaccine-preventable disease among children younger than 5 years old.

ETIOLOGY AND PATHOPHYSIOLOGY

• Pertussis is an infection of the respiratory tract produced by *Bordetella pertussis*. Less frequently, a similar illness is produced by *Bordetella parapertussis*, adenovirus, or *Chlamydia*. *B. pertussis* is spread by respiratory droplet transmission. Following inhalation, organisms attach to respiratory tract epithelial cells, multiply, and infiltrate the mucosa with inflammatory cells. Inflammatory debris in the lumen of the bronchi and peribronchial lymphoid hyperplasia obstruct the smaller airways, causing atelectasis. Attack rates in susceptible household contacts approach 100 percent, with an incubation period of 7 to 14 days.

- Infection with pertussis confers lifelong immunity. Vaccination is highly protective for 3 years and then declines in effectiveness over 12 years, after which, no protection may be evident. There is no passive immunization in utero and infants are not considered fully immunized until they have received three doses of the vaccine.

CLINICAL PRESENTATION

- Pertussis is characterized by three stages: the initial or catarrhal stage, characterized by upper respiratory tract symptoms that last for 7 to 10 days; the paroxysmal phase, characterized by episodic bouts of staccato cough that lasts 2 to 4 weeks; and the convalescent stage, characterized by a gradual resolution of symptoms. Infants in the paroxysmal phase will have intermittent coughing spells, frequently followed by posttussive emesis. There may be associated cyanosis. The paroxysms tend to be provoked by feeding or exertion and can be elicited when using a tongue blade to examine the throat. The staccato cough allows little or no inspiration between coughs and the paroxysm is followed by a prolonged, slow inspiration. Beyond infancy, inspiration through a partially closed glottis produces the characteristic whoop. This feature is absent in infants and, in those younger than 6 months, silent paroxysms may occur. In teenagers and adults, a persistent cough may be the only clue to infection with pertussis.
- Subconjunctival hemorrhages may be present secondary to the force of the coughing.

LABORATORY AND RADIOGRAPHIC FINDINGS

- Cultures of the nasopharynx plated on Bordet-Gengou agar may grow *B. pertussis*, however, this method is insensitive, time consuming, and not useful for diagnosis. Fluorescent antibody testing is the most utilized confirmatory test, but it has a low sensitivity and poor predictive value. The polymerase chain reaction test has a much higher sensitivity but is not commonly used.
- In infants older than 6 months pertussis produces an extreme leukocytosis (20,000 to 50,000) with a predominance of lymphocytes.
- Radiographs may be normal or demonstrate a shaggy right heart border.

DIAGNOSIS

- Diagnosis is usually based on history and physical examination. In an outbreak of pertussis, a cough lasting for 14 or more days is considered a case. For a sporadic diagnosis, the patient must meet the cough criterion and also have paroxysms, whoop, or posttussive emesis.
- Many cases of whooping cough are atypical, especially in partially immunized infants and older patients. Laboratory testing may be helpful.

TREATMENT

- Treatment is primarily supportive: oxygen and intravenous fluids may be required. Erythromycin, started in the incubation period or early catarrhal stage, will shorten the course of the disease. Initiation of therapy after the onset of paroxysms is ineffective. The dose is 40 to 50 mg/kg/day in four divided doses for 14 days. Although not proven to be effective, erythromycin prophylaxis is recommended for close contacts.

DISPOSITION AND OUTCOME

- Complications and death due to pertussis infection are greater in infants younger than 1 year old and these children should be admitted and monitored. Complications include apnea (especially in infants less than 6 months old), seizures, encephalopathy, and secondary bacterial pneumonia.

BIBLIOGRAPHY

Black S: Epidemiology of pertussis. *Pediatr Infect Dis J* 1:S85–S89, 1997.

Dodhia H, Miller E: Review of the evidence for the use of erythromycin in the management of persons exposed to pertussis. *Epidemiol Infect* 120:143–149, 1998.

Hallander HO: Microbiological and serological diagnosis of pertussis. *Clin Infect Dis* 28S:S99–S106, 1999.

Hampl SD, Olson LC: Pertussis in the young infant. *Semin Respir Infect* 10:58–62, 1995.

Hewlett EL: Pertussis current concepts of pathogenesis and prevention. *Pediatr Infect Dis J* 16S:S78–S84, 1997.

QUESTIONS

1. The etiologic agent in pertussis is:
   A. *Hemophilus influenzae*
   B. *Bartenella pertussis*
   C. *Bordetella pertussis*
   D. *Corynebacterium diphtheriae*
   E. *Pseudomonas aeruginosa*

2. Which of the following persons most likely has immunity to pertussis?
   A. A 15-year-old male who had pertussis at age 9 months
   B. A 2-week-old female whose mother had pertussis as a child
   C. A 15-year-old male who completed his series of pertussis vaccinations as an infant
   D. A 6-month-old who has had 2 doses of pertussis vaccine
   E. A 30-year-old who was fully immunized as a child and completed a series of three doses of vaccine

3. A 3-month-old child presents with a history of a persistent cough and a brief episode of apnea and cyanosis. On examination with a tongue blade, a staccato like cough is noted. Pertussis is suspected as the etiology of the disease. Which of the following is true of this presentation?
   A. The patient is experiencing stage I, or catarrhal stage, of pertussis.
   B. The patient is presenting in stage II, or paroxysmal phase, of pertussis.
   C. The patient is presenting in stage III, or quiescent period, of pertussis.
   D. The patient is presenting in IV, or the apneic stage, of pertussis.
   E. The patient is presenting in stage V, or the convalescent stage, of pertussis.

4. During an outbreak of pertussis, pertussis is diagnosed if a child presents with which of the following symptoms?
   A. A fever greater than 101°F
   B. An upper respiratory infection with a cough and posttussive emesis
   C. A cough of greater than 14 days duration
   D. An elevated white blood cell count with lymphocytosis
   E. A chest radiograph with a lobar infiltrate

ANSWERS

1. C. Pertussis is an infection produced by *Bordetella pertussis*. Less frequently, a similar illness is produced by *Bordetella parapertussis*, adenovirus, or *Chlamydia*.

2. A. Infection with pertussis confers lifelong immunity. Vaccination is highly protective for 3 years and then declines in effectiveness over 12 years, after which, no protection may be evident. There is no passive immunization in utero and infants are not considered fully immunized until they have received three doses of the vaccine.

3. B. Pertussis is characterized by three stages. The initial, or catarrhal, stage is characterized by upper respiratory tract symptoms that last for 7 to 10 days, followed by the paroxysmal phase, which is characterized by episodic bouts of staccato cough that lasts 2 to 4 weeks, and then is followed by the convalescent stage, or gradual resolution of symptoms.

4. C. Diagnosis is usually based on history and physical examination. In an outbreak of pertussis, a cough lasting for 14 or more days is considered a case.

30 BRONCHOPULMONARY DYSPLASIA

Kathleen Brown
Kemedy K. McQuillen
Patricia Lee

EPIDEMIOLOGY

- Bronchopulmonary dysplasia (BPD) is a chronic lung disease that can follow any neonatal lung disease that requires prolonged mechanical ventilation. Children with residual lung disease after 28 days of age are said to have BPD. An oxygen requirement at 36 weeks' corrected postgestational age predicts the development of the disease. The overall rate of BPD is about 15 percent for premature infants requiring mechanical ventilation. Low birth weight, male gender, and white race are risk factors.
  - BPD is characterized by:
  - Respiratory distress
  - Supplemental oxygen requirement
  - Radiologic abnormalities
  - Blood gas abnormalities

PATHOPHYSIOLOGY

- The pathogenesis of BPD is not fully understood. Factors thought to play a role in its development include host susceptibility, primary or secondary lung injury, and the lung response to injury. The principal histologic lung finding is a fibroproliferative response in excess of what is required for repair of lung damage.

CLINICAL PRESENTATION

- The spectrum of BPD disease ranges from mild asymptomatic disease to crippling cardiopulmonary dysfunction. Patients may be on home oxygen, bronchodilators, apnea monitors, and other medications.
- Exacerbation of lung disease secondary to a viral upper respiratory infection is a common reason for seeking ED care. Patients may have increased respiratory distress, poor feeding, lethargy or irritability, and an increased oxygen requirement.
- On physical examination, infants will usually be small-for-age with an increased anterior-posterior diameter of the chest. They will have tachypnea, rales, wheezes, or areas of decreased breath sounds. They may have signs of an upper respiratory infection.

LABORATORY AND RADIOGRAPHIC FINDINGS

- A chest radiograph will reveal hyperinflation with cystic or fibrotic areas. Old films should be used for comparison.
- Check oximetry on all patients with BPD and use baseline levels to interpret the results.
- Although children with BPD will often have hypercarbia and hypoxia at baseline, blood gas results can be helpful in assessing a severely symptomatic patient.
- RSV testing will identify patients who may need ribavirin therapy.

DIFFERENTIAL DIAGNOSIS

- Many BPD exacerbations are triggered by an upper respiratory infection and involve reactive airways as part of the pathology. Findings of an exacerbation may be confused with pneumonia, asthma, or bronchiolitis, however, these problems may also be coexistent and the cause of the exacerbation.

TREATMENT

- The treatment of a BPD exacerbation is mainly supportive.

- Provide oxygen and intravenous fluid if indicated.
- Consider mechanical ventilation for recurrent apnea spells, worsening hypercarbia, or refractory hypoxemia.
- Bronchodilators may be effective and should be used as they are for asthma. Systemic corticosteroids are effective in acute exacerbations, but their chronic use is associated with many side effects. The efficacy of inhaled steroids in patients not on ventilators has not been demonstrated. Parenteral diuretics may improve lung function and survival in some patients.
- BPD patients with RSV are candidates for ribavirin.

OUTCOME AND DISPOSITION

- Some patients with a BPD exacerbation due to an upper respiratory infection can be managed at home. Parents may have difficulty coping with a BPD exacerbation and this should be considered when making a disposition decision. Indications for admission include increased respiratory distress, increasing hypoxia or hypercarbia, new pulmonary infiltrates, and RSV infection.

BIBLIOGRAPHY

Bancalari E: Corticosteroids and neonatal lung disease. *Eur J Pediatr* 157S1:S31–S37, 1998.

Barrington KJ, Finer NN: Treatment of bronchopulmonary dysplasia. *Clin Perinatol* 25:177–202, 1998.

Brion LP, Primhak RA, Yong W: Aerosolized diuretics for preterm infants with chronic lung disease. *Cochrane Database of Systematic Reviews.* Issue 4, 2000.

Byrne BJ, Mellon BG, Lindstrom DP, Cotton RB: Is the BPD epidemic diminishing? *Semin Perinatol* 26:461–466, 2002.

Farrell PA, Fiascone JM: Bronchopulmonary dysplasia in the 1990s: A review for the pediatrician. *Curr Probl Pediatr* 27:129–163, 1997.

Lister P, Iles R, Shaw B, et al: Inhaled steroids for neonatal chronic lung disease. *Cochrane Database of Systematic Reviews.* Issue 4, 2000.

McColley SA: Bronchopulmonary dysplasia: Impact of surfactant replacement therapy. *Pediatr Clin North Am* 45: 573–586, 1998.

Saugstad OD: Bronchopulmonary dysplasia and oxidative stress: Are we closer to an understanding of the pathogenesis of BPD? *Acta Pediatr* 86:1277–1282, 1997.

QUESTIONS

1. The development of bronchopulmonary dysplasia can be predicted based on a history of:
   A. Oxygen requirement at 36 weeks corrected post-gestational age
   B. Mechanical ventilation for 3 days after birth
   C. Prematurity of 38 weeks gestational age
   D. Pneumonia at 1 week of age
   E. Family history

2. A 5-month-old male with a history of prolonged mechanical ventilation and BPD is brought to the emergency department for evaluation of wheezing. An RSV aspirate is positive. Appropriate management for this child should be:
   A. Discharge home if improved on bronchodilators with close follow-up
   B. Discharge home if improved with antibiotics and close follow-up
   C. Admission for ribavirin
   D. Admission for antibiotic therapy
   E. Admission for observation

ANSWERS

1. A. BPD is a chronic lung disease that can follow any neonatal lung disease that requires prolonged mechanical ventilation. Children with residual lung disease after 28 days of age are said to have BPD. An oxygen requirement at 36 weeks corrected postgestational age predicts the development of the disease.

2. C. Indications for admission include increased respiratory distress, increasing hypoxia or hypercarbia, new pulmonary infiltrates, and RSV infection. BPD patients with RSV are candidates for ribavirin.

31   CYSTIC FIBROSIS

Kathleen Brown
Kemedy K. McQuillen
Patricia Lee

EPIDEMIOLOGY

• Cystic fibrosis (CF), a generalized defect in exocrine gland secretions, is the most common lethal inherited disease among Caucasians in the United States, occurring in 1 in 2500 live, Caucasian births.

ETIOLOGY AND PATHOPHYSIOLOGY

• CF is inherited as an autosomal recessive condition. The CF gene is on the long arm of chromosome 7: DeltaF508 is the most common mutation that causes CF but more than 600 other causative mutations have been identified. The product of the defective gene is the cystic fibrosis transmembrane conductance regulator (CFTR), which controls fluid balance across epithelial cells. Alterations in chloride, sodium, and water transport result in viscous secretions that are associated with luminal obstruction and exocrine duct destruction and scarring. Clinically, most CF patients have malabsorption from pancreatic insufficiency and abnormal intestinal mucins and biliary tract secretions, elevated sweat electrolytes, and chronic pulmonary infections resulting in hyperinflation, bronchiectasis, atelectasis, and respiratory failure complicated by cor pulmonale. There is considerable variation in the severity of the disease.

CLINICAL PRESENTATION

• Patients not yet been diagnosed with CF may present with:
  ○ Failure to thrive
  ○ Chronic respiratory problems
  ○ Chronic gastrointestinal problems, especially diarrhea
  ○ Atypical asthma (especially with clubbing, bronchiectasis, or purulent sputum)
  ○ Recurrent respiratory infections
• Malabsorption may lead to hypoproteinemia or symptoms of vitamin deficiencies.
• Patients with clinical findings suggestive of CF should be referred for diagnostic evaluation.
• Patients with known CF most commonly present with a pulmonary exacerbation, hemoptysis, or cor pulmonale.
  ○ Patients with a pulmonary exacerbation present with worsening of their chronic lung disease, often preceded by an upper respiratory infection. They will have signs of respiratory distress, may be cyanotic, and may progress to respiratory failure. Chest examination will reveal diffuse rales, rhonchi, or wheezing and may show decreased breath sound and hyperresonance suggestive of a pneumothorax. Many patients with CF will have intermittent blood-streaked sputum, however, significant hemoptysis (30 to 60 mL) can result from erosion of a bronchial vessel. Less commonly, patients with CF will cough up blood from bleeding esophageal varices secondary to advanced cirrhosis. Pulmonary hypertension

and right ventricular hypertrophy may result from chronic lung disease and congestive heart failure may develop during a respiratory exacerbation.

- Acute nonpulmonary complications of CF include meconium ileus, rectal prolapse (usually in children under 3 years old), intestinal obstruction, and electrolyte abnormalities.

  ○ A neonate with meconium ileus will have a distended abdomen and a history of no or minimal meconium production. They may also have visible peristaltic waves or a palpable abdominal mass. Meconium ileus equivalent, or an intestinal obstruction secondary to dry abnormal stool, can occur in older children. Meconium ileus and meconium ileus equivalent can lead to volvulus, intussusception, or intestinal perforation.

  ○ As patients reach adulthood, they may develop diabetes mellitus, obstructive biliary tract disease, and obstructive azoospermia.

  ○ The elevated sweat electrolyte content gives patients with CF a salty taste and can lead to acute or chronic electrolyte depletion.

LABORATORY AND RADIOGRAPHIC FINDINGS

- The pilocarpine iontophoresis sweat test should be done in any patient suspected of having CF. It is used to identify high sweat chloride concentrations.
- Additionally, DNA probes are available for detection of some patients and carriers.
- Obtain sputum cultures for patients with known CF who present with a pulmonary exacerbation. Past sputum culture results are helpful in guiding initial antibiotic therapy.
- Blood cultures may be indicated in febrile or toxic appearing patients.
- Electrolyte determination will usually reveal low serum sodium and chloride levels. Bicarbonate levels and serum pH are usually elevated and are seen when the kidneys compensate for the increased salt loss in the sweat. Dehydration and symptomatic electrolyte deficiencies occur more commonly during hot weather.
- Obtain a hematocrit, type and crossmatch, and prothrombin time in patients with significant hemoptysis.
- Check oximetry in any patient with worsening pulmonary symptoms. Obtain a blood gas for patients with respiratory failure.
- Typical chest radiograph findings include diffuse peribronchial thickening, hyperinflation, and variable fluffy infiltrates. Comparison with previously obtained radiographs is necessary. Patients with a sudden change in pulmonary condition should have a chest radiograph to rule out a pneumothorax. Those with cor pulmonale will have a large heart, as opposed to the narrow heart usually seen in patients with CF, and prominent pulmonary vasculature.
- Patients with meconium ileus or meconium ileus equivalent will have dilated loops of bowel on an abdominal film and may have a bubbly, granular density in the lower abdomen representing the meconium or fecal mass.

DIFFERENTIAL DIAGNOSIS

- CF can present in many different ways because of the variability in the expression of its genetic defect. Patients who should be considered for a CF evaluation are discussed above.

TREATMENT

- Administer oxygen if indicated.
- Therapy for pulmonary exacerbations is aimed at relieving mucus plugging and obstruction and treating infection. The obstructive airway disease in CF is multifactorial and only partially reversible. β-Adrenergic and anticholinergic bronchodilators are often effective in the short term. Doses are the same as for asthmatic patients. Methylxanthines are sometimes used to treat acute pulmonary exacerbations unresponsive to other therapies. If they are used, it is important to remember that patients with CF have increased clearance, require larger or more frequent doses, and should have drug levels monitored.
- If recent sputum culture results are unavailable, begin empiric therapy aimed at *Staphylococcus aureus*, nontypable *Haemophilus influenzae*, and gram-negative bacilli in infants and young children, and *Pseudomonas aeruginosa* by the end of the first decade of life. Consider inhaled antibiotics, particularly tobramycin, in an acute exacerbation.
- Mucoactive agents, particularly recombinant human deoxyribonuclease (Pulmozyme), are not useful in acute exacerbations. Chest physiotherapy and postural drainage are well accepted but not proven to be effective for clearing secretions in patients with CF.
- Antiinflammatory medications may be helpful in the long-term management of patients with CF. Chronic oral steroids (1 to 2 mg/kg on alternate days) are

effective in slowing the progression of lung disease in CF but are associated with the development of cataracts and growth retardation. Continue patients on their chronic steroids and consider higher doses for adrenal suppression. Chronic high-dose ibuprofen and inhaled corticosteroids are commonly used, however, their efficacy is not proven.

- Treat a small (<10 percent) pneumothorax with tube thoracostomy and a tension pneumothorax with needle aspiration followed by tube thoracostomy.
- Admit patients with significant hemoptysis (>30 to 60 mL) for observation. Give vitamin K if the prothrombin time is prolonged. If bleeding persists, guidelines for replacement are the same as for bleeding from other sources. Massive hemoptysis (>300 mL) may compromise the airway and ligation or embolization of the bleeding vessel should be attempted with the help of a bronchoscopist and/or thoracic surgeon.
- Treat cor pulmonale with oxygen and diuretics while treating the underlying pulmonary disease.
- Patients with CF and respiratory failure do not respond as well to mechanical ventilation and have even more complications than do patients with other forms of chronic obstructive pulmonary disease. Factors that should be considered include the patient's baseline pulmonary function, the course of the patient's disease, and the expectations of the patient and their parents. In some cases, mechanical ventilation is not warranted. This decision should be made in conjunction with the patient's chronic care provider and/or the patient and the patient's parents.
- Recently, a number of patients with CF have undergone heart-lung transplants, with 3-year survival rates higher than 50 percent.
- Treat patients with uncomplicated meconium ileus or meconium ileus equivalent with saline or gastrografin enemas to relieve the obstruction. Laparotomy is indicated for perforation, volvulus, or intussusception, or if medical management is unsuccessful.
- Treat dehydrated patients or those presenting with electrolyte abnormalities with isotonic saline. Frequently check serum electrolytes to guide fluid therapy.

OUTCOME

- Many more CF patients are now surviving to adulthood due to effective antibiotics, earlier diagnosis, and prompt recognition and treatment of complications.

BIBLIOGRAPHY

Cheng K, Ashby D, Smythg R: Oral steroids for cystic fibrosis. *Cochrane Database of Systematic Reviews* Issue 4, 2000.

Dezateux C, Crighton A: Oral non-steroidal anti-inflammatory drug therapy for cystic fibrosis. *Cochrane Database of Systematic* Reviews Issue 4, 2000.

Dezateux C, Walters S, Balfour-Lynn I: Inhaled corticosteroids for cystic fibrosis. Cochrane *Database of Systematic Reviews* Issue 4, 2000.

Konstan MW: Therapies aimed at airway inflammation in cystic fibrosis. *Clin Chest Med* 19:101–113, 1998.

Marshall BC, Samuelson WM. Basic therapies in cystic fibrosis. Does standard therapy work? *Clin Chest Med* 19:487–504, 1998.

Ramsey BW: Drug therapy: Management of pulmonary disease in patients with cystic fibrosis. *N Engl J Med* 335:179–188, 1996.

Rosenstein BJ, Zeitlin PL: Cystic fibrosis. *Lancet* 351: 227–282, 1998.

Wark PA, McDonald V: Nebulized hypertonic saline for cystic fibrosis. *Cochrane Database of Systematic Reviews* Issue 4, 2000.

QUESTIONS

1. An 8-month-old boy presents with complaints of upper respiratory infection, cough, and diarrhea. On examination, you notice that he appears to be small for his age and has scattered bilateral wheezes. Chest radiograph reveals bilateral pneumonia. Electrolytes reveal hyponatremia and hypochloremic metabolic alkalosis. Appropriate management of this child should be all of the following **EXCEPT**:
   A. Admission for intravenous antibiotics
   B. Pilocarpine iontophoresis sweat test
   C. Sputum culture
   D. RSV aspirate
   E. Discharge home with oral cephalosporin
2. An 11-month-old female presents with rectal prolapse. Appropriate diagnoses to be considered should be:
   A. Giardia
   B. Proctitis
   C. Crohn's
   D. Cystic fibrosis
   E. Rotavirus
3. Which of the following is a frequent infectious agent causing pneumonia in a 14-year-old child with cystic fibrosis?
   A. *Staphylococcus aureus*
   B. *Neisseria gonorroheae*

C. *Psudomonas aeruginosa*
D. *Streptococcus pneumoniae*
E. *Klebsiella pneumoniae*

ANSWERS

1. E. This child is suspicious for cystic fibrosis. Patients with CF may present with failure to thrive, chronic respiratory problems, chronic gastrointestinal problems, atypical asthma, and recurrent respiratory infections. In addition to the evaluation of CF using the sweat test, treatment of the bilateral pneumonia should be admission for intravenous antibiotics, sputum cultures if possible, and RSV aspirate testing.

2. D. Acute nonpulmonary complication of cystic fibrosis include meconium ileus, rectal prolapse (usually in children under 3 year old), intestinal obstruction, and electrolyte disturbances.

3. C. *Pseudomonas aeruginosa* is a frequent cause of pneumonia in the older child (>10 years of age).

32 CONGENITAL HEART DISEASE

Kelly D. Young
Kemedy K. McQuillen
Gary R. Strange
Valerie A. Dobiesz

EPIDEMIOLOGY

- Congenital heart disease (CHD) occurs in approximately 8 in 1000 live births in the United States. This figure does not include common lesions such as bicuspid aortic valve (1 to 2 percent of the population) or mitral valve prolapse.
- Many genetic syndromes and teratogens are associated with a higher risk of specific congenital heart lesions.
- Most patients present during infancy (Table 32-1).

PHYSIOLOGY

FETAL CIRCULATION

- Oxygenated blood from the placenta enters the fetus through the umbilical vein, flows into the IVC either directly or via the ductus venosus, and passes through the *foramen ovale* into the left atrium, with 90 percent of blood bypassing the right heart and pulmonary circulation. The highly oxygenated blood in the left atrium mixes with pulmonary venous return, enters the left ventricle and the ascending aorta, and perfuses the brain. Deoxygenated blood returns from the cerebral circulation via the superior vena cava and enters the right atrium, right ventricle, and pulmonary artery. Because pulmonary vascular resistance is high in the fetus, most of this blood then flows through the

TABLE 32-1   Common Presentations by Age

AGE	PRESENTATION
0–2 weeks	Ductal-dependent circulatory failure
	Hypoplastic left heart syndrome
	Aortic coarctation, severe
	Aortic stenosis, severe
	Cyanosis
	Tetralogy of Fallot
	Transposition of the great arteries
	Total anomalous pulmonary venous return
	Truncus arteriosus
	Tricuspid atresia and other tricuspid anomalies
2–6 weeks	Congestive heart failure
	Ventricular septal defect, large
	Patent ductus arteriosus
	Atrioventricular canal defect
	Cyanosis
	Truncus arteriosus
	Tetralogy of Fallot
	Tricuspid atresia
6 weeks–6 months	Congestive heart failure
	Ventricular septal defect
	Atrial septal defect
	Atrioventricular canal defect
	Cyanosis
	Tetralogy of Fallot
Childhood–adulthood	Murmur
	Ventricular septal defect
	Atrial septal defect
	Patent ductus arteriosus
	Aortic stenosis
	Pulmonic stenosis
	Hypertension
	Aortic coarctation
	Syncope/exercise intolerance
	Aortic stenosis
	Pulmonic stenosis
	Eisenmenger's syndrome
	Arrhythmias
	Atrial septal defect
	Cyanosis
	Eisenmenger's syndrome

ductus arteriosus and enters the descending aorta, bypassing the pulmonary circulation. Two thirds of this descending aorta outflow returns to the placenta via the umbilical arteries, and one-third perfuses the lower part of the fetus.

NEONATAL CIRCULATION

- In the first hours of life, the pulmonary vascular resistance falls, allowing for increased pulmonary blood flow. Additionally, separation from the low-resistance placental circuit results in an increased systemic vascular resistance, further reducing blood flow through the ductus arteriosus. Increased blood P_{O_2} causes the smooth muscle of the ductus to constrict, functionally closing the ductus by 15 h of life. In the normal infant, the ductus becomes the ligamentum arteriosum by 2 to 3 weeks of age and the foramen ovale closes by 3 months of age.
- The physiology of neonates and young infants is one of rate-dependent cardiac output (to increase cardiac output, the heart rate must increase), increased oxygen consumption, and lower systolic reserve, resulting in a higher propensity for congestive heart failure. Other differences include shunting via the patent foramen ovale or ductus arteriosus, pulmonary vascular resistance that is higher and responsive to oxygen (decreases resistance), and a prominent right ventricle (right axis deviation on the electrocardiogram).

EVALUATION

HISTORY

- Assess general health including growth, development, and susceptibility to respiratory illnesses. Ask about symptoms of congestive heart failure: poor feeding, longer feeding times than the average infant, poor growth or failure to thrive, sweating with feeding, irritability or lethargy, weak cry, increased respiratory effort, dyspnea, tachypnea, and coughing. Ask about cyanosis and its alleviators or exacerbators: cardiac cyanosis is often worse with crying secondary to increased cardiac output, while respiratory cyanosis improves with crying and alveolar recruitment. Record pregnancy, birth, and family histories to elucidate genetic or teratogenic etiologies.

PHYSICAL EXAMINATION

- Check vital signs, including four-extremity blood pressures, and assess pulses in each extremity.

- Assess color to help classify the lesion into one of three categories:
  - Pink: congestive heart failure with L → R shunt
  - Blue: cyanotic heart disease with R → L shunt
  - Gray: outflow obstruction, hypoperfusion, and shock.
- Peripheral cyanosis, or acrocyanosis, may be seen in normal newborns so when looking for the central cyanosis that is seen in CHD, assess the nailbeds and mucous membranes. The presence of cyanosis requires 3 to 5 g of deoxygenated hemoglobin (correlating to an oxygen saturation of 80 to 85 percent), therefore, if a child is anemic, cyanosis may not be easily recognized.
- Auscultate for murmurs, S1 and S2, and extra sounds. Murmurs are commonly heard in normal children (Table 32-2). Benign cardiac murmurs tend to be softer, lower pitched, and early to midsystolic compared with pathologic murmurs. Diastolic, late systolic, or pansystolic murmurs are generally pathologic.
- Examine the abdomen for hepatomegaly: the liver in a normal infant is palpable 1- to 3-cm below the right subcostal margin.
- Examine the child for dysmorphic features.

ANCILLARY TESTS

- Chronically cyanotic children usually compensate with polycythemia.
- Do the *hyperoxia test* to differentiate between cardiac and respiratory cyanosis. Administer 100 percent oxygen for several min. With respiratory disease, there should be improvement in the P_{O_2} or oxygen saturation while, with cardiac cyanosis due to intracardiac right-to-left shunting, there will be no improvement.
- Obtain a *chest radiograph* (CXR) to evaluate pulmonary vascularity and the size and shape of the heart.
- Evaluate an *electrocardiogram* (ECG) for conduction and rhythm disturbances, chamber forces, and ischemic changes. ECGs vary greatly by age so consult a pediatric handbook for normal values. Some basic principles are listed in Tables 32-3 and 32-4.

CLASSIFICATION

- Lesions are usually classified as cyanotic or acyanotic and sub classified according to whether pulmonary blood flow (PBF) is increased, normal, or decreased.
  - Cyanotic lesions can be remembered by the "5 T's": tetralogy of Fallot (TOF), tricuspid anomalies

TABLE 32-2   Normal Benign Cardiac Murmurs

MURMUR	AGE	CHARACTER	POSITIONING	ETIOLOGY	DIFFERENTIAL DIAGNOSIS
Still's vibratory	Most common benign in children 2–6 yr old, can occur infant to adolescent	I–III/VI early systolic ejection murmur, left lower sternal border to apex, twanging musical quality	Louder when patient supine	Postulated to be from ventricular false tendons	VSD murmur is harsher
Pulmonary flow murmur	Child to young adult	II–III/VI crescendo-decrescendo, early to midsystolic, left upper sternal border, second intercostal space	Louder when patient supine, increased on full expiration	Flow in the pulmonary outflow tract	ASD has fixed split S2; pulmonic stenosis has higher pitched, longer murmur, ejection click
Peripheral pulmonic stenosis	Newborn to 1 yr old	I–II/VI low pitched, early to midsystolic ejection murmur in the pulmonic area and radiating to axillae and back	Increased with viral respiratory infections, lower heart rate, decreased with tachycardia	Turbulence at the peripheral pulmonary artery branches due to narrow angles in infants	Significant branch pulmonary artery stenosis in Williams syndrome; congenital rubella has higher pitched murmur, extends beyond S2; older child
Supraclavicular or brachio-cephalic	Child to young adult	Crescendo-decrescendo, systolic, low-pitched, above the clavicles, radiating to neck, abrupt onset and brief	Decreases with rapid hyperextension of the shoulders	Flow through the major brachiocephalic vessels arising from the aorta	Idiopathic hypertrophic subaortic stenosis: louder with Valsalva and softer with rapid squatting. Aortic stenosis: higher pitched, ejection click
Venous hum	Child	Faint to grade VI, continuous, humming, low anterior neck to lateral sternocleido-mastoid muscle to anterior chest infraclavicular	Louder when sitting, looking away from murmur; softer when lying, with compressed jugular vein or head turned toward murmur	Turbulence from the internal jugular and subclavian veins entering the superior vena cava	Patent ductus arteriosus has machinery murmur, not compressible, bounding pulses
Mammary souffle	Pregnant, lactating, rarely adolescent	High-pitched, systole into diastole, anterior chest over breast, varies day to day		Plethora of vessels over chest wall	Patent ductus arteriosus has machinery murmur, does not vary day to day

TABLE 32-3   Duration of ECG Intervals (Values in Seconds)

AGE	P-R LIMITS	QRS LIMITS	QTc LIMITS
0–7 d	0.08–0.12	0.04–0.10	0.34–0.54
7–30 d	0.08–0.12	0.04–0.07	0.30–0.50
1–3 mo	0.08–0.16	0.05–0.08	0.32–0.47
3–6 mo	0.08–0.12	0.05–0.08	0.35–0.46
6–12 mo	0.08–0.14	0.04–0.08	0.31–0.49
1–3 yr	0.08–0.16	0.04–0.08	0.34–0.43

SOURCE: Modified from Dittmer DS, Grebe RM: *Handbook of Circulation*. Philadelphia: WB Saunders, 1959, p 141.

TABLE 32-4   Age-Specific QRS Axis

AGE	RANGE	MEAN
1–7 d	80–160	125
1–4 weeks	60–160	110
1–3 mo	40–120	80
3–6 mo	20–80	65
6–12 mo	0–100	65
1–3 yr	20–100	55

SOURCE: From Hakim SN, Toepper WC: Cardiac disease in children, in Rosen P, Barkin RM (eds): *Emergency Medicine: Concepts and Clinical Practice II*. St. Louis, MO: Mosby-Year Book, 1992, p 546.

including tricuspid atresia and Ebstein's anomaly, truncus arteriosus, total anomalous pulmonary venous return (TAPVR), and transposition of the great arteries (TGA). Tetralogy of Fallot and the tricuspid anomalies have decreased PBF, whereas truncus arteriosus, TAPVR, and TGA have increased PBF.

○ Hypoplastic left heart syndrome (HLHS) also causes cyanosis and increased PBF.

○ Acyanotic lesions causing increased PBF often present with congestive heart failure (CHF); such lesions are ventricular septal defect (VSD), atrial septal defect (ASD), patent ductus arteriosus (PDA), and atrioventricular septal defect or AV canal defect. Acyanotic lesions with normal or decreased PBF include pulmonary stenosis (PS), aortic stenosis (AS), and aortic coarctation.

BRIEF SURVEY OF INDIVIDUAL LESIONS

- **Tetralogy of Fallot** is the most common cyanotic CHD in children older than 4 years. It has four components: right ventricular (RV) outflow obstruction, right ventricular hypertrophy (RVH), a large VSD, and an overriding aorta. Patients have a loud, harsh, pansystolic murmur in the left sternal border, and often a single S2. CXR shows a boot-shaped heart (coeur en sabot), decreased PBF, and in 25 percent of cases a right-sided aortic arch. ECG shows right axis deviation (RAD) and RVH. Severity depends on the degree of RV outflow obstruction.
- **Tricuspid atresia** must be accompanied by a right-to-left shunt at the level of the atria. It is rare and its findings depend on the presence or absence of a VSD and RV. **Ebstein's anomaly** is a displacement of the tricuspid valve into the RV: severity depends on the degree of displacement.
- **Truncus arteriosus** involves a single arterial trunk supplying both pulmonary and systemic circulations. A VSD is usually present and there may be no or mild cyanosis until right- and left-sided pressures mature. A murmur is detected in the first few days, pulses are bounding, and there is a single S2. The patient may have symptoms of CHF and recurrent pulmonary infections. CXR shows cardiomegaly and increased PBF. ECG shows left ventricular hypertrophy (LVH), RVH, or both.
- **(Total) anomalous pulmonary venous return** varies depending on whether it is total or partial (from one to four veins connecting to a location other than the left atrium) and where the veins connect. Cyanosis depends on the amount of mixing between right and left circulations and is usually mild to moderate. The S2 is widely split. CXR may show a "snowman" appearance, and ECG may show RVH, RAD, and right atrial enlargement (RAE).
- **Transposition of the great arteries** is the most common cyanotic lesion to present in the first week of life. The right ventricle feeds the aorta, whereas the left ventricle feeds the pulmonary artery. Mixing must occur, as the pulmonary and systemic circulations are in parallel. Symptoms include cyanosis and tachypnea in the first days of life; there is often no murmur.

CXR may be normal or may have an "egg on a string" appearance. ECG shows RAD and RVH but may be normal in the first days of life. If there is a large VSD to allow mixing, the infant may not present with CHF and cyanosis until 2 to 6 weeks of age.
- In **hypoplastic left heart syndrome** the right ventricle perfuses both circulations via the pulmonary artery. The systemic circulation is perfused through the PDA. Management varies depending on the parents' choice and resources available.
- **Ventricular septal defects,** accounting for 20 percent of CHD, is the most common congenital heart lesion. Small VSDs have a high rate of spontaneous closure. A harsh pansystolic murmur is present at the left lower sternal border. If the defect is large, respiratory symptoms and congestive heart failure develop in the first 3 months of life as pulmonary vascular resistance decreases and the left-to-right shunt increases. CXR may be normal or show signs of CHF. ECG may show LVH, RVH, and left atrial enlargement (LAE) if the defect is large.
- **Atrial septal defects** account for 12 percent of congenital heart lesions. Many patients are undiagnosed until adulthood. A soft systolic ejection murmur of increased pulmonic flow is heard in the left upper sternal border, and S2 is widely split and fixed. CXR shows right-sided chamber enlargement and increased PBF. ECG may show an RSR' in lead V1, a right bundle branch block (RBBB), and an increased PR interval.
- **Patent ductus arteriosus** occurs in 8:1000 premature infants and 2:1000 full-term infants. A continuous machinery-like murmur is heard in the left second intercostal space, first appearing at 2 to 5 days of age when falling pulmonary vascular resistance allows left-to-right shunting through the ductus. Because of the diastolic runoff into the PDA, pulses are bounding. Infants may develop CHF or may compensate with myocardial hypertrophy and present later with exercise intolerance. CXR shows increased PBF and, sometimes, cardiomegaly. ECG may show LVH. Treatment is with indomethacin or surgical ligation.
- **Atrioventricular septal defect or AV canal** is associated with Down's syndrome. CHF symptoms predominate. CXR shows increased PBF and cardiomegaly. ECG shows an increased PR interval, RAE and/or LAE, and RVH. The axis is often superior with extreme left axis deviation.
- **Pulmonary stenosis** is often recognized only when a murmur is noted during routine physical examination. An ejection click may be heard in the left second to third intercostal space. If the stenosis is moderate to severe, there may be cyanosis on exertion, syncope,

RV failure, and even sudden death. CXR shows a prominent main pulmonary artery and normal to decreased PBF. ECG may be normal or show RVH.

- **Aortic stenosis** may be asymptomatic or present as shock in infancy. Once symptomatic, patients complain of dyspnea on exertion, fatigue, abdominal pain, increased sweating, and exertional syncope (indicative of critical aortic stenosis). An ejection click is heard before the systolic ejection murmur in the right upper sternal border, radiating into the neck. There may be a left ventricular thrill or heave. CXR shows normal PBF. ECG shows LVH.
- **Aortic coarctation** accounts for 10 percent of CHD. The narrowing most commonly occurs just distal to the left subclavian artery branch. Symptoms range from CHF in infancy to hypertension in childhood or adulthood. Blood pressure is elevated in the upper extremities compared with the lower extremities, and femoral pulses are weak or absent. Children may complain of pain in the legs after exercise. A systolic ejection murmur at the apex radiates to the interscapular back. There may also be a diastolic murmur of aortic regurgitation. In some patients, a thrill is felt in the suprasternal notch. CXR is normal initially, but may show notching of ribs 3 through 8 posteriorly, as collateral circulation develops. ECG may show LVH. Children may present with complications of hypertension, including intracranial hemorrhage.

COMMON PRESENTATIONS

- Although knowledge of specific lesions is not necessary to effectively care for patients with CHD, recognition and prompt treatment is imperative.

DUCTAL-DEPENDENT LESIONS AND CARDIOGENIC SHOCK

- Lesions completely dependent on a patent ductus arteriosus for systemic or pulmonary blood flow present with acute onset circulatory failure and shock when the ductus closes, typically within the first week of life. Ductal-dependent lesions should be suspected in any infant with hypoperfusion, hypotension, severe acidosis, and cyanosis in the first 2 weeks of life; infants rarely present beyond 2 weeks old. The mainstay of therapy is prostaglandin E_1 (PGE_1) infusion to maintain ductal patency. A bolus of $0.1\,\mu g/kg$ is followed by an infusion of $0.1\,\mu g/kg/min$. Adverse

effects include hyperthermia, apnea, hypotension, rash, tremors, focal seizures, and bradycardia. Other etiologies for shock, such as sepsis, must be considered and treated. After immediate pediatric cardiology consultation, admit the patient to an intensive care unit.

CONGESTIVE HEART FAILURE

- Congestive heart failure (CHF) typically presents in the first 6 months of life in children with left-to-right shunts (VSD, PDA, AV canal, ASD) or excessive pressure load from a left sided obstruction (aortic stenosis or coarctation). Other causes include myocardial dysfunction (eg, cardiomyopathies) and dysrhythmias.
- Symptoms are gradual in onset and may include poor feeding (increased time to feed), poor growth, sweating, irritability or lethargy, weak cry, increased respiratory effort, dyspnea, tachypnea, chronic cough or wheeze, and increased frequency of respiratory infections.
- Physical examination may reveal tachypnea, retractions, nasal flaring, wheezing, rales (although less commonly than in adults), tachycardia, poor peripheral pulses, hepatomegaly (a cardinal sign of CHF in infants), or a gallop rhythm, murmur, or hyperactive precordium. Jugular venous distension and peripheral edema are rarely seen in young children. If present, edema is best appreciated in the eyelids, sacrum, and legs.
- CXR shows cardiomegaly (cardiothoracic ratio > 0.55 in infants, > 0.50 for children over 1 year old) and increased pulmonary vascularity.
- ECG findings depend on the lesion.
- Treatment includes fluid and sodium restriction, furosemide (1 mg/kg intravenously), and oxygen to keep saturations about 95 percent: over-oxygenating can lead to pulmonary vascular dilation and worsened failure. Keep the infant in a semireclined position, as if in a car seat. After consulting a pediatric cardiologist, consider starting the patient on digoxin. Be prepared for endotracheal intubation and ventilatory support in the event that they are needed. Nasal continuous positive airway pressure (CPAP) may also be used. If the patient is in shock, administer fluids judiciously: inotropic support with dopamine or dobutamine may be more appropriate.
- Assess a complete blood count, chemistry panel, calcium level, bedside glucose test, and arterial blood gas.
- Provide continuous monitoring of blood pressure, heart rate and rhythm, and oxygen saturation.

HYPOXEMIC "TET" SPELLS

- Sudden onset episodes of increased cyanosis may occur in young children with tetralogy of Fallot or other complex lesions with decreased PBF. A sudden increase in right-sided or decrease in left-sided pressures, worsens right-to-left shunting. The increased right-to-left shunting results in hypoxemia, cyanosis, and acidosis. In an attempt to increase cardiac output, hyperventilation and decreased systemic vascular resistance (SVR) ensues. Decreased SVR and increased venous return result in further shunting and a vicious cycle of ongoing shunting and hypoxemia occurs.
- Clinically, children present with a sudden increase in cyanosis, hyperpnea, restlessness, irritability or lethargy, and, occasionally, syncope. Left-to-right shunting murmurs may disappear during a spell. Spells are most common in children younger than 2 years and often occur when SVR is naturally decreased: in the morning after awakening, after a feeding, after defecation, or a bout of crying. The "tet spell" may occur in a previously acyanotic patient and may be the first sign of CHD.
- Spells must be differentiated from seizures, CHF, respiratory disease, and diabetic ketoacidosis.
- To treat a "tet spell" keep the child calm, administer oxygen, and place the child in a knee-chest position (to simulate squatting) to increase SVR. Older children can squat on their own to abort spells. If the spell is not improving, administer morphine, 0.1 to 0.2 mg/kg, intravenously or subcutaneously. Intravenous normal saline (10 mL/kg) should be given to counteract the vasodilating effects of morphine and to ensure adequate preload and pulmonary flow. Improved pulse oximetry, decreased cyanosis, decreased hyperpnea, and a calmer child signify successful therapy. If the above therapies are unsuccessful, give propranolol (0.1 to 0.2 mg/kg by slow intravenous push) or phenylephrine (0.1 mg/kg intravenously followed by an infusion of 2 to 10 μg/kg/min). Consider pediatric cardiology consultation prior to giving these medications. If all else fails, general anesthesia may be necessary.

PRESENTATIONS IN OLDER CHILDREN AND ADULTS

- Patients with an ASD, small VSD, PDA, PS, AS, or aortic coarctation may not be diagnosed until later in life when a murmur is heard on routine examination. Patients with an unrepaired ASD may present with atrial arrhythmias and a fixed split S2. Those with a PDA or AS may present with dyspnea on exertion and fatigue. Patients with critical AS may present with syncope. Patients with critical PS may present with cyanosis on exertion, right-sided heart failure, or syncope. Patients with aortic coarctation may be diagnosed when they are found to have hypertension or when they present with symptoms resulting from hypertension (headache, intracranial hemorrhage, dizziness, palpitations, and epistaxis). They may also have lower extremity claudication from hypoperfusion of the lower extremities.

EISENMENGER'S SYNDROME

- Patients with a large left-to-right shunt left unrepaired gradually develop pulmonary vascular disease due to the increased volume overload. When pulmonary hypertension becomes severe enough, the direction of shunting will reverse to right to left, and cyanosis ensues. This typically occurs in adolescence to early adulthood. Patients may complain of decreased exercise tolerance, dyspnea on exertion, hemoptysis, palpitations due to atrial arrhythmias, and symptoms of hyperviscosity due to chronic polycythemia (vision disturbances, fatigue, headache, dizziness, paresthesias, and cerebrovascular accident). Brain abscesses can occur with right-to-left passage of an infected embolus. On examination, there may or may not be a murmur and there is a loud S2. CXR shows decreased pulmonary vasculature (pruned pattern), and ECG shows RVH. The only definitive therapy is a heart-lung transplant. Patients with **Eisenmenger's syndrome** should avoid dehydration, heavy exertion, altitude, vasodilators, and pregnancy. Symptoms of hyperviscosity may be treated with phlebotomy. Ongoing care with a cardiologist should be arranged.

CARE OF THE POSTCARDIAC SURGERY CONGENITAL HEART PATIENT

CATEGORIES OF REPAIR

- Complete CHD repairs are successful for ASD, VSD, PDA, aortic coarctation, and TGA (switch procedure). Patients generally lead a normal life after a complete repair.
- Repairs of TOF, AV canal, and valve obstructions typically result in anatomic repairs with residual lesions; late complications may occur.

- Repairs requiring prosthetic materials will require replacement of the prosthetic material due to growth of the child or degeneration of the material.
- Physiologic repairs improve the patient's blood flow physiology but do not result in normal cardiac anatomy. These palliative repairs, which include the Fontan, Senning, and Mustard operations, invariably produce late complications.

POSTOPERATIVE COMPLICATIONS

- **Arrhythmias** are the most common problem and may present with palpitations, decreased appetite, emesis, and decreased exercise tolerance. Arrhythmias may result from the surgical repair, the underlying lesion, or medical therapy. Supraventricular tachycardia (SVT) is the most common clinically significant arrhythmia and is seen in lesions repaired with atriotomy (Senning, Mustard, Fontan, ASD repair, TAPVR repair). Bradycardia due to sinoatrial nodal disease is seen in 20 percent of patients status post Fontan repair, and first-degree block may occur after AV canal repair. Ventricular arrhythmias are rare. Premature ventricular contractions are benign if isolated and unifocal (order a 24-h Holter monitor test); consult a cardiologist if they are frequent, coupled, or multifocal. Isolated, infrequent premature atrial contractions are common in normal and postcardiac surgery patients. RBBB is common after VSD, TOF, and AV canal repairs.
- **Residual or recurrent lesions** occur as a complication of repair, due to incomplete success of the repair, from outgrowing prosthetic materials, or from conduit stenosis. Coarctations recur in 10 percent of repaired patients. Recurrent stenosis after PS or AS repair is common, as is aortic insufficiency after AS repair. Recurrent stenosis may be recognized by a new murmur or a change in exercise tolerance. A residual small VSD around the borders of the patch is present in 15 to 25 percent of patients after VSD or TOF repair; most close spontaneously within 6 to 12 months.
- **Endocarditis** is seen in congenital heart patients before and after surgical repair. Unrepaired complex congenital heart disease carries the highest risk, at 1.5 percent per patient-year. ASDs of the ostium secundum type are the lowest risk lesions and do not require antibiotic prophylaxis for procedures, even if unrepaired. Patients with repaired ASD, VSD, PDA, aortic coarctation, and PS (no mechanical valve) without residual lesions, and patients status post heart transplantation or pacemaker insertion also carry a low risk and do not require prophylaxis. Patients status post AS or TOF repair and those with prosthetic valves require prophylaxis.
- Antibiotic prophylaxis should be given prior to invasive procedures likely to produce bacteremia (Table 32-5).
- Other complications include poor growth, electrolyte disturbances due to medications, cerebral embolus in patients with right-to-left shunts, and increased susceptibility to respiratory illnesses. Cardiac patients may have a particularly difficult time with respiratory syncytial virus infections.

TABLE 32-5   Endocarditis Prophylaxis

Procedures For which Prophylaxis Is Recommended

Dental and periodontal procedures
Replacement of avulsed teeth
Tonsillectomy and/or adenoidectomy
Surgery involving respiratory mucosa
Rigid bronchoscopy
Sclerotherapy for esophageal varices
Esophageal stricture dilation
Endoscopic retrograde cholangiography
Biliary tract surgery
Surgery involving intestinal mucosa
Prostatic surgery
Cystoscopy
Urethral dilation

Prophylactic Regimens

Amoxicillin 50 mg/kg (maximum 2 g) orally 1 h before procedure
  If unable to take oral medication:
    Ampicillin 50 mg/kg (maximum 2 g) IM or IV 30 min before procedure
  If allergic to penicillin:
    Clindamycin 20 mg/kg (maximum 600 mg) orally 1 h before procedure
    Cephalexin or cefadroxil 50 mg/kg (maximum 2 g) orally 1 h before procedure
    Azithromycin or clarithromycin 15 mg/kg (maximum 500 mg) orally 1 h before procedure
  If unable to take oral medication and allergic to penicillin:
    Clindamycin 20 mg/kg (maximum 600 mg) IV 30 min before procedure
    Cefazolin 25 mg/kg (maximum 1 g) IM or IV 30 min before procedure
  For genitourinary and gastrointestinal (excluding esophageal) procedures, high-risk patient
    Ampicillin 50 mg/kg (maximum 2 g) *and* gentamicin 1.5 mg/kg (maximum 120 mg) IM or IV within 30 min of procedure. Six h later, ampicillin 25 mg/kg (maximum 1 g) IM or IV *or* amoxicillin 25 mg/kg (maximum 1 g) orally
  For genitourinary and gastrointestinal (excluding esophageal) procedures, high-risk patient allergic to pencillin
    Vancomycin 20 mg/kg (maximum 1 g) IV over 1–2 h *and* gentamicin 1.5 mg/kg (maximum 120 mg) IM or IV; complete within 30 min of procedure
  For genitourinary and gastrointestinal (excluding esophageal) procedures, moderate-risk patient
    Amoxicillin or ampicillin as above
  For genitourinary and gastrointestinal (excluding esophageal) procedures, moderate-risk patient allergic to penicillin:
    Vancomycin as above (without gentamicin)

BIBLIOGRAPHY

Brickner ME, Hillis LD, Lange RA: Medical progress: Congenital heart disease in adults (part 1). *N Engl J Med* 342:256, 2000.

Brickner ME, Hillis LD, Lange RA: Medical progress: Congenital heart disease in adults (part 2). *N Engl J Med* 342:334, 2000.

Clyman RI: Ibuprofen and patent ductus arteriosus. *N Engl J Med* 343:728–730, 2000.

Gewitz MH, Vetter VL: Cardiac emergencies. In: Fleischer GR, Ludwig S, eds. *Textbook of Pediatric Emergency Medicine*, 4th ed. Philadelphia: Lippincott Williams & Wilkins, 659–700, 2000.

Gidding SS, Anisman P: What pediatric residents should learn (or what pediatricians should know) about congenital heart disease. *Pediatr Cardiol* Jan 28, 2003 (epub ahead of print).

O-Laughlin MP: Congestive heart failure in children. *Pediatr Clin North Am* 46:263, 1999.

Overmeire BV, Smets K, Lecoutere D, et al: A comparison of ibuprofen and indomethacin for closure of patent ductus arteriosus. *N Engl J Med* 343:674–681, 2000.

Pelech AN: Evaluation of the pediatric patient with a cardiac murmur. *Pediatr Clin North Am* 46:167, 1999.

Rosenkranz ER: Pediatric surgery for the primary care pediatrician, part I: Caring for the former pediatric cardiac surgery patient. *Pediatr Clin North Am* 45:907, 1998.

Toepper WC, Hakim SN: Cardiac disorders. In: Rosen P, Barkin R, eds. *Emergency Medicine: Concepts and Clinical Practice*, 4th ed. St. Louis: Mosby-Year Book, 1159–1168, 1998.

Woolridge DP, Love JC: Congenital heart disease in the pediatric emergency department. *Pediatr Emerg Med Reports* 7: 69–92, 2002.

QUESTIONS

1. A 1-week-old infant is brought to the ED after suddenly becoming ill. The infant's skin is cool and pale-to-cyanotic. He is tachycardic with a weak pulse. Blood pressure is 60 systolic. What is the mainstay of therapy for this problem?
   A. Packed red cells or whole blood immediately
   B. Ceftriaxone, 100 mg/kg IV immediately
   C. Prostaglandin E_1, 0.1 µg/kg bolus, followed by 0.1 µg/kg/min infusion
   D. Epinephrine, 0.01 mg/kg IV bolus
   E. Dopamine, 5 to 10 µg/kg/min infusion

2. A 5-year-old child is found to have a blood pressure of 140/90 as he is evaluated by his pediatrician due to a complaint of bilateral leg pain with running. His femoral pulses are found to be weak bilaterally. He has a systolic ejection murmur at the apex and a thrill is palpable in the suprasternal notch. Chest x-ray shows notching of ribs 3 through 8, posteriorly. ECG shows LVH. These findings are most likely due to which of the following lesions?
   A. Coarctation of the aorta
   B. Aortic stenosis
   C. Pulmonary stenosis
   D. Patent ductus arteriosus
   E. Transposition of the great arteries

3. Which of the following is a characteristic associated with benign cardiac murmurs?
   A. Early to mid-systolic
   B. High pitched
   C. Late systolic
   D. Diastolic
   E. Pansystolic

4. A lesion that produces a left-to-right shunt will present as which of the following syndromes?
   A. Cyanotic heart disease
   B. Hypoperfusion and shock
   C. Asymptomatic; identified on routine physical examination
   D. Congestive heart failure
   E. Hypertension

5. A 2-year-old child with known congenital heart disease is brought to the ED while traveling with his parents. No medical records are available and the parents do not know the nature of the disease. The child has some degree of cyanosis all the time but today he became very cyanotic and this was associated with restlessness, irritability, and one episode of near syncope. He has a loud pansystolic murmur at the left sternal border. ECG shows RAD and RVH. Which of the following interventions is most likely to help in this situation?
   A. Dobutamine
   B. Morphine
   C. Trendelenburg position
   D. Isoproterenol
   E. Nitroprusside

6. Congenital heart disease can be classified as cyanotic and acyanotic types. Which of the following is classified as an acyanotic cardiac lesion?
   A. Tetralogy of Fallot
   B. Tricuspid anomalies
   C. Truncus arteriosus
   D. Ventricular septal defect
   E. Transposition of the great vessels

7. A 3-month-old infant with a history of ventricular septal defect, presents with the onset over 1 week of poor feeding, breathing difficulty, and cough. Physical examination reveals tachypnea, retractions, tachycardia, poor peripheral pulses, and hepatomegaly. Which of the following is true regarding this patient?
   A. The etiology is from a viral illness.

B. Jugular venous distension and peripheral edema are common in infants.

C. The CXR will show cardiomegaly and increased pulmonary vascularity.

D. Treatment includes a fluid bolus of 20 cc/kg of normal saline.

E. Supplemental oxygenation is detrimental in these patients.

8. A 1-week-old neonate is brought in to the ED for evaluation of poor feeding and cyanosis. The newborn has a pulse oximetry reading of 85% and appears cyanotic. You administer 100% oxygen for several minutes. Which of the following is correct regarding this patient?

A. If respiratory disease, there should be improvement in P_{O_2}.

B. If respiratory disease, there should be no change in the P_{O_2}.

C. If cardiac cyanosis from right-to-left shunting, a deterioration in the P_{O_2}.

D. This test does not help distinguish the etiology of cyanosis.

E. If cardiac cyanosis from right-to-left shunting, there should be improvement in P_{O_2}.

9. Which of the following is true regarding Eisenmenger's syndrome?

A. Typically occurs in the first 6 months of life.

B. Is seen in left-to-right shunts left unrepaired that develop pulmonary hypertension, reversal of the shunt, and cyanosis.

C. The definitive treatment is surgical repair of the cardiac lesion.

D. Vasodilators are beneficial in these patients.

E. The CXR shows increased pulmonary vascularity.

10. Which of the following is a correct statement regarding congenital heart lesions?

A. Transposition of the great arteries is the most common cyanotic lesion to present in the first week of life.

B. All ventricular septal defects must be repaired.

C. Tetralogy of Fallot involves a single arterial trunk supplying both pulmonary and systemic circulations.

D. Aortic coarctation results in elevated blood pressure in the lower extremities compared to upper extremities.

E. Atrial septal defects are typically diagnosed in the first month of life.

ANSWERS

1. C. Lesions completely dependent on a patent ductus arteriosus for systemic or pulmonary blood flow present with acute onset circulatory failure when the ductus closes, typically within the first week of life. The mainstay of therapy is prostaglandin E_1 infusion, which maintains the patency of the ductus.

2. A. These are the classic findings of aortic coarctation. Coarctation accounts for 10 percent of congenital heart lesions. The median age of detection is 5 to 8 years. Children may present with complications of hypertension, including intracranial hemorrhage.

3. A. Benign cardiac murmurs are usually softer, lower pitched and early to mid-systolic compared to pathologic murmurs. They are virtually never late systolic, diastolic, or pansystolic.

4. D. Lesions that produce a left-to-right shunt will typically result in CHF. Right-to-left shunts result in cyanotic heart disease. Outflow obstructions result in hypoperfusion and shock. Coarctation results in hypertension. Many lesions may be clinically inapparent and are discovered on routine physical examination. Examples include ASD, small VSD, PDA, PS, AS, and aortic coarctation.

5. B. This child most likely has tetralogy of Fallot and this is a hypoxemic "tet" spell. The cause is uncertain but the classic explanation is sudden increase in right ventricular outflow obstruction, leading to right-to-left shunting. Morphine, 0.1 to 0.2 mg/kg IV is the traditional first-line medical therapy. A fluid bolus of 10 mL/kg normal saline should be given concomitantly to counteract the vasodilatation caused by the morphine. The knee-chest position may be helpful and older children will often spontaneously squat when they have an attack. If the above therapies do not work, propranolol or phenylephrine may be used, usually in consultation with a pediatric cardiologist.

6. D. Cyanotic lesions are the "5 T's": tetralogy of Fallot, tricuspid anomalies, truncus arteriosus, total anomalous pulmonary venous return, and transposition of the great arteries. Acyanotic lesions include VSD, ASD, and patent ductus arteriosus.

7. C. This infant is presenting in CHF, which typically presents within the first 6 months of life in children with left-to-right shunts. Jugular venous distension and peripheral edema are rarely seen in young children. The CXR shows cardiomegaly and increased pulmonary vascularity. The treatment includes fluid and sodium restriction, furosemide, and oxygen to keep saturations about 95 percent.

8. A. This is the hyperoxia test that helps differentiate between cardiac and respiratory cyanosis. With respiratory disease, there should be improvement in the P_{O_2} or oxygen saturation while, with cardiac cyanosis due to intracardiac right-to-left shunting, there will be no improvement.

9. B. Patients with a large left-to-right shunt left unrepaired gradually develop pulmonary vascular disease due to the increased volume overload. When pulmonary HTN becomes severe, the direction of the shunting reverses and cyanosis develops. This typically occurs in adolescence to early adulthood. The definitive therapy is a heart-lung transplant. Vasodilators should be avoided. The CXR will show decreased pulmonary vasculature.

10. A. Transposition of the great arteries is the most common cyanotic lesion to present in the first week of life. Small VSDs have a high rate of spontaneous closure. Truncus arteriosus involves a single arterial trunk supplying both pulmonary and systemic circulations. Aortic coarctation results in blood pressure elevation in the upper extremities compared with the lower extremities. Many atrial septal defects are undiagnosed until adulthood.

33 CONGESTIVE AND INFLAMMATORY HEART DISEASES

William C. Toepper
Joilo Barbosa
Kemedy K. McQuillen
Gary R. Strange
Valerie A. Dobiesz

CONGESTIVE HEART FAILURE

- Congestive heart failure (CHF), the physiologic state in which cardiac output is unable to meet tissue metabolic demands, has many etiologies (Table 33-1).
- Cardiac output is determined by *preload*, or filling volume, (increased in left-to-right shunts), *afterload*, or the resistance the ventricles face upon ejection of blood (important in outlet obstruction or systemic hypertension), *contractility* (altered in cardiomyopathy), and *rate* (too slow results in inadequate output and too fast decreases diastolic filling).
- The features of CHF are due to end-organ hypoperfusion (Table 33-2). Initially, decreased renal blood flow results in renin/angiotensin-based salt and water retention, an increased circulating volume, and a rise in blood pressure due to angiotensin-2, a potent vasoconstrictor. Sympathetically mediated contractility results from decreased oxygen delivery. Redistribution of blood from skin and skeletal muscle to heart, brain, and kidney improves vital function. As

TABLE 33-1 Etiologic Basis of Congestive Heart Failure

Preload (Volume Overload)

Left-to-right shunt: VSD, PDA, AV fistula
Anemia: iron deficiency, sickle cell, thalassemia
Iatrogenic

Afterload (Increased SVR)

Congenital: coarctation of the aorta, aortic stenosis
Systemic hypertension

Contractility

Inflammatory: infectious (myocarditis)
Rheumatic: rheumatic fever, early Kawasaki, SLE
Toxin: digoxin, Ca^{2+} channel/β-blocker, cocaine
Traumatic: cardiac tamponade, myocardial contusion
Metabolic: electrolyte abnormality, hypothyroidism

VSD, ventricular septal defect; PDA, patent ductus arteriosus; AV, arteriovenous; SLE, systemic lupus erythematosus.

TABLE 33-2 Symptom-Based Assessment of Congestive Heart Failure

SIGNS/SYMPTOMS	MECHANISM	TREATMENT
Pulmonary Venous Congestion		
Tachypnea	L → R shunt	Diuresis
Wheezing	Pulmonary edema	Oxygen
Rales	Poor oxygenation	Sedation
Poor feeding		
Irritability		
Systemic Venous Congestion		
Hepatomegaly	Increased right-sided	Diuresis
Peripheral edema	filling pressure	(spironolactone)
Impaired Cardiac Output		
Decreased pulses	Decreased contractility	Digoxin
	and perfusion	Pressors
Delayed capillary		Afterload
refill		reduction

the disease process worsens, physiologic mechanisms are unable to keep up and overcompensation produces symptoms: salt and water retention produces edema, increased adrenergic response and tachycardia cause inadequate diastolic filling, decreased skin perfusion results in mottling and pallor, and increased systemic vascular resistance increases myocardial demand, causing hypertrophy or dilation. Diaphoresis during feeding is secondary to catecholamine release. Valve insufficiency or myocardial ischemia can further decrease cardiac output.

- Clinically, infants in CHF are irritable, feed poorly, are diaphoretic when eating, and have poor weight gain. An acute weight gain may be due to edema. They may have tachycardia, tachypnea, high or low blood pressure, poor capillary refill, and cough or chest congestion. Signs of CHF include adventitial lung sounds, a gallop rhythm, or hyperactive precordium. Displaced PMI, right ventricular lift, or palpable murmur is strongly suggestive of CHF. There may be hepatomegaly, a common finding in pediatric CHF. Pedal edema and neck vein distention are rare and facial edema and anasarca are late findings. The chest radiograph may show increased pulmonary vascular markings, interstitial fluid, or pulmonary edema. The ECG, in addition to assessing chamber enlargement or hypertrophy, is useful in picking up dysrhythmia or ST/T-wave changes. Echocardiography and/or pulmonary artery catheterization are diagnostic.

- The treatment of CHF is directed toward the cause:
  - Interventional techniques for obstructive lesions
  - Exchange transfusion for profound anemia
  - Pericardiocentesis for cardiac tamponade
- Empiric therapy includes:
  - Positioning
  - Sedation (morphine sulfate)
  - Supplemental oxygen
  - Intravenous fluids to relieve the work of feeding
- Pharmacologic therapy is directed at the specific cause:
  - Furosemide for fluid overload
  - Digoxin to improve cardiac contractility, slow rate, and relieve diaphoresis.

- Digoxin is contraindicated in myocarditis-associated CHF because of its arrhythmogenic effects on the irritable myocardium.
- Dosing is outlined in Table 33-3.
  - Amrinone, a positive inotrope that decreases pulmonary vascular resistance, may be beneficial in digoxin-refractory patients. It may cause hypotension.
  - β-Blockers may also have a role in chronic CHF by "upregulating" cell wall receptors and increasing contractility.
  - The decision to begin digoxin, amrinone, or β-blockers should be made in consultation with a pediatric cardiologist.
- Consider dopamine to increase contractility and blood pressure, dobutamine for its pronounced effect on contractility, and epinephrine to improve blood pressure (Table 33-4).
- In the setting of low output with increased systemic resistance, reduce afterload with an angiotensin-converting enzyme (ACE) inhibitor; however, do not use ACE inhibitors in patients with renal insufficiency or right-to-left shunts. In right-to-left shunt, the systemic circulation may improve at the expense of the pulmonary circulation. In severe cases, such as myocarditis with cardiogenic shock, the weakened myocardium ineffectively pumps against increased afterload. Vasodilators such as sodium nitroprusside may be helpful (Table 33-5).
- An algorithmic approach to CHF is presented in Fig. 33-1.
- Admit the child in moderate to severe CHF to an intensive care unit. Intubate if needed to improve oxygenation and provide positive end-expiratory pressure (PEEP).

MYOCARDITIS AND PERICARDITIS

- Can be subtle early in their presentation.
- Etiologies of myocarditis and pericarditis include viruses (enterovirus, varicella, and mumps), bacteria (*Haemophilus influenzae*, *C. diphtheria*, and

TABLE 33-3 Oral Dosing Guidelines for Digoxin[a]

AGE AND WEIGHT	ACUTE DIGITALIZATION (µg/kg)[b]	MAINTENANCE
Premature infant	20	5 µg/kg/day
Full-term infant	30	4–5 µg/kg q12h
2–24 mo	40–50	5–10 µg/kg q12h
>24 mo	30–40	4–5 µg/kg q12h

[a]IV dose is 75% of PO dose.
[b]Daily dose = 1/2 given initially, then 1/4 given at 8 h and 1/4 given at 16 h.

TABLE 33-4 Inotropic Agents: Dosage and Pharmacologic Effects

DRUG	DOSE (µg/kg/min)	INCREASED HR	INCREASED CONTRACTILITY	INCREASED AFTERLOAD	VASODILATION
Dopamine	1–5	1+	1+	0	renal
	6–20	2–3+	3+	1–3+	0
Dobutamine	2–10	1+	3+	0	1+
Epinephrine	0.05–1	3+	3+	0–3+	0–2+
				(dose dependent)	
Norepinephrine	0.05–0.5	2+	3+	4+	0
Isoproterenol	0.1	3+	2+	2+	0
				(bronchial smooth muscle)	

TABLE 33-5   Load-Altering Agents

DRUG	DOSE	COMMENTS
Nitroprusside	1–10 µg/kg/min IV	Cyanide toxicity
Captopril	Infants: 0.1–2.0 mg/kg PO q8–12h	Neutropenia, cough, proteinuria
Nitroglycerin	2–10 µg/kg/min IV	Use not well established in children
Amrinone	0.5–2 mg/kg, then 5–10 µm/kg/min IV	Hypotension

M. tuberculosis), rickettsia, fungus, parasites, and inflammatory disorders (Lyme disease, acute rheumatic fever, and collagen vascular disease). Most cases are idiopathic. Additional causes of myocarditis include toxins (cocaine), anomalous origin of the coronary arteries, and HIV.

- Signs and symptoms of **myocarditis** are primarily those of CHF: gallop rhythm, hyperactive precordium, hepatomegaly, wheezing, grunting, and tachypnea. There may also be fever with muscle or joint tenderness. Presentation is often fulminant, with cardiogenic shock, acidosis, or syncope secondary to dysrhythmia. Chest radiography may demonstrate cardiomegaly and pulmonary vascular congestion.

ECG findings include diffuse ST/T-wave changes, low voltage, interval prolongation, and ectopy. Ventricular ectopy signals diffuse myocardial involvement with risk of sudden death. Prognostic indicators include the presence of pulmonary vascular congestion, the acuity of onset of CHF, a cardiac index below 3 L/min, and a northwest axis. An arterial blood gas, acute viral serologies, and cardiac enzymes may be helpful. Consider emergent echocardiography. The definitive diagnostic procedure is a right-sided endocardial biopsy. Myocarditis carries a grave prognosis, with 35 percent mortality.

- ○ Initial management includes the treatment of CHF: bed rest, oxygen, fluid restriction, diuresis, and inotropic support may be necessary. Invasive monitoring should be considered.
- ○ Do not use digoxin because of its potential to cause dysrhythmia.
- ○ Anticipatory management of dysrhythmias may prevent sudden death: closely monitor and correct acid–base derangements, metabolic abnormalities, and fluid status.
- ○ Corticosteroids and immunosuppressants are rarely used to treat myocarditis and transplantation may be required for end-stagecardiomyopathy.

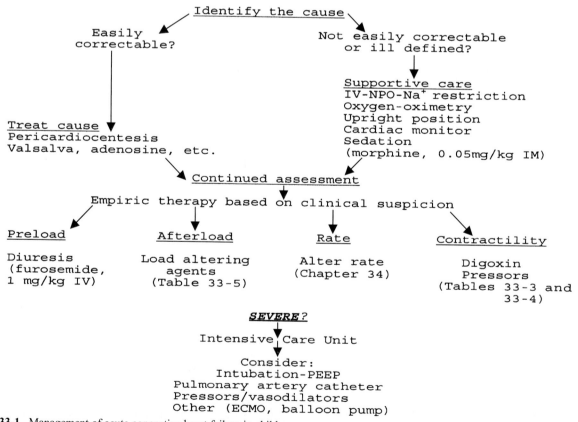

FIG. 33-1. Management of acute congestive heart failure in children.

- Rejection and infection maycomplicate the initial posttransplant period: suspect rejection in the setting of lethargy, poor feeding, fever, CHF, and dysrhythmia. Echocardiogram or biopsy may be necessary to confirm the diagnosis.
  - Infection should be approached individually: cytomegalovirus and *Pneumocystis carinii* infections are most common early after transplantation, when immunosuppression is highest.
- Unlike myocarditis, most cases of **pericarditis** are self-limited and follow a benign clinical course. Findings include pleuritic or positional chest pain, abdominal pain, dyspnea, fever, a pericardial friction rub and tachycardia. Sitting forward can often relieve the pain. The ECG can be diagnostic, with diffuse ST-segment elevation and PR depression. Low voltage and electrical alternans signal significant effusion. Treatment is supportive and directed toward the cause. Treat inflammation and pain with nonsteroidal antiinflammatory agents. Consider hospitalization and cardiology consultation in all cases. If a child appears ill or has a large effusion, admit them to an intensive care setting.
- In the setting of a significant effusion with an ill appearing child, consider **constrictive pericarditis**. Constrictive pericarditis is usually bacterial (*Staphylococcus aureus, H. influenzae,* and *Streptococcus pneumoniae*) and treatment consists of antibiotics, emergent pericardiocentesis, and an operative pericardial window.
- In some cases, effusion is minimal, but a thickened stiff pericardium results in **cardiac tamponade**. It is rare in viral or idiopathic pericarditis but should be considered when heart sounds are distant, or in the presence of pulsus paradoxus or jugular venous distention.

ENDOCARDITIS

- **Bacterial endocarditis** can complicate congenital heart disease, central venous catheters, or intravenous drugs and seeding can occur via dental caries, skin infections, and manipulation of the airway, gastrointestinal tract, or genitourinary tract. Staphylococcal and streptococcal species predominate, with HACEK organisms (*Hemophilus, Actinobacillus, Cardiobacterium, Eikenella,* and *Kingella*) and *Candida* as occasional offenders. Findings may include fever, weakness, myalgia, arthralgia, congestive heart failure secondary to valvular insufficiency, petechiae, or new neurologic findings. A new murmur is present in fewer than 50 percent of cases and Janeway lesions or Osler nodes are rare.

- Blood culture will identify the organism in 90 percent of cases. The white blood cell count and erythrocyte sedimentation rate may be elevated and anemia, hematuria, or embolic infiltrates may be present. In 70 to 80 percent of cases, echocardiography is diagnostic.
- If possible, start antibiotic therapy after an organism is recovered from blood cultures. In the sickest patients, though, empiric broad-spectrum coverage may be required before the organism is known. Removal of the vegetation or valve replacement may be indicated for persistent bacteremia, threatened or recurrent embolization, severe valve failure, recalcitrant arrhythmia secondary to vegetation, or myocardial abscess.
- Because of the high mortality rate (6 to 14 percent), prevention of endocarditis is vital. Indications for endocarditis prophylaxis are dynamic and current American Heart Association guidelines are summarized in Tables 32-5 and 33-6.

ACUTE RHEUMATIC FEVER

- The **carditis of acute rheumatic fever** is characterized by valve involvement. The acute phase begins 2 to 3 weeks after a group A streptococcal infection. Diagnosis is based on the Jones criteria (Table 33-7). Carditis can involve all three layers of the heart and a

TABLE 33-6   Endocarditis Prophylaxis in Cardiac Conditions[a]

Endocarditis Prophylaxis Recommended

High risk
   Prosthetic valves
   Previous bacterial endocarditis
   Complex cyanotic malformations
   Surgical systemopulmonary shunts

Moderate risk
   Rheumatic or acquired valvular dysfunction
   Hypertrophic cardiomyopathy
   MVP with regurgitation or thickened leaflets
   Most other complex cardiac malformations

Endocarditis Prophylaxis Not Recommended

Isolated secundum ASD
Repaired secundum ASD, VSD, PDA, without residua after 6 mo
Innocent murmurs
Previous Kawasaki syndrome without valvular dysfunction
Previous rheumatic fever without valvular dysfunction
Cardiac pacemakers and implanted defibrillators

ASO, atrial septal defect; VSD, ventriculoseptal defect; PDA, patent ductus arteriosus; MVP, mitral valve prolapse.
[a]This table lists selected conditions but is not meant to be all inclusive.

SOURCE: Adapted from Dajani AS, Taubert KA, Gerber MA, et al: prevention of bacterial endocarditis: Recommendations by the American Heart Association. *JAMA* 277:1794, 1997.

TABLE 33-7 Guidelines for the Diagnosis of Initial Attack of Rheumatic Fever (Jones Criteria, 1992 Update)

Major Manifestations

Carditis
Polyarthritis
Chorea
Erythema marginatum
Subcutaneous nodules

Minor Manifestations

Clinical findings
  Arthralgia
  Fever
Laboratory findings
  Elevated acute phase reactants
    Erythrocyte sedimentation rate
    C-reactive protein
  Prolonged PR interval

Supporting Evidence of Antecedent Group A Streptococcal Infection

Positive throat culture or rapid streptococcal antigen test
Elevated or rising streptococcal antibody titer
If supported by evidence of a preceding group A streptococcal infection, the presence of two major manifestations or of one major and two minor manifestations indicates a high probability of acute rheumatic fever.

benign acute phase can be followed years later with valvular insufficiency. Mitral insufficiency is most common and is characterized by a holosystolic, high-pitched, blowing apical murmur that radiates to the axilla. Aortic insufficiency may also occur and presents with a mid-diastolic, high-pitched, blowing murmur located at the base and radiating into the neck. The incidence of valve involvement is reduced with early aggressive management. Other cardiac findings include tachycardia, gallop rhythm, pericardial rub, or congestive heart failure. The ECG may demonstrate PR prolongation, conduction delays, left ventricular hypertrophy (LVH), or dysrhythmia. Echocardiography is used diagnostically and in follow-up.

- Treatment during the acute phase includes hospitalization, bed rest, high-dose aspirin, and penicillin or erythromycin to eradicate residual streptococci. Corticosteroid use is controversial but may have a role in the treatment of carditis or chorea. Long-term follow-up includes cardiac rehabilitation, surveillance for recurrence, endocarditis prophylaxis, and treatment of chronic failure.

CHEST PAIN IN CHILDREN AND ADOLESCENTS

- The cause of chest pain in the pediatric population is usually benign and includes musculoskeletal, pulmonic (pneumonitic, pleuritic, or asthmatic), traumatic, or gastrointestinal pain. The cases most concerning for cardiac pain are those involving children with known cardiac disease, chest pain during exercise, syncope, or children with abnormal vital signs or dysrhythmias. Cardiac chest pain may be caused by myocarditis or pericarditis (reviewed previously), aortic stenosis, hypertrophic cardiomyopathy, or ischemia. Aortic stenosis or hypertrophic cardiomyopathy are suggested by chest pain and a new murmur. These patients may present with exertional pain, dyspnea, ischemia, or syncope and should be screened for LVH: those with LV strain or ST/ T-wave abnormalities are at higher risk for ischemia or sudden death. Myocardial ischemia is rare but can occur in patients with a history of Kawasaki disease, in those who use cocaine, sniff glue, or take steroids chronically, or in patients with familial hyperlipidemia, familial hypercholesterolemia, or collagen vascular disease (particularly systemic lupus erythematosus). It can also occur with structural abnormalities of the heart and coronary arteries.

- Evaluation includes a thorough history and physical examination. Ancillary tests, such as chest radiography and ECG, may be helpful.

- Most children with chest pain can be safely discharged. A logical explanation for the pain and plans for follow-up should be provided. Prescribe nonsteroidal antiinflammatory agents or acetaminophen and explain activity level and back-to-school expectations.

BIBLIOGRAPHY

Bruns LA, Canter CE: Should beta-blockers be used for the treatment of pediatric patients with chronic heart failure. *Paediatr Drugs* 4:771–778, 2002.

Chinnock R, Sherwin T, Robie S, et al: Emergency department presentation and management of pediatric heart transplant recipients. *Pediatr Emerg Care* 11:355–369, 1995.

Dajani AS, Taubert KA, Gerber MA, et al: Prevention of bacterial endocarditis: Recommendations by the American Heart Association. *JAMA* 277:1794, 1997.

Feldman AM, McNamara D: Medical progress: Myocarditis. *N Engl J Med* 343:1388–1398, 2000.

O'Laughlin MP: Congestive heart failure in children. *Pediatr Clin North Am* 46:263–273, 1999.

Shannon KM: Arrhythmias in congenital heart disease. *Curr Treat Options Cardiovascular Med* 1:373–379, 1999.

QUESTIONS

1. A 2-month-old infant is brought to the ED by the mother who reports that the infant has been fussy for the past several days. He is taking less formula than previously and yesterday the mother noted him to be sweating profusely during feeding. He is afebrile with heart rate of 200 and respiratory rate of 60. What is the most likely cause of these complaints?
   A. Myocarditis
   B. Pericarditis
   C. Endocarditis
   D. Congestive heart failure
   E. Acute rheumatic fever

2. On physical examination, the child described above has rales and a hyperactive precordium associated with a gallop. There is hepatomegaly but no pedal edema or neck vein distention. Chest x-ray shows pulmonary edema. Which of the following is true regarding the most appropriate management?
   A. The child is kept at strict bed rest in the supine position.
   B. Sedation is contraindicated since it will result in respiratory depression.
   C. Oxygen can be given but concentrations are limited to <50%.
   D. Digoxin is contraindicated due its arrhythmogenicity.
   E. Fluid overload is treated with furosemide, 1 mg/kg/dose IV.

3. An infant presents with all of the symptoms and signs described above, but is also noted to be febrile and to have wheezing throughout the lung fields. Treatment with bronchodilators is ineffective. What etiology should be suspected?
   A. Myocarditis
   B. Pericarditis
   C. Endocarditis
   D. Acute rheumatic fever
   E. Kawasaki disease

4. An 8-year-old child presents with pleuritic chest pain that is partially relieved in the sitting position, leaning forward. On examination, there is tachycardia and a friction rub. On ECG, there is diffuse ST elevation and PR depression. What is the prognosis for this child?
   A. Grave, with 35 percent mortality
   B. Usually benign
   C. There is a high mortality rate without early antibiotic therapy
   D. There is a benign acute phase that may be followed years later with severe heart disease
   E. Benign unless there is an infectious etiology

5. The risk for development of bacterial endocarditis is high enough to warrant prophylaxis with all of the following cardiac conditions **EXCEPT**?
   A. Previous bacterial endocarditis
   B. Rheumatic valvular dysfunction
   C. Complex cyanotic malformations
   D. Previous rheumatic fever without valvular dysfunction
   E. Hypertrophic cardiomyopathy

6. Diagnosis of acute rheumatic fever can be based on which of the following?
   A. Two major or three minor manifestations of the Jones criteria.
   B. Supporting evidence of antecedent group A streptococcal infection and any of the manifestations of the Jones criteria.
   C. Supporting evidence of antecedent group A streptococcal infection and two major manifestations or one major and two minor manifestations of the Jones criteria.
   D. Jones criteria are no longer used in the diagnosis of rheumatic fever; diagnosis is made whenever there is preceding streptococcal infection followed by development of a murmur.
   E. Supporting evidence of antecedent group A streptococcal infection and complaint of chest pain.

7. A 10-year-old male presents with the complaint of a 1-day history of chest pain. Which of the following is true regarding this patient?
   A. The cause of chest pain in children is usually cardiac in etiology and serious.
   B. Concerning chest pain includes chest pain during exercise.
   C. Aortic stenosis typically presents without a murmur.
   D. Myocardial ischemia does not occur in children.
   E. A CXR and ECG are not helpful in the work-up.

8. Which of the following is true regarding the carditis of acute rheumatic fever?
   A. Is characterized by valve involvement.
   B. If asymptomatic during the acute phase, valvular insufficiency will not occur.
   C. Aortic insufficiency is the most common valvular abnormality.
   D. No change in incidence of valve involvement if treated early.
   E. Echocardiography is not useful in the work-up.

9. A 6-year-old female with a history of congenital heart disease presents after a dental procedure with complaints of fever, arthralgias, weakness, and petechiae. Which of the following is true regarding this patient?
   A. The predominant organisms are *Haemophilus* and *Cardiobacterium*.

B. Blood cultures will identify the organism in only 20% of cases.

C. The mortality rate is between 6 and 14%.

D. Echocardiography is diagnostic in 10% of cases.

E. Janeway and Osler nodes are common.

10. Which of the following is true regarding myocarditis?
   A. Most cases are caused by bacteria.
   B. Signs and symptoms are primarily those of cardiogenic shock.
   C. The definitive diagnostic procedure is echocardiography.
   D. Typically self-limited and benign.
   E. Transplantation may be required for end-stage cardiomyopathy.

ANSWERS

1. D. Clinically, children in CHF are irritable, feed poorly, and have poor weight gain. An acute weight gain may be due to edema. Diaphoresis during feeding is especially suggestive of CHF. Volume overload may present with respiratory symptoms. The lack of fever helps to differentiate from infection. Abnormal vital signs, such as unexplained tachycardia or tachypnea with normal temperature, may suggest cardiac disease.

2. E. Fluid overload is treated with furosemide. Upright positioning may be used as part of supportive care. Oxygen therapy need not be limited in the acute situation. Digoxin is contraindicated in CHF associated with myocarditis due to its arrhythmogenic effect on the irritable myocardium, but is indicated in other patients.

3. A. Myocarditis should be suspected in the wheezing, febrile child who does not respond to bronchodilators. CHF and cardiomegaly on chest radiography also suggest this diagnosis.

4. B. This child has pericarditis. Most cases are self-limited and will follow a benign course. Hospitalization and cardiology input are suggested. Occasionally, admission to an intensive care setting is necessary in an ill-appearing child or one with a large effusion.

5. D. Because of the high mortality rate, prevention of endocarditis is key. Prophylaxis is indicated for most complex cardiac malformations but is not recommended for previous rheumatic fever or Kawasaki disease without valvular dysfunction.

6. C. Diagnosis of the initial attack of rheumatic fever is based on the Jones criteria and requires supporting evidence of antecedent group A streptococcal infection and two major manifestations or one major and two minor manifestations of the Jones criteria.

7. B. The cause of chest pain in children is usually benign and includes musculoskeletal, pulmonic, traumatic, or gastrointestinal. The chest pain cases most concerning for cardiac abnormalities are those associated with known cardiac disease, exertional chest pain, syncope, or children with abnormal vital signs or dysrhythmia. Aortic stenosis usually presents with chest pain and a new murmur. Myocardial ischemia is rare but can occur in children. An ECG or CXR can be helpful in the evaluation of chest pain.

8. A. The carditis of ARF is characterized by valve involvement. A benign acute phase can be followed years later with valvular insufficiency. Mitral insufficiency is most common. The incidence of valve involvement is reduced with early aggressive management. Echocardiography is used diagnostically and in follow-up.

9. C. The predominant species are staphylococcal and streptococcal species. Blood cultures will identify the organism in 90 percent of cases. The mortality rate is high at 6 to 14 percent. Echocardiography is diagnostic in 70 to 80 percent of cases. Janeway lesions or Osler nodes are rare.

10. E. Most cases of myocarditis are idiopathic. Signs and symptoms of myocarditis are primarily those of CHF. The definitive diagnostic procedure is a right-sided endocardial biopsy. Myocarditis carries a grave prognosis, with a 35 percent mortality rate. Transplantation may be required for end-stage cardiomyopathy.

34 DYSRHYTHMIAS IN CHILDREN

William C. Toepper
Kemedy K. McQuillen
Valerie A. Dobiesz

EPIDEMIOLOGY

- Dysrhythmias in children are usually the result of cardiac lesions. Other causes include hypoxia, electrolyte imbalance, toxins, inflammatory disease, and cardioactive drugs, such as digoxin or over-the-counter cold remedies. A dysrhythmia associated with structural heart disease has a poorer prognosis than a one in a structurally normal heart. Evaluation of the child with idiopathic or unexplained dysrhythmia includes an echocardiogram.

- Age is an important consideration in the child with dysrhythmia. Some ventricular dysrhythmias disappear with age; other conditions associated with an escape pacemaker, worsen with age. Age is also a factor in the clinical presentation of the dysrhythmia. The infant may present with poor feeding, tachypnea, irritability, or signs of a low output state. The older child will have specific symptoms, such as syncope, chest pain, or palpitations. Active adolescents with syncope, palpitations, or exertional chest pain should be investigated promptly.
- The emergency management of dysrhythmias is dependent on rate, QRS width on a 12-lead ECG, and clinical stability, as determined by heart rate and blood pressure (Table 10-4). Children are tolerant of most rhythm disturbances, providing ample time for precise interpretation.

SLOW RATES

SINUS BRADYCARDIA

- **Sinus bradycardia** can be a manifestation of serious underlying disease or a normal physiologic variant. Serious causes include hypoxia, hypothyroidism, increased intracranial pressure, or calcium channel blocker, beta-blocker, or digoxin toxicity. Treat the underlying condition to correct the rate. If the cause is unclear and oxygenation and ventilation are adequate, give an unstable patient epinephrine (1:10,000, 0.01 mg/kg IV/IO) and atropine (0.02 mg/kg IV/IO).

ATRIOVENTRICULAR BLOCKS

- **Complete atrioventricular (AV) block** may be congenital or acquired. Congenital block associated with structural abnormalities has a poorer prognosis than AV block associated with maternal collagen vascular disease. Rates of 50 to 80 bpm are typical in complete AV block and rates above 50 are rarely symptomatic. Complete AV block is suspected in utero in the setting of sustained fetal bradycardia, polyhydramnios, and congestive heart failure (CHF). Treatment of neonatal symptomatic bradycardia due to AV block includes control of CHF, atropine or isoproterenol, and temporary transcutaneous, transthoracic, or umbilical transvenous pacing.
- **Acquired third degree block** is associated with myocarditis, endocarditis, rheumatic fever, cardiomyopathy, Lyme disease, or tumor. Postoperative blocks, which are less common today because of intraoperative mapping, may last for years or occur years after surgery. Unlike congenital third degree block, QRS complexes are usually wide. Treatment is similar, except patients with syncope must be paced immediately.

PACEMAKERS IN CHILDREN

- The indications for pediatric pacemakers include:
  ○ Symptomatic bradycardia (most common)
  ○ Prolonged Q T syndrome
  ○ Cardioinhibitory syncope lasting longer than 10 s
- Most permanent pediatric pacemakers are transvenous, with epicardial units being reserved for premature infants and those with right-to-left shunts. Choice of mode depends on disease. Most units can be programmed to sense, demand, or inhibit at the atrial or ventricular level, depending on the needs of the child. They may also be programmed to sense motion or breathing.
- Syncope or palpitations in a child with a pacemaker suggests malfunction. Chest radiography may reveal wire fracture or lead displacement. Most malfunctions are not mechanical and require external reprogramming. Uncaptured paced beats outside the refractory period require investigation. If the problem is not easily resolved, the patient should be admitted.
- Most temporary pacing in children is transcutaneous. If transcutaneous pacing is ineffective, a 3- to 6-F transvenous pacemaker can be placed via a femoral sheath. Atrial lead placement is preferred to avoid perforation or valve incompetence. After proper positioning, the catheter is connected to the pacemaker and maximum current is chosen. Upon successful capture, current is then decreased until capture is lost. This is the threshold current. The current is then set at 200 percent threshold. Sensitivity can be adjusted to allow for asynchronous pacing (low sensitivity) or overriding by native sinus pacemaker (high sensitivity).

FAST RATES

PAROXYSMAL SUPRAVENTRICULAR TACHYCARDIA

- The most common dysrhythmia in children is **paroxysmal supraventricular tachycardia** (PSVT). PSVT is differentiated from sinus tachycardia by:
  ○ Abrupt onset
  ○ Rate higher than 230 bpm
  ○ Absence of normal P waves

○ Little rate variation
- In infants, symptoms include ill appearance, poor feeding, tachypnea, and irritability.
- Although it may be associated with fever, infection, drug exposure, or congenital heart disease, PSVT is usually caused by one of two mechanisms: younger children are more likely to have accessory pathway tachycardia. Adolescents may have AV nodal reentry.
  ○ Accessory pathway tachycardia is usually orthodromic, with antegrade AV conduction and retrograde accessory pathway conduction (Fig. 34-1). Conduction during sinus rhythm can be via the accessory pathway, resulting in a short PR interval and appearance of a delta wave. This characterizes the Wolff–Parkinson–White (WPW) syndrome. Some accessory pathways only conduct retrograde during bouts of PSVT and are termed "concealed" because they are not apparent on surface ECG.
  ○ AV nodal reentry PSVT, is more common in adults, but may cause one third of cases of PSVT in adolescents. Within the AV node, fast pathways with long refractory periods are blocked during a PAC, allowing for anterograde conduction down the slow tract. The impulse then propagates up the fast tract, initiating reentry.
  ○ Distinguishing nodal from accessory pathway PSVT is difficult during episodes of PSVT.
    ▪ Negative P waves in II, III, and avF, may indicate retrograde conduction through the accessory pathway but they are usually buried in the QRS complex.
    ▪ Pointed or peaked T waves suggest retrograde P waves. P waves are almost never seen in AV nodal reentry.
    ▪ Lack of delta wave during sinus rhythm does not rule out concealed accessory tracts.
- Unstable PSVT is treated with synchronized cardioversion, 0.5 J/kg, increasing to 2 J/kg as needed. If unsuccessful, esophageal overdrive pacing may be necessary.

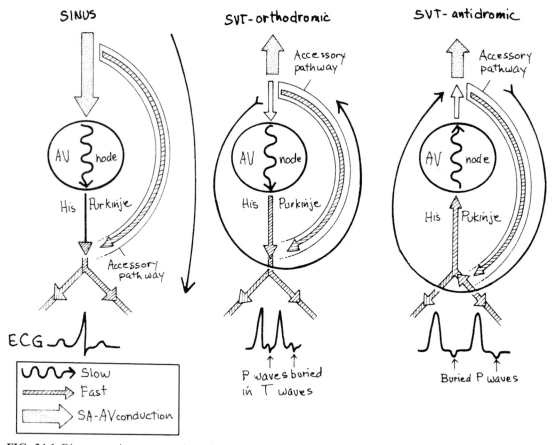

FIG. 34-1 Diagrammatic representation of accessory pathway disease during sinus rhythm and PSVT. Sinus–Short PR, delta wave, characteristic of WPW; Orthodromic-fast retrograde conduction through accessory pathway leads to reentry. His–Purkinje conduction is normal, complexes are narrow. Retrograde P waves are abnormally directed and buried in T wave; Antidromic (rare)–fast antegrade conduction through accessory pathway leads to abnormal His–Purkinje conduction and wide complexes. Retrograde P waves are abnormally directed and buried in T waves.

- Stable PSVT can be treated with vagal maneuvers by placing a bag of ice with some water over the nose and forehead for 15 to 20 s.
  - Ocular pressure and nasogastric tube manipulation are discouraged.
  - If ice water fails, adenosine, 0.1 mg/kg, followed by 0.3 mg/kg, is recommended. Adenosine terminates nodal and accessory pathway tachycardia. Transient side effects include headache, flushing, chest pain, apnea, bronchospasm, and asystole.
    - Adenosine can be used in hypotension but should be avoided in the patient on theophylline. Immediate recurrence rate approaches 50 percent.
  - Digitalis is commonly used to prolong AV nodal conduction and refractoriness of fast and slow tracts (see Table 33-3). It may precipitate ventricular tachycardia (VT) and should be used under the supervision of a pediatric cardiologist. Digoxin may take hours to work and, if cardioversion is necessary, there is a risk of ventricular fibrillation.
  - Verapamil is reserved for children older than 2 to 3 years of age. Hypotension, cardiovascular collapse, and death have occurred in infants. Older children with stable but recalcitrant PSVT may respond to IV verapamil, 0.1 mg/kg, slowly.
    - Calcium chloride, 10 mg/kg, and IV saline should be available to treat hypotension.
  - If the above measures fail, procainamide or propranolol may be useful.
    - Procainamide is preferred in narrow complex tachycardia thought to be ventricular. A 5- to 15-mg/kg bolus is given over 20 to 30 min, watching for hypotension.
    - Propranolol, 0.1 mg/kg IV, is useful in WPW or other accessory pathway diseases.
- Rhythm disturbances, such as atrial fibrillation, accelerated ventricular rhythm, and wide-complex tachycardia, may require resuscitation.
- Any infant with new onset PSVT should be hospitalized and structural heart disease ruled out. Electro physiologic studies (EPS) and surgical ablation may be necessary.

ATRIAL FLUTTER AND FIBRILLATION

- **Atrial flutter** and **fibrillation** in children are rare. Children with congenital heart disease, rheumatic fever, or dilated cardiomyopathy are at highest risk. Patients with atrial flutter or fibrillation, in combination with an accessory pathway or hypertrophic cardiomyopathy, are at high risk for sudden death. Cardiovert unstable patients with 0.5 J/kg. If not effective, attempt overdrive pacing 10 to 20 bpm faster than the flutter rate. Patients with long-standing atrial disease associated with a diseased sinus node are at risk for bradycardia or asystole on termination. Pacing must be available.

PREMATURE VENTRICULAR CONTRACTIONS

- **Premature ventricular contractions** (PVCs) in the infant and young child are rare: unifocal PVCs begin appearing in healthy children during adolescence. The patient is usually asymptomatic and has a normal physical examination, chest x-ray, and ECG. Unusual morphology, such as multifocal PVCs, coupling, or the "R on T" phenomenon, are rarely cause for emergency intervention in the asymptomatic child with a normal Q T interval. PVCs that diminish during exercise or stress are benign and require no therapy. Patients with myocarditis, cardiomyopathy, congenital heart disease, those who are postoperative from cardiac surgery, or those who have syncope or exercise-induced PVCs, are at greater risk and may require treatment. Lidocaine, procainamide, propranolol, or amiodarone may be useful using guidelines similar for ventricular tachycardia.

ACCELERATED IDIOVENTRICULAR RHYTHM

- **Accelerated idioventricular rhythm** (AIVR) is a benign pediatric dysrhythmia that has the appearance of ventricular tachycardia. It begins gradually with fusion beats and is a monomorphic, wide-complex rhythm that originates from an accelerated ventricular focus with rates that are rarely faster than 150 bpm. Patients with AIVR are stable. AIVR rarely responds to medication and can be a warning of a residual hemodynamic abnormality associated with corrected congenital heart disease.

VENTRICULAR TACHYCARDIA

- **Ventricular tachycardia** (VT) is rare in children. It is distinguished from PSVT by wide QRS complexes, more than 0.08 to 0.09 s, depending on age (complexes as narrow as 0.06 s have been noted in infantile VT). Wide complexes can also be seen in PSVT if conduction is antegrade through an accessory pathway. Rates averaging 250 bpm are rarely helpful in differentiating PSVT from VT. AV dissociation with P wave and QRS independence helps distinguish VT from PSVT.

Idiopathic ventricular tachycardia can be seen in a child with a normal heart who is completely asymptomatic: it is usually not treated. Causes of VT include electrolyte disturbance, toxins, myocarditis, structural heart disease, tumor, cardiomyopathy, or long QT syndrome. Recurrent exercise-induced syncope is often due to VT and the initial work-up may be negative. EPS or biopsy may be necessary to guide treatment.

- Regardless of etiology, unstable wide-complex tachycardia should be synchronously cardioverted with 2 to 4 J/kg. Any patient in cardiorespiratory arrest should be defibrillated. Upon conversion, lidocaine is begun, 1 to 2 mg/kg bolus, followed by a 15 to 50 μg/kg/min infusion. Lidocaine is also the treatment for stable VT. Amiodarone, 5 mg/kg over 1 h, may also be useful. Procainamide may be useful for wide-complex tachycardia of uncertain origin because of its effect both above and below the AV node. An initial dose of 10 to 15 mg/kg over 30 to 45 min is followed by 20 to 80 μg/kg/min. Adenosine is safe and may be useful in the rare case of PSVT with aberrancy.

VENTRICULAR FIBRILLATION

- Ventricular fibrillation is treated with defibrillation, at 2 J/kg and then 4 J/kg. Correction of precipitating factors, such as acidosis, hypoxia, or metabolic derangements, aids in conversion.

OTHER CARDIAC CONDITIONS ASSOCIATED WITH DYSRHYTHMIAS

LONG QT SYNDROME

- Jervell and Lange-Nielsen first described the association of syncope, sudden death, deafness, and **long QT interval** in 1957. In 1963, Romano described the syndrome in normal-hearing patients. Congenital long QT syndrome (LQTS) is an inherited syndrome characterized by paroxysmal ventricular tachycardia and torsades de pointes. It can progress to ventricular fibrillation and sudden death. There may be a family history of syncope, sudden death, unusual seizures, drop attacks, or congenital deafness.
- Acquired QT prolongation associated with type IA antiarrhythmics, drugs, anorexia nervosa, bulimia, and electrolyte derangements can also predispose to dysrhythmia. A QTc longer than 0.44 s is a sign of delayed repolarization; more than 0.5 s is highly associated with sudden death. T wave alternans is also seen. Treatment includes β-blockers to help control sympathetic rushes and decrease the incidence of syn-

cope, ganglionectomy or pacing. Magnesium is used to treat torsades de pointes. Mortality from untreated congenital LQTS approaches 50 percent.

HYPERTROPHIC CARDIOMYOPATHY

- **Hypertrophic cardiomyopathy** (HC) is characterized by a hypertrophied, nondilated left ventricle.
  ○ Symptoms include chest pain, dyspnea, syncope, CHF, or sudden death. Some patients are asymptomatic.
  ○ Dysrhythmias include atrial fibrillation and ventricular tachyarrhythmia, the leading causes of sudden death.
    ▪ Atrial fibrillation associated hypertrophic cardiomyopathy puts a child at high risk for 1:1 conduction, ventricular tachycardia, and sudden death.
  ○ Outflow obstruction is rare.
  ○ A late systolic murmur and paradoxical splitting of S2 may be present.
  ○ Risk factors for sudden death include:
    ▪ Presence in infancy
    ▪ Advanced symptoms at diagnosis
    ▪ LV dysfunction
    ▪ Family history of sudden death
  ○ LV or septal hypertrophy on ECG is a poor prognostic sign.
  ○ Echocardiogram is diagnostic.
  ○ Therapy depends on the clinical manifestation:
    ▪ β-Blockers are used for CHF but have no effect on rates of sudden death.
    ▪ Amiodarone can control atrial fibrillation but may cause sudden death; implantable defibrillators may be preferred.
    ▪ Surgical myectomy may be necessary for significant outflow obstruction.

BIBLIOGRAPHY

Ganz LI, Friedman PL: Supraventricular tachycardia. *N Engl J Med* 332:162–173, 1995.

Hofffman TM, Wernovsky G, Wieand TS: The incidence of arrhythmias in a pediatric intensive care unit. *Pediatr Cardiol* 23:598–604, 2002.

Kugler JD, Danford DA: Management of infants, children and adolescents with paroxysmal supraventricular tachycardia. *J Pediatr* 129:324–338, 1996.

MacLellan-Tobert SG, Porter CJ: Accelerated idioventricular rhythm: A benign arrhythmia in childhood. *Pediatrics* 96:122–125, 1995.

Meldon SW, Brady WJ, Berger S, Mannenbach M: Pediatric ventricular tachycardia: A review with 3 illustrative cases. *Pediatr Emerg Care* 10:294–300, 1994.

Roden DM, George AL: The cardiac ion channel: Relation to management of arrhythmias. *Annu Rev Med* 47:135–148, 1996.

Sacchetti A, Moyer V, Baricella R: Primary cardiac arrhythmias in children. *Pediatr Emerg Care* 15:95–98, 1999.

Spirito P, Seidman CE, McKenna WL, Maron BJ: The management of hypertrophic cardiomyopathy. *N Engl J Med* 336:775–785, 1997.

QUESTIONS

1. What is the most common dysrhythmia in children?
   A. Sinus bradycardia
   B. Atrioventricular block
   C. Paroxysmal supraventricular tachycardia
   D. Atrial flutter
   E. Premature ventricular contractions

2. Unstable PSVT in an infant is best treated with which of the following?
   A. Verapamil, 0.1 mg/kg slow IV push
   B. Digitalis, 30 µg/kg IV slow IV for acute digitalization
   C. Vagal maneuvers, such as placing a bag of ice water over the nose and forehead
   D. Adenosine, 0.1 mg/kg IV push followed by 0.3 mg/kg, if needed.
   E. Synchronized cardioversion, 0.5 J/kg, increasing to 2 J/kg as needed

3. A 16-year-old boy presents with syncope while playing basketball. He has no medical history and was fine prior to this episode. He presents without current complaints. On questioning of his mother, you find that her brother was a victim of sudden death for unexplained reasons 20 years before. His ECG is normal except for a QTc of 0.55 s. What is the prognosis?
   A. The findings are a sign of delayed repolarization and unlikely to cause any significant problem.
   B. This patient has congenital long QT syndrome (LQTS) and may experience recurrent syncope but is not at risk of significantly increased mortality.
   C. β-Blockers are contraindicated.
   D. Mortality of untreated congenital LQTS approaches 10 percent.
   E. QTc prolongation of more than 0.5 s is highly associated with sudden death.

4. A 10-year-old child presents after a syncopal episode. He reports progressive dyspnea on exertion. He is noted to have a late systolic murmur and paradoxical splitting of S2. On questioning, his uncle died a sudden death at age 25 years. Which of the following is correct regarding this patient?
   A. Digoxin and nitrates are the treatment of choice.
   B. An echocardiogram is the diagnostic study of choice.
   C. The murmur may be increased by squatting or forceful hand gripping.
   D. It is not hereditary.
   E. This patient may be safely discharged.

5. Which of the following is not a cause of sinus bradycardia in children?
   A. Hypoxia
   B. Hypothyroidism
   C. Increased intracranial pressure
   D. Fever
   E. Digoxin toxicity

6. Which of the following is true regarding pacemakers in children?
   A. The most common indication is symptomatic bradycardia.
   B. Most are epicardial units.
   C. Syncope in a child with a pacemaker suggests overmedication.
   D. The mode is programmed to sense at the atrium.
   E. A CXR is not indicated in a child with a pacemaker malfunction.

7. What is the most common cause of dysrhythmias in children?
   A. Hypoxia
   B. Cardiac lesions
   C. Electrolyte imbalances
   D. Toxins
   E. Inflammatory disease

8. Which of the following is not a cause of acquired third degree block?
   A. Myocarditis
   B. Rheumatic fever
   C. Hypothyroidism
   D. Lyme disease
   E. Cardiomyopathy

9. A 15-year-old male with a history of hypertrophic cardiomyopathy (HCM) presents with the complaint of palpitations. His ECG reveals atrial fibrillation at a rate of 170. Which of the following is true regarding this patient?
   A. This patient is at high risk for sudden cardiac death.
   B. If unstable, the patient should be treated with adenosine.
   C. Atrial fibrillation is common in children.
   D. Cardioversion should be attempted at 4J/kg.
   E. Pacing is never indicated in these patients.

ANSWERS

1. C. The most common dysrhythmia in childhood is PSVT. PSVT is differentiated from sinus tachycardia by its abrupt onset, rates higher than 230 bpm, the absence of normal P waves, or by little rate variation during stressful activities, such as phlebotomy. Symptoms include poor feeding, tachypnea, and irritability.

2. E. Unstable PSVT is treated with cardioversion. If unsuccessful, esophageal overdrive pacing may be necessary. Vagal maneuvers may be used to convert stable patients. Adenosine is effective but immediate recurrence rates approach 50 percent. Digitalis is best used in the well-known stable patient with AV nodal reentry. A pediatric cardiologist should be consulted prior to administration. Verapamil can cause hypotension, cardiovascular collapse, and death in infants and its use is not recommended for infants under 2 to 3 years of age.

3. E. QTc prolongation of more than 0.5 s is highly associated with sudden death. Mortality of untreated congenital LQTS approaches 50 percent. β-Blockers decrease the incidence of syncope and reduce mortality.

4. B. This patient has hypertrophic cardiomyopathy. Digoxin and nitrates should be avoided. Echocardiography is the diagnostic study of choice. The murmur decreases with squatting and forceful hand gripping. It is hereditary. Patients with syncope should be admitted.

5. D. Causes of sinus bradycardia include hypoxia, hypothyroidism, increased intracranial pressure, or calcium channel blocker, beta-blocker, or digoxin toxicity.

6. A. The most common indication for pediatric pacemakers is symptomatic bradycardia. Most permanent pediatric pacemakers are transvenous. Choice of mode depends on the disease and can be programmed to sense, demand, or inhibit at the atrial or ventricular level. A CXR may reveal wire fracture or lead displacement.

7. B. The most common cause of dysrhythmias in children is cardiac lesions. A dysrhythmia associated with structural heart disease has a poorer prognosis than one in a structurally normal heart.

8. C. Acquired third degree heart block is associated with myocarditis, endocarditis, rheumatic fever, cardiomyopathy, Lyme disease, or tumor.

9. A. Patients with atrial fibrillation in combination with HCM are at high risk for sudden death. Unstable patients should be cardioverted with 0.5 J/kg. If not effective, overdrive pacing should be attempted. Atrial fibrillation is rare in children.

35 PERIPHERAL VASCULAR DISEASE

William C. Toepper
Joilo Barbosa
Kemedy K. McQuillen
Valerie A. Dobiesz
Gary R. Strange

HYPERTENSION

- Blood pressure in children is age, gender, and height dependent (Table 35-1). **Severe hypertension,** or systolic or diastolic blood pressures consistently above the 95th percentile, requires evaluation, therapy, and consultation. **Significant hypertension,** or blood pressure between the 90th and 95th percentile, requires observation, follow-up, and nonpharmacologic therapy. In the very young child, it requires prompt evaluation.

- Hypertension in children is usually due to an underlying illness. Neonatal hypertension is commonly due to renovascular disease, coarctation of the aorta, or kidney malformation. Renal artery thrombosis from an umbilical catheter is not uncommon. In children younger than 6 years old, renal parenchymal disease, coarctation, or renovascular disease is usually the

TABLE 35-1 Classification of Severe Hypertension

AGE (yr)		MALE AT 50TH PERCENTILE HEIGHT[a] (95TH PERCENTILE BP)	FEMALE AT 50TH % HEIGHT[a] (95TH PERCENTILE BP)
1			
	Systolic BP	>102	>104
3			
	Systolic BP	>109	>107
	Diastolic BP	>65	>66
6			
	Systolic BP	>114	>111
	Diastolic BP	>74	>73
10			
	Systolic BP	>117	>119
	Diastolic BP	>80	>78
15			
	Systolic BP	>131	>128
	Diastolic BP	>83	>83

[a] Normal blood pressures (BPs) in very tall children will be higher than the values presented. Normal BPs in short children will be lower. All-inclusive tables are referenced in the above Task Force report.

SOURCE: Adapted from National Heart, Lung and Blood Institute: Report of the Task Force on Blood Pressure Control in Children—1987. *Pediatrics* 79:1–25, 1987.

cause. Essential hypertension emerges between the ages of 6 and 10 years and is the leading cause of hypertension in the adolescent.

- Blood pressure is measured in a comfortable seated position. The infant should be lying down and quiet. It should be measured in both arms and one leg with an appropriate cuff. The bladder should encircle the limb without overlapping by more than 2 cm, and the bladder width should be at least 40 percent of the limb circumference: small cuffs falsely elevate blood pressure, and large cuffs falsely underestimate blood pressure.
  - Systolic pressure is determined at the onset of the first sound and the disappearance of sound determines diastolic pressure.
  - If auscultation is difficult, Doppler or oscillometric methods can be used. Automated devices are reliable.
  - In the older child, manual blood pressure should be taken several times over several weeks before chronic hypertension is diagnosed.

NEONATAL HYPERTENSION

- Causes of hypertension are listed in Table 35-2. **Neonatal hypertension** deserves additional comment. Unlike older children and adults, hypertensive neonates tend to be symptomatic with irritability, poor feeding with failure to thrive, respiratory distress if CHF is present, or seizures. Infants younger than 1 month with

TABLE 35-2 Causes of Hypertension in Children

Drugs and Poisons	**Central Nervous System**
Cocaine	Increased intracranial pressure
Sympathomimetic agents	Encephalitis
Amphetamines	**Cardiac**
Phencyclidine	Coarctation of the aorta
Corticosteroids	Aortic insufficiency
Cyclosporine	
Lead	**Metabolic**
Antihypertensive medication withdrawal	Hypercalcemia
	Hypernatremia
Renal	**Miscellaneous**
Glomerulonephritis	Essential hypertension
Henoch–Schönlein purpura	Anxiety and pain
Hemolytic-uremic syndrome	Preeclampsia
Congenital malformation	Porphyria
Polycystic kidneys	Systemic lupus erythematosus
Renovascular	Bronchopulmonary dysplasia
Renal artery stenosis	
Renal vein thrombosis	
Endocrine	
Pheochromocytoma	
Congenital adrenal hyperplasia	
Oral contraceptives	

systolic readings higher than 100 mm Hg may be hypertensive; those with readings above 110 mm Hg require aggressive evaluation and treatment.

ESSENTIAL HYPERTENSION

- Many factors contribute to the development of **essential hypertension:** obesity, poor physical fitness, and family history are risk factors. Sodium intake does not correlate with hypertension in children, but reductions are recommended for early hypertension. The adolescent with essential hypertension should be counseled about drugs that may elevate blood pressure and the use of birth control pills.

CLINICAL MANIFESTATIONS

- Most hypertensive children are asymptomatic.
- Signs and symptoms may suggest the etiology:
  - Glomerulonephritis may present with hematuria or weakness.
  - Coarctation of the aorta is suspected with diminished femoral pulses, collateral circulation, and a hyperactive precordium.
  - Renovascular anomalies are associated with bruits, blunt abdominal trauma, or café-au-lait spots.
- Acute or severe elevations of blood pressure may lead to hypertensive emergencies, or an elevation of blood pressure that results in end-organ damage, including encephalopathy, congestive heart failure, nephropathy, eye ground changes, and seizures. Symptoms include headache, dizziness, visual changes, nausea, emesis, or altered level of consciousness. Blood pressure reduction must begin immediately and should proceed cautiously.

ASSESSMENT

- The initial evaluation of the hypertensive child depends on the age and clinical picture. The likelihood of identifying a cause is directly related to the blood pressure and indirectly related to the age of the child.
  - Young children with significant hypertension should have a complete blood count, electrolytes, renal functions, uric acid, urinalysis, and renal ultrasound. Chest radiograph, electrocardiogram, and echocardiogram may be helpful.
  - Older children with mildly elevated blood pressure should have urinalysis and measurement of renal functions. A lipid profile may be helpful.

- Older children with symptoms or a significantly elevated blood pressure may require further evaluation.
- Hospitalization is indicated for hypertensive emergencies and for acute hypertension due to serious diseases such as hyperthyroidism.

MANAGEMENT

- The management of mild hypertension in children begins with weight loss, exercise, and a low-sodium diet.
- A hypertensive emergency with acutely elevated blood pressure and end-organ injury requires prompt, controlled reduction (Table 35-3). The goal of treatment with parenteral therapy is an initial 20 percent decrease with complete control by 2 to 3 days. A search for any underlying cause such as drug ingestion, glomerulonephritis, or pheochromocytoma, must be done. Acutely elevated blood pressure due to high intracranial pressure may not require immediate reduction.
- Hypertensive urgency is defined as a minimally symptomatic elevation of blood pressure with the potential for end-organ damage. Treatment is with an oral medication that provides a slow reduction in blood pressure over 24 to 48 h. Slow reduction prevents hypotension and rebound tachycardia. Agents are listed in Table 35-4. The most commonly used antihypertensives are listed in Table 35-5. A brief discussion follows, with the agents most useful in hypertensive emergencies given in boldface.

TABLE 35-3 Therapy for Hypertension in Children

Indications for Nonpharmacologic Intervention Strategies

Systolic or diastolic blood pressure (BP) >90th percentile (high-normal)

Indications for Initiation of Antihypertensive Drugs

Significant diastolic hypertension
Evidence of target organ injury
Symptoms or signs related to elevated BP

Use of Parenteral Therapy

Indicated in acute severe hypertension, such as with acute glomerulonephritis, hemolytic-uremic syndrome, head injuries, or any risk of target organ damage

Therapeutic Goals

Diastolic BP <90th percentile
Minimal side effects
Use of the least amount of drug necessary to effectively reduce BP
High degree of patient compliance

SOURCE: Adapted from the National Heart, Lung and Blood Institute: Report of the Task Force on Blood Pressure Control in Children—1987. *Pediatrics* 79:1–25, 1987.

TABLE 35-4 Drugs Useful in Pediatric Hypertensive Crises

DRUG	DOSE
Nitroprusside	0.5–1 mcg/kg/min up to 8 mcg/kg/min
Labetalol	0.2–2 mg/kg IV
Nifedipine	0.25–0.5 mg/kg po
Esmolol	0.5 mg/kg IV over 1–2 min, then 0.2 mg/kg/min
Diazoxide	1–5 mg/kg/dose IV up to 150 mg
Hydralazine	0.2–0.4 mg/kg IV; repeat twice prn

- **Angiotensin-converting enzyme (ACE) inhibitors** interfere with the formation of angiotensin II, a potent vasoconstrictor, resulting in decreased aldosterone and norepinephrine, and reducing renal vascular resistance, increasing renal blood flow and benefiting cardiac function. Captopril and enalapril are effective in young children. Side effects include dry cough, rash, angioedema, neutropenia, proteinuria, hyperkalemia, and elevation of creatinine. ACE inhibitors are contraindicated in bilateral renal artery stenosis and pregnancy.
- **Calcium channel blockers** reduce blood pressure by inhibiting calcium influx and decreasing smooth muscle contraction. Side effects include tachycardia and negative inotropy that normalize within weeks, constipation, somnolence, peripheral edema, and headache. **Nifedipine** is most commonly used in children. Sublingual routes may be used for hypertensive emergency when intravenous access is impossible: significant hypotension can result. Oral administration yields a more predictable response.
- **Diuretics** decrease intra- and extravascular volumes. Homeostatic mechanisms neutralize this effect, quickly leading to resistance. The most commonly used agents are loop diuretics, thiazides, and potassium-sparing diuretics for aldosterone-dependent hypertension. These are the safest medications for initial use. Side effects of loop diuretics include hypercalcemia, hyperlipidemia, and hypokalemia. Thiazides cause calciuria, hyperlipidemia, and hypokalemia.
- α-**Adrenergic blocking agents:** Peripheral α-antagonists, such as **prazosin**, result in smooth muscle relaxation with minimal reflex tachycardia. Central α-agonists, such as clonidine, act by decreasing sympathetic activity. Their peripheral effects on the presynaptic α_2-receptors cause a decrease in norepinephrine release. Side effects include dry mouth and sedation. Clonidine should be tapered to prevent the development of severe rebound hypertension.
- β-**Adrenergic blocking agents** bind cardiovascular, renin/angiotensin, and central nervous system receptors, causing an immediate decrease in heart rate and cardiac output and a short lived, mild increase in the blood pressure due to unopposed α-effect. They are well absorbed orally but have considerable first-pass

TABLE 35-5 Pharmacologic Management of Hypertension in Children

	INITIAL DOSE (mg/kg/DOSE)	MAXIMUM/DAY (mg/kg)	FREQUENCY
ACE Inhibitors			
Captopril	1.5	6	tid
Enalapril	0.15	1	bid
Calcium Channel Blockers			
Nifedipine	0.25	3	tid–qid
Diuretics			
Hydrochlorothiazide	1	2–3	bid
Furosemide	1	12	bid–qid
Spironolactone	1	3	bid–qid
α-Adrenergic Agents			
Prazosin	0.05–0.1	0.5	tid–bid
Clonidine	0.05–0.1	0.5–0.6	qid
β-Blockers			
Propranolol	1	8	bid
Atenolol	1	8	bid–qd
Vasodilators			
Minoxidil	0.1–0.2	1	bid

effect. Side effects, less common in children, include bradycardia, bronchospasm, and sleep disturbances. They can also adversely affect glucose metabolism and cause elevation of triglyceride levels.

- **α- and β-Adrenergic blocking agents: Labetalol** has both α- and β-blocking effects. The β-effects predominate. It is well absorbed orally but has a high first-pass drug metabolism. It is indicated mainly for intravenous use in hypertensive crises.

- **Vasodilating agents** include **minoxidil** and **hydralazine**. Minoxidil is highly effective but is limited by side effects of fluid retention and compensatory tachycardia, controlled by diuretics and β-blockers, and hypertrichosis. **Nitroprusside** is a powerful vasodilator that is very useful in the treatment of hypertensive emergencies. It has a prompt onset of action and short duration. Cyanide toxicity can result from prolonged use or in the very young infant. Thiocyanate levels should be monitored. **Diazoxide**, a potent arterial smooth muscle dilator, can cause hypotension, coma, or renal failure. A safe, controlled reduction is achieved by using 1- to 2 mg/kg boluses every 10 min.

THROMBOEMBOLIC DISEASE IN CHILDREN

- **Virchow's triad** (increased viscosity, decreased flow, and disruption of endothelial integrity) allows for pathologic clotting in children and adolescents. Thromboembolic (TE) disease may go undetected in children because they tolerate incidents that might be devastating to the adult.

- Risk factors for thrombophlebitis, deep vein thrombosis (DVT), and pulmonary embolism overlap (Table 35-6). Most children with TE complications have underlying disease, such as liver disease or nephrotic syndrome. The single greatest risk factor is an indwelling central venous catheter. Another risk is a congenital predisposition, which may play a factor in 25 percent of cases. Hypercoagulability is most often caused by activated protein C resistance, but it may also be due to deficiency of antithrombin or proteins S or C. These conditions may be unmasked by oral contraceptives or minor trauma. The homozygote will present in the first few hours with purpura fulminans, a rapidly progressive hemorrhagic dermal necrosis that is devastating and often fatal. It is treated with fresh frozen plasma. The heterozygote may go unrecognized until challenged by one of many risk factors. Early recognition is detected by a thorough family history for clotting disorders. Diagnosis of a congenital hypercoagulable state during a TE event is difficult because large thromboses cause temporary deficiencies of clotting factors. When congenital hypercoagulability is suspected, certain drugs (OCPs) must be avoided.

- **Deep vein thrombosis** (DVT) in children is most often related to indwelling catheters. Many central

TABLE 35-6   Major Risk Factors for Thromboembolic Disease

ADOLESCENTS	CHILDREN	ADULTS
Oral contraceptives	Hydrocephalus	Oral contraceptives
Trauma	Trauma	Trauma
Elective abortion	Congenital heart disease	Pregnancy
Surgery	Infection	Surgery
Prolonged immobilization	Neoplasia	Neoplasia
Collagen vascular disease	Prolonged immobilization	Heart disease
Intravenous drug abuse	Surgery	Collagen vascular disease
Rheumatic heart disease	Dehydration	Protein S deficiency
Dehydration	Protein S deficiency	
Obesity		
Renal transplantation		
Protein S deficiency		

line clots are asymptomatic. Findings, if present, include a swollen, tender, warm, and red extremity. Symptoms of upper extremity central line thrombus include headache, facial swelling, and difficulty with infusion. DVTs not related to central lines most commonly affect the iliofemoral vein and can extend into the vena cava. Venogram is the diagnostic study of choice although Doppler ultrasound flow studies are approaching the sensitivity of a venogram and may be utilized. Central line dye infusions are unreliable for determining the extent of a catheter-related thrombus.

- **Right atrial thrombosis** is usually related to a central line, but may occur in congenital heart disease. Patients are often asymptomatic or symptoms may include central line malfunction, fever, or congestive heart failure. Diagnosis is made on echocardiogram. Treatment may be medical or surgical depending on the size of the thrombus.
- **Pulmonary embolism** (PE) is reported in around 4 percent (1/1000 hospital admissions) of pediatric autopsies: approximately one-third may have contributed to mortality. PEs in children are almost always associated with endothelial integrity disruption. Disruption is usually proximal and includes central venous catheters or congenital heart disease with endocarditis. Only 42 percent of PEs in children are associated with DVT. Emboli need not be massive to cause problems: catheter-associated pulmonary hypertension from chronic seeding is also devastating. Disease patterns in adolescents are similar to those in adults. Presenting symptoms include pleuritic chest pain (84 percent), dyspnea (58 percent), cough (47 percent), and hemoptysis (32 percent). Objective findings include hypoxia ($P_{O_2} < 80$ percent), abnormal chest x-ray (50 percent), tachypnea (42 percent), or fever (32 percent). A classic presentation is rare in children. Diagnosis is with a ventilation/perfusion scan or chest CT with IV contrast. Pulmonary angiography is diagnostic when other studies are equivocal.

TREATMENT OF THROMBOEMBOLIC DISEASE

- Initial treatment of TE disease is anticoagulation.
  - Heparin, 75 U/kg intravenous bolus, is followed by an infusion of 20 U/kg/h and adjusted to maintain the APTT at 60 to 85 s. Therapy continues for 5 to 10 days. Protamine can reverse the effects of heparin and is dosed based on the most recent heparin administration (1 mg/100 U heparin).
  - Low-molecular weight heparin is also used and is easier to administer, more predictable, may be more effective, and has fewer bleeding complications. Dose is age adjusted, with newborns requiring the greatest dose per weight.
  - Oral warfarin is begun at 0.2 mg/kg and adjusted to attain an international normalized ratio (INR) of 2 to 3. Maintenance for the first TE lasts 3 to 6 months. Local recurrence and postphlebitic syndrome (persistent pain, swelling, pigmentation, induration, and ulceration) may occur.
- Thrombolytic therapy is used to restore catheter patency. Urokinase is preferred to streptokinase to avoid allergic phenomena with repeated dosing. The dose of urokinase is 0.3 mL (15,000 U) over 2 to 4 h. Thrombolytic therapy for massive PE or DVT is occasionally indicated, but safety and efficacy have not been determined.
- Children with previous thromboembolic events, strong family histories of hypercoagulability, dilated cardiomyopathy, or indwelling catheters should be considered for prophylaxis: use heparin flushes for catheter prophylaxis and low-dose heparin, 5000 U/dose, for inpatient DVT prophylaxis in adolescents. There is no evidence that perioperative prophylaxis is beneficial in children.

BIBLIOGRAPHY

Andrew M, Michelson AD, Bovill E, et al: Guidelines for antithrombotic therapy in pediatric patients. *J Pediatr* 132: 575–588, 1998.

David M, Andrew M. Venous thromboembolic complications in children. *J Pediatr,* 123:337–346, 1993.

Evans DA, Wilmott RW: Pulmonary embolism in children. *Pediatr Clin North Am* 41:569–584, 1994.

Flynn JT, Pasco DA: Calcium channel blockers: Pharmacology and place in therapy of pediatric hypertension. *Pediatr Nephrol* 15:302–316, 2000.

National High Blood Pressure Education Program Working Group on Hypertension Control in Children and Adolescents: Update on the 1987 Task Force Report on High Blood Pressure in Children and Adolescents: A working group report from the National High Blood Pressure Education Program. *Pediatrics* 98:649–658, 1996.

Sinaiko AR: Hypertension in children. *N Engl J Med* 335:1968–1973, 1996.

Temple ME, Nahata MC: Treatment of pediatric hypertension. *Pharmacotherapy* 20:140–150, 2000.

Vavilala MS, Nathens AB, Jurkovich GJ, et al: Risk factors for venous thromboembolism in pediatric trauma. *J Trauma* 52:922–927, 2002.

QUESTIONS

1. When a hypertensive urgency is diagnosed, the goal of treatment is which of the following?
   A. Improvement over a 24- to 48-h period
   B. No treatment is necessary in the acute setting if there is no evidence of end-organ damage
   C. Immediate reduction of blood pressure to the normal range
   D. Assure that the blood pressure is checked daily for the next 3 days
   E. Immediate amelioration with intravenous drugs, followed by initiation of oral therapy

2. When a hypertensive emergency is diagnosed, the goal of treatment is which of the following?
   A. Improvement over a 24- to 48-h period
   B. No treatment is necessary in the acute setting if there is no evidence of end-organ damage
   C. Immediate reduction of blood pressure to the normal range
   D. Assure that the blood pressure is checked daily for the next 3 days
   E. Use parenteral agents to gradually reduce the blood pressure by 20 percent, then plan to achieve complete control within 2 to 3 days

3. Which of the following is true regarding blood pressure elevation in children?
   A. Hypertension is diagnosed as a systolic blood pressure >120 or diastolic >90.
   B. Hypertension in children is most commonly idiopathic.
   C. A blood pressure cuff that is too small may falsely elevate blood pressure.
   D. Automated blood pressure machines are not reliable.
   E. Chronic hypertension may be diagnosed in older children with one elevated blood pressure measurement.

4. A 10-year-old female with a history of leukemia is undergoing chemotherapy. She presents with a complaint of headache, facial swelling, and right arm swelling, tenderness, and erythema. She denies fever or any recent illness. Her blood work is unremarkable. Which of the following is correct regarding this patient?
   A. The cause in children is most often related to indwelling central catheters.
   B. The diagnostic study of choice is a CXR.
   C. Central line dye infusions are helpful in diagnosis.
   D. Treatment is with broad spectrum antibiotics.
   E. Prophylaxis does not prevent this condition.

5. An 8-year-old male presents to the ED with a complaint of headache. He is noted to have a blood pressure of 140/90. On physical examination, he is noted to have an abdominal bruit and café-au-lait spots on his skin. What is the most likely cause of this patient's hypertension?
   A. Glomerulonephritis
   B. Coarctation of the aorta
   C. Renal artery thrombosis
   D. Renovascular anomalies
   E. Down's syndrome

6. Which of following is not associated with a child presenting with a hypertensive emergency?
   A. Headache
   B. Visual changes
   C. Altered mental status
   D. Shortness of breath
   E. Dysuria

7. A 16-year-old male with a history of hypertension is being treated in the PICU for a hypertensive emergency with an IV nitroprusside drip with good control of his blood pressure. He begins to complain of feeling nervous, short of breath, and having tinnitus. His pulse oximetry reading is 100 percent. He has a metabolic acidosis on laboratory testing. Which of the following is correct regarding this patient?
   A. He has developed hypertensive encephalopathy.
   B. The thiocyanate levels should be monitored.
   C. A carboxyhemoglobin level should be ordered.
   D. A pulmonary embolism should be suspected.

E. Blood draws would reveal chocolate-colored venous blood.

8. Which of the following is not a risk factor for thromboembolic disease in children?
   A. Nephrotic syndrome
   B. Indwelling central venous catheter
   C. Erythema nodosum
   D. Protein C deficiency
   E. Antithrombin deficiency

ANSWERS

1. A. The goal is improvement over 24 to 48 h. Slow reduction with oral agents prevents hypotension and rebound tachycardia. Overly aggressive reduction may result in end-organ hypoperfusion from loss of cerebral autoregulation. Nifedipine, clonidine, and atenolol are commonly used agents.

2. E. By definition, a hypertensive emergency exists when there is evidence of end-organ damage. Blood pressure should be reduced immediately but in a controlled fashion, as outlined previously. Immediate reduction to normal may lead to hypoperfusion and further end-organ damage.

3. C. Blood pressure in children is age, gender, and height dependent. Hypertension in children is usually due to an underlying illness. A small cuff may falsely elevate blood pressure. Automated devices are reliable. In an older child, blood pressure should be repeated over several weeks before chronic hypertension is diagnosed.

4. A. This patient has an upper extremity deep venous thrombosis. The most common cause in children is related to indwelling catheters. A venogram or Doppler ultrasound flow study is the diagnostic study of choice. Central line dye infusions are unreliable. The treatment is with heparin. Prophylaxis in children with indwelling catheters using heparin flushes is recommended.

5. D. Signs and symptoms may suggest the etiology in hypertensive children. Renovascular anomalies are associated with bruits, blunt abdominal trauma, or café-au-lait spots.

6. E. Hypertensive emergencies result in end-organ damage including encephalopathy, CHF, nephropathy, eye ground changes, and seizures. Symptoms include headache, dizziness, visual changes, nausea, vomiting, or altered level of consciousness.

7. B. Nitroprusside may result in cyanide toxicity from prolonged use or in the very young infant. Thiocyanate levels should be monitored.

8. C. Most children with thromboembolic complications have underlying disease, such as liver disease or nephrotic syndrome. The single greatest risk factor is an indwelling central venous catheter. Hypercoagulability may be caused by protein C, S, or antithrombin deficiency.

NEUROLOGIC EMERGENCIES

36 AGE-SPECIFIC NEUROLOGIC EXAMINATION

Susan Fuchs
William R. Ahrens
Patricia Lee

INTRODUCTION

- The neurologic system in the infant is an evolving one and the evaluation changes with age. Most of the examination can be accomplished by observation alone.

GENERAL PHYSICAL EXAMINATION

- The evaluation of the child includes the measurement of head circumference and assessment of any dysmorphic features.

NEUROLOGIC EXAMINATION

- If the child has an altered mental status, a quick assessment is performed using the APVU system (see Table 10-9). A more formal infant Glasgow Coma Scale (GCS) has been developed to assess younger patients (see Table 10-8).
- Pupillary response to light is an indication of an intact second nerve, as this requires reception by the second nerve and outflow from the third nerve. The blink reflex does not appear until 3 to 4 months of age.
- Cranial nerves III, IV, and VI are evaluated by observing the size of the pupils, the eye position at rest, and the integrity of the extraocular muscles.
- Cranial nerve V is assessed by asking the patient to open and close the mouth.

- Cranial nerve VII is assessed by asking the child to smile or show the teeth and to close the eyes tightly against resistance. Upper motor neuron disorders affecting cranial nerve VII spare the upper part of the face, which receives innervation from both sides of the brain, whereas, lower motor neuron disorders produce both upper and lower facial weakness.
- Cranial nerve VIII is roughly evaluated by ringing a bell or clinking a set of keys and observing whether the infant or child turns to the sound.
- Evaluation of phonation and the gag reflex tests cranial nerves IX and X and watching the position of the tongue at rest and when extended, tests cranial nerve XII. With a lesion of cranial nerve XII, the tongue deviates to the affected side.
- Cranial nerve XI is tested by evaluating the patient's ability to rotate the head and shrug the shoulders.
- After testing mental status and cranial nerves, the child is evaluated for the presence of motor weakness. Observing the infant crawl or the child walk or run provides clues regarding which muscle groups require formal testing.
- Testing coordination involves assessment of cerebellar function. Even young children can perform finger-to-nose testing or rapid supination or pronation of the hand. Infants may be placed in a sitting position to test for the possibility of truncal ataxia.
- The Romberg test can be used to evaluate cerebellar function, as well as posterior column integrity.
- Many primitive reflexes are present at birth but disappear as the child grows. In certain neurologic diseases, these reflexes persist and serve as markers of pathology (Table 36-1).
- The Babinski reflex involves stimulation of the plantar surface of the foot from the heel along the lateral border of the sole, crossing over the distal end of the metatarsals to the big toe.

TABLE 36-1 Normal Reflexes

REFLEX	APPEARANCE	DISAPPEARANCE (mo)
Moro	Birth	5–6
Palmar grasp	Birth	6
Plantar grasp	Birth	8–15
Root response	Birth	3–4
Tonic neck	Birth	5–6

- ○ A positive response is dorsiflexion of the big toe with separation (fanning) of the other toes.
- ○ It indicates pyramidal tract pathology.
- ○ A positive Babinski reflex can be seen in most normal 1-year-old children and may exist until 2.5 years of age.

BIBLIOGRAPHY

Menkes JH: *Textbook of Child Neurology*, 5th ed. Baltimore, Williams & Wilkins, 1995.

Mickel HS: The neurologic exam in the emergency setting. In: Tintinalli JE, Krome RL, Ruiz E, eds. *Emergency Medicine: A Comprehensive Study Guide*, 5th ed. New York: McGraw- Hill, 1415–1422, 2000.

Swaiman KF: Neurologic examination after the newborn period until 2 years of age. In: Swaiman KF, Ashwal A, eds. *Pediatric Neurology: Principles & Practice*, 3d ed. St Louis: Mosby, 31–38, 1999.

QUESTIONS

1. A 10-month-old boy is brought by parents after he fell out of his carrier from a 3-ft height. On examination, the child opens his eyes spontaneously, has inconsolable crying, and withdraws to touch. A GCS evaluation score for this child would be:
   A. 11
   B. 12
   C. 13
   D. 14
   E. 15
2. Assessment of a 1-month-old's ability to visualize light is best done by:
   A. Blink reflex
   B. Pupillary light response
   C. Accommodation
   D. Tracking of objects
   E. Nystagmus
3. Cranial nerve VIII is best evaluated in an infant by:
   A. Observing for symmetry in smile
   B. Observing eye closure
   C. Clinking a set of keys
   D. Observing the tongue during phonation
   E. Observing the tracking of eye movements
4. A quick motor evaluation can be done on an infant by:
   A. Observation of crawl
   B. Testing for resistance to passive movements
   C. Observation of infant smile
   D. Observation of withdrawal from pain
   E. Observation of infant interaction with parents
5. A positive Babinski reflex is seen in an 18-month-old infant who rolled off the couch. This finding indicates:
   A. Upper motor neuron injury
   B. May be normal
   C. Lower motor neuron injury
   D. Need for immediate CT scan of brain
   E. Child abuse

ANSWERS

1. C. This child has spontaneous eye opening = 4, irritable crying = 4, and active withdrawing to touch = 5.
2. B. Pupillary response to light is an indication of an intact second nerve. The blink reflex does not appear until 3 to 4 months of age.
3. C. Cranial nerve VIII (auditory nerve) is best tested for by ringing a bell or clinking a set of keys and observing whether the infant or child turns to the sound.
4. A. Observing the infant crawl or the child walk or run provides clues regarding which muscle groups require formal testing.
5. B. A positive Babinski reflex can be seen in most normal 1-year-old children and may exist until 2.5 years of age.

37 ALTERED MENTAL STATUS AND COMA

Susan Fuchs
William R. Ahrens
Heather M. Prendergast

INTRODUCTION

- **Lethargy** is a state of reduced wakefulness in which the patient displays disinterest in the environment and is easily distracted but is easily arouseable and can communicate.

- **Delirium** is characterized by disorientation, delusions, hallucinations, fearful responses, irritability, and sensory misperception.
- **Obtundation** is severe blunting of alertness with a decreased response to stimuli.
- **Stupor** exists when the patient can only be aroused by extremely vigorous and repeated stimulation.
- **Coma** occurs when a profound reduction in neuronal function results in unresponsiveness to sensory stimuli.

PATHOPHYSIOLOGY

- In general, patients with altered mental status have suffered a diffuse insult to the brain. The more severe the insult, the greater the alteration in mental status.
- For coma to occur, the underlying abnormality must involve damage to either both cerebral hemispheres or to the ascending reticular activating system, which transverses the brainstem through the upper pons, midbrain, and diencephalon, and plays a fundamental role in arousal.
- Metabolic, infectious, and toxic etiologies tend to produce diffuse but symmetric deficits. Structural lesions result in focal deficits that progress in a predictable pattern.
- Supratentorial lesions produce focal findings that progress in a rostral–caudal fashion, whereas subtentorial lesions result in brainstem dysfunction followed by a sudden onset of coma, cranial nerve palsies, and respiratory disturbances. The causes of coma are listed in Table 37-1.

PHYSICAL EXAMINATION

- The presence of a Babinski response indicates an upper motor neuron lesion.
- In decorticate posturing, the arms are flexed and the legs extended. This position implies dysfunction of the cerebral hemispheres with preservation of the brainstem.
- Decerebrate posturing is characterized by extension of both upper and lower extremities with internal rotation, which may occur as a response to pain. It implies a lesion at the level of the midbrain.
- Flaccid paralysis implies a diffuse lesion involving both hemispheres and brainstem.
- Consistent hyperventilation can occur in lesions of the midbrain and lower pons. Cheyne–Stokes respiration is characterized by periods of tachypnea followed by apnea. It signifies a bilateral hemispheric abnormality with an intact brainstem.

TABLE 37-1 Etiology of Altered Mental Status Based on the Mnemonic "Tips from the Vowels"

MNEMONIC DEVICE	CATEGORY	CAUSE
A	Abuse	Head trauma
		Shock
E	Epilepsy (and other causes of seizures)	Hypernatremia
		Hypocalcemia
		Hypoglycemia
		Hyponatremia
		Postictal state
		Status epilepticus
	Endocrine	Addison's disease
		Hyperthyroidism
		Hypothyroidism
		Inborn errors of metabolism
	Electrolyte disorders	Hypercalcemia
		Hypernatremia
		Hyponatremia
I	Infection	Brain abscess
		Encephalitis
		Meningitis
		Sepsis
		Subdural empyema
	Intussusception	Neurologic presentation
O	Overdose	Alcohol
		Carbon monoxide
		Lead
		Opiates
		Salicylates
		Sedatives
U	Uremia (and other metabolic causes)	Hemolytic uremic syndrome
		Hepatic encephalopathy
		Hypoxia
		Renal failure
		Reye's syndrome
T	Trauma	Child abuse
	Tumor	Head trauma
		Hemorrhage
I	Insulin-related problems	Diabetic ketoacidosis
		Hyperglycemia
		Hypoglycemia
		Ketotic hypoglycemia
		Nonketotic hypoglycemia
P	Psychogenic	Diagnosis of exclusion
S	Shock	Anaphylactic
		Cardiogenic
		Hemorrhagic
		Hypovolemic
		Neurogenic
		Septic
	Stroke (and other CNS lesions)	Arteriovenous malformations
		Hemorrhage
	Shunt-related problems	Hydrocephalus
		Shunt dysfunction

- Ataxic breathing is characterized by an irregular rate and depth and can occur with lesions at the level of the pons and medulla.
- Small, reactive pupils imply metabolic lesions affecting the cerebral hemispheres, or a lesion in the medulla. Pinpoint, nonreactive pupils can result from a metabolic derangement or a lesion in the lower pons.
- Midposition and fixed pupils imply a lesion in the midbrain or upper pons. In the presence of coma, a unilateral dilated pupil can imply third nerve compression from uncal herniation.
- Bilateral fixed pupils can imply tectal herniation and can be seen in severe hypothermia. In some cases, they imply severe permanent brain damage.
- In the oculocephalic reflex, the head is passively moved from side to side. When brainstem function is intact, the eyes move together toward the side opposite that which the head is turned.

LABORATORY TESTING

- All patients with altered mental status should have a bedside glucose determination.
- Radiographic examination of the cervical spine is performed if there is any suspicion of trauma. If physical examination suggests a structural lesion, an emergent CT scan of the brain is performed.

THERAPY

- Intubation is required for patients with altered mental status who have lost protective airway reflexes and who are at risk for aspiration. Intubation is also indicated for patients with evidence of critically increased intracranial pressure (ICP).
- All patients receive oxygen, naloxone, and, if hypoglycemia is suspected, 0.5 to 1.0 g/kg of glucose.
- Hypotension is avoided, since it can result in cerebral hypoperfusion and ischemia. However, over-aggressive hydration is avoided in the presence of increased ICP.
- Hyperventilation produces vasoconstriction of the cerebral arteries and will reduce elevated ICP. The P_{CO_2} is not reduced below 30 to 35 torr because severe vasoconstriction and cerebral ischemia can result.
- Mannitol or furosemide may be useful adjuncts for patients with severely increased ICP.
- Some patients may benefit from elevating the head of the bed to 30 degrees, to facilitate venous drainage.

SPECIAL CONSIDERATIONS

LEAD ENCEPHALOPATHY

- Severe lead toxicity is a consideration in any child with profoundly altered mental status or coma. Lead encephalopathy can be associated with increased ICP and seizures. Patients with lead encephalopathy often have a history of pica.

INTUSSUSCEPTION

- There is a "neurologic presentation" of intussusception in which the child manifests a depressed level of consciousness that can range from lethargy to obtundation. The overall appearance of the patient can mimic shock or sepsis. There is often a history of vomiting.

REYE'S SYNDROME

- Reye's syndrome is a disorder characterized by the acute onset of encephalopathy, elevated liver enzymes and serum ammonia, and the presence of microvesicular fatty changes in the liver. Pathophysiology may involve the interaction of salicylates and certain viruses, especially influenza and varicella
- The syndrome begins with unremitting vomiting and can progress from lethargy to disorientation, combativeness, and, in severe cases, coma.
- Reye's syndrome has five stages of severity according to the degree of encephalopathy:
  - Stage 1: lethargy, with an otherwise normal neurologic examination.
  - Stage 2: stupor or combatativeness, with inappropriate verbal response.
  - Stages 3 to 5: increasing degrees of coma.
- Management is predicated on controlling increased intracranial pressure; patients who progress to stage 2 or 3 require intubation and hyperventilation. Mannitol may be useful. Hypoglycemia is common and is treated with intravenous D10.

INBORN ERRORS OF METABOLISM

- Numerous inborn errors of metabolism can present early in life with vomiting, seizures, and altered mental status; some are accompanied by metabolic acidosis. Laboratory diagnosis involves examination of urine and plasma for amino acids, organic acids, and carnitine.

BIBLIOGRAPHY

Orlowski JP: Whatever happened to Reye's syndrome? Did it ever really exist? *Crit Care Med* 27:1582–1587, 1999.

Sarnaik AP: Reye's syndrome: Hold the obituary. *Crit Care Med* 27:1674–1676, 1999.

Taylor DA, Ashwal S: Impairment of consciousness and coma. In: Swaiman KF, Ashwal S, eds. *Pediatric Neurology: Principles and Practice.* St Louis: Mosby, 861–872, 1999.

Vannucci RC, Wasiewski WW: Diagnosis and management of coma in children. In; Pellock JM, Myer EC, eds. *Neurologic Emergencies in Infancy and Childhood*, 2d ed. Boston: Butterworth-Heinemann, 103–122, 1993.

QUESTIONS

1. An 8-year-old child with Type I Diabetes is brought is to the Emergency Department for altered mental status. On arrival to the department, you find a moderately dehydrated child who can only be aroused by vigorous and repeated stimulation. Which of the following accurately describes the mental status of this child?
   A. Lethargy
   B. Delirium
   C. Obtundation
   D. Stupor
   E. Coma

2. A 14-year-old patient is brought to the Emergency Department for alcohol intoxication. On examination, you note the patient has moderate blunting of alertness and a decreased response to stimuli. Which of the following accurately describes the mental status of this patient?
   A. Lethargy
   B. Delirium
   C. Obtunded
   D. Stupor
   E. Coma

3. A 3-year-old child is brought to the Emergency Department for vomiting and diarrhea for 3 days. On examination, you find a severely dehydrated child lying quietly on the examination cart. The child is easily arouseable, and communicates without difficulty. The **BEST** description for the child's mental status would be which of the following?
   A. Depression
   B. Lethargy
   C. Normal mental status
   D. Delirium
   E. Stupor

4. Paramedics bring in an unresponsive child. The child is successfully intubated. Based on history and physical assessment, you suspect an intracranial structural lesion. Which of the following findings would be the **MOST** consistent with a lesion in the medulla?
   A. Pinpoint, nonreactive pupils
   B. Mid-position and fixed pupils
   C. Unilateral dilated pupils
   D. Bilateral fixed pupils
   E. Small, reactive pupils

5. A 2-year-old patient is brought to the ED by concerned parents. Parents report recent upper respiratory symptoms for the past week. Over the last 2 days, the child has had unremitting vomiting. A low-grade fever was treated with generic aspirin. On examination, you find a moderately dehydrated and lethargic child. A neurologic examination is normal. You suspect you may be dealing with Reye's syndrome. Which of the following **BEST** describes the degree of encephalopathy?
   A. Stage 1
   B. Stage 2
   C. Stage 3
   D. Stage 4
   E. Stage 5

ANSWERS

1. D. The child's mental status would be classified as stupor. This condition warrants aggressive investigation and intervention.

2. C. The patient's mental status would be classified as obtundation. As with any alteration in mental status, this condition requires aggressive attention to determining the etiology.

3. B. The child's mental status would be classified as lethargy. Lethargy is a state of reduced wakefulness in which the patient displays disinterest in the environment and is easily distracted, but is easily arouseable and able to communicate.

4. E. Small, reactive pupils imply metabolic lesions affecting the cerebral hemispheres, or a lesion in the medulla.

5. A. Reye's syndrome is divided into five stages of severity according to the degree of encephalopathy. Stage 1 is characterized by lethargy and an otherwise normal neurologic examination. Patients can rapidly deteriorate from lethargy to disorientation to combativeness, and coma. The mainstay of treatment is controlling increased intracranial pressure.

38 SEIZURES

Susan Fuchs
William R. Ahrens
Heather M. Prendergast

INTRODUCTION

- A **seizure** results from a paroxysmal electrical discharge of neurons within the brain. **Epilepsy** is defined as two or more unprovoked seizures.

CLASSIFICATION

- Seizures are fundamentally classified as partial or general. Partial seizures were formerly known as focal seizures.
- In **partial simple seizures**, there is no impairment of consciousness. In complex partial seizures, consciousness is impaired. In general, simple partial seizures involve one cerebral hemisphere. Abnormalities in **complex partial seizures** can be unilateral or bilateral.
- **Generalized seizures** involve both hemispheres of the brain and are characterized by convulsions. **Clonic** seizures are characterized by rhythmic jerking and flexor spasms of muscles, **tonic** seizures by sustained muscle contraction resulting in rigidity, and **tonic-clonic** seizures by a combination of both.
- **Petit mal (absence) seizures** are nonconvulsive and are characterized by an abrupt and brief loss of awareness, associated with staring or blinking.
- **Benign childhood epilepsy**, also known as **Rolandic epilepsy**, has an onset between 3 and 13 years of age, often occurs upon awakening, and consists of facial movements, grimacing, and vocalizations.
- **West syndrome** involves infantile spasms, characterized by sudden tonic contractions of the extremities, head, and trunk. The classic EEG finding is hypsarrhythmia.
- **Lennox-Gastaut syndrome** has its onset at 1 to 8 years of age and consists of multiple seizure types. These children often have seizures every day.

FIRST SEIZURE AND RECURRENT SEIZURES

- Aside from fever, the most common causes of seizures in children (Table 38-1) include:
  - Infections
  - Trauma

TABLE 38-1 Etiology of Childhood Seizures

Infections	**Inborn Errors of Metabolism**
Meningitis	
Meningoencephalitis	**Vascular**
Brain abscess	Intracranial hematoma
	Embolism
Trauma	Infarction
Hemorrhage: epidural, subdural	Hypertensive encephalopathy
Posttraumatic	
	Tumor
Intoxication	
Lead	**Psychological**
Cocaine	Hyperventilation
PCP	Breath-holding spells
Amphetamine	
Aspirin	**Congenital**
Carbon monoxide	Malformations
Theophylline	Birth asphyxia
	Neurocutaneous syndromes
Drug Withdrawal	
(Anticonvulsants)	**Other**
	Status post DPT immunization
Metabolic	
Hypoglycemia	**Seizure Disorder**
Hyponatremia	Noncompliance
Hypernatermia	Inadequate drug level
Hypocalcemia	
Hypomagnesemia	

  - Toxic exposures
  - Failure to take prescribed anticonvulsants
- In addition, childhood seizures are often idiopathic.

LABORATORY EVALUATION

- A bedside glucose check is performed on all patients who have had a seizure. Other laboratory studies are individualized. If the child has been on anti seizure medication, a drug level is obtained.

RADIOLOGIC EVALUATION

- For most patients with a generalized seizure, no focal findings on physical examination, and no history of trauma, there is little use for a CT scan. Neuroimaging is reserved for those with a focal seizure, an abnormal neurologic examination, a suspected intracranial mass lesion, or infection. Magnetic resonance imaging (MRI) is preferable to a CT scan as small tumors, hamartomas, or temporal lobe lesions are better visualized.

ELECTROENCEPHALOGRAM (EEG)

- An EEG is the study of choice in the evaluation of childhood seizures; it should be performed a few days to weeks after the seizure. An abnormal EEG (diffuse or focal) is the most important predictor of seizure recurrence. A normal EEG does not rule out a seizure disorder.

DISPOSITION

- Any child who experiences a first focal seizure or who has an abnormal neurologic examination should be considered for hospital admission. If the child has a first generalized seizure, a negative ED workup, and is stable, further workup can be performed on an outpatient basis. There is no way to absolutely predict seizure recurrence.
- Many anticonvulsants are available, some of which have efficacy for certain types of seizures (Table 38-2).

NEONATAL SEIZURES

- Neonatal seizures occur during the first 28 days of life, although most occur shortly after birth. Because

TABLE 38-2   Anticonvulsant Choice—Daily Oral Medications

SEIZURE TYPE	DRUG OF CHOICE (IN ORDER OF PREFERENCE)
Absence	Ethosuximide (Zarontin) 15–40 mg/kg/d bid Valproic acid (Depakene) or divalproex (Depakote) 10–45 mg/kg/d bid or qid Clonazepam (Klonopin) 0.05–0.3 mg/kg/d tid Lamotrigine (Lamictal) 5–15 mg/kg qd or bid if given alone; 1–5 mg/kg qd or bid when given with valproic acid
Atonic	Valproic acid, clonazepam, ethosuximide
Myoclonic	Valproic acid, clonazepam, lamotrigine
Partial	Carbamazepine (Tegretol/Carbatrol) 10–30 mg/kg/d bid or qid Phenytoin/fosphenytoin 4–8 mg/kg/d bid Valproic acid Phenobarbital 2–8 mg/kg/d qd/bid Primidone (Mysoline) 12–25 mg/kg/d bid/qid Gabapentin (Neurontin)[a] 30–45 mg/kg/d tid Oxcarazepin (Trileptal)[a] 20–40 mg/kg/d bid Tiagabine (Gabatril)[a] 1–2 mg/kg/d bid/qid
Generalized, tonic-clonic	Carbamazepine, phenytoin, phenobarbital, primidone, valproic acid, lamotrigine, topiramate (Topamax)[a] (5–10 mg/kg/d bid)
Infantile spasms	ACTH, prednisone

[a] Drug not FDA approved for children.

TABLE 38-3   Causes of Neonatal Seizures

Hypoxia/Anoxia (Intrauterine or Perinatal)

Cerebral Ischemia (Secondary to Hypoxia/Anoxia)

Hemorrhage
 Subarachnoid (birth trauma)
 Subdural (birth trauma)
 Intraventricular/intracerebral (prematurity)

Infection
 Meningitis: group B streptococci, *Escherichia coli*
 Meningoencephalitis: herpes, cytomegalovirus, toxoplasmosis

Metabolic
 Hypoglycemia (especially first day of life)
 Hypocalcemia (days 3–14)
 Pyridoxine (vitamin B$_6$) deficiency

Drug Withdrawal
 Narcotics

Inborn Errors of Metabolism (Days 4–7)
 Aminoacidurias
  Maple syrup urine disease
  Phenylketonuria
 Urea cycle defects: citrullinemia
 Organic acidurias: proprionic acidemia

Structural Anomalies
 Lissencephaly

Hereditary Disorders
 Tuberous sclerosis

the cerebral cortex is immature, seizures in neonates can be extremely subtle, consisting only of lip smacking, eye deviation, or apnea. Motor activity can appear normal.

- Neonatal seizures are commonly related to:
  - Perinatal asphyxia
  - Metabolic abnormalities, especially hypoglycemia and hypocalcemia
  - Central nervous system infections
  - Perinatal hemorrhage
  - Table 38-3 lists the causes of neonatal seizures.
- Less commonly, seizures are related to inherited metabolic abnormalities, including urea cycle defects and abnormalities in amino acid metabolism. These defects often become apparent after the infant begins feeding and usually cause lethargy, vomiting, and poor feeding as well as seizures. A rare cause of refractory seizures in neonates is inherited pyridoxine deficiency.
- Phenobarbital (10 to 20 mg/kg intravenously) is the drug of choice for neonatal seizures, with phenytoin (10 to 15 mg/kg) the second choice.
- In refractory seizures, pyridoxine (50 to 100 mg intravenously) is indicated, to treat potentially pyridoxine-dependent seizures. Other metabolic abnormalities

such as hypocalcemia (<7 mg/dL) and hypomagnesemia are corrected.

FEBRILE SEIZURES

- A **febrile seizure** is a seizure accompanied by a fever without evidence of intracranial infection, intracranial abnormality, or toxin. Febrile seizures usually occur between 6 months and 5 years of age. Most febrile seizures are self-limited, generalized, and last for less than 15 min, in which case, they are classified as simple.
- A complex or atypical febrile seizure:
  - Lasts more than 15 min
  - Occurs more than once in a 24-h period
  - Has a focal component
- Following a febrile seizure, children will usually have a postictal period during which they are lethargic, irritable, or confused.
- Approximately 2 to 5 percent of all children will have a febrile seizure. They occur most commonly in children younger than 2 years old. Twenty-five to 30 percent of children who have one febrile seizure will have a recurrence.
- A complete physical examination focuses on determining the etiology of the fever, with particular attention to excluding central nervous system infection. In a febrile seizure, the neurologic examination is normal.

DIAGNOSTIC EVALUATION

- For the first simple febrile seizure, there are no required laboratory studies.
- The greatest controversy surrounds the need to perform a lumbar puncture in a child who has had a febrile convulsion. A child over 18 months old who is nontoxic, with a normal mental status, and who has no evidence of neck pain or stiffness does not require a lumbar puncture. In a child who is still postictal or noncommunicative (younger than 12 months) or who has received prior antibiotics, a lumbar puncture should be considered.
- Other studies, such as CT scan and EEG, are not warranted after the first simple febrile seizure.

THERAPY

- Treatment with anticonvulsants is not indicated after a first febrile seizure.
- Patients with repeated febrile seizures may subsequently require treatment.

DISPOSITION

- Patients with febrile seizures may be discharged with follow-up by their primary care provider unless an underlying infection precludes discharge.
- Parental reassurance and education regarding the benign nature of febrile seizures, the low risk of recurrence, and the low incidence of subsequent epilepsy are part of the discharge instructions.

STATUS EPILEPTICUS

- **Status epilepticus** is a seizure lasting longer than 30 min or two or more seizures without recovery of consciousness in between. Status can develop with either generalized or partial seizures.
- Initial therapy consists of:
  - Meticulous attention to maintaining patency of the airway and adequacy of oxygenation and ventilation
  - Pulse oximetry is monitored continuously.
  - High-flow oxygen is administered to all patients via mask or bag-valve-mask ventilation.
  - Venous access is secured as soon as possible.
  - Cardiac status is continuously monitored.
- Benzodiazepines are the first-line treatment for an actively seizing patient.
  - Lorazepam (Ativan) has an onset of action of 2 to 3 min and a relatively long half-life of 12 to 24 h.
    - Side effects include respiratory depression and sedation.
    - The dose is 0.05 to 0.10 mg/kg, up to a maximum of 8 mg.
  - Diazepam (Valium) is useful for control of seizures.
    - It has an onset of action of 1 to 3 min, but its half-life of 15 to 20 min means that repeated doses are often required.
    - The dose is 0.1 to 0.3 mg/kg, administered slowly by intravenous push.
    - Side effects include respiratory depression, hypotension, sedation, and bradycardia.
    - Diazepam can also be given rectally, using the intravenous formulation in a dose of 0.5 mg/kg for the first dose and 0.25 mg/kg for any subsequent doses, to a maximum of 20 mg. There is also a rectal gel form of diazepam (Diastat) available, with the dose via this formulation of 0.5 mg/kg for children 2 to 5 years of age, 0.3 mg/kg for those 6 to 11 years, and 0.2 mg/kg for children over 12 years of age. (It is available in several premeasured sizes: 2.5, 5.0, and 10 mg.)
  - Midazolam (Versed) is a benzodiazepine that is rapidly absorbed after intramuscular injection and is an alternative to other benzodiazapines when it is

impossible to obtain intravenous or intraosseous access.

- The dose is 0.1 mg/kg, with an onset of action in approximately 15 min.
- A long-acting anticonvulsant is indicated after seizures are controlled with benzodiazepines.
  - Phenytoin, when given intravenously, has rapid brain deposition.
    - The loading dose is 20 mg/kg, which must be given slowly, 50 mg/min in adults or 1 mg/kg/min in children less than 50 kg.
    - Side effects include hypotension and cardiac conduction disturbances.
  - Fosphenytoin is a new water-soluble prodrug of phenytoin.
    - It is dosed according to phenytoin equivalents (PE). The intravenous loading dose is 20 mg PE/kg, which can be given at a rate of 3 mg PE/kg/min up to 150 mg PE/min.
    - The only side effects are pruritus and paresthesias.
    - It can also be given intramuscularly (same dose as intravenously); however, peak levels are reached in 3 h.
  - Phenobarbital is still a useful drug for treating status epilepticus, and it remains the drug of choice for neonatal seizures.
    - Peak brain levels are reached in 10 to 20 min, and its duration of action is over 48 h.
    - The loading dose is 20 mg/kg IV given slowly at 100 mg/min.
    - Side effects include respiratory depression (additive with benzodiazepines), sedation, and occasionally hypotension.
- For refractory status, pentobarbital, diazepam, or midazolam may be given as continuous infusions.
  - Pentobarbital is given as a loading dose of 5 to 20 mg/kg intravenously, followed by an infusion of 0.5 to 3 mg/kg/h, to keep the level between 20 to 50 μg/mL and to produce burst suppression on the EEG, or cessation of epileptic activity. Hypotension is common; vasopressors are often needed with pentobarbital coma.
  - Diazepam is infused at a rate or 2 mg/kg/h, or midazolam is given initially as a loading dose of 0.15 mg/kg, then 0.5 to 1 μg/kg/min, and titrated upward (up to 4 μg/kg/min) over 60 min until there is cessation of seizures or burst suppression on the EEG.
- Other options status epilepticus include the use of:
  - Intravenous propofol (3 to 6 mg/kg/h)
  - Inhalation anesthetics, such as isoflurane
- Therapy of nonconvulsive status epilepticus is similar to that of convulsive status, using a benzodiazepine, phenytoin, or fosphenytoin.

BIBLIOGRAPHY

American Academy of Pediatrics, Committee on Quality Improvement, Sub-Committee on Febrile Seizures: Practice parameter: Long-term treatment of the child with simple febrile seizures. *Pediatrics* 103:1307–1309, 1999.

American Academy of Pediatrics: Provisional Committee on Quality Improvement, Subcommittee on Febrile Seizures: Practice parameter: The neurodiagnostic evaluation of the child with a first simple febrile seizure. *Pediatrics* 97:769–775, 1996.

Baumann RJ, Duffner PK: Treatment of children with simple febrile seizures: The AAP practice parameter. Pediatr Neurol 23:11–17, 2000.

Camfield PR, Camfield CS: Pediatric epilepsy: An overview. In: Swaiman KF, Ashwal S, eds. *Pediatric Neurology: Principles and Practice*, 3d ed. St. Louis: Mosby, 629–633, 1999.

Dreifuss FE: Partial seizures (focal and multifocal). In: Swaiman KF, Ashwal S, eds. *Pediatric Neurology: Principles and Practice*, 3d ed. St. Louis: Mosby, 646–660, 1999.

Haafiz A, Kissoon N: Status epilepticus: Current concepts. *Pediatr Emerg Care* 15:119–129, 1999.

Holmes GL, Riviello JJ: Midazolam and pentobarbital for refractory status epilepticus. *Pediatr Neurol* 20:259–264, 1999.

Kriel RL, Birnbaum AK, Cloyd JC: Antiepileptic drug therapy in children. In: Swaiman KF, Ashwal S, eds. *Pediatric Neurology: Principles and Practice*, 3d ed. St. Louis: Mosby, 682–718, 1999.

Meek PD, Davis SN, Collins DM, et al: Guidelines for nonemergency use of parenteral phenytoin products: Proceedings of an expert panel consensus process. *Arch Intern Med* 159:2639–2644, 1999.

Pellock JM: Status epilepticus. In: Swaiman KF, Ashwal S, eds. *Pediatric Neurology: Principles and Practice*, 3d ed. St. Louis: Mosby, 683–691, 1999.

Sabo-Graham T, Seay AR: Management of status epilepticus in children. *Pediatr Rev* 19:306–309, 1998.

Stafstrom CE: The pathophysiology of epileptic seizures: A primer for pediatricians. *Pediatr Rev* 19:342–351, 1998.

Tasker RC: Emergency treatment of acute seizures and status epilepticus. *Arch Dis Child* 79:78–83, 1998.

Warden CR, Zibulewsky J, Mace S, et al: Evaluation and management of febrile seizures in the out-of-hospital and emergency department settings. *Ann Emerg Med* 41:215–222, 2003.

QUESTIONS

1. Approximately 6 months following a severe head injury during a football game, a 14-year-old is brought to the ED for evaluation of a "focal" seizure. To accurately classify his seizures as simple partial, which of the following must be **TRUE**?
   A. Involvement of staring or blinking
   B. No impairment of consciousness

C. Nonconvulsive in nature
D. Brief loss of awareness
E. Onset between the ages of 3 and 13 years of age.

2. A 10-year-old child is brought to the ED for evaluation of a seizure. The child has a history of a previous seizure 1 year ago. Seizures occur on awakening and consist of facial movements and vocalizations. A computed tomography scan of the brain is unremarkable. Which of the following would accurately describe the seizure disorder?
   A. Petit mal
   B. West syndrome
   C. Benign childhood epilepsy
   D. Complex partial seizures
   E. Simple partial seizures

3. A 7-year-old child is brought to the emergency department for evaluation of a generalized seizure. The child has no previous history of seizures. On arrival, the child is postictal. Assessment of oxygenation and ventilation indicate that they are adequate. Which of the following is a management priority in this patient?
   A. Cardiac monitor
   B. Urinalysis
   C. Neurologic examination
   D. Bedside glucose
   E. Rectal temperature

4. A 22-month-old child is brought to the ED for evaluation of fever and generalized seizure activity. The duration was less than 10 min, with spontaneous resolution. On arrival, the toddler has a fever of 103.5° F. She is active and nontoxic appearing. Which of the following is MOST appropriate for management and disposition?
   A. Lumbar puncture, antibiotics, and admission for observation
   B. Parental reassurance
   C. Computed tomography of the brain
   D. Antibiotics and admission for observation
   E. Extended ED observation and discharge

5. A 9-year-old child with a known seizure disorder is brought to the ED for evaluation of vomiting. Shortly after arrival, the child has two consecutive seizures without recovery of consciousness in between. You determine that the airway is patent and the remainder of the vitals are within normal limits. Which of the following pharmacologic agents is the most appropriate for initial use?
   A. Lorazepam
   B. Diazepam
   C. Midazolam
   D. Phenytoin
   E. Phenobarbital

ANSWERS

1. **B.** In simple partial seizures, there is no impairment of consciousness. They involve one cerebral hemisphere. Partial seizures were formerly known as focal seizures. Petit mal seizures are nonconvulsive.

2. **C.** Benign childhood epilepsy, also known as Rolandic epilepsy, has an onset between 3 and 13 years of age. These seizures often occur on awakening and consist of facial movements, grimacing, and vocalizations.

3. **D.** It is important that a bedside glucose assessment is performed on all patients who have had a seizure. Hypoglycemia can be corrected by administration of dextrose.

4. **B.** Febrile seizures usually occur between 6 months and 5 years of age. Most seizures are self-limited, generalized, and last for less than 15 min. For the first simple febrile seizure, there are no required laboratory studies. In a child over 18 months old who is nontoxic, with a normal mental status, and has no evidence of neck pain or stiffness, a lumbar puncture is not required. Patients with febrile seizures may be discharged with follow-up. Parental reassurance is a must regarding the benign nature of febrile seizures.

5. **A.** Benzodiazepines are the first-line treatment for an actively seizing patient. Lorazepam has an onset of 2 to 3 min and a relatively long half-life of 12 to 24 h. Diazepam is also useful for control of seizures. A long-acting anticonvulsant is indicated after seizures are controlled with benzodiazepines.

39   SYNCOPE

Susan Fuchs
William R. Ahrens
Patricia Lee

INTRODUCTION

• **Syncope** refers to a sudden and transient loss of consciousness and postural tone. Fifteen to fifty percent of children will have experienced a syncopal episode by age 18 years.

PATHOPHYSIOLOGY

• The pathophysiology of syncope varies with etiology (Table 39-1), but it always results from momentarily inadequate delivery of oxygen and glucose to the brain.

TABLE 39-1   Causes of Syncope

Neurocardiogenic (Vasodepressor)

Orthostatic hypotension
Environmental triggers
Excess vagal tone
Situational syncope
Reflex syncope (pallid breath-holding spells)

Cardiac

Arrhythmias
   Supraventricular tachycardias
   Atrial flutter
   Wolfe–Parkinson–White syndrome
   Ventricular tachycardia
   Ventricular fibrillation
   Conduction disturbances
      Atrioventricular block
      Prolonged QTc
      Sick sinus syndrome
Obstructive lesions
   Aortic stenosis
   Pulmonic stenosis
   Idiopathic hypertrophic subaortic stenosis
   Mitral stenosis
   Coarctation of the aorta
   Tetralogy of Fallot
   Anomalous origin of the left coronary artery
   Tumors
Other
   Myocarditis
   Pericarditis
   Cardiac tamponade
   Cardiomyopathy
   Pulmonary hypertension

Noncardiac

Metabolic
   Hypoglycemia
   Hypocalcemia
   Hypomagnesemia
Toxic
Seizures
Psychogenic
   Hyperventilation
   Hysteria

- Syncope can result from inadequate cardiac output, which can be secondary to obstruction of blood flow, or to an arrhythmia. It can also result from inappropriate autonomic compensation for the normal fall in blood pressure that occurs on rising from a sitting or supine position.

HISTORY

- The first component in the evaluation of a patient with syncope is to determine that momentary loss of consciousness actually occurred. It is common for patients to confuse acute dizziness or vertigo with loss of consciousness. A sudden change in posture, emotional excitement, respiratory difficulty, palpitations, and any history of trauma are essential information.
- An important consideration in any patient with a history of loss of consciousness is the possibility that the patient may have suffered a seizure. Convulsions are unusual during syncopal episodes, except during very severe events.

PHYSICAL EXAMINATION

- Particular attention is paid to vital signs, especially to pulse and orthostatic blood pressure. A positive "tilt test" is a decrease in systolic blood pressure by 20 mm Hg accompanied by an initial elevation in heart rate (20 beats per min), which can be followed rapidly by bradycardia and syncope.

DIAGNOSTIC STUDIES

- The selection of laboratory studies of use in the evaluation of the syncope patient is largely guided by the history and physical examination. Blood glucose is indicated in most patients, as is a hemoglobin.
- For all patients with a history of syncope, a 12-lead electrocardiogram is indicated.
  - Special attention is paid to determination of the corrected QT interval (QTc), since prolonged QT syndrome is a cause of syncope in children.
  - If abnormalities are seen, or if a cardiac abnormality is strongly suspected, further evaluation will include a 24-h ambulatory (Holter) monitor and cardiology consultation.

SPECIFIC ETIOLOGIES OF SYNCOPE

NEUROCARDIOGENIC (AUTONOMIC, VASODEPRESSOR, VASOVAGAL) SYNCOPE

- The most common syncope in children is **neurocardiogenic** (vasodepressor or vasovagal) syncope. There is a sudden, brief loss of consciousness due to vasodilatation and decreased peripheral resistance, resulting in decreased arterial pressure, hypotension, bradycardia, and then decreased cerebral blood flow (Bezold–Jarisch reflex).
- A tilt-table test can be performed by a cardiologist to diagnose true neurocardiogenic syncope. A positive tilt-table test response, consisting of an initial increase in heart rate followed by bradycardia and syncope, may warrant drug therapy if frequent episodes occur.
- Another autonomic cause of syncope is excess vagal tone, which can imitate cardiac causes of syncope, as

the children will have a low resting heart rate, junctional rhythms, and depressed sinoatrial node function. Exercise can increase this vagal tone and lead to syncope.

- Breath-holding spells are another example of reflex syncope. The age of onset of breath-holding spells is 6 to 18 months. Pallid breath-holding spells are usually provoked by some mild antecedent trauma (usually to the head). The child may gasp and cry, then become quiet, lose postural tone and consciousness, and become pale. The child may have clonic movements in more severe episodes. They regain consciousness in less than 1 min.
- A cyanotic breath-holding spell is often precipitated by anger or frustration. The child cries, becomes quiet and holds the breath in expiration. This apnea is associated with cyanosis and there may be a loss of consciousness, limpness, or opisthotonic posturing, with recovery usually within 1 min.

CARDIAC SYNCOPE

- **Cardiac syncope** is can result from arrhythmia, obstruction, and cyanosis.
- Arrhythmias that can cause syncope include supraventricular tachycardia (SVT), atrial tachycardia, Wolff–Parkinson–White syndrome, atrial flutter, ventricular tachycardia, and ventricular fibrillation.
- Conduction abnormalities, such as AV block, sick sinus syndrome, and long QT syndrome (QTc greater than 440 msec), can all cause syncope.
- Obstructive lesions can impair cardiac output and cerebral blood flow, leading to syncope. These include congenital lesions such as aortic stenosis, pulmonic stenosis, idiopathic hypertrophic subaortic stenosis (IHSS), mitral stenosis, coarctation of the aorta, tetralogy of Fallot, and anomalous origin of the left coronary artery.
- Acquired lesions include cardiac tumors and conditions secondary to myocarditis, pericarditis, cardiac tamponade, and cardiomyopathy.

NONCARDIAC SYNCOPE

- Hypoglycemia is the main metabolic disorder that can cause syncope. Prior to a loss of consciousness, there is often a period of confusion and weakness.
- Psychological causes of syncope include hyperventilation and hysteria. Hyperventilation results in hypocapnia, which causes cerebral vasoconstriction and decreased cerebral blood flow.

DISPOSITION

- Most patients with syncope can be discharged from the emergency department with appropriate follow-up.
- Those who require admission have conditions with a cardiac origin that require urgent evaluation. Patients with arrhythmias precipitated by drugs require inpatient monitoring for at least the half-life of the offending agent.

BIBLIOGRAPHY

Chaves-Carbello E: Syncope and paroxysmal disorders other than epilepsy. In: Swaiman KF, Ashwal S, eds. *Pediatric Neurology.* St. Louis: Mosby, 763–772, 1999.

Kapoor WN: Syncope. *N Engl J Med* 343:1856, 2000.

Khan IA: Long QT syndrome: Diagnosis and management. *Am Heart J* 143:7–14, 2002.

Lewis DA, Dhala A: Syncope in the pediatric patients: A cardiologist's perspective. *Pediatr Clin North Am* 46:205, 1999.

Prodinger RJ, Reisdorff EJ: Syncope in children. *Emerg Med Clin North Am* 16:617, 1998.

Roddy SM: Breath-holding spells and reflex anoxic seizures. In: Swaiman KF, Ashwal S, eds. *Pediatric Neurology.* St. Louis: Mosby, 759–762, 1999.

QUESTIONS

1. What percentage of children will have experienced a syncopal episode by the age of 18 years?
   A. 2 to 5
   B. 5 to 10
   C. 15 to 50
   D. 30 to 80
   E. over 80
2. Evaluation of a patient with syncope should include all of the following **EXCEPT**:
   A. ECG
   B. Glucose level
   C. Hemoglobin level
   D. Potassium level
   E. Vital sign evaluation
3. The most common cause of syncope in children is:
   A. Vasovagal
   B. Arrhythmia
   C. Hypoglycemia
   D. Hyperventilation
   E. Congenital cardiac lesion
4. A 15-month-old girl is brought by parents who state that she was crying following a fall from a sitting

position and suddenly became limp, pale, and stopped breathing for 15 to 30 s until they shook her. On physical examination, the child is alert and normal appearing. Characteristics of this type of syncope include all the following **EXCEPT**:
  A. Clonic movements
  B. Common to ages 6 to 18 months of age
  C. No cyanosis
  D. Loss of postural tone
  E. Lasts 2 to 3 min before recovery
5. Common arrhythmias that can result in syncope in children include all of the following **EXCEPT**:
  A. Wolff–Parkinson–White syndrome
  B. Sinus tachycardia
  C. Atrial tachycardia
  D. Ventricular fibrillation
  E. Supraventricular tachycardia

ANSWERS

1. C. Fifteen to fifty percent of children will have experienced a syncopal episode by age 18 years.
2. D. Particular attention should be paid to vital signs, especially to pulse and orthostatic blood pressure. Blood glucose and hemoglobin levels are indicated in the evaluation of syncope in most patients. For all patients with a history of syncope, a 12-lead electrocardiogram is indicated. Prolonged QT syndrome is a cause of syncope in children.
3. A. The most common syncope in children is neurocardiogenic (vasodepressor or vasovagal) syncope. There is a sudden, brief loss of consciousness due to vasodilatation and decreased peripheral resistance, resulting in decreased arterial pressure, hypotension, bradycardia, and then decreased cerebral blood flow.
4. E. The breath-holding spell usually lasts less than 1 min.
5. B. Sinus tachycardia is generally well tolerated in pediatric patients.

40 ATAXIA

Susan Fuchs
William R. Ahrens
Valerie A. Dobiesz

INTRODUCTION

• Ataxia is a disorder of intentional movement characterized by impaired balance and coordination. It can variably affect the trunk or extremities.

PATHOPHYSIOLOGY

• Ataxia can result from a variety of lesions, including damage to:
  ○ Peripheral nerves
  ○ Spinal cord
  ○ Cerebellum
  ○ Cerebral hemispheres
• Metabolic and systemic disorders can also cause ataxia. One of the most common etiologies is drug intoxication, especially with alcohol or phenytoin.

EVALUATION

• Findings of cerebellar dysfunction include:
  ○ Nystagmus
  ○ Staggering
  ○ Wide-based gait
• Damage to the spinal cord can cause ataxia when the patient stands with the eyes closed, which is referred to as a Romberg's sign.
• Specific neurologic tests to evaluate ataxia include:
  ○ Finger-to-nose and heel-to-shin maneuvers
  ○ Rapid alternating hand movements
  ○ Heel and toe walking
  ○ Tandem gait
• For diagnostic purposes, it is useful to categorize ataxia as acute, intermittent, or chronic. Chronic ataxia is further categorized as progressive or nonprogressive (Table 40-1).

ACUTE ATAXIA

• Acute ataxia generally has an onset of less than 24 hours.
• Drug toxicity and infections are the most common etiologies. Specific toxins include:
  ○ Anticonvulsants
  ○ Alcohol
  ○ Sedative-hypnotics
• Acute metabolic processes, such as hypoglycemia, are also implicated, although they are usually accompanied by multiple systemic manifestations.
• Central nervous system infections can uncommonly cause acute ataxia.

ACUTE CEREBELLAR ATAXIA

• A common cause of ataxia in children younger than 5 years of age.

TABLE 40-1   Causes of Ataxia

Acute

Postinfectious
   Acute cerebellar
   Polymyoclonus/opisthotonos
Posttraumatic
   Hematoma
   Mass
Infection
   Meningitis
   Encephalitis
Polyneuritis
Posterior fossa tumors
Intoxications
   Alcohol
   Anticonvulsants
   Cyclic antidepressants
   Sedative-hypnotics

Chronic

Progressive
   Tumor
   Abscess
   Hydrocephalus
   Degenerative
Intermittent
   Migraine
   Seizures
   Metabolic
   Multiple sclerosis
Nonprogressive
   Cerebral palsy
   Sequelae of
      Head trauma
      Lead poisoning
      Cerebellar malformations
         Dandy–Walker cysts
         Agenesis
         Hypoplasia

- The onset of ataxia is insidious and predominantly affects the gait, although dysmetria, nystagmus, and dysarthria can occur.
- Acute cerebellar ataxia is thought to be a postinfectious phenomenon.
- It is a self-limiting illness with an excellent prognosis.

MYOCLONIC ENCEPHALOPATHY OF INFANCY

- This syndrome of acute ataxia occurs in association with occult neuroblastoma or aseptic meningitis.
- It is differentiated from acute cerebellar ataxia by its association with rapid, chaotic conjugate eye movements (opsoclonus).

CHRONIC INTERMITTENT ATAXIA

- The most common cause of intermittent ataxia is a migraine headache that involves the basilar artery. It

is essential to exclude an acute infectious process, toxic ingestion, or mass lesion.

CHRONIC PROGRESSIVE ATAXIA

- Chronic progressive ataxia has an insidious onset and progresses slowly over weeks to months. The differential diagnosis consists of:
  ○ Brain tumors
  ○ Hydrocephalus
  ○ Neurodegenerative disorders
- The combination of ataxia, headache, irritability, and vomiting in a child younger than 6 years old is characteristic of a medulloblastoma.
- Hydrocephalus, whether congenital or acquired, can cause ataxia due to stretching of frontopontocerebellar fibers. It is often accompanied by headache and vomiting and, when the patient presents late in the course of illness, can be associated with critically increased intracranial pressure.
- Neurodegenerative diseases are a group of inherited disorders that can cause spinocerebellar degeneration and progressive ataxia.

BIBLIOGRAPHY

Swaiman KF: Muscle tone and gait disturbances. In: Swaiman KF, Ashwal S, eds. *Pediatric Neurology: Principles and Practice*, 3d ed. St. Louis: Mosby, 54–62, 1999.

Swaiman KF: Movement disorders and disorders of the basal ganglia. In: Swaiman KF, Ashwal S, eds. *Pediatric Neurology: Principles and Practice*, 3d ed. St. Louis: Mosby, 801–831, 1999.

Swaiman KF: Cerebellar dysfunction and ataxia in childhood. In: Swaiman KF, Ashwal S, eds. *Pediatric Neurology: Principles and Practice*, 3d ed. St. Louis: Mosby, 787–800, 1999.

QUESTIONS

1. Which of the following conditions is not generally associated with ataxia?
   A. Phenytoin toxicity
   B. Acute cerebellar ataxia
   C. Alcohol intoxication
   D. Myoclonic encephalopathy of infancy
   E. Dermatomyositis
2. Damage to which of the following structures is most likely to lead to ataxia?
   A. Peripheral nerves
   B. Heart

C. Kidneys
D. Skin
E. GI tract
3. Which of the following is the most useful test in the evaluation of ataxia?
   A. Postural vital signs
   B. Gait evaluation
   C. Kernig's and Brudzinski signs
   D. Cremasteric reflex evaluation
   E. Evaluation of the nail beds
4. The most common cause of chronic intermittent ataxia is which of the following?
   A. Cerebellar bleed
   B. Neuroblastoma
   C. Aseptic meningitis
   D. Hydrocephalus
   E. Migraine headache involving the basilar artery

ANSWERS

1. E. Drug intoxications especially with phenytoin or alcohol intoxication may cause ataxia as well as acute cerebellar ataxia and myoclonic encephalopathy of infancy. Dermatomyositis is not typically associated with ataxia.
2. A. Ataxia can result from a variety of lesions, including damage to peripheral nerves, spinal cord, cerebellum, and cerebral hemispheres, as well as metabolic and systemic disorders.
3. B. A complete examination is necessary of a patient that presents with ataxia but in particular certain tests should be done, such as finger-to-nose and heel-to-shin maneuvers, rapid alternating hand movements, gait evaluation, such as heel and toe walking, tandem gait. The Romberg test will evaluate spinal cord injury.
4. E. The most common cause of intermittent ataxia is a migraine headache that involves the basilar artery.

41   WEAKNESS

Susan Fuchs
William R. Ahrens
Valerie A. Dobiesz

INTRODUCTION

- The term "weakness" can refer to a general phenomenon that affects all or most of the body or may refer to a specific area, such as an extremity. The primary focus in this chapter is on weakness arising from neuromuscular lesions.

PATHOPHYSIOLOGY

- Paresis implies a complete or partial weakness.
- Paralysis is a loss of function.
- Paraplegia is paralysis of the lower half of the body, while quadriplegia involves all four limbs; both usually result from a spinal cord lesion.
- Hemiplegia, involving one side of the body, generally results from a lesion in the brain.
- Abnormalities of the neuromuscular system are further classified as arising from an upper or lower motor neuron unit.
  ○ Upper motor neuron diseases usually present with asymmetrical weakness that is contralateral to the lesion and are associated with hyperreflexia, increased muscle tone, and the absence of atrophy or fasciculations.
  ○ Lower motor neuron diseases present with symmetrical weakness that can be isolated to specific muscle groups and are associated with findings of decreased muscle tone and depressed reflexes.
- Involvement of bulbar muscles is manifested by cranial nerve findings, facial muscle weakness, and chewing or swallowing difficulties.
- Neuropathies are disorders of nerves and tend to produce more prominent distal muscle weakness, hypesthesias or paresthesias, and decreased reflexes, especially early in the disease.
- Myopathies are disorders of muscle and can be inflammatory or congenital.

DIAGNOSIS

HISTORY

- It is vital to distinguish between acute and chronic disorders. Slowly progressive symptoms imply a chronic or congenital disorder. The loss of developmental milestones implies a degenerative disorder.

PHYSICAL EXAMINATION

- Motor strength in the extremities is evaluated and rated on a scale of 1 to 5, as follows:
  ○ 0, total lack of contraction
  ○ 1, trace contraction
  ○ 2, active contraction without gravity
  ○ 3, movement against gravity
  ○ 4, movement against resistance
  ○ 5, normal motor strength
- Hyperreflexia or sustained clonus indicates an upper motor neuron lesion, whereas absent or decreased

reflexes imply a problem in a lower motor distribution.
- An abnormality of touch and position on one side and pain and temperature on the other suggests a cord lesion.
- The unilateral loss of all sensations suggests a brain lesion.
- A stocking and glove distribution of sensory loss suggests a peripheral neuropathy.

LABORATORY EVALUATION

- The laboratory and radiographic evaluation are based on the provisional diagnosis.
- Electromyography and nerve conduction studies are indicated if lower motor neuron disease is suspected, but they are not emergency department (ED) procedures.

SPECIFIC CAUSES OF WEAKNESS

GUILLAIN-BARRÉ SYNDROME

- Also known as acute inflammatory demyelinating polyradiculoneuropathy, Guillain-Barré syndrome occurs in both children and adults. The pathogenesis is unknown.
- The syndrome often starts with nonspecific muscular pain, most often in the thighs, followed by weakness, which is most often symmetric and distal. Weakness progresses upward and, in some cases, results in total paralysis within 24 hours. Cranial nerve involvement is common. Deep tendon reflexes are usually absent, but plantar responses remain downgoing.
- Autonomic involvement can produce labile changes in blood pressure and bowel and bladder incontinence.
- The degree of weakness and the rate of progression of disease vary considerably.
- Spinal fluid analysis may reveal a high protein.
- The treatment for Guillain-Barré syndrome is supportive care. Mechanical ventilation may be necessary. Steroids and other immunosuppressive agents are of questionable value. Plasmapheresis may shorten the course of disease, as may therapy with intravenous gammaglobulin.

TRANSVERSE MYELITIS

- Transverse myelitis is a syndrome characterized by acute dysfunction at a level of the spinal cord. The onset is usually over 24 to 48 hours. Patients may initially complain of paresthesias and weakness of the lower extremities. Progressive weakness usually results and a sensory level develops.
- Flaccid paralysis and decreased reflexes are characteristic early in the process but are later followed by increased muscle tone.
- It is imperative to exclude a treatable mass lesion. This is usually done by MRI or contrast myelography.
- Most patients with transverse myelitis recover some function. Corticosteroids may benefit some patients.

TICK PARALYSIS

- Tick paralysis is caused by a tick that produces a neurotoxin that prevents liberation of acetylcholine at neuromuscular junctions. Small children are at particular risk. Several days after the tick attaches, the patient begins to experience ataxia and difficulty walking. If the tick is not removed, flaccid paralysis and death can result.
- Removal of the tick is curative.

BOTULISM

- Infection with *Clostridium botulinum* can produce three neurologic diseases. Symptoms result from a toxin generated from spores of the bacteria that inhibits release of acetylcholine at the prejunction of terminal nerve fibers.
  - Food-borne botulism results from ingestion of toxin contained in improperly canned foods. Diarrhea and vomiting are followed by neurologic symptoms, often secondary to cranial nerve dysfunction. Blurred vision, dysarthria, and diplopia can occur and can be followed by weakness of the extremities. Deep tendon reflexes may be weak or absent. Antitoxin may be effective in food-borne botulism.
  - Wound botulism results from infection of a contaminated wound. It is usually indistinguishable from food-borne botulism. Treatment includes wound debridement and antibiotic therapy. Antitoxin may be useful.
  - Infant botulism is caused by colonization of the intestinal tract by spores of *Clostridium botulinum*.
    - It has been related to the ingestion of contaminated honey.
    - A prominent manifestation is constipation.
    - The infant can develop difficulty sucking and swallowing and can become hypotonic.
    - Symmetrical paralysis can develop, with involvement of cranial nerves.

- Diagnosis is by isolating the toxin in the infant's stool.
- Electromyography is also useful.
- The management of infant botulism is supportive. Treatment with antitoxin and antibiotics does not seem to be of benefit.

MYASTHENIA GRAVIS

- The three basic categories of myasthenia gravis in the pediatric population are:
  - Transient neonatal variety
  - Persistent neonatal form
  - Juvenile myasthenia gravis
- Neonatal transient myasthenia gravis occurs in infants born to mothers with the disease and is caused by maternal antiacetylcholine receptor antibodies that cross the placenta. In its severe form, it can cause problems with sucking and swallowing and ventilatory insufficiency. Treatment is with neostigmine or pyridostigmine. The disease usually improves in 4 to 6 weeks.
- Persistent neonatal myasthenia gravis may be autoimmune in nature or of a hereditary variety. Symptoms usually appear on the first day of life and, in more severe cases, include ptosis, swallowing difficulties, and respiratory insufficiency. Pharmacologic therapy is with anticholinesterase agents.
- Juvenile myasthenia gravis commonly has its onset at around 10 years of age. Ptosis, ophthalmoplegia, and weakness of other facial muscles are commonly present. The disease tends to become worse throughout the day. Both remissions and exacerbations are common, and up to 50 percent of affected children may develop seizures.
- The primary treatment is with anticholinesterase agents. In refractory or severe cases, immunosuppressive agents, plasmapheresis, or thymectomy may be necessary. Erythromycin therapy can exacerbate symptoms and is avoided.

MYASTHENIC CRISIS
- Occasionally, exacerbations of symptoms can occur that result in profound weakness, difficulty swallowing secretions, and respiratory insufficiency. This can be associated with antibiotic therapy, central nervous system depressants, antiarrhythmics, and hypokalemia.

CHOLINERGIC CRISIS
- Overdose of cholinergic medication can cause a "cholinergic crisis," which has similar manifestations to an exacerbation of the disease (myasthenic crisis).

BELL'S PALSY

- Bell's palsy is a condition that results in unilateral facial weakness. It is thought to result from swelling and edema of cranial nerve VII.
- In most cases, Bell's palsy is idiopathic. However, associated conditions include otitis media, Lyme disease, and temporal bone trauma.
- Symptoms may begin with ear pain, followed by the development of facial weakness, characterized by a drooping mouth and inability to close the eye on the affected side. Inability to close the mouth can make eating and drinking difficult.
- Bell's palsy affects the muscles of the forehead on the side of the lesion. In a lesion of the central nervous system, the forehead is spared, because it receives innervation from both sides of the brain.
- The prognosis of Bell's palsy is generally good, with recovery usually beginning in 2 to 4 weeks. Steroid therapy may be beneficial if started early in the course of illness.
- Treatment includes lubricating solutions for the eye on the affected side to maintain moisture of the cornea. Patients with inability to close the eye may require patching. In young children, ophthalmologic consultation may be advisable.

MYOPATHIES

- Myopathies are diseases that affect skeletal muscle. Many myopathies are congenital.

MUSCULAR DYSTROPHIES
- Muscular dystrophies are disorders associated with progressive degeneration of muscle, resulting in relentlessly increasing weakness. The most common is Duchenne muscular dystrophy, usually an X-linked recessive disorder.
- Clinical manifestations usually become apparent at about age 3 years, when patients begin to develop weakness of the hip girdle and shoulder muscles. The disease is characterized by a progressive loss of muscle strength.
- In the later stages, cardiomyopathy is common and scoliosis can result in pulmonary insufficiency. Survival beyond early adulthood is rare.

PERIODIC PARALYSIS
- Periodic paralysis is an example of a metabolic myopathy that results in muscle weakness. There are three varieties, characterized by associated hypokalemia, hyperkalemia, and normokalemia.

- Episodes of hypokalemic periodic paralysis have their onset during the first or second decade of life. Paralysis usually begins proximally and spreads distally. The episode can last for many hours. Serum potassium during an attack is usually decreased. Treatment with potassium during an attack may be helpful.
- Hyperkalemic periodic paralysis is associated with intermittent attacks beginning in the first or second decade of life. Attacks can be provoked by periods of rest following heavy exertion. Weakness can develop rapidly and last for hours.
- The respiratory muscles are usually spared. Some patients develop myotonia during attacks. The degree of hyperkalemia varies. In severe cases, standard therapy for malignant hyperkalemia is indicated.
- Normokalemic periodic paralysis can be provoked by exposure to cold, activity, and alcohol. The serum potassium does not change during an attack. Treatment with sodium during an attack may improve weakness.

BIBLIOGRAPHY

Cox N, Hinkle R: Infant botulism. *Am Fam Physician* 65:1388–1392, 2002.

Leshner RT, Teasley JE: Pediatric neuromuscular emergencies. In: Pellock JM, Myer EC, eds. *Neurologic Emergencies in Infancy and Childhood*, 2d ed. Boston: Butterworth-Heinemann, 242–261, 1993.

Shannon S, Meadow S, Horowitz SH: Are drug therapies effective in treating Bell's palsy? *J Fam Pract* 52:156–161, 2003.

Sharshar T, Chevret S, Bourdain F, et al: Early predictors of mechanical ventilation in Guillain-Barré syndrome. *Crit Care Med* 31:278–283, 2003.

Swaiman KF (ed): *Pediatric Neurology: Principles and Practice*, 2d ed. St. Louis: Mosby, 1385–1520, 1994.

QUESTIONS

1. Which of the following findings is most indicative of bulbar muscle weakness?
   A. Asymmetrical weakness, hyperreflexia, swallowing difficulties
   B. Distal muscle weakness, increased reflexes, facial muscle weakness
   C. Symmetrical proximal muscle weakness, decreased muscle tone, depressed reflexes
   D. Hypesthesias, cranial nerve findings, decreased reflexes
   E. Cranial nerve findings, facial muscle weakness, swallowing difficulties

2. A 5-year-old boy presents with a complaint of weakness to his lower extremities. He is noted to have bilateral hyperreflexia and slight clonus. What do these findings indicate?
   A. An upper motor neuron lesion
   B. A lower motor neuron lesion
   C. A myopathy
   D. A tendon injury
   E. A radiculopathy

3. Which of the following neurologic findings is matched correctly with the source of the abnormality?
   A. Stocking and glove sensory loss – spinal cord lesion
   B. An abnormality of touch and position on one side and temperature on the other – brain lesion
   C. A unilateral loss of all sensation – brain lesion
   D. Hemiplegia – spinal cord lesion
   E. Paraplegia – brain lesion

4. A 10-year-old male presents with a history of symmetric lower extremity weakness that is progressing proximally. He had a recent upper respiratory tract infection 2 weeks ago but has been well since. He has absent deep tendon reflexes in the lower extremities. Which of the following is true regarding this condition?
   A. The etiology is bacterial.
   B. It is an acute inflammatory demyelinating neuropathy.
   C. Cranial nerve involvement is rare.
   D. Autonomic dysfunction is not associated with this disorder.
   E. Treatment is with high dose steroids.

5. A 6-year-old girl is brought in by her parents with a complaint of restlessness, paresthesias of her feet, and weakness to her legs. She has had no recent illnesses and is afebrile. She is noted to be ataxic and have decreased deep tendon reflexes. The family just returned from a camping trip. She denies headache, arthralgias, or rashes. Which of the following is true regarding the treatment of this patient?
   A. Electromyography is indicated to elucidate the cause.
   B. Spinal fluid analysis may reveal a low protein.
   C. Corticosteroids are beneficial in the treatment.
   D. The treatment is tick removal.
   E. It is a progressive demyelinating disease.

6. Which of the following is true regarding botulism?
   A. There is only one form of the disease.
   B. It causes symmetric ascending paralysis.
   C. Infants may present with poor sucking, listlessness, constipation, and weakness.
   D. Altered mental status is a hallmark.
   E. Antibiotics are the treatment of choice.

7. Which of the following is true regarding myasthenia gravis in children?
   A. Juvenile myasthenia gravis occurs at birth and is transient.
   B. Persistent neonatal myasthenia gravis is treated with anticholinesterase agents.
   C. Erythromycin is the antibiotic of choice in juvenile myasthenia gravis.
   D. Exacerbations of the disease are easily distinguishable from overdose of cholinergic medications.
   E. Neonatal transient myasthenia gravis is caused by perinatal infections.

8. A 14-year-old female presents with the complaint of unilateral facial weakness. She has a drooping mouth and is unable to close her eye on the affected side. The remainder of her physical examination is normal. Which of the following is true regarding this condition?
   A. This is a lesion of the central nervous system.
   B. The prognosis is poor.
   C. It is a cranial nerve V palsy.
   D. A stat CT scan should be ordered.
   E. Treatment includes eye lubricants.

ANSWERS

1. E. Bulbar muscle involvement is manifested by cranial nerve findings, facial muscle weakness, and chewing or swallowing difficulties.

2. A. Hyperreflexia or sustained clonus indicates an upper motor neuron lesion, whereas absent or decreased reflexes imply a lower motor distribution.

3. C. A unilateral loss of all sensation suggests a brain lesion. Stocking and glove sensory loss suggests peripheral neuropathy. Crossed sensory findings is suggestive of spinal cord injury. Hemiplegia generally results from a brain lesion. Paraplegia is from a spinal cord lesion.

4. B. This patient has Guillain-Barré syndrome, an acute inflammatory demyelinating neuropathy of unknown etiology. Cranial nerve involvement is common. Autonomic involvement can produce labile changes in blood pressure and bowel and bladder incontinence. Treatment is supportive care. Steroids are of questionable value. Plasmapheresis may be beneficial.

5. D. This patient has tick paralysis caused by a tick that produces a neurotoxin preventing the liberation of acetylcholine at neuromuscular junctions. The treatment is tick removal. If untreated, it may progress to flaccid paralysis and death.

6. C. There are three forms: food-borne, wound, and infantile types. Early findings involve optic and bulbar musculature and progress to descending weakness and respiratory insufficiency. The patient has normal mentation. The treatment is supportive.

7. B. There are three basic types of myasthenia gravis in the pediatric population: transient neonatal, persistent neonatal, and juvenile myasthenia gravis. Juvenile myasthenia gravis has its onset at ~ age 10 years and is associated with remissions and exacerbations. Both persistent neonatal myasthenia gravis and juvenile myasthenia gravis are treated with anticholinesterase agents. Erythromycin therapy can exacerbate symptoms and is avoided. Exacerbations of symptoms (myasthenic crisis) have a similar presentation to overdose of cholinergic medication (cholinergic crisis). Neonatal transient myasthenia gravis is caused by maternal antiacetylcholine receptor antibodies that cross the placenta.

8. E. This patient has a Bell's palsy, an idiopathic mononeuritis of CN VII. The prognosis is generally good with recovery beginning in 2 to 4 weeks. The treatment includes lubricating solutions for the eye to prevent corneal abrasions. Steroid and acyclovir therapy may be beneficial.

42 HEADACHE

Susan Fuchs
William R. Ahrens
Patricia Lee

INTRODUCTION

- Headaches can be classified as:
  - Organic
  - Vascular
  - Functional
  - Psychological

ORGANIC HEADACHES

- Organic headaches usually result from a process that causes increased intracranial pressure or from an inflammatory process that is usually infectious in nature. Organic headaches may be progressive, wake a patient from sleep, increase with straining or coughing, or may be associated with fever and meningeal findings.
- Lesions associated with increased intracranial pressure include:
  - Brain tumors
  - Hydrocephalus

- Hypertensive encephalopathy
- Pseudotumor cerebri
- Acute hemorrhage, both spontaneous and traumatic
- Infectious etiologies include:
  - Meningitis
  - Encephalitis
  - Sinusitis
  - Brain abscesses

PSEUDOTUMOR CEREBRI

- Pseudotumor cerebri causes headache associated with increased intracranial pressure in the absence of a mass lesion.
- It is associated with high doses of vitamin A and steroid therapy and is especially common in obese adolescent girls.
- Patients may have papilledema on examination.
- Lumbar puncture will reveal an opening pressure greater than 20 cm H_2O.
- Therapy includes serial lumbar punctures to relieve acute symptoms and acetazolamide to reduce the formation of CSF.

HYPERTENSIVE ENCEPHALOPATHY

- Severe elevation in blood pressure can cause headache and if untreated, can result in the development of encephalopathy and seizures.
- This should be suspected in a patient with a severe headache whose diastolic blood pressure is greater than the 95th percentile for age.
- In young children, the development of hypertension is often secondary to an acute illness, such as fulminant glomerulonephritis.

ACUTE HEMORRHAGE

- The child presenting with a severe headache of sudden onset may have suffered an intracranial hemorrhage.
- Spontaneous intracranial hemorrhage usually results from either a ruptured aneurysm or arteriovenous malformation.

MENINGITIS, ENCEPHALITIS, BRAIN ABSCESS

- The association of headache with a fever and stiff neck implies an infectious etiology.

- If there are focal neurologic abnormalities or signs of increased intracranial pressure, a CT scan or MRI of the brain is performed prior to a lumbar puncture to avoid the potential for herniation.

VASCULAR HEADACHES

- Migraine headache is an example of vascular headache. Several theories exist as to their etiology. The vascular hypothesis is that vasoconstriction results in focal neurologic signs or an aura, followed by vasodilation and pain.
- Migraines tend to be recurrent, with symptom-free intervals of varying lengths in between episodes.
- The headache tends to be unilateral, throbbing, or pulsating, is often associated with nausea and vomiting, and is relieved with sleep.
- There is a genetic predisposition to migraines, with a positive family history in 70 to 90 percent of cases.
- Boys are more commonly affected until puberty, when girls become more predisposed.
- Migraine with aura (previously called a classic migraine) occurs less frequently in children than in adults.
  - Visual symptoms include scotomas, blurring, and abnormalities in the perception of lights.
  - Somatosensory disturbances may consist of abnormal smells, distorted perception of images, or even focal motor weakness.
- Migraine without aura (common migraine) is the most common type of migraine in children. It is differentiated from the classic migraine by the lack of a definable aura.
- A complicated migraine is associated with transient neurologic disturbances, which include ophthalmoplegia and hemiparesis.
  - The deficits are thought to result from cerebral vasoconstriction resulting in ischemia and edema, and they resolve spontaneously.
- A variant of vascular headache fairly common in childhood is the basilar artery migraine, which results in ataxia and vertigo, at times accompanied by visual disturbances.
- Benign paroxysmal vertigo can also be considered a migraine variant.
  - Occurs in children 2 to 6 years old
  - Consists of sudden, brief episodes when the child cannot stand upright without support
  - Episodes last for several minutes, and then the child recovers completely.
- ED treatment of migraines consists of providing analgesia and treating associated symptoms, such as nausea, during the acute attack.

○ Once a migraine is ongoing, gastric motility and absorption of medications are reduced, so parenteral medications may be more effective.

FUNCTIONAL HEADACHES

TENSION-TYPE HEADACHES

- Tension-type headaches (muscle contraction or stress headache) tend to be chronic and nonprogressive in nature.
- Pain is described as band-like, bilateral, or generalized.
- There is no accompanying aura, and nausea is rare.

PSYCHOGENIC HEADACHES

- Psychogenic headaches tend to be chronic and nonprogressive.
- Characterized by vague complaints and nonspecific symptoms.
- May result from stress, adjustment reactions, conversion reactions, depression, and malingering.

BIBLIOGRAPHY

Annequin D, Tourniare B, Massiou H: Migraine and headaches in childhood and adolescence. *Pediatr Clin North Am* 47:617–631, 2000.

Forsyth R, Farrell K: Headache in childhood. *Pediatr Rev* 20:39–45, 1999.

Lewis DW, Ashwal S, Dahl G, et al: Practice parameter: evaluation of children and adolescents with recurrent headaches: Report of the Quality Standards Subcommittee of the American Academy of Neurology and the Practice Committee of the Child Neurology Society. *Neurology* 59:490–498, 2002.

Rothner AD: Headaches. In: Swaiman KF, Ashwal S, eds. *Pediatric Neurology: Principles & Practice*, 3d ed. St, Louis: MO: Mosby, 747–758, 1999.

Winner PK: Headaches in children. *Postgrad Med* 101:81–90, 1997.

QUESTIONS

1. Lesions associated with increased intracranial pressure include:
   A. Tumors
   B. Hydrocephalus
   C. Hypertensive encephalopathy
   D. Sinusitis
   E. Pseudotumor cerebri

2. A 12-year-old obese female presents with a complaint of severe headache. A CT scan is done and is negative for mass effect or intracerebral lesions. A lumbar puncture is done and the opening pressure is 42 cm H_2O. Appropriate treatment for this condition would be all of the following **EXCEPT**:
   A. Admission for antibiotics
   B. Examination for papilledema
   C. Further history to determine vitamin A exposure or steroid use
   D. Serial lumbar punctures
   E. Acetazolamide

3. Common characteristics of migraines include all of the following **EXCEPT**:
   A. Boys are more commonly affected until puberty.
   B. Migraines with aura occur less frequently in children than adults.
   C. Migraines are rarely relieved by sleep.
   D. Ophthalmoplegia and hemiparesis may be a feature of migraine.
   E. Ataxia and vertigo accompanied by visual disturbances may be a migraine.

ANSWERS

1. D. Sinusitis alone does not result in increased intracranial pressure.
2. A. Pseudotumor cerebri is associated with high doses of vitamin A and steroid therapy and is especially common in obese adolescent girls. Patients may have papilledema on examination. Therapy for pseudotumor cerebri includes serial lumbar punctures to relieve acute symptoms and acetazolamide to reduce the formation of CSF.
3. C. Migraines are usually relieved by sleep.

43 HYDROCEPHALUS

Susan Fuchs
William R. Ahrens
Valerie A. Dobiesz

INTRODUCTION

- Hydrocephalus refers to the excess accumulation of cerebrospinal fluid (CSF). This can occur due to obstruction of CSF flow, reduced absorption, or excess production. Most CSF is produced by the choroid plexus. It absorbed by the arachnoid villi and granulations.

- Most cases of hydrocephalus result from congenital or acquired obstructions to the flow of CSF from the brain to the spinal canal. Congenital malformations include the Arnold–Chiari malformation, which is elongation and downward displacement of the medulla into the fourth ventricle, and the Dandy–Walker syndrome, which causes obstruction at the outlet of the fourth ventricle.
- Beyond the neonatal period, the most common causes of acquired hydrocephalus are mass lesions, which include tumors, cysts, and abscesses. Other acquired causes of hydrocephalus are meningitis, encephalitis, posthemorrhagic adhesions, and vascular malformations.

CLINICAL PRESENTATION

- The clinical presentation of hydrocephalus depends on the age of the patient and the rate at which it develops. Rapidly developing hydrocephalus can cause sudden neurologic decompensation.
- Infants with hydrocephalus are often diagnosed on routine examination by finding head circumference disproportionately large for age or splitting of the cranial sutures.
- When intracranial pressure becomes severely elevated, the infant develops vomiting and lethargy, which can signal impending herniation. Dysfunction of cranial nerve III may result in loss of upward gaze, or the "sundown or setting-sun" sign.
- Older children with hydrocephalus will usually complain of headache, which is often progressive in nature, worse in the morning, awakens the patient from sleep, and is exacerbated by lying down or straining. Gait disturbances can occur, especially ataxia, which is characteristic of children with posterior fossa tumors.
- As with infants, older children develop vomiting as intracranial pressure begins to become severely elevated. Papilledema is a late finding in children and is rarely found in infants, but it implies a severe increase in intracranial pressure.

MANAGEMENT

- The primary goal of management of the child with hydrocephalus is the assessment and control of elevated intracranial pressure. Patients may be quite stable or in imminent danger of herniation.
- Patients who are lethargic on presentation, those with a Glasgow Coma Scale score less than 8, or those who

deteriorate in the emergency department are intubated following rapid sequence induction procedures.
- Intubated patients are ventilated to achieve a P_{CO_2} of 30 to 35 torr. Patients who do not respond with an improved mental status to intubation and ventilation may benefit from diuretic therapy with mannitol (0.25 to 1 g/kg) or furosemide (1 mg/kg).
- It is appropriate to elevate the head of the bed 15 to 30 degrees.
- After the patient is stabilized, a computed tomography scan or magnetic resonance image of the brain is performed to define the lesion and plan definitive treatment.
- Therapy usually includes placement of an intracranial pressure monitoring device by a neurosurgeon. In dire circumstances, a percutaneous ventricular tap may be performed.

BIBLIOGRAPHY

Ashwal S: Congenital structural defects. In: Swaiman KF, Ashwal S, eds. *Pediatric Neurology: Principles and Practice*, 3d ed. St Louis: Mosby, 234–273, 1999.

Kotagal S: Increased intracranial pressure. In: Swaiman KF, Ashwal S, eds. *Pediatric Neurology: Principles and Practice*, 3d ed. St Louis: Mosby, 945–953, 1999.

QUESTIONS

1. What is the most common cause of hydrocephalus?
   A. Reduced absorption of CSF
   B. Excess production of CSF
   C. Obstructions of CSF flow
   D. Anencephaly
   E. Birth trauma
2. An Arnold–Chiari malformation is best described as:
   A. Elongation and downward displacement of the medulla into the fourth ventricle
   B. Posthemorrhagic adhesions
   C. A vascular malformation
   D. Dysplasia of the choroid plexus
   E. Pleomorphism of the arachnoid villi
3. Which of the following would best describe the clinical presentation of a child with hydrocephalus?
   A. An acute neurologic decompensation
   B. Depends on the age of the patient and the rate at which it develops
   C. Vomiting, lethargy, and dysfunction of cranial nerve III
   D. Headaches, gait disturbances, and ataxia
   E. Nausea, vomiting, and papilledema

4. An 8-year-old female with a history of Dandy–Walker syndrome presents to the ED complaining of headache exacerbated by lying down, nausea, vomiting. She is noted to be lethargic, have papilledema on funduscopic examination, and a dilated left pupil. Which of the following should not be used in the treatment of this patient?
   A. Elevation of the head of the bed
   B. Intubation and ventilation to achieve a P_{CO_2} of 15 to 20 torr
   C. Mannitol
   D. CT scan or MRI when stabilized
   E. Placement of an intracranial pressure monitoring device by a neurosurgeon

ANSWERS

1. C. Most cases of hydrocephalus result from congenital or acquired obstruction to the flow of CSF from the brain to the spinal canal.
2. A. Arnold–Chiari malformations are congenital malformations with an elongation and downward displacement of the medulla into the fourth ventricle.
3. B. The clinical presentation of hydrocephalus depends on the age of the patient and the rate at which it develops. Infants may be diagnosed on routine examination of head circumference or may have sudden neurologic decompensation.
4. B. This patient has evidence of increased intracranial pressure and impending herniation. Dandy–Walker syndrome causes obstruction at the outlet of the fourth ventricle. Measures that can be used to decrease ICP would include: elevating the head of the bed, intubation using RSI and ventilation to achieve a P_{CO_2} of 30 to 35 torr, diuretic therapy with mannitol or furosemide, a CT scan or MRI after stabilization to plan definitive treatment, and placement of an intracranial pressure monitoring device by a neurosurgeon. Ventilating to a P_{CO_2} of 15 to 20 torr would be detrimental to the patient.

44 CEREBRAL PALSY

Susan Fuchs
William R. Ahrens
Valerie A. Dobiesz

INTRODUCTION

• The brain injury that results in cerebral palsy (CP) can occur during the antepartum, peripartum, or postnatal period. The actual cerebral injury is a hypoxic-ischemic insult.

CLINICAL PRESENTATION

• The major disorder is of muscle tone, but there can also be neurologic disorders, such as seizures, vision disturbances, and impaired intelligence.
• Spastic CP is the most common variant; it is characterized by a generalized increase in muscle tone, deep tendon reflexes, and rigidity of the limbs on both flexion and extension. Many children have pseudobulbar involvement, resulting in swallowing difficulties and recurrent aspiration. Intellectual impairment is severe, and half have a tonic-clonic seizure disorder.
• Spastic diplegia is characterized by bilateral spasticity, with greater involvement of the lower extremities than the upper. Other manifestations include convergent strabismus, delayed speech development, and seizure disorders. Intellectual impairment parallels the motor deficit.
• Spastic hemiparesis is a unilateral paresis that usually affects the upper extremity more than the lower. Some degree of spasticity and flexion contracture usually results.
• Another classification of CP is extrapyramidal or dyskinetic, which accounts for 10 to 15 percent of cases. Dyskinesia is difficulty performing voluntary movements.

COMPLICATIONS

• The most common problem in CP patients presenting to the emergency department is breakthrough seizures. Anticonvulsant drug levels are often subtheraputic.
• Chronic aspiration can result in reactive airway disease and, for some patients, chronic hypoxia and hypercarbia. Acute pneumonia is common after aspiration; diagnosis may be difficult, as chronic changes are often present on chest radiograph. In many cases, functional lung impairment mandates a low threshold for hospital admission.
• Many children with cerebral palsy have significant feeding difficulties that require placement of a gastrostomy tube or button. Problems with feeding tubes are common.
• Many patients with CP who are significantly impaired are vulnerable to urinary tract infections and perineal skin breakdown that can result in infection. Most febrile CP patients require a urinalysis and urine culture.

BIBLIOGRAPHY

Davis DW: Review of cerebral palsy, part I: Description, incidence and etiology. *Neonatal Network* 16:7–11, 1997.

Perlman JM: Intrapartum hypoxic-ischemic cerebral injury and subsequent cerebral palsy: Medicolegal issues. *Pediatrics* 99:851–859, 1997.

Swaiman KF, Rusman BS: Cerebral palsy. In Swaiman KF, Ashwal S, eds. *Pediatric Neurology: Principles & Practice*, 3d ed. St. Louis, MO: Mosby, 312–324, 1999.

QUESTIONS

1. What is the underlying brain injury that occurs in the peripartum period resulting in cerebral palsy?
   A. Cerebral edema
   B. Intraventricular bleeding
   C. Hypoxic-ischemic insult
   D. Hyperosmolarity
   E. Hypopituitarism
2. Which of the following is not typically associated with cerebral palsy?
   A. Spasticity
   B. Seizures
   C. Impaired intelligence
   D. Vision disturbances
   E. Hypothyroidism
3. What is the most common problem in cerebral palsy patients that present to the ED?
   A. Reactive airway disease
   B. Aspiration pneumonia
   C. Gastrostomy tube problems
   D. Breakthrough seizures
   E. Urinary tract infections

ANSWERS

1. C. The brain injury that results in cerebral palsy is a hypoxic-ischemic insult and can occur during the antepartum, peripartum, or postnatal period.
2. E. The major disorder is of muscle tone and spastic CP is the most common variant. Neurologic disorders can also occur such as seizures, vision disturbances, and impaired intelligence.
3. D. Although all these problems may be seen in patients with cerebral palsy, the most common problem is breakthrough seizures. Anticonvulsant drug levels are often subtherapeutic.

45 CEREBROVASCULAR SYNDROMES

Susan Fuchs
William R. Ahrens
Heather M. Prendergast

INTRODUCTION

- Both ischemic and hemorrhagic strokes are less common in children than adults. Ischemic strokes can be divided into arterial ischemic strokes and sinovenous thrombosis. In children, hemorrhagic strokes are as common as ischemic strokes.
- Ischemic strokes are caused by vascular occlusion of an artery, usually due to thromboembolism, or occlusion of venous sinuses or cerebral veins (sinovenous thrombosis). The ratio of arterial ischemic stroke (AIS) to sinovenous thrombosis (SV) is 3:1.
- In children, risk factors associated with AIS include cardiac disease, coagulation disorders, dehydration, infection, vasculitis, cancer, metabolic disorders, moyamoya, sickle cell anemia, and perinatal complications.
- Sinovenous thrombosis can occur due to thrombophlebitis, hemoconcentration, or coagulation abnormalities. Risk factors associated with SV are prothrombotic disorders, dehydration, systemic infection, head and neck infections (otitis, mastoiditis, and sinusitis), hematologic disorders, drugs, cardiac disease, cancer, and perinatal complications.
- The underlying diseases that cause AIS and SV are listed in Table 45-1.
- Hemorrhagic strokes involve the rupture of cerebral blood vessels with leakage of blood into the brain parenchyma, subarachnoid space, or ventricular system.
- Intracerebral hemorrhage occurs when arteries or veins rupture into intracerebral areas or brain parenchyma. The greatest risk factor is head trauma, followed by aneurysms and vascular malformations.
- Subarachnoid hemorrhage results from rupture of an aneurysm or an arteriovenous malformation (AVM). Risk factors include disorders associated with vascular malformations, aneurysms, and hypoxia in neonates. These conditions are summarized in Table 45-2.

DIAGNOSIS

- Arterial ischemic strokes usually have a rapid onset, and present with focal neurologic deficit.
- An older child with a sinovenous thrombosis may present with slowly progressive signs, such as fever, vomiting, or headache. A young infant may have

TABLE 45-1   Predisposing Conditions for Ischemic Stroke

Cardiac

Congenital heart disease
Rheumatic heart disease
Bacterial endocarditis
Arrhythmias
Cardiomyopathy
Prosthetic heart valves
VSD/ASD
Patent foramen ovale

Infection

Meningitis
Encephalitis (especially
    varicella)

Vasculopathy

Moyamoya disease
Postradiation vasculopathy

Systemic Disorders

Systemic lupus erythematosus
Polyarteritis nodosa
Leukemia
Nephrotic syndrome
Inflammatory bowel disease
Takayasu's arteritis
Dermatomyositis
Rheumatoid arthritis
Diabetes mellitus

Hematologic Disorders

Sickle cell disease
Protein S and C deficiencies
Antithrombin III deficiency
Polycythemia
Hemolytic uremic syndrome
Thrombotic uremic syndrome
Thrombotic thrombocytopenic
    purpura
Idiopathic thrombocytopenic
    purpura

Acquired Prothrombotic States

Lupus anticoagulant/
    anticardiolipin antibodies
Plasminogen deficiency

Trauma

Head injury
Neck injury
Intraoral trauma
Child abuse

Drugs

Cocaine
Oral contraceptives
Antineoplastic agents
    (eg, L-asparaginase)
Steroids
LSD
Amphetamines
Alcohol

Metabolic Disorders

Homocystinuria
Hypoglycemia
Mitochondrial
    encephalomyopathy
    (MELAS)
Hyperlipidemia

Neurocutaneous Syndromes

Neurofibromatosis
Sturge–Weber syndrome
Tuberous sclerosis

Hereditary Disorders

Ehlers–Danlos syndrome
Fabry's disease

Vasospastic Disorders

Migraine

VSD, Ventriculoseptal defect; ASD, atrial septal defect.

TABLE 45-2   Conditions Predisposing to Hemorrhagic Stroke

Vascular Malformations

Aneurysms
Arteriovenous malformations
Cavernous malformation

Coagulation Defects

Hemophilia
Disseminated
    intravascular coagulation
Idiopathic thrombocytopenic
    purpura
Vitamin K deficiency
Anticoagulation treatment
Leukemia
Aplastic anemia
Factor deficiencies

Systemic Disorders

Hypertension
Hepatic failure
Sickle cell disease

Drugs

Amphetamines
Phenylpropanolamine
Cocaine

Head Trauma

Child abuse

Brain Tumors

Infection

Herpes simplex
Varicella

Congenital Syndromes

Ehlers–Danlos Syndrome
Neurofibromatosis
Tuberous sclerosis

- Neurocutaneous disorders, such as neurofibromatosis, Sturge–Weber syndrome, and tuberous sclerosis are all associated with both ischemic and hemorrhagic strokes.

DIAGNOSTIC EVALUATION

- An electrocardiogram (ECG) and an echocardiogram should be performed on all children in whom underlying heart disease is suspected.
- Although magnetic resonance imaging (MRI) is more sensitive in detecting infarcts, especially smaller ones and infarcts of the brain stem and cerebellum, a computed tomography (CT) scan is superior to the MRI in detecting hemorrhage acutely (less than 12 hours).
- The CT scan with contrast may also miss small hemorrhage, AVMs, or aneurysms, and may even be normal within the first 12 hours after an ischemic stroke.
- Magnetic resonance angiography (MRA) can be done at the time of the MRI to visualize the flow through the cerebral arteries and does correlate well with angiography. MRI can also be used with MR venography to diagnose sinovenous thrombosis.
- The gold standard to visualize intracranial and extracranial vessels is cerebral angiography.
- For patients in whom a hemorrhagic stroke is suspected and in whom the CT scan is negative, a lumbar puncture is indicated. The cerebrospinal fluid (CSF) is evaluated for the presence of red blood cells, which indicates hemorrhage. In some cases, the CSF may appear xanthochromic, which is also consistent with hemorrhage.

dilated scalp veins, eyelid swelling, and a large anterior fontanelle.

- An older child with a hemorrhagic stroke may have a history of severe headache or neck pain.
- A history of cardiac disorders, especially complex congenital heart disease or a prosthetic heart valve, should raise suspicion of an embolic phenomenon.
- Twenty-five percent of patients with sickle cell disease will develop cerebrovascular problems.
- The presence of systemic lupus erythematosus and other forms of vasculitis, such as polyarteritis nodosa, mixed connective tissue disease, or Takayasu's arteritis, have all been associated with arterial ischemic and sinovenous thrombosis.

TREATMENT

- Specific therapy is directed at the etiology of the stroke, such as correction of clotting abnormalities, antibiotics for infections, antiepileptic medication for seizures, and surgery for evacuation of a hematoma.
- In patients with sickle cell disease, exchange transfusion is indicated for ischemic stroke.
- Steroids may be indicated in patients with underlying vasculitis who have suffered a stroke.

BIBLIOGRAPHY

DeVeber G: Cerebrovascular disease in children. In: Swaiman KF, Ashwal S, eds. *Pediatric Neurology: Principles and Practice.* St. Louis: Mosby, 1099–1124, 1999.

Gabis LV, Yangala R, Lenn NJ: Time lag to diagnosis of stroke in children. *Pediatrics* 110:924–928, 2002.

Scott PA, Barsan WG: Stroke, transient ischemic attack, and other central focal conditions. In: Tintinalli JE, Kelen GD, Stapczynski JS, eds. *Emergency Medicine: A Comprehensive Study Guide,* 5th ed. New York: McGraw-Hill, 1430–1440, 2000.

Solomon GE: Acute therapy of childhood stroke. In: Pellock JM, Myer EC, eds. *Neurologic Emergencies in Infancy and Childhood,* 2d ed. Boston, Butterworth-Heinemann, 179–207, 1993.

QUESTIONS

1. Which of the following is **NOT** a risk factor for the development of an arterial ischemic stroke in the pediatric population?
   A. Sickle cell anemia
   B. Sepsis
   C. Dehydration
   D. Sinusitis
   E. Vasculitis

2. In children, ischemic strokes are divided into arterial ischemic strokes and sinovenous thrombosis. Which of the following accurately reflect the rate of occurrence?
   A. 1:1
   B. 2:1
   C. 3:1
   D. 4:1
   E. 5:1

3. A 6-year-old girl is brought to the Emergency Department for evaluation of fevers vomiting, and headache. The mother states that the symptoms have gradually worsened over the last 2 to 3 days. Which of the following would **NOT** heighten the index of suspicion of sinovenous thrombosis in this child?
   A. Sickle cell anemia
   B. Multiple episodes of otitis and sinusitis
   C. History of complex congenital heart disease
   D. Vasculitis
   E. History of thrombophlebitis

4. You suspect a neurologic event in a 7-year-old boy with a history of sickle cell anemia. The child is brought to the ED within 1 hour of the onset of symptoms. The child is awake and responsive, however, demonstrates a focal neurologic deficit. A diagnostic priority in this child would be which of the following?
   A. Electrocardiogram
   B. Echocardiogram
   C. Computed tomography
   D. Magnetic resonance Imaging
   E. Magnetic resonance angiography

ANSWERS

1. D. Risk factors associated with arterial ischemic stroke include cardiac disease, coagulation disorders, dehydration, infection, vasculitis, and sickle cell anemia. Sinusitis is most often a risk factor for development of sinovenous thrombosis.

2. C. Ischemic strokes are less common in children than adults and are the result of vascular occlusion of the artery or occlusion of venous sinuses or cerebral veins. The ratio of arterial ischemic stroke to sinovenous thrombosis is 3:1.

3. A. Sickle cell anemia is more commonly a risk factor associated with arterial ischemic stroke.

4. C. Although MRI is more sensitive in detecting infarcts, a CT is superior to the MRI in detecting hemorrhage acutely. The etiology of stroke in this patient is initially unclear. Twenty-five percent of patients with sickle cell anemia develop cerebrovascular problems.

46 THE FEBRILE CHILD

Nattasorn Plipat
Suchinta Hakim
William R. Ahrens
Gary R. Strange
Valerie A. Dobiesz

The authors would like to thank Dr. Stanford Shulman for his gracious review of this chapter.

INTRODUCTION

- Fever is a centrally mediated increase in body temperature that results when some stimulus causes an upward adjustment in the "set point" of the thermoregulatory center. Fever is produced by pyrogens, released from leukocytes and other phagocytic cells.
- Fever is usually considered to be present with a rectal temperature greater than 38.0°C (100.4°F). Children tend to have a higher temperature than adults. Body temperature is highest in the afternoon.
- During infection, moderate fever is probably beneficial because it enhances host-defense reactions. Rapidly rising temperature, however, may be associated with febrile convulsions.
- Hyperpyrexia, defined as a core temperature greater than 41.1°C (106°F), can result in complications such as central nervous system damage and rhabdomyolysis.
- Neonates and young infants are considered to be deficient in the ability to localize and neutralize bacterial infections. The exact age at which the developing immune system reaches adequate maturity is unknown.
- Although predictable organisms tend to affect different age groups, there is significant crossover.

AGE GROUPS

- Neonates younger than 28 days old are susceptible to organisms from maternal flora, especially group B streptococcus, *Escherichia coli*, and *Listeria monocytogenes.*
- Because they are presumed to localize bacterial infections poorly, virtually any bacterial infection in these patients is considered to be capable of disseminating and causing serious bacterial infection (SBI).
- The traditional approach to febrile infants in this age group has usually included an aggressive workup to search for bacterial illness, followed by hospitalization and empiric antibiotic therapy until cultures of blood, cerebrospinal fluid (CSF), and urine are negative.
- In many centers, management now includes an effort to define a subgroup of these patients as being at particularly low risk for a serious bacterial infection and, therefore, candidates for outpatient management.
- Patients between 3 and 36 months of age constitute the next traditional age group. Up to 2 percent of patients in this age group, with temperatures greater than 39°C, who appear well and have no focus of infection on physical examination, will have positive blood cultures—a situation referred to as occult bacteremia.
- After 36 months of age, the management of the non immunocompromised, febrile pediatric patient is similar to that of the healthy adolescent and adult.

PRESENTATION

- A temperature measured by a caretaker familiar with a thermometer is much more accurate than a history noting that the patient "felt warm."
- Helpful information in neonates and infants includes the patient's general level of activity, feeding, and

interaction with the environment. In older patients, a history of play activity is helpful.

- A large percentage of infectious illnesses in the pediatric population involve the respiratory tract. The combination of rhinorrhea, cough, and sore throat suggests upper respiratory infection.

- Vomiting or diarrhea usually indicate an infectious process involving the gastrointestinal tract, such as viral or bacterial gastroenteritis. However, vomiting and diarrhea can also occur as nonspecific findings in other infections.

- Stool that contains blood is associated with bacterial enteritis, which in neonates and young infants is a potentially serious infection.

- Many infectious illnesses are highly contagious and affect multiple members of a household. They range in severity from the benign common cold to serious diseases, such as tuberculosis.

- Treatment with outpatient oral antibiotics may mask symptoms of serious disease, as in the case of partially treated meningitis.

PHYSICAL EXAMINATION

- It is a fundamental principle that, in neonates and very young infants, the limited development of the patient makes clinical assessment more difficult, even for the experienced clinician. Attempts to apply reproducible scales of observation to this age group to predict the presence of SBI have met with mixed results.

- The most important factor to assess is the patient's mental status, which is evaluated by observing the patient's interaction with the environment. Older infants and children should recognize their parents and demonstrate curiosity about their surroundings.

- Patients who are inconsolable or appear worse when held or rocked by their parents are demonstrating true irritability, which may indicate central nervous system infection. Anxiousness and lethargy are also signs of serious illness.

- In a febrile patient in whom peripheral perfusion is diminished but who has no history compatible with fluid loss, septic shock is possible. In practice, most patients with significantly decreased perfusion also have depressed mental status.

- It is also important to realize that in neonates and infants, depressed mental status and signs of impaired perfusion can occasionally be intermittent. Any febrile pediatric patient with a history of even a momentary decrease in mental status or perfusion is presumed to have an overwhelming infection.

- Rales are infrequently heard in pediatric patients, especially infants, even in the presence of well-documented bacterial pneumonia. Percussion of the chest while listening with the stethoscope is more sensitive for determining an area of pneumonic consolidation.

- The extremities are evaluated for the presence of erythema or swelling, especially of the joints. In infants, range of motion is assessed. Both osteomyelitis and septic arthritis are more common in children than in adults; early diagnosis is imperative to avoid morbidity.

MANAGEMENT

SEPTIC-APPEARING OR TOXIC CHILD

- Sepsis is a clinical condition in which an infectious illness results in systemic toxicity and can ultimately result in irreversible shock. It is virtually always caused by a blood-borne bacterial illness. Bacterial sepsis is far more common in neonates and young infants than in healthy older children or adults.

- Neonates may present with a history of poor feeding, decreased activity, somnolence, respiratory difficulty, or apnea, or parents may merely complain that the baby "is not acting right."

- The failure of the child to recognize the parents is an ominous sign that signifies impaired perfusion of the central nervous system.

- The physical examination may reveal evidence of decreased peripheral perfusion, including capillary refill delay of greater than 2 s, cool, pale extremities, or diminished peripheral pulses.

- In the pediatric patient, blood pressure is an unreliable indicator of sepsis. In the initial stages, the blood pressure can be normal, the extremities warm, and the pulse bounding. As shock progresses, perfusion deteriorates. Only in the final stages does blood pressure fall. Petechiae or purpura are ominous findings that suggest fulminant meningococcemia.

- In relatively stable patients, supplemental oxygen and maintenance of hydration may suffice. In unstable patients, intubation, mechanical ventilation, and aggressive circulatory support, including massive volume resuscitation, invasive monitoring, and the use of pressors, may be necessary. Antibiotic therapy is tailored to the specific situation and is based on the most likely pathogen for the age group (Table 46-1).

TABLE 46-1   Most Common Pathogens in Childhood Bacterial Sepsis

AGE GROUP	PATHOGENS (PENDING CULTURES)	ANTIMICROBIAL	INITIAL DOSE (mg/kg)
0–1 mo	Group B *Streptococcus*, Enterobacteriaceae, *Staphylococcus aureus*, *Listeria monocytogenes*, *Staphylococcus epidermidis*	Ampicillin + gentamicin *or* ampicillin + cefotaxime	50–100 2.5 50–100 50
1–3 mo	Group B *Streptococcus*, *S. aureus*, *Streptococcus pneumoniae*, *Hemophilus influenzae*	Ampicillin + cefotaxime *or* ampicillin + ceftriaxone *or* ampicillin + chloramphenicol[a]	50–100 50 50–100 50–100 50–100 25
3–24 mo	*S. pneumoniae*, *Neisseria meningitidis*, *H. influenzae*, *S. aureus*	Cefotaxime *or* ceftriaxone *or* ampicillin + chloramphenicol[a]	50 50–100 50–100 25
>24 mo	*S. pneumoniae*, *H. influenzae*, *S. aureus*, *N. meningitidis*	Cefotaxime *or* ceftriaxone *or* ampicillin + chloramphenicol[a]	50 50–100 50–100 25
Immunocompromised	*S. aureus*, *Proteus*, *Pseudomonas*, Enterobacteriaceae	Vancomycin + ceftazidime + ticarcillin *or* tobramycin *or* gentamicin	15 50 75 2.5 2.5

[a] Primarily used in parts of the world in which cephalosporins are unavailable.

FEBRILE INFANTS YOUNGER THAN 28 DAYS OLD

- The management of the febrile patient younger than 28 days old is based on the assumption that the patient's immune system is inherently unable to localize and contain a bacterial infection.
- Another fundamental assumption is that in this age group, even the most experienced clinician is unable to distinguish the patient in the early stages of sepsis from the patient with a benign febrile illness.
- Blood-borne pathogens include group B streptococcus, *E. coli*, and *Listeria monocytogenes*.

- It is assumed that even patients with a focus of bacterial infection may be bacteremic and the organism has potentially seeded their CSF.
- The laboratory evaluation of the febrile neonate includes a complete blood count and cultures of blood, CSF, and urine.
- It is imperative that the urine culture be obtained by catheterization or by suprapubic tap, since a bag specimen is unreliable and can obscure the diagnosis.
- In the neonatal period, the urinalysis may be unremarkable in up to 50 percent of children with a documented positive urine culture.

- Patients with diarrhea or a history of bloody or mucoid stool require a stool culture. Stool microscopy is considered significant if there are more than 5 red blood cells (RBCs) or white blood cells (WBCs) per high-powered field.
- Treatment of the febrile patient younger than 28 days of age includes hospitalization and empiric therapy with ampicillin and either an aminoglycoside or a cephalosporin, such as cefotaxime or ceftriaxone, until all cultures are negative.

FEBRILE INFANTS 28 DAYS TO 3 MONTHS OLD

- Essentially the same principles apply to this age group as for neonates. However, clinical experience has shown that:
  - Most well-appearing febrile infants from 28 days to 2 to 3 months of age do not have documentable bacterial infections.
  - Those who have appropriately treated bacterial infections do well.
  - Many patients admitted under a "rule-out sepsis" protocol suffer iatrogenic complications.
- These observations have resulted in efforts to identify patients with an exceedingly low probability of having a SBI who would be candidates for outpatient management.
- Current data support the following approach to the well-appearing febrile patient between 28 days and 3 months of age.
  - Any bacterial infection, except otitis media, is considered to be an SBI.
  - Infants with evidence of infection of the soft tissue, joint, or bone are pan-cultured and admitted for appropriate antibiotic therapy.
  - If no source of infection is found, laboratory data are obtained in an effort to classify the infant as low or high risk for bacterial infection.
    - Low-risk criteria are somewhat debatable but in general include:
      - WBC count between 5000 and 15,000/mm^3
      - band count below 1500/mm^3
      - normal urinalysis
      - normal CSF
      - in patients with diarrhea, stool microscopy with less than 5 WBCs per high powered field; WBCs in the stool reflect the potential for *Salmonella* enteritis
  - Infants who are classified as low risk appear to have a low probability of having an SBI (less than 1 percent). There is currently support for discharging these patients from the ED provided that there is

close follow-up. Some favor empiric therapy with ceftriaxone, which can be administered intramuscularly at a dose of 50 mg/kg. Patients receiving ceftriaxone should return in 24 h for a second dose.
  - Given the extremely low risk of an SBI in this group, another management option is discharging the patient without antibiotic treatment, with a presumed diagnosis of viral infection. Close follow-up is necessary. In this management strategy, a lumbar puncture may not be necessary, because the risk of partially treating occult meningitis by the empiric administration of antibiotics is not a consideration.
  - Especially if there is any question regarding the reliability of follow-up, inpatient treatment should be strongly considered.

INFANTS 3 TO 36 MONTHS OF AGE

FEVER WITH A FOCUS OF INFECTION

- Infants who are older than 3 months presumably have acquired sufficient immunologic integrity that the risk of dissemination of a bacterial infection is low. The management of these patients is based on the nature of the infection.
- Certain focal bacterial infections are associated with a high likelihood of bacteremia. This is especially true in infections caused by *Haemophilus influenzae* type B. Blood cultures are indicated, and a lumbar puncture should be strongly considered. The incidence of *H. influenzae* B infection has dramatically decreased since the introduction of HIB vaccine.
- Other infections often associated with bacteremia are soft tissue infections secondary to *Staphylococcus aureus* and *Salmonella* enteritis, which can be especially problematic in younger infants.

FEVER WITHOUT A FOCUS OF INFECTION

- The major concern in this group is the phenomenon of occult bacteremia, the clinical situation in which a relatively well-appearing febrile infant with no focus of bacterial infection has a positive blood culture.
- Seeding of the bloodstream with bacteria is presumably a result of colonization of the nasopharynx with offending organisms. Bacteremia often provokes a fever but may be clinically silent and the patient may appear well.
- Occult bacteremia occurs primarily in patients with a temperature of greater than 39°C. At lower temperatures, the risk of bacteremia is much lower. Beyond 39°C, there is a direct correlation between the height of fever and the probability of bacteremia.

- Prior to the use of HIB vaccine, the prevalence of occult bacteremia ranged from 2.8 to 11.6 percent. The most common cause was *Streptococcus pneumoniae*, which accounted for 60 to 85 percent of cases. The second most common was *H. influenzae* type B, which accounted for 5 to 20 percent.
- Since the first HIB vaccine was licensed in 1987, the incidence of invasive *H. influenzae* infections in children younger than 5 years has decreased by more than 96 percent. In most recent studies in the post-HIB vaccine era, the current rate of occult bacteremia is 1.6 to 1.9 percent.
- The most common pathogen remains *S. pneumoniae* (85 to 92 percent of cases). Other agents are *Salmonella, Neisseria meningitidis*, group A streptococcus, and group B streptococcus.
- There is no laboratory test for definitely diagnosing or excluding bacteremia, however, the likelihood of bacteremia is directly correlated with the degree of elevation of the WBC count. The combination of a temperature greater than 40°C and a WBC greater than 15,000 mm³ increases the probability of bacteremia from about 2.6 to 11 percent.
- Attempts to correlate the erythrocyte sedimentation rate and C-reactive protein with bacteremia have had limited success.
- Urinary tract infections account for up to 7 percent of male patients younger than 6 months of age and 8 percent of female infants younger than 1 year of age who have fever without focus.
- Chest x-rays are unlikely to be helpful in febrile pediatric patients without pulmonary findings, such as cough and tachypnea. Stool cultures are likely to be useful only for patients who have bloody diarrhea or more than 5 WBCs per high powered field.
- Untreated bacteremia with *S. pneumoniae* appears to uncommonly result in morbidity, with perhaps a 6 percent risk for subsequent development of meningitis. Although *N. meningitidis* is an infrequent cause of occult bacteremia, up to half of the affected patients develop meningitis or sepsis.
- Evidence suggests that treatment with parenteral antibiotics is beneficial in preventing meningitis for patients with occult bacteremia, when compared with no treatment at all or treatment with oral antibiotics, which are effective against *S. pneumoniae* but not *H. influenzae*.
- Ceftriaxone has the advantage of providing coverage against *H. influenzae*, which is 40 percent penicillin and amoxicillin resistant. Ceftriaxone also provides antibiotic effect for 24 h and penetrates the CSF.
- One management strategy in the well-appearing infant who is 3 to 36 months of age with a temperature above 39°C is to obtain a screening complete blood count. Those patients with a WBC count greater than 15,000/mm³ are at increased risk for occult bacteremia and should have a blood culture sent.
- Male infants younger than 6 months of age and females younger than 2 years of age undergo a urinalysis and urine culture.
- Any patient who appears toxic has a lumbar puncture performed. Empiric therapy with ceftriaxone is then administered.
- An alternative management strategy is to obtain a blood culture on all patients with a temperature greater than 39°C and initiate empiric therapy with ceftriaxone. This would result in a large number of patients at low risk of bacteremia receiving treatment, because of the lack of a screening WBC.
- Patients who have blood cultures positive for *N. meningitides* or *H. influenzae* should be recalled to the ED and hospitalized for treatment. If a lumbar puncture was not performed on the initial visit, it should be done on the patient's arrival.
- Children with a blood culture positive for *S. pneumoniae* who are afebrile and look well receive a second dose of ceftriaxone and a follow-up course of oral penicillin. Patients with pneumococcemia who have persistent fever or are ill-appearing require admission for parenteral antibiotics.
- In February 2000, a seven-valent pneumococcal conjugate vaccine was licensed for use among infants and young children. This vaccine covers almost 90 percent of pneumococcal serotypes responsible for invasive diseases in the United States. The approach to the fully immunized, nontoxic-appearing febrile children will most likely change dramatically as use of the vaccine becomes widespread.
- Although the vaccine does not have efficacy against serotypes not included in the vaccine, to date there are no data indicating an increase in disease with nonvaccine serotypes in vaccinated children. Another potential benefit of this vaccine is providing herd immunity.
- The management of the febrile patient between 3 and 36 months of age will remain controversial until such time as bacteremia can be excluded. Some authorities believe that neither laboratory evaluation nor empiric antibiotic therapy is indicated in well-appearing febrile children with no focus of infection.
- All authorities agree that regardless of the ED treatment, close follow-up is the most important factor in ensuring a good outcome.

FEBRILE CHILD OLDER THAN 36 MONTHS OF AGE

- Beyond 36 months of age, the immune system of the healthy child has developed to the point where disseminated bacterial infection is much less common. Even bacteremic patients very uncommonly seed their meninges or develop full-blown sepsis. An exception to this is meningococcemia, which remains a serious disease at all ages.

• Blood counts and cultures are usually not indicated, except in ill-appearing children. Most older febrile patients have viral illness and require no workup.

TREATMENT OF FEVER

• Despite the great frequency of the problem, whether to treat fever with antipyretics remains controversial. The majority of patients with fever do well, and lowering the body temperature may obviate some of the potentially beneficial effects of fever.

• Patients who definitely require aggressive treatment are those with a history of febrile seizure and those who are physiologically unstable; in these patients, the increased basal metabolic rate can further compromise cardiopulmonary function.

• Pharmacologic therapy of fever predominantly consists of treatment with acetaminophen and nonsteroidal antiinflammatory drugs. Because of a likely link with Reyes' syndrome, the American Academy of Pediatrics does not recommend aspirin use in febrile children.

• Body temperature can also be reduced by external cooling, which in small children is easily achieved by bathing. Water temperature should be tepid and not cold enough to induce shivering.

BIBLIOGRAPHY

Alpern ER, Alessandrini EA, Bell LM, et al: Occult bacteremia from a pediatric emergency department: Current prevalence, time to detection, and outcome. *Pediatrics* 106: 505, 2000.

Baraff LJ: Management of fever without source in infants and children. *Ann Emerg Med* 36:602–614, 2000.

Baraff LJ, Bass JW, Fleisher GR, et al: Practice guideline for the management of infants and children 0–36 months of age with fever without source. *Ann Emerg Med* 22:1198, 1993.

Centers for Disease Control: Preventing pneumococcal disease among infants and young children: Recommendations of the Advisory Committee on Immunization Practices (ACIP). *MMWR* 49:1, 2000.

Fleisher GR, Rosenberg N, Vinci R, et al: Intramuscular versus oral antibiotic therapy in young, febrile children. *J Pediatr* 124:504, 1994.

Hausdorff WP, Bryant J, Paradiso PR, et al: Which pneumococcal serogroups cause the most invasive disease: Implications for conjugate vaccine formulation and use, Part I. *CID* 30:100, 2000.

Hausdorff WP, Bryant J, Kloek C, et al: The contribution of specific pneumococcal serogroups to different disease manifestations: Implications for conjugate vaccine formulation and use, Part II. *CID* 30:122, 2000.

Lee GM, Harper MB: Risk of bacteremia for febrile young children in the post-*Haemophilus influenzae* type B era. *Arch Pediatr Adolesc Med* 152:624, 1998.

Lieu TA, Ray GT, Black SB, et al: Projected cost-effectiveness of pneumococcal conjugate vaccination of healthy infants and young children. *JAMA* 283:1460, 2000.

McCarthy PL: Fever without apparent source on clinical examination. *Curr Opin Pediatr* 15:112–120, 2003.

Scolnik D, Kozer E, Jacobson S, et al: Comparison of oral versus normal and high-dose rectal acetaminophen in the treatment of febrile children. *Pediatrics* 110:553–556, 2002.

QUESTIONS

1. Neonates younger than 28 days old are susceptible to organisms from maternal flora and these include which of the following?
   A. *Escherichia coli*
   B. *Staphylococcus aureus*
   C. *Mycoplasma pneumoniae*
   D. *Streptococcus pneumoniae*
   E. *Neisseria meningitides*

2. Which of the following statements is true regarding infections in neonates $\leq$ 28 days of age?
   A. Serious bacterial infections are typically associated with high fevers.
   B. Height of fever correlates well with the seriousness of the infection.
   C. Virtually any bacterial infection in these patients is considered to be capable of disseminating and causing serious bacterial infection.
   D. Hypothermia is unlikely after the first few days of life.
   E. Due to maternal antibodies, neonates are able to localize most bacterial infections.

3. In the age group of 28 days to 3 months, which of the following criteria can be used in defining a group at low risk for serious bacterial infection and therefore eligible for outpatient management?
   A. WBC count $< 15,000/mm^3$
   B. Band count $< 2500/mm^3$
   C. Urinalysis consistent with infection
   D. CSF with < 100 WBC/mm^3
   E. For patients with diarrhea, stool microscopy with no WBCs

4. For patients between the ages of 3 and 36 months, occult bacteremia has been considered to be a risk for patients with temperature >39°C. The use of WBC counts, blood cultures, and empiric antibiotics in these children is controversial and may be unnecessary due to which of the following factors?
   A. Demonstrated effectiveness of parental education in the skills needed to identify evidence of SBI.
   B. Widespread use of vaccines for *Hemophilus influenzae* and *Streptococcus pneumoniae*.
   C. Expanded broad-spectrum effectiveness or oral antibiotics.
   D. Lower level of resistance to quinolone antibiotics than to cephalosporins.
   E. New evidence showing lack of correlation between temperature elevation and seriousness of infection.

5. A 3-month-old infant is brought by his mother who says that her baby has had two episodes where he appeared to stop breathing. These occurred over the past 24 h, during which, he has had a tactile fever. You find an alert infant with temperature of 102°F and no focus of infection. He is breathing quietly at a rate of 24/min. What do you do?
   A. Reassure the mother regarding the respiratory status, initiate antibiotics and arrange for 24-h follow-up.
   B. Perform a septic work-up and admit the patient for observation.
   C. Perform a septic work-up and, if negative, discharge on empiric antibiotics.
   D. Observe for 6 h in the ED and if no evidence of apnea, discharge on empiric antibiotics.
   E. Perform a septic work-up and, if negative, discharge on no antibiotics, pending results of blood cultures.

6. Children who are inconsolable or appear worse when held or rocked by their parents are suspected of which of the following conditions?
   A. Occult bacteremia
   B. Child abuse
   C. Septic arthritis
   D. Central nervous system infection
   E. Intussusception

7. A 10-year-old child presents with a high fever associated with widespread petechiae and purpura. This presentation is suggestive of which of the following problems?
   A. Idiopathic thrombocytopenic purpura
   B. Staphylococcal scalded skin syndrome
   C. Toxic shock syndrome
   D. Fulminant meningococcemia
   E. Rocky Mountain spotted fever

ANSWERS

1. A. Neonates are susceptible to organisms from the maternal flora and these include *E. coli*, group B streptococcus, and *Listeria monocytogenes*.

2. C. Because they are presumed to localize bacterial infections poorly, virtually any bacterial infection in these patients is considered to be capable of disseminating and causing serious bacterial infection (SBI).

3. A. Low-risk criteria are somewhat debatable but in general include:
   1. WBC count between 5000 and 15,000/mm³
   2. Band count below 1500/mm³
   3. Normal urinalysis
   4. Normal CSF
   5. In patients with diarrhea, stool microscopy with less than 5 WBCs per high powered field. WBCs in the stool reflect the potential for *Salmonella* enteritis.

4. B. Widespread use of these vaccines has markedly reduced the incidence of SBI due to *Haemophilus influenzae* and pneumococcus. Many authorities believe that neither laboratory evaluation nor empiric antibiotic therapy is indicated in well-appearing febrile children in this age group with no focus of infection.

5. B. Especially in infants, overwhelming infection can cause apnea. It is important to realize that apnea can be intermittent and that the patient may appear stable between episodes.

6. D. Children with true irritability are suspected of having central nervous system infection.

7. D. Petechiae and purpura in association with high fever are very suggestive of meningococcemia. This illness often has a fulminant course and antibiotics should be administered immediately.

47 MENINGITIS

Gary R. Strange
John Marcinak
Steve Lelyveld
Valerie A. Dobiesz

EPIDEMIOLOGY

• The epidemiology of bacterial meningitis has changed significantly over the past 20 years. Bacterial meningitis is now predominantly a disease of adults.

The most important contributor to this change has been the decrease in frequency of *Haemophilus influenzae* type b since the introduction of the conjugate vaccine against this organism.

- *Streptococcus pneumoniae* is now the major cause of bacterial meningitis in infants 1 month to 2 years of age in the United States. A heptavalent pneumococcal conjugate vaccine was introduced in the year 2000 that covers about 80 percent of invasive serotypes and is expected to prevent over 12,000 cases of meningitis and bacteremia, annually.
- Over half of all cases of meningitis are aseptic, and most of these cases have a benign outcome.

PATHOPHYSIOLOGY

- Most pathogens enter the subarachnoid space by hematogenous spread. In addition, they may enter through a mechanical disruption, as in a fracture of the base of the skull, or by direct extension from an infection in the ear, mastoid air cells, sinuses, orbit, or other adjacent structure.
- Many of the pathologic changes of meningitis are not primarily due to infection but result from the response of the human immune system to the infection.

PRESENTATION

- The "classic" signs and symptoms of meningitis include headache, photophobia, stiff neck, change in mental status, bulging fontanelle, nausea, and vomiting.
- The Brudzinski sign occurs when the irritated meninges are stretched, with neck flexion causing the hips and knees to flex involuntarily. The Kernig sign of nerve root irritation is present when the hip is flexed to 90 degrees and the examiner is unable to passively extend the leg fully.
- Children with meningeal irritation often resist walking or being carried. Signs and symptoms of meningeal irritation are reasonably reliable in older infants and children, but their absence does not rule out intracranial infection.
- The younger the child, the less obvious the signs and symptoms until late in the course of the disease. Neonates and young infants are likely to present with poor feeding, irritability, inconsolability, or listlessness.
- The course of meningitis may be either insidious (90 percent) or fulminant (10 percent). If the course is insidious, the patient has a high likelihood of presenting to a physician with a nonspecific illness, especially when the pathogen is pneumococcus.
- Meningococcal disease typically presents with a more fulminant course. Concomitant meningococcal bacteremia rapidly progresses to petechiae, purpura fulminans, and cardiovascular collapse. As other causes of pediatric meningitis have been contained, meningococcal disease has become a leading infectious cause of death.

DIFFERENTIAL DIAGNOSIS

- In the early phases, meningitis may be confused with a number of acute febrile illnesses. As the disease progresses, alteration of mental status becomes more prominent. The differential diagnosis is broad (Table 47-1).

MANAGEMENT

UNSTABLE PATIENTS

- The ABCs must not be neglected while performing diagnostic procedures, such as lumbar puncture. In the unstable child, lumbar puncture should be withheld until after stabilization and antibiotic administration.
- Shock is treated with rapid intravenous or intraosseous infusion of crystalloid solution in 20-mL/kg aliquots.

TABLE 47-1   Differential Diagnosis for Meningitis

Acute febrile illnesses
  Cerebral abscess
  Cervical adenitis
  Encephalitis
  Gastroenteritis
  Otitis media
  Peritonsillar abscess
  Pneumonia
  Pyelonephritis
  Retropharyngeal abscess
  Septicemia
  Upper respiratory infection
  Viral syndromes

Diabetic ketoacidosis and other altered metabolic states
Hypothyroidism
Reye's syndrome
Seizure disorders
Subarachnoid or subdural hemorrhage with or without direct
  trauma or abuse
Torticollis
Toxic ingestions

However, careful assessment of the need for continuing fluid resuscitation should be used, since fluid overload can lead to worsening of cerebral edema. Once the patient is stabilized, fluid should be given at the usual maintenance rate.

• Signs of increased intracranial pressure (worsening mental status, papilledema, full fontanelle, and widening of sutures) should be treated with elevation of the head at 30 degrees and initiation of controlled ventilation to keep the Pa_{CO_2} between 30 and 35 mm Hg. Patients who do not respond to controlled ventilation may benefit from the use of diuretic therapy with mannitol (0.25 to 1 g/kg) or furosemide (1 mg/kg).

• Infants and children are generally treated with a cephalosporin (ceftriaxone, 100 mg/kg/dose qd or cefotaxime 50 mg/kg/dose tid). In areas where cephalosporins are of limited availability, the combination of ampicillin, 100 mg/kg/dose qid, and chloramphenicol, 25 mg/kg/dose bid, is an option.

• If the organism is known to be *S. pneumoniae* or if gram-positive cocci are seen on Gram's stain of the CSF, penicillin and cephalosporin resistance is possible. Vancomycin is the only antibiotic to which all strains of pneumococci are susceptible, and it is, therefore, added to a broad-spectrum cephalosporin for comprehensive therapy (vancomycin, 15 mg/kg/dose bid and cefotaxime, 50 mg/kg/dose tid).

STABLE PATIENTS

• Phlebotomy for diagnostic studies is followed promptly by lumbar puncture in stable patients with manifestations suggestive of meningitis. The initial workup includes a complete blood count (CBC), electrolytes, glucose, renal functions, and blood culture.

• Normal CSF laboratory parameters are age-related (Table 47-2). A low white blood cell count, with a predominantly mononuclear cell type, and normal glucose and protein point to a viral etiology. High protein, low sugar, and elevated polymorphonuclear leukocytes (PMNs) point to a bacterial etiology.

ANTIBIOTIC TREATMENT

• Newborns are generally treated with an initial dose of ampicillin, 100 mg/kg, and an aminoglycoside, such as gentamicin, 2.5 mg/kg. Based on local sensitivities, a cephalosporin active against gram-negative bacilli, such as cefotaxime, 50 mg/kg, may be substituted for the aminoglycoside.

CORTICOSTEROID TREATMENT

• Dexamethasone, 0.15 mg/kg intravenously, when given prior to the antibiotic, decreases intracranial pressure, cerebral edema, and CSF lactate concentrations. Dexamethasone significantly decreases hearing loss and other neurologic sequelae in meningitis caused by *Haemophilus influenzae* type b. Clinical trials and meta analyses suggest that dexamethasone therapy improves the outcome for patients with bacterial meningitis due to other agents, but the evidence is not yet conclusive.

SEQUELAE

• The majority of children with aseptic meningitis have a self-limited illness without subsequent problems. In spite of modern antibiotic treatment, the mortality of *H. influenzae* type b meningitis is 5 to 10 percent, and for *S. pneumoniae* meningitis, it is 20 to 40 percent. Up to 20 percent of survivors will have some long-term sequelae.

TABLE 47-2   Normal Cerebrospinal Fluid (CSF) Values

PARAMETER	PRETERM INFANT	TERM INFANT	CHILD
Cell count (WBC/mm^3)	9 (0–25) 57% PMNs	8 (0–22) 61% PMNs	0–7 0% PMNs
Glucose	24–63 mg/dL (mean 52)	34–119 mg/dL (mean 52)	40–80 mg/dL
CSF/blood glucose Ratio	55–105%	44–128%	50%
Protein	65–150 mg/dL (mean 115)	20–170 mg/dL (mean 90)	5–40 mg/dL

BIBLIOGRAPHY

Aronin SI: Bacterial meningitis: Principles and practical aspects of therapy. *Curr Infect Dis Rep* 2:337–344, 2000.

Bonsu B, Harper M: Fever interval before diagnosis, prior antibiotic treatment and clinical outcome for young children with bacterial meningitis. *Clin Infect Dis* 32:566–572, 2001.

Nathan BR, Scheld WM: New advances in the pathogenesis and pathophysiology of bacterial meningitis. *Curr Infect Dis Rep* 2:332–336, 2000.

Quagliarello VJ, Scheld WM: Treatment of bacterial meningitis. *N Engl J Med* 336:708–716, 1997.

Schuchat A, Ropbinson K, Wenger JD, et al: Bacterial meningitis in the United States in 1995. *N Engl J Med* 337:970–976, 1997.

Short WR, Tunkel AR: Changing epidemiology of bacterial meningitis in the United States. *Curr Infect Dis Rep* 2:327–331, 2000.

Tunkel AR, Scheld WM: Corticosteroids for everyone with meningitis? *N Engl J Med* 347:1613–1615, 2002.

Willoughby RE, Polack FS: Meningitis: What's new in diagnosis and management. *Contemp Pediatr* 15:49–70, 1998.

QUESTIONS

1. Which of the following is true regarding meningitis?
   A. The majority of all cases of meningitis are bacterial in origin.
   B. *Haemophilus influenza* type B is the major cause of bacterial meningitis in infants 1 month to 2 years of age.
   C. Bacterial meningitis is now primarily a disease of adults.
   D. Most pathogens enter the subarachnoid space via direct extension.
   E. The majority of aseptic meningitis results in some type of long-term sequela.

2. The Brudzinski sign in bacterial meningitis is which of the following?
   A. When the neck is flexed, the hips and knees flex involuntarily.
   B. When the neck is flexed, there is severe pain in the hips and knees.
   C. When the hip is flexed to 90 degrees, the examiner is unable to passively extend the leg fully.
   D. When the hip is flexed to 90 degrees, the neck flexes involuntarily.
   E. Neck and back stiffness with inability to flex the neck.

3. Which of the following is true regarding the management and treatment of bacterial meningitis?

A. A lumbar puncture should be performed before treatment in all patients suspected of having this diagnosis.
B. Newborns should be treated with a cephalosporin, such as ceftriaxone or cefotaxime.
C. Dexamethasone should be administered immediately after antibiotics in order to be effective.
D. The mortality of *Streptococcus pneumoniae* meningitis is < 1 percent with the prompt administration of antibiotics.
E. Up to 20 percent of survivors will have some long-term sequelae.

4. Which of the following is true regarding the administration of dexamethasone in the treatment of bacterial meningitis?
   A. The appropriate dose is 1 mg/kg intravenously every 12 h.
   B. When given prior to antibiotics, it decreases intracranial pressure, cerebral edema, and CSF lactate concentrations.
   C. It has been shown to significantly decrease hearing loss and other neurologic sequelae when meningitis is caused by any of the common bacteria.
   D. The mechanism of action is cerebral vasoconstriction.
   E. Administration should be withheld until the bacterial etiology has been determined.

5. A 5-year-old male presents with a history of fever, headache, vomiting, neck stiffness, and photophobia. A lumbar puncture is done and the CSF reveals high protein, low sugar, and elevated polymorphonuclear leukocytes. While in the ED, the patient deteriorates and develops worsening mental status and papilledema. His vitals are as follows: BP is 80/40; P 90; T 102°F. All of the following are indicated in the management of this patient **EXCEPT**:
   A. Elevate the head to 30 degrees
   B. Initiate controlled ventilation
   C. Administer a fluid bolus of normal saline at 20 mL/kg
   D. Administer mannitol or furosemide
   E. Ensure that antibiotics have been administered

ANSWERS

1. C. Over the past 20 years, there has been a significant change in the epidemiology of bacterial meningitis secondary to the introduction of the conjugate vaccine against this organism. It is now predominantly a disease of adults. *Streptococcus pneumoniae* is now the major cause of bacterial meningitis in infants

1 month to 2 years of age in the United States. Over half of all cases of meningitis are aseptic, and most of these cases have a benign outcome.

2. A. The Brudzinski sign occurs when the irritated meninges are stretched with neck flexion causing the hips and knees to flex involuntarily. The Kernig sign of nerve root irritation occurs when the hip is flexed to 90 degrees and the examiner is unable to passively extend the leg fully. Signs and symptoms of meningeal irritation are reasonably reliable in older infants and children but their absence does not rule out intracranial infection.

3. E. In spite of modern antibiotic treatment, the mortality of *H. influenzae* type b meningitis is 5 to 10 percent, and for *S. pneumoniae* meningitis, it is 20 to 40 percent. Up to 20 percent of survivors will have some long-term sequelae. In an unstable child, lumbar puncture should be withheld until after stabilization and antibiotic administration. Newborns are generally treated with an initial dose of ampicillin, 100 mg/kg, and an aminoglycoside, such as gentamycin, 2.5 mg/ kg. Dexamethasone should be administered prior to antibiotics for the antiinflammatory effects.

4. B. Dexamethasone should be administered prior to antibiotics for the antiinflammatory effects, such as decreasing intracranial pressure, cerebral edema, and CSF lactate concentrations. The dose is 0.15 mg/kg intravenously. Dexamethasone significantly decreased hearing loss and other neurologic sequelae in meningitis caused by *Haemophilus influenza* type b. Clinical trials and meta analyses suggest that dexamethasone therapy improves the outcome for patients with bacterial meningitis due to other agents, but the evidence is not yet conclusive.

5. C. This patient presents with the classic signs and symptoms of meningitis. The LP results are indicative of a bacterial etiology. An LP with a low white blood cell count with a predominantly mononuclear cell type and normal glucose and protein is indicative of a viral etiology. He then develops signs of increased intracranial pressure (worsening mental status, papilledema, full fontanelle, and widening of sutures). The management of increased ICP includes elevating the head to 30 degrees and initiating controlled ventilation to keep the Pa_{CO_2} between 30 and 35 mm Hg. Patients who do not respond to controlled ventilation may benefit from the use of diuretic therapy with mannitol (0.25 to 1 g/kg) or furosemide (1 mg/kg). Only patients in shock should be administered a fluid bolus. Fluid overload can lead to worsening cerebral edema and is contraindicated in this patient with evidence of increased intracranial pressure.

48 TOXIC SHOCK SYNDROME

Shabnam Jain
Gary R. Strange
Heather M. Prendergast

ETIOLOGY AND PATHOGENESIS

- Toxic shock syndrome (TSS) is a rare acute febrile disease characterized by high fever, diffuse desquamating erythroderma, vomiting, abdominal pain, diarrhea, myalgia, and nonspecific neurological abnormalities. It can progress rapidly to hypotension, multisystem dysfunction, and death.
- The Centers for Disease Control and Prevention have formulated a case definition (Table 48-1). In the absence of a definitive laboratory marker, the strict application of the case definition undoubtedly excludes many subclinical cases.
- Most cases of TSS have been directly associated with *Staphylococcus aureus*, of which 67 percent are phage type 1. A disease that is clinically indistinguishable from TSS can be caused by group A streptococcus,

TABLE 48-1   Toxic Shock Syndrome: Criteria for Diagnosis

Fever:	Temperature ≥38.9°C
Rash:	Diffuse macular erythroderma, with subsequent desquamation, particularly of palms and soles
Hypotension:	Systolic blood pressure ≤90 mm Hg for adults and for children, systolic blood pressure <5th percentile for age
	Syncope

Involvement of ≥3 of the following organ systems clinically or by abnormal laboratory tests:

Gastrointestinal:	Vomiting or diarrhea at onset of illness
Muscular:	Severe myalgia or CPK > twice normal
Mucous membranes:	Vaginal, conjunctival, or oropharyngeal hyperemia
Renal:	BUN or serum creatinine > twice normal or pyuria in the absence of a urinary tract infection
Hematologic:	Platelet count <100,000/mm³
Hepatic:	Evidence of hepatitis (total bilirubin, SGOT, or SGPT > twice normal)
Central nervous system:	Disorientation without focal neurologic signs when fever and hypotension are absent

Negative results on the following tests, if obtained:

	Blood, throat, or CSF culture
	Serologic tests for rocky mountain spotted fever, leptospirosis, or measles

Streptococcus pneumoniae, or *Pseudomonas aeruginosa*. The pathogenesis is thought to be related to production of a toxin, currently referred to as toxic shock syndrome toxin-1.

- The most impressive aspect of the pathophysiology of TSS is the massive vasodilatation and rapid movement of serum proteins and fluid from the intravascular to the extravascular space.

EPIDEMIOLOGY

- The Centers for Disease Control and Prevention have reported a decrease in the annual incidence of TSS, presumably from the increased awareness of risk associated with tampon use.
- Although TSS is most often seen in menstruating women, cases are reported in nonmenstruating women, children, and men. Nonmenstrual cases occur in a variety of clinical settings, chiefly associated with postpartum or cutaneous/subcutaneous *Staphylococcus aureus* infections, with predisposing factors including burns, abrasions, abscesses, and nasal packing.

CLINICAL MANIFESTATIONS

- TSS can mimic many common diseases and should be considered in any patient who has unexplained fever, rash, and a toxic condition out of proportion to local findings. There is sudden onset of high fever associated with chills, vomiting, diarrhea, myalgia, dizziness, hypotension, and rash. The skin findings may be dramatic and present as a severe erythroderma and erythema of mucus membranes, which fades within 3 days of its appearance and is followed by full-thickness desquamation.
- Abnormal laboratory values reflect the multi-system involvement in TSS.

DIFFERENTIAL DIAGNOSIS

- Kawasaki disease is characterized by fever, conjunctival hyperemia, and erythema of mucous membranes with desquamation. Although it is clinically similar, it lacks many of the features of TSS, including diffuse myalgia, vomiting, abdominal pain, diarrhea, azotemia, thrombocytopenia, and shock. Kawasaki disease occurs typically in children under 5 years of age.
- Staphylococcal scarlet fever is also very similar to TSS, with both illnesses caused by toxin-producing staphylococcus.

- Streptococcal scarlet fever is rare after the age of 10 years. The "sandpaper" rash of scarlet fever is distinct from the macular rash of TSS.
- Septic shock must always be considered in the differential diagnosis of TSS. The appearance of a rash and the laboratory abnormalities associated with TSS will aid in distinguishing these two entities.

MANAGEMENT

- Management depends on prompt recognition, as well as on the identification of the infectious focus. The focus must be drained and foreign material, such as nasal packing or retained tampon, promptly removed.
- A β-lactamase–resistant antistaphylococcal antibiotic, such as oxacillin or nafcillin, has been the recommended treatment, but clindamycin has recently been recommended as having greater efficacy in TSS. Alternative antibiotics for patients allergic to penicillin include clindamycin, erythromycin, rifampin, and trimethoprim-sulfamethoxazole.
- The most important initial therapy is aggressive volume replacement. Crystalloids or fresh frozen plasma may be used for the management of hypotension, with pressors added if fluids alone are not sufficient.
- Corticosteroids are recommended, but have not been shown conclusively to affect outcome. There is some evidence that methylprednisolone, 30 mg/kg, may reduce the severity of the illness if administered early.

RECURRENCES

- More than half of the patients not treated with a β-lactamase–resistant antibiotic have recurrences. Most recurrent episodes occur by the second month following the initial episode, on the same day of menses as the prior attack. In the majority of patients, the initial episode is the most severe.

BIBLIOGRAPHY

Andrews MM, Parent EM, Barry M, Parsonnet J: Recurrent nonmenstrual toxic shock syndrome: Clinical manifestations, diagnosis, and treatment. *Clin Infect Dis* 32:1470–1479, 2001.

Centers for Disease Control: Defining the group A streptococcal toxic shock syndrome. *JAMA* 269:390–391, 1993.

Herzer CM: Toxic shock syndrome: Broadening the differential diagnosis. *J Am Board Fam Pract* 14:131–136, 2001.

Kniffin W, Smith R, Stashwick C: Toxic shock syndrome in three adolescent males. *J Adolesc Health Care* 10:166–169, 1990.

Meadows M: Tampon safety: TSS now rare, but women still should take care. *FDA Consum* 2000;34:20–24.

Reiss MA: Toxic shock syndrome. *Prim Care Update Ob-Gyn* 7:85–90, 2000.

Russell NE, Pachorek RE: Clindamycin in the treatment of streptococcal and staphylococcal toxic shock syndromes. *Ann Pharmacother* 34:936–939, 2000.

Vincent JM, Demers DM, Bass JW: Infectious exanthems and unusual infections. *Adolesc Med* 11:327–358, 2000.

QUESTIONS

1. Which of the following is a true statement regarding toxic shock syndrome (TSS)?
   A. It is most commonly caused by group A streptococcus.
   B. Antistaphylococcal antigen is the definitive laboratory marker
   C. The pathogenesis is thought to be related to a toxin; toxic shock syndrome toxin-1.
   D. The pathophysiology includes a massive vasoconstriction.
   E. Corticosteroids have been shown to be the treatment of choice.
2. The appropriate management of TSS would include the administration of which of the following?
   A. Broad spectrum antibiotics
   B. Beta-lactamase–resistant antistaphylococcal antibiotic
   C. A third-generation cephalosporin antibiotic
   D. A fluororoquinolone antibiotic
   E. A macrolide antibiotics
3. Which of the following is correct regarding TSS?
   A. The annual incidence is increasing.
   B. Is most often seen in males with nose bleeds.
   C. It can rapidly progress to hypotension, multisystem dysfunction, and death.
   D. TSS is easily diagnosed having a distinctive clinical presentation.
   E. TSS is an immune-mediated vasculitis.
4. A 26 yo G2P2 female presents with a 3-day history of high fever, chills, vomiting, diarrhea, myalgia, dizziness, hypotension, and rash that has since faded and is now desquamating. Her last normal menstrual period was 1 week ago. Her pregnancy test is negative. The most appropriate management of this patient would be:
   A. Removal of any foreign material (tampon, nasal packing), naficillin, crystalloid volume replacement, and corticosteroids
   B. Aspirin, immunoglobulin, crystalloid volume replacement, corticosteroids

   C. Crystalloid volume replacement, antipyretics, and penicillin
   D. Crystalloid volume replacement, vasopressors, and supportive measures
   E. Crystalloid volume replacement, dapsone, and corticosteroids
5. Which of the following statements regarding TSS is correct?
   A. The most important initial therapy is administration of antibiotics.
   B. More than half of the patients not treated with β-lactamase–resistant antibiotic have recurrences.
   C. The rash has characteristic target lesions.
   D. Septic shock should not be considered in the differential of TSS.
   E. It is a common acute febrile illness.

ANSWERS

1. C. Most cases of TSS have been directly associated with *Staphylococcus aureus*. The pathogenesis is thought to be related to production of a toxin, currently referred to as toxic shock syndrome toxin-1. There is no definitive laboratory marker in making the diagnosis but is made according to the CDC case definition. The most impressive aspect of the pathophysiology of TSS is the massive vasodilatation and rapid movement of serum proteins and fluid from the intravascular to the extravascular space. Corticosteroids are recommended, but have not been shown conclusively to affect outcome. There is some evidence that methylprednisolone, 30 mg/kg, may reduce the severity of the illness if administered early.
2. B. A β-lactamase–resistant antistaphylococcal antibiotic, such as oxacillin or nafcillin, has been the recommended treatment, but clindamycin has recently been recommended as having greater efficacy in TSS. Alternative antibiotics for patients allergic to penicillin include clindamycin, erythromycin, rifampin, and trimethoprim-sulfamethoxazole.
3. C. The Centers for Disease Control and Prevention have reported a decrease in the annual incidence of TSS, presumably from the increased awareness of risk associated with tampon use. TSS is most often seen in menstruating women, cases are reported in nonmenstruating women, children, and men. TSS can progress rapidly to hypotension, multisystem dysfunction, and death. TSS can mimic many common diseases and should be considered in any patient who has unexplained fever, rash, and a toxic condition out of proportion to local findings. The differential diagnosis may include Kawasaki disease, Staphylococcal scarlet fever, Streptococcal scarlet

fever, and septic shock. The pathogenesis is thought to be related to production of a toxin and not an immune mediated vasculitis.

4. A. This patient is presenting with a clinical presentation consistent with TSS. Management of this patient with TSS depends on prompt recognition, as well as on the identification of the infectious focus. The focus must be drained and foreign material, such as nasal packing or retained tampon, promptly removed. A β-lactamase–resistant antistaphylococcal antibiotic, such as oxacillin or nafcillin, crystalloid volume replacement, and corticosteroids are all recommended in the management.

5. B. The most important initial therapy is aggressive volume replacement. Crystalloids or fresh frozen plasma may be used for the management of hypotension. More than half of the patients not treated with a β-lactamase–resistant antibiotic have recurrences. Most recurrent episodes occur by the second month following the initial episode, on the same day of menses as the prior attack. In the majority of patients, the initial episode is the most severe. The skin findings may be dramatic and present as a severe erythroderma and erythema of mucous membranes, which fades within 3 days of its appearance and is followed by full-thickness desquamation. Septic shock must always be considered in the differential diagnosis of TSS. The appearance of a rash and the laboratory abnormalities may help in distinguishing these two entities. TSS is a rare acute febrile disease.

49 KAWASAKI SYNDROME

Gary R. Strange
Shabnam Jain
Heather M. Prendergast

ETIOLOGY AND PATHOGENESIS

- Kawasaki syndrome (KS), or mucocutaneous lymph node syndrome, is an acute, self-limited, multisystem vasculitis of unclear etiology. KS is the leading cause of acquired heart disease in children in the United States and Japan.

- The disease may occur sporadically or in mini-epidemics. In the United States, cases occur throughout the year with no definite seasonal occurrence. The peak incidence is in children 18 to 24 months of age, with 80 to 85 percent of cases occurring under the age of 5 years.

- KS appears to be caused by either an infectious agent or the immune response to an infectious agent. Inherent immaturity of the immune system resulting in T-cell unresponsiveness has recently been hypothesized.

CLINICAL FINDINGS

- Since there are no pathognomonic laboratory findings, the diagnosis is established clinically. Fever and at least four of five other clinical findings (Table 49-1) are required to establish the diagnosis.

- The acute or febrile phase lasts 7 to 15 days and is the period when most diagnostic clinical features occur. Fever is universal, often high, and usually sustained.

- The subacute phase lasts for approximately 2 to 4 weeks and begins with resolution of fever and elevation of the platelet count. It ends with the return of platelet counts to near normal levels.

- The subacute phase is dominated by desquamation that may have already begun before the disappearance of fever. Desquamation is a constant feature of KS. It is noted first in the periungual region, with peeling underneath the finger and toenails.

- Thrombocytosis is another constant feature of the subacute phase, with platelet counts in the range of 500,000 to 3,000,000/mm^3.

- It is during the subacute phase that complications, such as coronary artery aneurysms and hydrops of the gallbladder, develop.

- The recovery or convalescent phase may last months to years. It is during this phase that coronary artery disease may be recognized.

- Laboratory findings are nonspecific in KS. The complete blood count often shows an elevated white blood cell count with a left shift. A mild hemolytic anemia may be present. Elevated platelet counts occur in the

TABLE 49-1 Diagnostic Criteria for Kawasaki Syndrome

Fever persisting for ≥5 days
and
At least four of the following findings:
Bilateral, painless bulbar conjunctival injection without exudate
Mucous membrane changes of the upper respiratory tract, including injected, dry, fissured lips, oral mucosal and pharyngeal injection, and "strawberry tongue"
Peripheral extremity changes, including erythema and edema of hands and feet in the acute phase and periungual and generalized desquamation in the convalescent phase
Polymorphous truncal exanthem
Acute, nonpurulent cervical lymphadenopathy
Findings cannot be explained by some other known disease process

subacute phase but are usually normal in the acute phase.

- The electrocardiogram may show dysrhythmias, prolonged PR or QT intervals, and nonspecific ST-T wave changes. Two-dimensional echocardiography may demonstrate coronary artery dilation or aneurysms, pericardial effusion, or decreased contractility.

DIFFERENTIAL DIAGNOSIS

- The differential diagnosis is extensive because of the nonspecific nature of the clinical features (Table 49-2). Most viral exanthems can be eliminated based on the clinical course, absence of diagnostic features, epidemiologic considerations, and immunization status.

COMPLICATIONS

- The most serious manifestation of KS is cardiac involvement, which may result in coronary aneurysms, valvular insufficiency, congestive heart failure, myocardial infarction, dysrhythmias, rupture of aneurysms, and pericardial effusion. It is assumed that during the acute febrile phase, a pancarditis occurs, with a variable number of children developing coronary vasculitis with necrosis of blood vessel wall, aneurysm formation, or thrombosis.
- Echocardiography is the most sensitive technique for delineating proximal coronary aneurysms, with a diagnostic sensitivity of 80 to 90 percent. In selected cases, angiography may demonstrate lesions of the peripheral cardiac vessels. Dilatation of the coronary

TABLE 49-2 Differential Diagnosis for Kawasaki Syndrome

Viral illnesses

  Rubeola
  Rubella
  Epstein–Barr virus infection
  Adenovirus infection
  Enterovirus infection

Bacterial infections

  Toxic shock syndrome
  Scarlet fever

Rickettsial diseases

  Rocky Mountain spotted fever

Rheumatologic disease

  Juvenile rheumatoid arthritis
  Systemic lupus erythematosus
  Acute rheumatic fever

arteries due to vasculitis is recognized in about 50 percent of patients, beginning on day 7 to 8 of the illness.

- The most common cause of early death in KS is myocardial infarction, occurring in the subacute phase.
- Hydrops of the gallbladder is an acalculous cholecystitis that is noted in the subacute phase of the illness. Hydrops is a self-limited condition that occurs in 3 percent of the patients and is a functional rather than obstructive distension.
- Other complications include iridocyclitis or anterior uveitis (in about 80 percent of patients), mastoiditis, necrotic pharyngitis, renal infarcts, gangrene of the fingers and toes, encephalopathy, and subarachnoid hemorrhage.

MANAGEMENT

- All patients diagnosed with KS should be hospitalized immediately for administration of intravenous gamma globulin (IVGG), aspirin therapy, and cardiac evaluation. Routine testing includes complete blood count with platelets, urinalysis, electrolytes, liver profile, chest radiograph, electrocardiogram, and echocardiogram.
- Bed rest, coupled with close cardiac monitoring, is essential. Only by detecting the initial stages of cardiac complications can appropriate critical measures be taken to save the life of a severely affected child.
- Early in the course of the illness, IVGG may help decrease the inflammatory response and decrease the incidence of coronary artery aneurysm. The dose of IVGG is 2 g/kg infused over 8 to 12 h.
- Aspirin appears to be another particularly important therapeutic modality. Although it does not have an immediate antipyretic effect, aspirin can reduce the height and duration of fever and may serve as an important antithrombotic factor. It is given in a sequential dosage regimen: a high dose (100 mg/kg/day divided into 4 doses) until the 14th day of illness, followed by a low dose (3 to 5 mg/kg/day as a single-day dose).
- Corticosteroids were considered to be contraindicated in KS due to unfavorable results in early studies. However, there is growing evidence of their beneficial effect in immunoglobulin-resistant disease.

PROGNOSIS

- The overall mortality rate of KS in American children is below 1 percent. It is higher in infants younger than 1 year.

BIBLIOGRAPHY

Dale RC, Saleem MA, Daw S, et al: Treatment of severe complicated Kawasaki disease with oral prednisolone and aspirin. *J Pediatr* 137:723, 2000.

Kuijpers TW, Wiegman A, Van Lier RA, et al: Kawasaki disease: A maturational defect in immune responsiveness. *J Infect Dis* 180:1869, 1999.

Rowley AH, Shulman ST: Kawasaki syndrome. *Pediatr Clin North Am* 46:313, 1999.

Shingadia D, Shulman ST: New perspectives in the drug treatment of Kawasaki disease. *Pediatr Drugs* 1:291, 1999.

Shinohara M, Sone K, Tomomasa T, et al: Corticosteroids in the treatment of the acute phase of Kawasaki disease. *J Pediatr* 135: 465, 1999.

Win MT, Minich LL, Bohnsack JF, et al: Kawasaki disease: More patients are being diagnosed who do not meet American Heart Association criteria. *Pediatrics* 104:10, 1999.

Yunagawa H, Tuohong Z, Oki I, et al: Effects of gammaglobulin on the cardiac sequelae of Kawasaki disease. *Pediatr Cardiol* 20:248, 1999.

QUESTIONS

1. Which of the following are typically associated with presentations of Kawasaki syndrome?
   A. Persistent, low-grade fever lasting 3 to 5 days followed by diffuse maculopapular rash.
   B. Pathognomonic laboratory findings are leukocytosis and microcytic anemia.
   C. Recovery time for most patients is 3 to 4 weeks.
   D. Thrombocytosis is characteristic of the subacute phase.
   E. Pethichiae and purpura are present during the acute phase.
2. A 24-month old child is brought to the Emergency Department for evaluation of prolonged fevers and a rash. Clinical examination reveals desquamation of the fingertips. You suspect the patient may have Kawasaki syndrome. Of the following, the most useful diagnostic test is:
   A. Arterial blood gas
   B. Angiography
   C. Echocardiogram
   D. Visual acuity and fluorescein staining
   E. Coagulation times
3. Which of the following is the **MOST** typical ECG finding in patients with Kawasaki syndrome?
   A. Nonspecific ST-T wave changes
   B. Sinus arrhythmia
   C. Sinus bradycardia
   D. Shortened QT intervals
   E. Supraventricular tachycardia
4. In a patient diagnosed with Kawasaki syndrome, which of the following is **NOT** recommended for management?
   A. Initial high-dose aspirin therapy
   B. Intravenous gamma globulin
   C. Intravenous methylprednisolone
   D. Intravenous hydration
   E. Bed rest
5. A 5 year-old girl presents to the emergency department and is diagnosed with Kawasaki syndrome in the subacute phase. Potential complications during this phase would include which of the following?
   A. Pancreatitis
   B. Acalculous cholecystitis
   C. Nephrolithiasis
   D. Optic neuritis
   E. Hepatitis

ANSWERS

1. D. Patients with Kawasaki syndrome usually present during either the acute or subacute phase. The acute phase is characterized by persistent high fevers lasting from 7 to 15 days. There are no pathognomonic laboratory findings therefore, the diagnosis is primarily clinical. In the subacute phase, a thrombocytosis is a constant feature.
2. C. The most serious manifestation of Kawasaki syndrome is coronary aneurysm. Echocardiography has a sensitivity of 80 to 90 percent for detecting proximal aneurysms and should be attempted first. Angiography may also detect lesions of the peripheral cardiac vessels; however, it has the disadvantage of being invasive. Ocular evaluation is warranted because of the increased incidence of iridocyclitis or anterior uveitis; however, the evaluation should not take priority over the cardiac evaluation.
3. A. Various ECG findings can be seen in Kawasaki syndrome patients. Findings include prolonged PR and QT intervals and dysrhythmias. The majority of ECG in patients will demonstrate nonspecific ST-T wave changes.
4. C. Corticosteroids are considered to be contraindicated in the treatment of Kawasaki syndrome. There have been recent studies demonstrating a benefit for patients with immunoglobulin-resistant disease.
5. B. In the subacute phase, patients may develop hydrops of the gallbladder, which represents an acalculous cholecystitis. This condition is usually self-limited and represents a functional distension.

50 COMMON PARASITIC INFESTATIONS

Gary R. Strange
Steven Lelyveld
Valerie A. Dobiesz

INTRODUCTION

- In spite of advances in sanitation throughout the world, new medications, and the heightened awareness of health care providers, between one-fourth and one-half of the world's population has a parasitic infestation at any given time. An increasingly mobile society has made disease containment nearly impossible.
- The oral exploratory behavior of the child, coupled with a poor capacity to avoid arthropods, place him or her at particular risk for acquiring parasites. Important factors to be sought in the history are listed in Table 50-1.
- Three major groups of parasites cause human disease:
  ○ Protozoa
  ○ Helminths
    ▪ Nematodes (roundworms)
    ▪ Cestodes (flatworms)
    ▪ Trematodes (flukes)
  ○ Arthropods

NEMATODES (ROUNDWORMS)

- *Ascaris lumbricoides* is the largest and most prevalent human nematode, with an estimated 1 billion cases worldwide. Although it is most commonly found in tropical and subtropical climates, it is present throughout the United States. Ascariasis is most common in preschool and early school age children.
  ○ Albendazole (400 mg orally as a single dose) or pyrantyl pamoate (11 mg/kg orally as a single dose; maximum 1 g) is curative. Piperazine salts (50 to 75 mg/kg for 2 days) are recommended for ascariasis complicated by intestinal or biliary obstruction, since they cause relatively rapid expulsion of the worms.
  ○ There is controversy with regard to the clinical significance of *Ascaris* infestation. However, about 20,000 deaths annually are attributed to it, mostly due to intestinal obstruction. Preventive therapy in endemic areas may be considered.
- *Enterobius vermicularis* (pinworm) is present in all parts of the United States and affects individuals of all ages and socioeconomic levels.

TABLE 50-1 Symptoms of Parasitic Disease

SYMPTOM	POSSIBLE CAUSE
Abdominal pain	*Ascaris, Clonorchis, Diphyllobothrium, Entamoeba, Fasciola, Giardia.* hookworm, *Hymenolepsis, Schistosoma, Taenia, Trichuris*
Anemia	*Babesia, Diphyllobothrium,* hookworm, *Leishmania donovani, Plasmodium* species, *Trichuris*
Asthma	*Ascaris, Strongyloides, Toxocara*
Conjunctivitis and keratitis	*Filariae (Onchocerca volvulus), Taenia, Trichinella, Trypanosoma*
Diarrhea	*Dientamoeba, Entamoeba, Fasciola, Fasciolopsis, Giardia,* hookworm, *Hymenolepsis, L. donovani, Palantidium, Schistosoma, Strongyloides, Taenia, Trichinella, Trichuris*
Edema	*Fasciolopsis, Filariae (Wuchereria bancrofti), Trichinella, Trypanosoma*
Eosinophilia	*Ascaris, Dracunculus, Fasciola, Filariae (W. bancrofti, Brugia malayi),* fluke *(Paragonimus westermani, Chlonorchis sinensis, Fasciolopsis leuski), Hymnenolepsis,* hookworm, *Schistosoma, Strongyloides, Taenia, Toxocara, Trichinella, Trichuris*
Fever	*Ascaris, Babesia, Entamoeba, Fasciola, Filariae (W. bancrofti),* fluke *(C. sinensis), Giardia, L. donovani, Plasmodium* species, *Toxocara, Trichi, Trichuris, Trypanosoma*
Hemoptysis	*Ascaris, Echinococcus, Paragonimus*
Hepatomegaly	Fluke *(C. sinensis, Opisthorchis viverrini, Fasciola), L. donovani, Plasmodium* species, tapeworm *(Echinococcus), Schistosoma, Toxocara, Trypanosoma*
Intestinal obstruction	*Ascaris, Diphyllobothrium,* fluke *(Fasciolopsis buski), Strongyloides, Taenia*
Jaundice	Fluke *(C. sinensis, O. viverrini), Plasmodium* species
Meningitis	*Acanthamoeba,* malaria *(Plasmodium falciparum), Naegleria,* primary amebic meningoencephalitis, *Toxocara, Trichinella, Trypanosoma*
Myocardial disease	*Taenia, Trichinella, Trypanosoma (T. cruzi)*
Nausea and vomiting	*Ascaris, Entamoeba, Giardia, Leishmania, Taenia, Trichinella, Trichuris*
Pneumonia	*Ascaris, Filariae (W. bancrofti, B. malayi),* fluke *(P. westermani), Strongyloides, Trichinella*
Pruritus	*Dientamoeba, Enterobius, Filariae (O. volvulus), Trichuris*
Seizures	*Hymenolepsis, Trichinella, Paragonimus,* tapeworm *(Echinococcus, Cysticercus)*
Skin ulcers	*Dracunculus,* hookworm, *L. donovani, Trypanosoma*
Splenomegaly	*Babesia, Toxoplasma, Plasmodium*
Urticaria	*Ascaris, Dracunculus, Fasciola, Strongyloides, Trichinella*

○ Cellophane tape, placed sticky side to perianal skin when the child first awakens and then viewed under low power, is usually diagnostic, but repeated examination may be necessary.

○ Treatment is with albendazole, 400 mg orally. Pyrantel pamoate (11 mg/kg) or mebendazole (100 mg) may also be used. Each drug is given as a single dose, with a repeat dose given 2 weeks later to remove secondary hatchings.

- *Trichuris trichiura* (whipworm) is found in southern Appalachia, southwest Louisiana, and other warm rural areas.

  ○ Albendazole (400 mg) as a one-time dose may be sufficient, but in heavy infestations, the course of treatment should be extended to 3 days. Mebendazole (100 mg bid for 3 days) may also be used.

- *Trichinella spiralis*, the causative agent for trichinosis, is found throughout the United States, with increasing prevalence in the Northeast and Mid-Atlantic states.

  ○ When ingested, digestive enzymes liberate the encysted larvae, which lodge in the duodenum and jejunum, grow, and, within 2 days, mature and copulate. The females give birth to living larvae that bore through the mucosa, become blood-borne, and migrate to striated muscle, heart, lung, and brain.

  ○ Treatment with aspirin and steroids is initially aimed at reducing the inflammatory symptoms. Mebendazole (200 to 400 mg tid for 3 days and then 400 mg tid for 10 days) is indicated for severe disease but may not be effective after encystment.

- The hookworms, *Necator americanus* and *Ancylostoma duodenale*, are found between 36° north and 30° south latitude and are one of the most prevalent infectious diseases of humans, with an estimated 1 billion individuals affected.

  ○ The eggs hatch in the soil, releasing rhabditiform larvae that feed on bacteria and organic debris. They double in length, molt, and may survive as filariform larvae for several weeks.

  ○ Upon contact, they burrow through the skin, causing pruritus (ground itch), enter the blood, travel to the lung, and are ingested.

  ○ Albendazole (400 mg bid for 2 to 3 days), mebendazole (100 mg bid for 3 days), or pyrantel pamoate (11 mg/kg qd for 3 days) is recommended. Cutaneous larva migrans is usually self-limited, but topical application of 10 percent thiabendazole, ivermectin (150 to 200 μg orally), or albendazole (400 mg qd for 3 days) may hasten resolution.

- *Strongyloides stercoralis* (threadworm) is found in southern Appalachia, Kentucky, and Tennessee. Like the hookworm, it penetrates the skin, producing pruritus and cutaneous larva migrans.

○ Thiabendazole (50 mg/kg/day divided bid, maximum 3 g/day) for 2 days is recommended. An alternative drug is ivermectin, 200 μg qd for 1 to 2 days. In disseminated strongyloidiasis, treatment may need to continue for up to 2 weeks.

TREMATODES (FLUKES)

- Flukes are oval, flat worms with a ventral sucker for nutrition and attachment. Eggs are shed in the stool of definitive hosts, hatch into miracidia, and enter an intermediate host, such as a snail or other crustacean, fish, or bird. They develop into cercariae, which leave the intermediate host to become free living prior to infesting the definitive host on contact with contaminated water.

- *Fasciolopsis buski* infests the gut; *Fasciola hepatica, Opisthorchis sinensis*, and *Schistosoma mansoni* the liver; *Schistosoma haematobium* the bladder; and *Paragonimus westermani* the lung.

- Praziquantel (40 mg/kg/day divided into 2 doses for 1 or 2 days) is recommended for *S. haematobium, S. mansoni*, and *S. intercalatum*. A higher dose, 60 mg/kg/day divided into 3 doses for 1 day, is recommended for *S. japonica* and *S. mekongi*.

- Of particular interest in pediatric emergency medicine is the avian schistosome, *Trichobilharzia ocellata*. Spread by migratory birds to the freshwater lakes of the northern United States, the cercariae cause dermatitis, known as swimmer's itch. The intense reaction produced by host defenses is treated with heat and antipruritics. Severe cases are treated with thiabendazole cream.

CESTODES (FLATWORMS AND TAPEWORMS)

- Cestodes attach to the gut of the definitive host with hooks or suckers at the head (scolex), from which grow segmented proglottids. Each proglottid is equipped to produce large volumes of eggs. These eggs, along with terminal proglottids, pass in the stool and are ingested by the intermediate host.

- *Taenia solium* (pork tapeworm) and *Taenia saginatum* (beef tapeworm) infestations are generally asymptomatic and are diagnosed when a parent brings a proglottid to the emergency department for identification.

- *Diphyllobothrium latum* (fish tapeworm) is becoming more prevalent with the increased popularity of raw fish. Because *D. latum* absorbs 50 times more vitamin B_{12} than *Taenia*, it causes pernicious anemia.

- *Echinococcus granulosus* (sheep tapeworm) is found in agricultural countries. Most reported cases are from the southeastern United States. Symptomatology is secondary to hydatid cyst formation with mass effect.

- Most tapeworms are treated with praziquantel (5 to 25 mg/kg once). *Echinococcus* infection and cysticercosis respond best to albendazole (15 mg/kg/day divided tid for 28 days).

PROTOZOA

- *Entamoeba histolytica* is a water-borne, single-cell organism. It is found in epidemic proportion after heavy rain in areas of suboptimal sanitation and among closely confined populations. In addition to ingestion of contaminated water, it can be spread by direct human contact, both sexually and in breast milk.
  - Most patients carry amebas asymptomatically in the cecum and large intestine. Heavy infestations of *E. histolytica* produce a colitis-like picture (gay bowel). These patients may present with nausea, vomiting, bloating, pain, bloody diarrhea, and leukocytosis without eosinophilia.
  - Metronidazole (35 to 50 mg/kg/day divided tid for 10 days) followed by iodoquinol (40 mg/kg/day divided tid for 20 days) is recommended to eradicate infestation.
- *Dientamoeba fragilis* is a flagellate that lives in the cecum and proximal large bowel. It has worldwide distribution. It is generally not invasive, does not form cysts, and closely resembles *Trichomonas*, except for the lack of a flagellum.
  - It may be found in children in day care, causing mucosal irritative symptoms of abdominal pain, decreased appetite, diarrhea, and eosinophilia. It is diagnosed when trophozoites are found in the stool, after the use of permanent stains.
  - The treatment is iodoquinol (40 mg/kg/day divided tid for 20 days).
- *Giardia lamblia* is a flagellate that thrives in the relatively alkaline pH of the duodenum and proximal small bowel. Infestation occurs after ingestion of contaminated water or other fecal-oral behavior. It is commonly found in day care centers; among travelers, immunocompromised children, and patients with cystic fibrosis; and in association with hepatic or pancreatic disease.
  - Flatulence, nonbloody diarrhea or constipation, abdominal distension, and pain are common symptoms. Fever, weight loss, and fat, carbohydrate, and vitamin malabsorption can occur.
  - Metronidazole (15 mg/kg/day divided tid for 5 days) is recommended.

- Over the past 10 years, the number of cases of malaria reported by the Centers for Disease Control and Prevention has remained stable at about 1000 a year, with one-fourth occurring in children. Two-thirds of cases are imported from subSaharan Africa.
  - With a high index of suspicion, one looks for the parasite on thick and thin blood smears. *Plasmodium falciparum* is characterized by a predominance of ring forms within the red blood cells, banana-shaped gametocytes, and the absence of mature trophozoites and schizonts. *Plasmodium malariae, Plasmodium vivax,* and *Plasmodium ovale* have round gametocytes with mature trophozoites and schizonts on smear.
  - To prevent infestation in travelers, prophylaxis is recommended beginning 1 week before departure and continuing for 4 to 6 weeks after return. Resistance of *P. falciparum* and *P. vivax* to chloroquine is now spreading. If a person is traveling to a sensitive area, chloroquine (5 mg/kg of base, maximum 300 mg) given once a week, is recommended.
  - Once someone is infected, chloroquine (10 mg/kg of base, maximum 600 mg, followed by 5 mg/kg of base, maximum 300 mg at 6, 25, and 48 h) or quinine sulfate (25 mg/kg/day divided tid for 3 to 7 days) and pyrimethamine sulfadoxine (number of tablets based on age) given on the last day of quinine are recommended. As *P. vivax* and *P. ovale* infestations tend to recur, they should, when identified, also be treated with primaquine phosphate (0.3 mg/kg/day for 14 days).
- *Babesia microti* has an erythrocytic phase similar to that of malaria. It is transmitted by the deer tick *Ixodes dammini* from a rodent reservoir and is, therefore, found in the same geographic distribution as Lyme disease (northeastern states, Wisconsin, and Minnesota).
  - Treatment is with clindamycin (20 to 40 mg/kg/day divided tid) and quinine (25 mg/kg/day divided tid) for 7 days. Alternatively, a 7-day regimen of atovaquone (750 mg q 12 h) and azithromycin (500 mg on day 1 and 250 mg thereafter) has been shown to be effective and to have fewer adverse reactions.
- *Pneumocystis carinii* has a low virulence and is found in the latent phase in a large percentage of the American population. When the host is immunocompromised, trophozoites replicate in alveolar spaces and spread through the vascular and lymphatic beds. It is found in more than 60 percent of patients with HIV infection.
  - Treatment is with trimethoprim (15 to 20 mg/kg/day) and sulfamethoxazole (75 to 100 mg/kg/day) in 3 or 4 divided doses orally or pentamidine (3 to 4 mg/kg/day) intravenously for 2 to 3 weeks.

- *Cryptosporidium, Isospora belli,* and *Toxoplasma gondii* belong to the protozoan subclass *Coccidia,* which also includes *Plasmodium.* Modes of transmission include direct human contact and ingestion of fecally contaminated food and water. *Toxoplasma* is also transmitted transplacentally, with blood transfusion and organ transplantation. Intermediate hosts include farm animals (*Cryptosporidium*), cats (*Toxoplasma*), and other mammals.
  - Although some children harbor *Cryptosporidium* and *Isospora* asymptomatically, both organisms can cause a secretory, cholera-like diarrhea after a 2-week incubation. Large volumes of watery, non-bloody, leukocyte-free stool may produce significant dehydration.
  - The trophozoites of *Toxoplasma gondii* have a predilection for the brain, heart, and bone, although they can invade any nucleated cell. Approximately 2500 infants are born annually in the United States with congenital disease, 10 percent of which have the *Toxoplasma* triad of hydrocephalus, chorioretinitis, and intracranial calcifications. The long-term prognosis is poor.
  - Acquired toxoplasmosis in the immune-competent host is asymptomatic but may produce a subclinical reaction in the reticuloendothelial system. For patients with AIDS and other types of immunocompromise, reactivation produces severe central nervous system involvement and dissemination to the heart and lungs.
  - Prompt treatment with pyrimethamine (2 mg/kg/day for 3 days and then 1 mg/kg/day for 4 weeks) and sulfadiazine (100 to 200 mg/kg/day for 4 weeks) is recommended. However, there is a high fatality rate once *Toxoplasma* becomes reactivated.
- The parasites *Pediculus humanus capitus* (head louse), *Pediculus humanus corporis* (body louse), and *Phthirus pubis* (pubic or crab louse) attach eggs (nits) firmly to hair shafts, close to the skin. Lice are transmitted by direct human contact or the sharing of clothing or other personal articles.
  - A 10-min rinse with 1-percent permethrin (Nix) has been reported to kill adult lice and 90 percent of nits. It may, however, exacerbate the pruritus and erythema. It is too toxic to use near the eyes, where petrolatum is recommended to suffocate the lice.
  - Resistance to permethrin is now common, with reported insecticidal activity down 28 percent in one study. The combination of 1-percent permethrin with trimethoprim/sulfamethoxazole has recently been reported to be 95 percent effective, compared to 80 percent for permethrin alone.
- *Sarcoptes scabiei* (scabies) are transmitted by direct close and prolonged human contact. Following a 3- to 6-week incubation, the scabies mite burrows between the fingers and toes as well as in the groin, external genitalia, and axillae, depositing eggs in the tunnel as she goes.
  - The itch is worse at night, with infants sleeping poorly and rubbing their hands and feet together. Small red, raised papules are formed, which may progress to vesicles and pustules.
  - A single application of 5-percent permethrin cream is curative for children over 2 months. Younger children may be treated with sulfur precipitated in petrolatum. The long incubation period makes treating the entire family advisable.

BIBLIOGRAPHY

Beigel Y, Greenburg Z, Ostfeld I: Clinical problem-solving: Letting the patient off the hook. *N Engl J Med* 342:1658, 2000.

Georgiev VS: Chemotherapy of enterobiasis. *Expert Opin Pharmacother* 2: 267, 2001.

Georgiev VS: Necatoriasis: Treatment and developmental therapeutics. *Expert Opin Pharmacother* 9:1065, 2000.

Georgiev VS: Pharmacotherapy of ascariasis. *Expert Opin Pharmacother* 2:223, 2001.

Hipolito RB, Mallorca FG, Zuniga-Macaraig ZO, et al: Head lice infestation: Single drug versus combination therapy with one percent permethrin and trimethoprim/sulfamethoxazole. *Pediatrics* 107:E30, 2001.

Krause PI, Lepore T, Sikand VK, et al: Atovaquone and azithromycin for the treatment of babesiosis. *N Engl J Med* 343:1454, 2000.

QUESTIONS

1. A 6 year-old boy presents with a complaint of a pruritic rash for 1 week that is worse at night. The rash is noted between the fingers and toes, groin, and axillae. The rash has small, red raised papules with a few scattered vesicles. Several family members also have a similar rash. The most appropriate management is:
   A. Oatmeal baths, calamine lotion, and diphenhydramine
   B. Draw a CBC, blood cultures, and start broad spectrum antibiotics
   C. Apply cellophane tape in the perianal area for definitive diagnosis
   D. Mebendazole for 10 days
   E. A single dose of 5-percent permethrin cream and treatment of entire family

2. Which of the following is a true statement regarding *Ascaris lumbricoides*?
   A. It is most commonly found in cold climates.
   B. It is most commonly found in infants.
   C. Albendazole or pyrantyl pamoate in a single dose is curative.
   D. It is a rare, worldwide parasitic infestation.
   E. Infestation is caused by larvae burrowing through the skin entering the blood and migrating to the intestines.

3. The "Scotch-tape test" may be used to test for which type of parasitic infestation?
   A. *Enterobius vermicullaris* (pinworm)
   B. *Necatur americanus* (hookworm)
   C. *Trichuris trichiura* (whipworm)
   D. *Entamoeba histolytica*
   E. *Ascaris lumbricoides*

4. Which of the following parasitic infestations are associated with cutaneous larva migrans causing pruritus and a rash?
   A. *Enterobius vermicullaris* (pinworm)
   B. *Necatur americanus* (hookworm)
   C. *Trichuris trichiura* (whipworm)
   D. *Loa loa* (African eye worm)
   E. *Schistosoma haematobium* (blood flukes)

5. A 10 year-old boy from Mexico presents with a new-onset seizure. He had no prodromal symptoms and was in excellent healthy prior to this. He denied any trauma or injury. What is the most likely etiology of the seizure?
   A. Idiopathic
   B. Cerebral edema
   C. *Taenia solium* (pork tapeworm)
   D. *Toxoplasm gondii*
   E. Child abuse

6. Which of the following is true regarding *Toxoplasma gondii* infestations?
   A. Domesticated dogs are reservoirs for infection.
   B. The congenital *Toxoplasma* triad includes hydrocephalus, chorioretinitis, and intracranial calcifications.
   C. They are transmitted by an arthropod vector.
   D. Immune-competent hosts will develop CNS infections.
   E. No known treatment is available.

ANSWERS

1. E. This child has scabies (*Sarcoptes scabiei*), which is transmitted by direct close and prolonged human contact. The distribution is typically between the fingers and toes, groin, external genitalia, and axillae, where the mite burrows and deposits eggs. Treatment is a single application of 5-percent permethrin cream. It is advisable to treat the entire family because of the long incubation period.

2. C. *Ascaris* is the largest and most prevalent human nematode with an estimated 1 billion cases worldwide. It is typically found in tropical and subtropical climates. It is most common in preschool and early school age children. Albendazole and pyrantyl pamoate in a single dose is considered curative. Infestation is caused by egg ingestion and worms reside in the small bowel.

3. A. The "Scotch-tape test" can be used to collect and observe the eggs of *Enterobius vermicullaris* by microscopy. The tape is placed sticky side to perianal skin when the child first awakens. The adult worms are small, and reside in the rectum. They will lay eggs around the rectum causing intense pruritus.

4. B. Cutaneous larva migrans is acquired when hookworm larvae penetrate the skin and cause pruritus and a rash and is usually self-limited. Application of 10% thiabendazole, ivermectin or albendazole may hasten resolution.

5. C. *Taenia solium* is associated with cysticercosis and is often responsible for new-onset seizures in Mexican immigrants or travelers to Mexico.

6. B. *Toxoplasm gondii* is a protozoan infestation, with the domestic cat being the reservoir for infection. The parasite can be transmitted transplacentally if the mother has never been exposed. The *Toxoplasma* triad is hydrocephalus, chorioretinitis, and intracranial calcifications. The long-term prognosis is poor. Acquired infection in immune-competent hosts is typically asymptomatic. The treatment is pyrimethamine and sulfadiazine.

51 GASTROENTERITIS

Elizabeth C. Powell
Sally L. Reynolds
William R. Ahrens
Heather M. Prendergast

INTRODUCTION

- In the United States, most children less than 5 years old have gastroenteritis two or three times per year, while children attending day care have approximately five illnesses per year.
- Although bacteria and parasites are sometimes isolated, viruses cause 80 percent of gastroenteritis in children in the United States.

ETIOLOGY

VIRUSES

- Rotavirus, the single most commonly identified cause of severe diarrhea in young children, accounts for 30 to 50 percent of cases. The peak age of incidence is between 3 and 15 months. Illness usually begins with fever and vomiting, followed by watery, nonbloody diarrhea. Symptoms last 5 to 7 days.
- Enteric adenovirus (serotypes 31, 40, and 41), the second most frequently identified cause of viral diarrhea in children, is responsible for 5 to 10 percent of gastroenteritis cases requiring hospital admission. Ill children have fever and watery diarrhea.
- The Norwalk virus causes epidemic gastroenteritis in older children during winter months. Illness is short, usually lasting less than 3 days. Fever and myalgia often accompany the gastrointestinal symptoms.

BACTERIA

- The usual organisms that cause bacterial gastroenteritis in U.S. children are:
  - *Campylobacter jejuni*
  - *Salmonella* spp.
  - *Shigella* spp.
  - *Yersinia enterocolitica*
  - *Clostridium difficile*
  - *Aeromonas*
- *Escherichia coli* (enterotoxigenic, enteropathogenic, and enteroinvasive), the pathogen responsible for most bacterial diarrhea worldwide, is an uncommon cause of diarrhea in the United States.
- In young children, *Salmonella* and *Shigella* infections are associated with specific complications.
- Salmonella gastroenteritis is associated with a 5 to 10 percent incidence of bacteremia in infants less than 1 year of age. Young infants and children who are immunocompromised or who have sickle cell disease are at risk for complications, which include pneumonia, meningitis, and osteomyelitis.
- *Shigella* gastroenteritis is associated with seizures in some affected children. Seizure activity may precede the diarrhea.
- *Yersinia* gastroenteritis can cause mesenteric adenitis or terminal ileitis, with symptoms that mimic appendicitis.

PARASITES

- *Giardia* is an identified pathogen in children attending day care. It is responsible for both acute and chronic diarrhea. It has a high rate of asymptomatic infection, and in untreated children, cysts can be shed for months.

• *Cryptosporidium* is spread from person to person. Transmission is aided by asymptomatic carriers and the organism's resistance to chlorine.

PATHOPHYSIOLOGY

• The symptoms and stool characteristics of viral, bacterial, and parasitic diarrhea are similar. Viral-induced diarrhea is noninflammatory.
• Bacterial infection is either noninflammatory, inflammatory, or penetrating (Table 51-1). In the United States, bacterial diarrhea is usually inflammatory. Bacteria infect the bowel wall, usually the colon.
• Noninflammatory bacterial diarrhea involves the small bowel. Stools are watery because infection alters fluid absorption at the villus tip (enteropathogenic *E. coli*) or because of endotoxin production (enterotoxigenic *E. coli*).
• Parasitic diarrhea is noninflammatory.

Table 51-1 Pathophysiology and Etiology of Diarrhea

NONINFLAMMATORY (WATERY)	INFLAMMATORY	PENETRATING
Vibrio cholera	*Shigella*	*Salmonella*
Escherichia coli (enterotoxigenic)	*Salmonella*	*typhi*
	Campylobacter	*Yersinia*
Staphylococcal food poisoning	*jejuni*	*Campylobacter*
Clostridium perfringens food poisoning	*Clostridium difficile*	*fetus*
	E. coli (invasive)	
Rotavirus		
Enteric adenovirus		
Norwalk-like virus		
Giardia		
Cryptosporidium		

HISTORY AND PHYSICAL EXAMINATION

• The history is focused on the quantity of stools and the presence of blood or mucus in the fecal matter. Approximately 10 percent of children have blood in their stools.
• Useful past history includes prior gastrointestinal surgery or inflammatory bowel disease, and other chronic illness or immunodeficiency. Information about current antibiotic use, as well as day care or school exposure, foreign travel, and diet, is helpful.
• Physical examination focuses on assessing hydration status (Table 51-2) and excluding a surgical abdomen.

DIAGNOSTIC EVALUATION

• Most children with uncomplicated gastroenteritis need no laboratory studies. Stool cultures are useful in febrile children with blood in their stools, during community outbreaks, and for those children who are immunosuppressed.
• The rotazyme assay, used to detect rotavirus, is helpful to cohort and avoid cross-contamination among inpatients. It is rarely indicated in managing outpatients.
• The electrolytes in children with diarrhea and dehydration frequently show abnormal bicarbonate levels (10 to 18 mEq/L).
• Infants less than 3 months old with *Salmonella* enteritis are more likely to have bacteremia when the leukocyte count is greater than $15,000/mm^3$.
• *Shigella* is associated with normal total leukocyte count, but an increased number of band forms.

TABLE 51-2 Clinical Assessment of Severity of Dehydration

SIGNS AND SYMPTOMS	MILD DEHYDRATION	MODERATE DEHYDRATION	SEVERE DEHYDRATION
General appearance and condition:			
Infants and young children	Thirsty, alert, restless	Thirsty, restless, lethargic, but irritable or drowsy	Drowsy, limp, cold, sweaty, cyanotic extremities, may be comatose
Older children and adults	Thirsty, alert, restless	Thirsty, alert, postural hypotension	Cold, sweaty, muscle cramps, cyanotic extremities, conscious
Radial pulse	Normal rate and strength	Rapid and weak	Rapid, sometimes impalpable
Respiration	Normal	Deep, ± rapid	Deep and rapid
Anterior fontanel	Normal	Sunken	Very sunken
Systolic BP	Normal	Normal or low	<90 mm Hg; may be unrecordable
Skin elasticity	Pinch retracts immediately	Pinch retracts slowly	Pinch retracts slowly (>2 s)
Eyes	Normal	Sunken	Sunken
Tears	Present	Absent	Absent
Mucous membranes	Moist	Dry	Very dry
Urine flow	Normal	Reduced amount, dark	None for several hours
Body weight loss (%)	3–5	6–9	10 or more
Estimated fluid deficit (mL/kg)	30–50	60–90	100 or more

Campylobacter and *Yersinia* infections are associated with leukocyte counts in the normal range.

TREATMENT

ORAL THERAPY

- Children estimated to be less than 5 percent dehydrated can usually be managed with oral solutions.
- Oral rehydration therapy, particularly in infants, should be done with a solution that contains an appropriate carbohydrate to sodium ratio. Fruit juices and decarbonated soda beverages often contain high-carbohydrate and low-sodium concentrations. Apple and white grape juice also contain sorbitol, which can exacerbate diarrhea.
- Oral solutions are also available commercially in flavored and frozen forms (ice pops); their use may improve compliance in toddlers. Breastfed infants should be nursed through the course of their illness, as breast milk is very well tolerated.
- Children who are not dehydrated should be fed an age-appropriate diet throughout their illness. Foods best tolerated are those that are easily digested and include bananas, applesauce, and other fruits and vegetables; yogurt; lean meats; and complex carbohydrates, such as cereal, rice, noodles, potatoes, or bread.
- Infants may be given formula after dehydration is corrected. Although some clinicians recommend initial refeeding with a lactose-free formula, current data do not show these formulas to be superior to milk-based formulas.

IV THERAPY

- Infants and children who are significantly dehydrated or who cannot tolerate oral therapy are candidates for intravenous treatment. The management is discussed in the section on fluid and electrolyte abnormalities.
- Toddlers and older children with mild to moderate dehydration, mild acidosis, and normal sodium values may be discharged from the emergency department after IV rehydration and oral intake.
- Patients with difficult IV access can be rehydrated by nasogastric tube with commercial rehydrating solutions; this is as effective as intravenous therapy.
- Antidiarrheal agents and antiemetics are not recommended in the treatment of infectious gastroenteritis.
- Data suggest that bismuth subsalicylate (Pepto-Bismol) may be of modest benefit in reducing the duration of diarrhea. Because of its cost and need for frequent administration, further confirmation of its practical efficacy is warranted.
- Although phenothiazines reduce emesis, extrapyramidal reactions limit their usefulness in children.
- *Salmonella* gastroenteritis is treated with antibiotics in infants younger than 3 months, in children with malignancy or who are recipients of immunosuppressive therapy, and in children with sickle cell disease. They are also indicated for severe colitis, focal infection (osteomyelitis and pneumonia) and bacteremia (Table 51-3). Recommended antibiotics are ampicillin and chloramphenicol. Trimethoprim-sulfamethoxazole is an alternate therapy.
- Uncomplicated *Salmonella* gastroenteritis in children and in healthy infants over 3 months of age does not require antibiotics, as they do not shorten the duration

TABLE 51-3   Antibiotics for Diarrhea

ORGANISM	ANTIBIOTIC	RECOMMENDATIONS
Salmonella	Ampicillin Amoxicillin Trimethoprim-sulfamethoxazole Cefotaxime Ceftriaxone Chloramphenicol Fluoroquinolones	Treatment of specific, high-risk patients Focal infections Prolonged carrier state
Shigella	Trimethoprim-sulfamethoxazole Ampicillin Ceftriaxone—for resistant strains	Treatment recommended for all cases
Campylobacter	Erythromycin Azithromycin	Treatment shortens illness and prevents relapse
Giardia	Metronidazole Furazolidone or albendazole—when suspension needed	Treatment recommended for symptomatic infections

of illness and may prolong the carrier state, during which organisms are excreted.

- In *Shigella* gastroenteritis, antibiotics shorten the course of illness and eliminate the organism from the stool, thus preventing spread, and are therefore recommended for susceptible strains. Ampicillin or trimethoprim-sulfamethoxazole is effective. Amoxicillin is less effective. If the susceptibility pattern is not known or if a resistant strain is isolated, parenteral ceftriaxone or a fluoroquinolone should be given.

- *Campylobacter* enteritis usually will resolve spontaneously without antibiotics. However, when given early during the infection, erythromycin and azithromycin shorten the duration of illness and prevent relapse. In some areas, erythromycin is not effective because of resistant organisms. Treatment is, then, based on sensitivity testing.

- Symptomatic infection with *Giardia* should be treated with metronidazole. In children who cannot swallow pills, furazolidone, which is available in a liquid suspension of 50 mg/15 mL, is an acceptable alternative.

- Albendazole is also an effective treatment of *Giardia* in children; it can be formulated into a suspension and given to children more than 2 years old. The dose is 400 mg by mouth each day for 5 days.

- *Escherichia coli* O157:H7 causes sporadic and epidemic gastrointestinal infections. In an estimated 15 percent of infected U.S. children, the hemolytic-uremic syndrome develops after the diarrhea. Data suggest that antibiotic treatment of children with *E. coli* O157:H7 infection increases the risk of the hemolytic-uremic syndrome.

BIBLIOGRAPHY

American Academy of Pediatrics, Subcommittee on Acute Gastroenteritis: Practice parameter: The management of acute gastroenteritis in young children. *Pediatrics* 97:424, 1996.

Cicirello HG, Glass RI: Current concepts of the epidemiology of diarrheal diseases. *Semin Pediatr Infect Dis* 5:163, 1994.

Duggan C, Nurko S: "Feeding the gut": The scientific basis for continued enteral nutrition during acute diarrhea. *J Pediatr* 131:801, 1997.

Figueroa-Quintanilla D, Salazar-Lindo E, Eyzaguirre-Maccan E, et al: A watery diarrheal disease. *N Engl J Med* 328:1653, 1993.

Nagar AL, Wang VJ: Comparison of nasogastric and intravenous methods of rehydration in pediatric patients with acute dehydration. *Pediatrics* 109:566, 2002.

Garcia Pena BM, Mandl KD, Kraus SJ, et al: Ultrasonography and limited computed tomography in the diagnosis and management of appendicitis in children. *JAMA* 282:1041, 1999.

Kapikian AZ: Viral gastroenteritis. *JAMA* 269:627, 1993.

Pickering LK (ed): *American Academy of Pediatrics Report of the Committee on Infectious Diseases*, 25th ed. 198, 253, 502–503, 511, 2000.

Wong CS, Jelacic S, Tarr PI, et al: The risk of the hemolytic uremic syndrome after antibiotic treatment of *Escherichia coli* O157:H7 infections. *N Engl J Med* 342:1930, 2000.

QUESTIONS

1. Parents bring a 12-month-old for evaluation of fevers, vomiting, and diarrhea. Symptoms have been present for 4 days. The infant recently began attending day care. To the parents' knowledge, there have been no similar symptoms or sick contacts within the day care. Parents describe the stools as watery and nonbloody. On examination, you find a nontoxic and well-hydrated infant. Which of the following is the **MOST** likely etiology of gastroenteritis in this infant?
   A. *Campylobacter jejuni*
   B. Rotavirus
   C. Norwalk virus
   D. Enteric adenovirus
   E. *Salmonella* spp.

2. An 8-year-old child is brought for evaluation of fevers, vomiting, and diarrhea. You learn that several of the child's classmates have similar symptoms. Parents are concerned about the "flu" because of the child's complaints about body aches. Which of the following is the **MOST** likely etiology of gastroenteritis in this child?
   A. *Campylobacter jejuni*
   B. Rotavirus
   C. Enteric adenovirus
   D. Norwalk virus
   E. *Salmonella* spp.

3. A 6-year-old child with a history of sickle cell disease is brought to the emergency department for evaluation of low-grade fevers, vomiting, and diarrhea. The parents state the last sickle cell crisis was 5 months ago. On examination, the child is nontoxic appearing but mildly dehydrated. The abdominal examination is benign. In addition to hydration, which of the following would be the **MOST** appropriate management and disposition for this patient?
   A. Perform a stat rotazyme assay, if negative then discharge to home
   B. Obtain electrolytes, if normal bicarbonate levels then discharge to home
   C. Oral rehydration therapy, if successful then discharge to home
   D. Begin antibiotics, obtain cultures and admit for observation
   E. Obtain cultures and admit for observation

4. Treatment of *Giardia* would **NOT** include which of the following?
   A. Metronidazole
   B. Chloramphenicol
   C. Albendazole
   D. Furazolidone
   E. Stool cultures

5. In which of the following conditions would stool culture **NOT** be mandatory?
   A. 8-month-old infant with suspected *Salmonella* gastroenteritis
   B. Febrile child with bloody diarrhea
   C. Community outbreaks
   D. 12-Month-old child with suspected rotavirus
   E. Immunosuppressed child

ANSWERS

1. **B.** Rotavirus is the single most commonly identified cause of severe diarrhea in young children. The peak age of incidence is between 3 months and 15 months. Illness usually begins with fever and vomiting, followed by watery, nonbloody diarrhea. Symptoms typically last 5 to 7 days.

2. **D.** The Norwalk virus causes epidemic gastroenteritis in older children during the winter months. Typically, the duration of symptoms is short lasting less than 3 days. Fever and myalgia often accompany the gastrointestinal symptoms.

3. **D.** Patients with sickle cell disease are more susceptible to *Salmonella* infections and are at increased risk for complications. *Salmonella* gastroenteritis should be treated with antibiotics in infants younger than 3 months, immunosuppressed children, and children with sickle cell disease. Recommended antibiotics are ampicillin and chloramphenicol.

4. **B.** Treatment for *Giardia* includes the following: metronidazole, albendazole, and furazolidone. Chloramphenicol is not useful for parasitic infections.

5. **D.** Most children with uncomplicated gastroenteritis do not need laboratory studies. Stool cultures are useful in febrile children with blood in their stools, during community outbreaks, and those children who are immunosuppressed.

52 NONSURGICAL GASTROINTESTINAL PROBLEMS

Tulika Singh
William R. Ahrens
Heather M. Prendergast

ABDOMINAL PAIN

- Abdominal pain is classified as either visceral or somatic.
  - **Visceral pain** is a result from distension of a hollow viscus or from an ischemic process. It can be severe and of sudden onset, with a colicky nature, and is often poorly localized.
  - **Somatic pain** arises from myelinated nerve fibers from the parietal peritoneum. It is often of gradual onset, and more sharply localized than visceral pain.
- Abdominal pain can also be referred to areas of the body that share innervation through the same afferent neural segments.
- Nonsurgical causes of abdominal pain are listed in Table 52-1.

TABLE 52-1   Nonsurgical Causes of Abdominal Pain

Age under 2 years
Gastroenteritis
Colic
Constipation
Lead poisoning
Ages 2 to 12 years
Psychosocial
Enterocolitis
Otitis media
Constipation
Child abuse
Sickle cell disease
Irritable bowel disease
Chronic recurrent abdominal pain
Urinary tract infection
Henoch–Schönlein purpura
Diabetic ketoacidosis
Mesenteric adenitis
Lead intoxication
Streptococcal pharyngitis
Age over 12 years
Idiopathic
Constipation
Chronic recurrent abdominal pain
Pregnancy
Urinary tract infection
Diabetic ketoacidosis
Pelvic inflammatory disease
Sickle cell disease
Streptococcal pharyngitis
Mesenteric adenitis
Psychosocial

HISTORY

- Persistent, nonremitting pain of less than several hours' duration indicates a high likelihood of a surgical etiology, as does pain that is localized to a specific area. Pain that wakes patients from sleep almost always indicates organic pathology, which can be surgical or medical.
- Crampy or colicky pain usually results from the distension of a viscus. It is most commonly due to gastroenteritis, but can also be seen in surgical emergencies, such as a bowel obstruction. Sharp, localized pain often indicates peritoneal inflammation.
- Patients with recurrent or chronic abdominal pain are particularly problematic. They are questioned regarding associated weight loss, fatigue, arthralgias, melena, or hemochezia, all of which indicate an inflammatory process.

PHYSICAL FINDINGS

- The examination begins with an assessment of the child's general appearance. Patients with peritoneal inflammation tend to lie still, whereas children with obstruction may be restless or writhe in pain.
- The examination of the abdomen includes assessment of bowel sounds, tenderness, guarding, rebound, and distension.
- If there is a history of gastrointestinal bleeding or a surgical emergency is suspected, a rectal examination is indicated and the stool is checked for occult blood.
- All pediatric patients with abdominal pain require a genital examination to rule out an incarcerated inguinal hernia as the etiology of the pain.

DIAGNOSTIC TESTING

- Ancillary laboratory tests are generally most helpful in supporting the clinical impression derived from the history and physical examination.
- An elevated leukocyte count indicates an inflammatory or infectious process. A urinalysis is helpful in excluding a urinary tract infection. If hepatitis or pancreatitis is suspected, liver function tests and pancreatic enzymes may be helpful.
- For patients with diarrhea accompanying abdominal pain, a microscopic stool examination revealing red or white blood cells indicates an inflammatory process, usually secondary to infectious enteritis.
- Abdominal radiographs can be helpful in cases of suspected bowel obstruction. Other diagnostic modalities are discussed as they apply to specific diseases.

VOMITING

- Vomiting most commonly results from a self-limited infectious illness, however, it may be secondary to serious systemic, metabolic, or central nervous system disorders.

HISTORY

- The presence of bile in the emesis is never "normal" and always suggests the possibility of an obstructive lesion, especially in infants, where it may signify a malrotation.
- The appearance of blood in the emesis can indicate a gastrointestinal hemorrhage, although true blood must always be distinguished from substances with which it is easily confused.
- Associated abdominal pain is especially worrisome if it is present in between episodes of vomiting.
- The association of headache with vomiting always raises the index of suspicion for intracranial pathology.

PHYSICAL FINDINGS

- Lethargy, papilledema, and, in infants, splitting of the sutures or a full anterior fontanel, indicate increased intracranial pressure.
- The abdomen is assessed for the presence of distension, the character of the bowel sounds is evaluated, and the presence of tenderness, guarding, or rebound is noted.
- If a surgical abdomen is considered, a rectal examination is indicated.

DIAGNOSTIC TESTING

- The history and physical examination direct the laboratory evaluation of individual patients. In cases where a self-limited infectious process is likely and patients do not appear dehydrated, no laboratory studies are necessary.
- The urine-specific gravity is useful as an indication of the status of the patient's hydration.
- For patients who appear dehydrated, serum electrolytes, creatinine, and blood urea nitrogen are indicated. For patients with suspected liver disease, a hepatic profile is helpful.
- Abdominal radiographs are only indicated in cases where bowel obstruction is suspected.

DIARRHEA

- The majority of patients with diarrhea are suffering from mild, self-limited infectious illness. However, diarrheal diseases remain a major cause of morbidity and mortality throughout the world.

HISTORY

- Diarrhea is characterized by an increase in the frequency and a decrease in the consistency of patients' stools.
- The presence of blood usually indicates an infectious etiology, which in children is often due to bacterial enteritis. However, life-threatening events can also cause bloody diarrhea. These include intussusception and the hemolytic uremic syndrome. For patients previously treated with antibiotics, pseudomembranous colitis is a consideration.
- True formula allergy can cause bloody diarrhea, but is not life-threatening.

PHYSICAL FINDINGS

- The physical examination of patients with diarrhea focuses on determining the etiology of the problem and assessing the hydration status of the patient.
- The presence of fever implies an infectious etiology.
- In the presence of bloody diarrhea, an abdominal mass indicates a high probability of an intussusception.
- If there is any history of bloody diarrhea or the patient is less than 2 to 3 months old with fever and diarrhea, a rectal examination is indicated and the stool is examined for the presence of red and white blood cells.

DIAGNOSTIC TESTING

- For patients with mild, nonbloody diarrhea, who do not appear dehydrated, no laboratory work-up is indicated.
- In febrile patients with bloody diarrhea, a stool specimen is sent for bacterial culture and evaluation for ova and parasites. Neonates with stools positive for white blood cells also have stool cultures performed to rule out *Salmonella*.
- For patients with bloody diarrhea who are not febrile, a life-threatening process, such as intussusception or hemolytic uremic syndrome, is excluded. For patients who have been treated with antibiotics, stool is sent for assay for *Clostridium difficile* toxin.

CONSTIPATION

- Constipation is a decrease in the frequency of stooling, often associated with a change in the character of the stool. There are few life-threatening diagnostic possibilities in pediatric patients with constipation.

HISTORY

- A detailed history is important to differentiate true from perceived constipation. It is a deviation from established bowel habits in which stool frequency decreases or consistency changes that indicates constipation.
- Especially in neonates, it is important to establish the pattern of stooling from birth, since delayed passage of meconium in the first 24 to 48 h is associated with organic pathology, especially Hirschsprung's disease.
- Organic causes of constipation can be associated with failure to thrive. Difficulties in making the transition from diapers can result in psychogenic constipation. Soliciting a history of fecal incontinence or encopresis is important.
- Associated symptoms to elicit include lethargy, poor feeding, fever, and vomiting. It is axiomatic that these do not result from functional constipation.

PHYSICAL FINDINGS

- The physical examination of constipated patients focuses on differentiating systemic etiology from an obstruction of the gastrointestinal tract.
- Infants are evaluated for the stigmata of hypothyroidism or the cranial nerve palsies of infantile botulism, both of which can cause constipation.
- True constipation may cause mild abdominal fullness, but significant distension is abnormal. Constipation should never cause peritoneal findings.
- Presence of impacted stool in the rectal vault suggests true constipation. Absence of stool in the rectal vault suggests proximal pathology, especially Hirschsprung's disease.

DIAGNOSTIC TESTING

- If there is any abnormality noted on the physical examination or the history is suggestive of a surgical emergency, an abdominal radiograph is indicated to rule out a bowel obstruction or severe colonic dilatation.

MANAGEMENT

- The mainstay of treatment of constipation consists of dietary manipulation to increase fiber and bulk, decrease fat content, and increase total fluid intake. In neonates and young infants, additional feedings of water in between formula or breast-feeding may be all that is necessary to break the cycle.
- Stool softeners, such as docusate and senna, are generally considered safe for children and may be useful until bowel habits have been reregulated. Although not considered a routine treatment, a one-time insertion of a glycerin suppository may be helpful.
- Disimpaction with oral medication has been shown to be highly effective when high doses of mineral oil, polyethylene glycol electrolyte solutions, or both are used.
- Rectal disimpaction may be performed with phosphate soda enemas, saline enemas, or mineral oil enemas followed by a phosphate enema. The use of soap suds, tap water, and magnesium enemas are not recommended because of their potential toxicity.
- Phosphate enemas are not indicated in children less than 2 years of age or for patients with conditions predisposing them to alteration in absorption and excretion of phosphate, including Hirschsprung's disease, imperforate anus, chronic renal failure, or renal dysplasia.

GASTROINTESTINAL BLEEDING

- Life-threatening gastrointestinal bleeding in children is uncommon, reflecting the relative infrequency of cirrhosis of the liver and gastrointestinal malignancies in the pediatric age group. Upper gastrointestinal hemorrhages occur proximal to the ligament of Treitz. Lower gastrointestinal hemorrhages occur distal to the ligament of Treitz, most commonly in the colon.

PRESENTATION

- Hematemesis, or the vomiting of blood, is almost always a manifestation of an upper gastrointestinal hemorrhage. The blood may be bright red or have a coffee-ground appearance. Twenty to forty percent of patients with upper gastrointestinal bleeding do not have hematemesis.
- Melena refers to the passage of dark, sticky, sweet-smelling stools. Melena usually results from an upper gastrointestinal hemorrhage. Hemochezia is the passage of bright red blood from the rectum. This usually involves a hemorrhagic process in the lower gastrointestinal tract. Blood mixed with the stool usually indicates an infectious or inflammatory process.

UPPER GASTROINTESTINAL HEMORRHAGE

GASTRITIS

- **Gastritis** in pediatric patients is often associated with severe physiologic stress, such as trauma, burns, and sepsis. The use of aspirin can also cause gastritis. Abdominal pain is a common presenting complaint, and vomiting can occur. In severe cases, hematemesis or melena can develop. Life-threatening hemorrhage is uncommon.
- The primary treatment consists of antacids and H_2 blockers.

ULCER DISEASE

- **Peptic ulcer disease** in children has somewhat similar manifestations to that in adults. Up to 70 percent of children with ulcers have a family history of the disease.
- While infection with *Helicobacter pylori* is rare in children in the United States, it is often associated with gastritis and duodenal ulcers in affected pediatric patients.
- Noninvasive tests such as *H. pylori* antigen immunoassay in the stool and the C-urea breath test (UBT) are becoming more widely available. Serologic methods are unreliable in young children. Treatment includes 7 to 14 days of a twice-daily, triple-drug regimen with omeprazole, clarithromycin, and amoxicillin.
- Older children are likely to have abdominal pain, with or without associated vomiting, and nighttime wakening. Preschool children often suffer gastrointestinal bleeding, obstruction, or perforation. Of these, bleeding is the most common symptom.
- Stress ulcers are common in pediatric patients with serious illness, such as sepsis, or after major trauma or extensive burns.
- Patients with known chronic ulcer disease are managed with antacids and H_2-blocking agents.

ESOPHAGEAL AND GASTRIC VARICES

- **Esophageal** and **gastric varices** are associated portal vein hypertension.
- Biliary atresia is the most common cause of variceal bleeding in children. Other causes of cirrhosis are complications of umbilical vein catheterization, neonatal

hepatitis, congenital hepatic fibrosis, and cystic fibrosis.
- Two thirds of pediatric patients with portal hypertension hemorrhage before 5 years of age. Bleeding varices are the most common cause of life-threatening upper gastrointestinal hemorrhage in children.

NEWBORNS
- In newborns, vitamin K deficiency can result in gastrointestinal hemorrhage. However, this problem has been largely eliminated by the use of prophylactic vitamin K. Maternal blood may be swallowed and confused with gastrointestinal bleeding in newborns.

MANAGEMENT
- In all patients with upper gastrointestinal hemorrhage, it is essential that the hemodynamic status of patients is aggressively assessed and managed.
- Blood is sent for an urgent type and cross-match for packed red blood cells and, if liver disease is present, fresh frozen plasma.
- Laboratory studies include a complete blood cell count, electrolyte levels, and renal functions. A coagulation profile is indicated in all cases of significant hematemesis. Liver function tests are indicated if hepatic insufficiency is suspected.
- Placement of a nasogastric tube is indicated in all patients with a history of hematemesis or an examination that reveals melena. A negative nasogastric aspirate does not conclusively rule out hemorrhage, since up to 16 percent of patients with clear drainage have active bleeding. The known or suspected presence of varices is not a contraindication to the insertion of a nasogastric tube.
- If the nasogastric aspirate reveals active bleeding, gastric lavage is indicated. Free water appears to be as safe as normal saline, and fears about inducing water intoxication exaggerated. The temperature of the water does not appear to influence the outcome.
- Nasogastric lavage clears the stomach of blood, which, in the presence of liver failure, can lead to hyperammonemia and possibly aggravated hepatic encephalopathy.
- In persistent hemorrhage due to esophageal varices, vasopressin in a dose of 0.1 to 0.4 U/min may control the bleeding. Somostatin is a hypothalamic extract that decreases splenic flow and may be more effective than vasopressin in controlling variceal hemorrhage. Experience in children is limited.
- A significant number of patients with varices will be bleeding from concomitant gastritis or ulcers. When performed within 24 h of the onset of bleeding, endoscopy can identify the lesion 90 percent of the time.

LOWER GASTROINTESTINAL BLEEDING
- Currently, it is possible to identify the etiology in 90 percent of children with lower gastrointestinal hemorrhage. Malignancies and diverticulitis are extremely rare.

NECROTIZING ENTEROCOLITIS
- However, up to 10 percent of cases occur in full-term infants, usually within the first 10 days of life. Early symptoms include lethargy, poor feeding, temperature instability, and apnea. As the disease progresses, either heme-positive or grossly bloody stools are seen.
- Abdominal radiographs may reveal air in the bowel wall (**pneumatosis intestinalis**). Patients have nothing by mouth, and broad spectrum antibiotic coverage is initiated.

COAGULOPATHY
- Coagulopathy resulting in GI hemorrhage in newborns is almost always due to vitamin K deficiency, which is now rare. However, any newborns with significant gastrointestinal bleeding should receive supplemental vitamin K.

ANAL FISSURES
- **Anal fissures** are the most common cause of rectal bleeding in infancy, most often in patients less than 1 year of age. Patients usually have blood-streaked stools. Infants may also appear to have pain with bowel movements. The fissure is often visible on inspection of the anus. The treatment is usually with stool softeners and sitz baths.

FORMULA INTOLERANCE OR ALLERGY
- Formula intolerance can result from a true allergy to cow's milk protein. The presentation varies from chronic diarrhea and failure to thrive to grossly bloody stools indicative of severe colitis. Vomiting can also occur and can at times be bloody.
- Up to 20 to 30 percent of patients intolerant to cow's milk are also intolerant to soy-based formulas.
- Infants with formula-induced enterocolitis can have elevated white blood cell counts, and fecal leukocytes. Eosinophilia may be present in both peripheral blood as well as in stool smears.
- Symptoms resolve within 48 h after withdrawal of the formula and recur if the formula is reintroduced.
- Infants with milk- or soy-induced colitis are treated with an elemental formula, such as nutramagen or pregestimil.

INFECTIOUS COLITIS

- Infectious colitis is a common cause of lower gastrointestinal bleeding worldwide. Certain bacterial organisms are strongly linked to bloody diarrhea. There is a detailed discussion in the chapter on gastroenteritis.

LYMPHONODULAR HYPERPLASIA

- **Lymphonodular hyperplasia** is a benign disorder seen in infants and preschoolers. It can be associated with bright red rectal bleeding, which is rarely severe. Diagnosis is made by sigmoidoscopy or air-contrast radiography.
- There is no treatment, and the disorder usually resolves within 3 months of onset.

MECKEL'S DIVERTICULUM

- **Meckel's diverticulum** is the result of incomplete obliteration of the omphalomesenteric duct, usually located within 10 cm of the ileocecal valve. The condition can result in massive, painless rectal bleeding, obstruction, perforation, and peritonitis, or may remain totally silent.
- Rectal bleeding results from acid secreted by ectopic gastric tissue that causes ulceration and erosion of tissue.

Sixty percent of complications from Meckel's diverticulum, including hemorrhage and obstruction, occur in patients less than 2 years of age. The diverticulum is confirmed by performing a technetium-99m scan that identifies ectopic gastric tissue. When symptomatic, the diverticulum is removed surgically.

JUVENILE POLYPS

- **Juvenile polyps** account for 90 percent of all polyps found in children. They are found primarily in children less than 8 years old. They have no malignant potential. In some cases, rectal bleeding is severe.

COLIC

- **Colic** is an imprecise term used to describe a combination of symptoms that occur in infants between the ages of 1 and 4 months. Symptoms include episodes of excessive crying, fussiness after feeding, and paroxysms of irritability.
- In many cases, persistent crying is the only manifestation of colic. Infants appear well and are afebrile. It is important to exclude serious manifestations of inconsolable crying before making the diagnosis of colic.
- Twenty to 40 percent of infants with colic respond to a milk-exclusion diet.

- Sedatives and anticholinergic medications are not indicated.

SPECIFIC DISEASE ENTITIES

GASTROESOPHAGEAL REFLUX

- **Gastroesophageal reflux** (GER) refers to the regurgitation of stomach contents into the esophagus. Most infants and children have physiologic reflux with no clinical consequences. Distal esophagitis is by far the most common complication.
- Severe GER can result in failure to thrive, esophageal strictures, Barrett's esophagus, gastrointestinal bleeding, recurrent aspiration pneumonia, reactive airway disease, and iron deficiency anemia.
- Infants with refractory regurgitation or those with associated symptoms require more extensive evaluation. Studies include barium swallow, esophageal pH monitoring, endoscopy, and scintiscanning with a ^{99}Tc-sulfurcolloid –labeled meal.
- Parents are encouraged to "burp" babies frequently during feeding. Placing infants in the prone position at 45 to 60 degrees after feeding may help more severe regurgitation.
- Medical management includes agents such as ranitidine (Zantac), bethanechol, which increases gastric motility; and metoclopramide, which increases tone in the lower esophageal sphincter and relaxes pyloric sphincter tone.
- Patients who do not respond to medical management may require surgical intervention, most commonly a Nissan fundoplication, in which the body of the stomach is wrapped around and sutured in front of the esophagus.

GALLBLADDER DISEASE

- Certain disorders can predispose children to gallstones and cholecystitis. Hemolytic anemias, especially sickle cell disease and the thallasemias predispose patients to the formation of pigmented stones. Patients with cystic fibrosis also have a relatively high incidence of gallstones, as do patients with ileal Crohn's disease.
- Cholelithiasis in children has a similar presentation to that of adults. Intermittent, colicky right upper quadrant pain that may radiate to the scapula is characteristic.
- Ultrasonography will demonstrate stones and can define the anatomy of the gallbladder wall and the width of the common bile duct. For patients with

cholecystitis, antibiotic therapy and surgical consultation are indicated.

PANCREATITIS

- Pancreatitis is uncommon in children, especially before the age of 10 years
- Blunt abdominal trauma is a frequent cause of pancreatitis in children. Viral illnesses, especially mumps, can cause pancreatitis, as can a multitude of drugs. It is also associated with congenital anomalies of the biliary tree and infrequently with gallstones that obstruct the pancreatic duct.
- Pancreatitis causes epigastric pain that may radiate to the back. In many cases, the onset of pain is gradual. Vomiting is usually present.
- The abdominal examination may reveal tenderness in the epigastrium; affected children tend to lie still, with their hips slightly flexed. Low-grade fever is present in 50 to 60 percent of cases.
- The laboratory work-up includes measurement of liver function tests, a complete blood cell count, and electrolyte, BUN, creatinine, glucose, and calcium levels.
- The quantitative amylase level is useful as a screening for pancreatic disease but does not correlate with the severity of illness. Somewhat more specific is an elevation in the amylase:creatinine clearance ratio. Serum lipase level may also be elevated.
- An ultrasound evaluation of the pancreas or a computed tomography of the abdomen may be useful.
- Therapy of pancreatitis consists of fluid resuscitation and maintenance of serum electrolyte level. Nasogastric suction may help to diminish pain. Analgesics are usually necessary for pain relief. Meperidine is the drug of choice; morphine or codeine should not be used because they increase spasm at the sphincter of Oddi.
- Complications include the formation of a pancreatic abscess or pseudocyst and the development of pleural effusion.

HEPATITIS

- **Hepatitis** is a common viral infection with clinical manifestations that range from asymptomatic infection to fulminant liver failure. Several distinct viral etiologic agents have been identified and are currently labeled hepatitis A, B, C, D, and E. Of these, hepatitis B is the most problematic.
- Transmission of hepatitis A in humans is usually via contact with infected fecal material. The incubation period is usually 2 to 4 weeks.

- Hepatitis A infection in children is usually mild and self-limited, although occasionally severe infection can occur. In young children, the illness is frequently asymptomatic and is usually not associated with jaundice.
- Symptomatic patients usually suffer an acute febrile illness characterized by nausea, anorexia, and fatigability.
- There may or may not be icterus or jaundice apparent on physical examination. If present, it generally does not appear until several weeks after exposure.
- Laboratory findings include elevation in serum transaminase levels that reflect liver injury. Both conjugated and unconjugated fractions of bilirubin are elevated.
- IgM antibody to hepatitis A is usually detectable 6 to 8 weeks after the illness. IgG develops later and persists for years.
- Treatment of hepatitis A is supportive. Hospitalization is indicated for patients who are unable to tolerate oral nutrition.
- Serum immune globulin treatment is indicated in household contacts of affected patients to prevent the spread of clinical hepatitis. Hepatitis A in pregnant patients does not infect the fetus. There is no carrier state in hepatitis A.
- There is now a vaccine available against hepatitis A, especially recommended for travelers to endemic countries.
- Hepatitis B virus (HBV) is transmitted through body secretions such as semen, cervical secretions, saliva, and exudative wound secretions. It can also be transmitted by infected blood or blood products. Hepatitis B virus can be transmitted from an infected mother to the newborn, perhaps at delivery.
- About 90 percent of infected newborns become chronic carriers of the infection. The incubation period of HBV is 2 to 5 months. Rarely, HBV results in severe, fulminant hepatitis.
- In many patients, especially infants and young children, infection with HBV is asymptomatic. Symptomatic infection produces nausea, vomiting, and malaise.
- It may also cause arthralgia and arthritis and can result in a papular acrodermatitis on the face, buttocks, and extensor surfaces of the arms and legs. Some patients can develop immunemediated glomerulonephritis.
- Hepatomegaly or splenomegaly may be present. By the time jaundice appears, children will probably be afebrile. The classic description of clay-colored stools may not be present in children.
- Laboratory findings reveal elevated serum transaminase levels and both conjugated and unconjugated bilirubin

values. Testing for the HBV is through a series of serum tests for antigen and antibody detection.

- Treatment of HBV infection is supportive. Hospital admission is indicated for patients in whom nausea and vomiting preclude adequate hydration and nutrition and for the rare patient with fulminant hepatitis.
- Infection with HBV is now preventable due to the development of a highly effective synthetic vaccine. Passive immunization is possible with hepatitis B immune globulin (HBIG).
- Previously described non-A non-B hepatitis is now identified as two separate etiologic agents.
- Parenterally acquired non-A non-B is now called hepatitis C. It is usually a mild infection of insidious onset, manifested by malaise and jaundice. It is more common in adults. The incidence of developing chronic liver disease approaches 50 percent.
- Enterically transmitted non-A non-B is now called hepatitis E. Transmission of hepatitis E closely resembles that of hepatitis A. Malaise and jaundice are presenting signs, with arthralgias, fever, and abdominal pain as additional associated symptoms. There are no serologic markers for HEV.
- Hepatitis D virus can only multiply in the presence of hepatitis B. It is usually transmitted parenterally. Infection with hepatitis D results in an increased incidence of chronic liver disease.

FULMINANT HEPATIC FAILURE

- **Fulminant hepatic failure** is a syndrome characterized by severe hepatic dysfunction and encephalopathy. It usually evolves over a period of less than 8 weeks and affects all organ systems.
- Any infectious cause of hepatitis can result in fulminant hepatic failure, though it is uncommon in hepatitis A. Hepatic failure can also result from toxic exposure, especially from acetaminophen or the mushroom *Amanita phalloides.*
- A predominant manifestation of hepatic failure is encephalopathy. In later stages, coma can develop. Cerebral edema may develop and may result in death.
- Failure to synthesize liver-dependent coagulation factors results in a bleeding diathesis.
- Laboratory findings reveal elevated transaminase and serum ammonia levels. The prothrombin time is increased. Serum albumin may be decreased. In the vast majority of cases, serum bilirubin level is increased. Hyponatremia may be present, but is usually dilutional. In some patients, renal failure develops.
- Management consists of supportive care. Hypoglycemia is especially common. The administration of fresh frozen plasma may help correct the coagulopathy.

- Oral lactulose causes watery diarrhea of a low pH and may decrease serum ammonia levels. Oral neomycin also may decrease the formation of ammonia.

JAUNDICE

- **Jaundice** is common in newborns, where some degree of hyperbilirubinemia is virtually universal. However, the appearance of jaundice beyond the immediate neonatal period is virtually always a manifestation of pathology.
- Bilirubin is largely formed by the destruction of red blood cells and the catabolism of heme proteins. After conjugation, bilirubin is excreted in the bile and from there, into the intestinal tract. At elevated levels, the unconjugate form is neurotoxic.

UNCONJUGATED HYPERBILIRUBINEMIA

Newborns and Young Infants
- In the immediate neonatal period, **unconjugated hyperbilirubinemia** is of great concern largely because of its association with **kernicterus**, an irreversible neurologic disorder that occurs when unbound bilirubin is deposited in the brain.
- In its early phases, kernicterus is characterized by lethargy, poor feeding, and, in some cases, opisthotonus. In its full-blown form, it ultimately results in choreoathetosis, extrapyramidal signs, and mental retardation.
- In full-term newborns, kernicterus is associated with levels of unconjugated serum bilirubin levels less than 20 mg/dL. In premature infants, lower levels can cause kernicterus.

Physiologic Jaundice
- The most common cause of unconjugated hyperbilirubinemia in the neonatal period is physiologic jaundice. It is thought to result from transiently impaired conjugation and excretion of bilirubin.
- Jaundice becomes visible on the second to third day of life and peaks around the fourth day. The maximum elevation is usually less than 6 mg/dL.
- Physiologic jaundice is a nonpathologic condition, with no neurologic sequelae.

Breast Milk Jaundice
- Jaundice is more common in breast-fed infants than it is in bottle-fed infants. This may be due, in part, to substances contained in breast milk that antagonize the conjugation and excretion of bilirubin.
- Rarely, breast-fed infants can develop elevations of unconjugated bilirubin starting in the first week of life that can reach 15 to 27 mg per 100 mL by the second or third week.

- The hyperbilirubinemia resolves with the cessation of breastfeeding and does not recur when it is resumed. A diagnosis of breast-milk jaundice assumes that other pathologic causes of hyperbilirubinemia have been considered.

Increased Hemolysis

- Increased hemolysis in newborn infants is the most common cause of hyperbilirubinemia severe enough to warrant phototherapy or exchange transfusion. It is usually secondary to maternal–fetal blood group incompatibility in either rhesus or ABO antigens. Jaundice usually appears in the first 24 h of life.
- Severe bruising or **cephalohematoma** secondary to trauma during delivery can also result in increased metabolism of heme proteins and unconjugated hyperbilirubinemia. Other causes of hemolysis include congenital diseases such as hereditary spherocytosis and glucose-6-phosphate dehydrogenase deficiency.

Miscellaneous

- Unconjugated hyperbilirubinemia can result from a variety of unusual causes. These include hypothyroidism, Down's syndrome, and pyloric stenosis or other high intestinal obstructions.
- Bacterial infections, including those from the urinary tract, can cause unconjugated hyperbilirubinemia, although there may also be a component of conjugated bilirubin.

Evaluation and Management

- Infants with unconjugated bilirubin greater than 5 to 6 mg/dL after 2 to 3 days of life merit investigation.
- Laboratory evaluation includes a complete blood cell count, reticulocyte count, and Coombs' test. If a bacterial infection is a consideration, cultures of blood, cerebrospinal fluid, and urine are obtained, in addition to a urinalysis.
- The diagnosis of breast-milk jaundice is made after pathologic causes of hyperbilirubinemia are excluded and serum bilirubin level decreases after breastfeeding is stopped.
- The majority of newborns with unconjugated hyperbilirubinemia do well with expectant management, with particular attention paid to maintaining adequate hydration.
- For patients with moderate to severe elevation, phototherapy is the treatment of choice. Indirect hyperbilirubinemia is reduced by exposure to high-intensity light.
- The criteria for the initiation of phototherapy vary according to gestational age and birth weight. Consultation with a neonatologist is indicated in full-term infants with values nearing 20 mg/dL. Infants with rapidly rising serum bilirubin who do not respond to phototherapy may require exchange transfusion.

Older Children

- In older children, unconjugated hyperbilirubinemia is most likely the result of a hemolytic process or an inherited defect in the conjugation of bilirubin.
- The work-up for hemolytic anemia includes a complete blood cell and reticulocyte count and a serum haptoglobin level. A common genetic defect in conjugation is Gilbert's syndrome, a deficiency in glucuronyl transferase that is associated with normal hepatic function.

CONJUGATED HYPERBILIRUBINEMIA

Newborns and Infants

- **Conjugated hyperbilirubinemia** is present when the conjugated fraction of bilirubin exceeds 20 percent of the total. It most commonly occurs secondary to intrahepatic cellular damage and is less often due to obstruction of biliary flow.
- Conjugated hyperbilirubinemia is always pathologic. Most infants with conjugated hyperbilirubinemia will present within the first month of life.

Infectious Causes

- Neonatal cholestasis can occur secondary to hepatic injury from a multitude of infectious causes. Cytomegalovirus, rubella, herpes simplex, varicella, coxsackie, and hepatitis B are common viral etiologies.
- Syphilis and toxoplasmosis are also implicated. Most of these result from intrauterine involvement and are often associated with congenital anomalies and hepatosplenomegaly.
- Bacterial sepsis can result in conjugated hyperbilirubinemia, although the unconjugated fraction is also usually increased. The urinary tract is a common site of infection and can involve gram-negative organisms, such as *Escherichia coli*. Jaundice often starts at 3 to 4 days of age and, in some instances, can be the only manifestation of infection.

Metabolic Causes

- Metabolic disorders that can cause conjugated hyperbilirubinemia include alpha1 antitrypsin deficiency, cystic fibrosis, and galactosemia. Most metabolic disorders will have clinical manifestations other than jaundice that will lead to the diagnosis.

Extrahepatic Diseases

- The major extrahepatic cause of conjugated hyperbilirubinemia in infancy is biliary atresia, a syndrome characterized by absence of the bile ducts anywhere between the duodenum and hepatic ducts. Patients present with jaundice, dark urine, and often with acholic stools.

- The evaluation of patients with suspected biliary atresia usually includes a liver biopsy, which may help to exclude neonatal hepatitis, a disorder of unknown etiology in which there is diffuse hepatocellular destruction.
- For patients in whom atresia extends to the portahepatis, the Kasai procedure, a hepatoportoenterostomy, may allow drainage of bile. A major complication of the Kasai procedure is the risk of ascending cholangitis.
- A choledochal cyst is a congenital saccular dilatation of the common bile duct. It can present with jaundice and a right upper quadrant mass or with symptoms of cholangitis, including fever and leukocytosis.

Older Children

- Conjugated hyperbilirubinemia in older children most commonly results from infectious hepatitis. Drug-induced liver injury is also fairly common.
- Less commonly, genetic or metabolic disorders can present with jaundice and conjugated hyperbilirubinemia. Relatively common metabolic defects include alpha1 antitrypsin deficiency and Wilson's disease.

BIBLIOGRAPHY

Baker SS, Liptak GS, Colletti RB, et al: Constipation in infants and children: Evaluation and treatment. *J Pediatr Gastroenterol Nutr* 29:612–626, 1999.

Braden B, Posselt H, Ahrens P, et al: New immunoassay in stool provides an accurate noninvasive diagnostic method of *Helicobacter pylori* screening in children. *Pediatrics* 106:115–117, 2000.

Dennery PA, Seidman DS, Stevenson DK: Neonatal hyperbilirubinemia. *N Engl J Med* 344:581–590, 2001.

Gupta R, Gernsheimer J, Golden J: Acute abdominal pain and vomiting in a 10-year-old girl. *Ann Emerg Med* 30:322–328, 1997.

Hardy S, Keel SB: Weekly clinicopathological exercises: Case 35-1999: A five-month-old girl with coffee-grounds vomitus. *N Engl J Med* 341:1597–1603, 1999.

Hill DL, Heine RG, Cameron DJS, et al: Role of food protein intolerance in infants with persistent distress attributed to reflux esophagitis. *J Pediatr* 136:641–647, 2000.

Hill D, Hosking CS: Infantile colic and food hypersensitivity. *J Pediatr Gastroenterol Nutr* 30(suppl):S67–S76, 2000.

Matsumoto T, Goto Y, Miike T: Markedly high eosinophilia and an elevated serum IL-5 level in an infant with cow milk allergy. *Ann Allergy Asthma Immunol* 82:252–256, 1999.

Peters JM: Management of gastrointestinal bleeding in children. *Curr Treat Options Gastroenterol* 5:399–413, 2002.

Weydert JA, Ball TM, Davis MF: Systematic review of treatments for recurrent abdominal pain. *Pediatrics* 111:e1–11, 2002.

Yachha SK, Chetri K, Saraswat VA, et al: Management of childhood pancreatic disorders: A multidisciplinary approach. *J Pediatr Gastroenterol Nutr* 36:206–212, 2003.

QUESTIONS

1. A 10-year-old boy is brought to the ED for evaluation of colicky abdominal pain. Which of the following would **NOT** be included in the differential?
   A. Gastroenteritis
   B. Bowel obstruction
   C. Incarcerated inguinal hernia
   D. Peritonitis
   E. Renal stone

2. A 7-year-old boy presents for evaluation of abdominal pain. The pain is localized to the right lower quadrant. On examination, the child is ill appearing and exhibits suprapubic and right lower quadrant tenderness. In addition to a thorough abdominal examination, which of the following is mandatory in including and excluding potential etiologies of the pain?
   A. A rectal examination
   B. A genital examination
   C. A urinalysis
   D. Stool for occult blood
   E. Nasogastric aspirate

3. An 18-month-old girl is brought by parents for evaluation of bloody diarrhea. You suspect an infectious etiology. Which of the following would **NOT** be included in the differential for bloody diarrhea?
   A. Intussusception
   B. Hemolytic uremia syndrome
   C. Hirschsprung's disease
   D. Formula allergy
   E. Bacterial enteritis

4. An 11-year-old girl is brought to the ED for evaluation of abdominal pain. You learn the child was recently hospitalized for extensive burns and smoke inhalation. She complains of nighttime awakenings and occasional vomiting. Which of the following is the **MOST** likely diagnosis in this patient?
   A. Stress ulcers
   B. Hepatitis
   C. Pancreatitis
   D. Small bowel obstruction
   E. Cholecystitis

5. Complications of gastroesophageal reflux include all of the following **EXCEPT**:
   A. Failure to thrive
   B. Chronic pancreatitis
   C. Reactive airway disease
   D. Iron deficiency anemia
   E. Gastrointestinal bleeding

6. An 11-year-old girl is brought to the ED for evaluation of epigastric pain that radiates to the back and vomiting. She reports the onset of pain was gradual and began following a fall from the monkey bars at the neighborhood park. Which of the following would the **MOST** specific in screening for pancreatic disease?
   A. Obstructive series
   B. Liver function tests
   C. Amylase
   D. Amylase:creatinine clearance ratio
   E. Calcium levels

7. Which of the following is the most common cause of hyperbilirubinemia requiring phototherapy or exchange transfusion?
   A. Cephalohematoma
   B. Breast milk jaundice
   C. Physiologic jaundice
   D. ABO antigens
   E. Pyloric stenosis

8. A 1-month-old baby is brought by parents for evaluation of jaundice and dark urine. The parents also noticed a change in the appearance of her stools. The differential diagnosis for this patient **WOULD** include which of the following?
   A. Hepatitis B infection
   B. Biliary atresia
   C. Maternal–fetal blood group incompatibility
   D. Hereditary spherocytosis
   E. Down's syndrome

ANSWERS

1. D. Crampy or colicky pain usually results from the distension of a viscus. It is most commonly due to gastroenteritis, but can also be seen in surgical emergencies, such as bowel obstruction and incarcerated inguinal hernia. Patients with peritoneal inflammation tend to have a sharp, localized constant pain.

2. B. All pediatric patients with abdominal pain require a genital examination to rule out an incarcerated inguinal hernia as the etiology of the pain. If there is a history of gastrointestinal bleeding or a surgical emergency is suspected, a rectal examination is indicated and the stool is checked for occult blood.

3. C. The presence of blood usually indicates an infectious etiology, which in children, is often due to bacterial enteritis. Other causes of bloody diarrhea include intussusception, hemolytic uremic syndrome, pseudomembranous colitis, and true formula allergy. Hirschsprung's disease causes constipation.

4. A. Stress ulcers are common in pediatric patients with serious illness, such as sepsis, or major trauma or extensive burns. Older children are likely to have abdominal pain, with or without associated vomiting, and nighttime wakening.

5. B. Gastroesophageal reflux (GER) refers to the regurgitation of stomach contents into the esophagus. Most infants and children have physiologic reflux with no clinical consequences. Severe GER can result in failure to thrive, esophageal strictures, Barrett's esophagus, gastrointestinal bleeding, recurrent aspiration pneumonia, reactive airway disease, and iron deficiency anemia.

6. D. Pancreatitis is relatively uncommon in children before the age of 10 years. Blunt abdominal trauma is a frequent cause of pancreatitis in children. The quantitative amylase level is useful as a screening for pancreatic disease but does not correlate with the severity of illness. An elevation in the amylase:creatinine ratio is more specific.

7. D. Increased hemolysis in newborn infants is the most common cause of hyperbilirubinemia severe enough to warrant phototherapy or exchange transfusion. Causes include maternal–fetal blood group incompatibility in either rhesus or ABO antigens.

8. B. Conjugated hyperbilirubinemia is often due to intrahepatic cellular damage or to obstruction of biliary flow. The major extrahepatic cause of conjugated hyperbilirubinemia in infancy is biliary atresia. Patients present with jaundice, dark urine, and with acholic stools.

53 ACUTE ABDOMINAL CONDITIONS THAT MAY REQUIRE SURGICAL INTERVENTION

Jonathan Singer
William R. Ahrens
Heather M. Prendergast

OBSTRUCTIONS

MALROTATION WITH MIDGUT VOLVULUS

- An arrest of the normal embryonic rotation of the alimentary tract may result in suspension of sections of bowel, including the vascular supply, by a narrow pedicle.
- The rotational anomaly will create a vague gastrointestinal symptom such as failure to thrive, chronic recurrent abdominal distension, episodic vomiting that may be bilious, or persistent unexplained diarrhea.

- With malrotations involving the duodenum, small bowel, and colon up to the midgut, a strangulating volvulus may occur. In over 75 percent of cases, this precipitous event occurs within the first month of life. Males are affected twice as often as females.
- Patients who develop midgut volvulus experience sudden abdominal discomfort and vomiting. The pain is intense and unremitting. The vomiting becomes repetitious and bile stained.
- If the volvulus is not recognized within hours, viability of the gut may be compromised and bloody vomiting or bloody stools with or without shock may occur. Affected children are acutely ill, pale, and distressed, and may have poor perfusion.
- If the obstruction is high and decompressed by repeated vomiting, abdominal distension is absent. A newborn with malrotation and midgut volvulus evaluated shortly after onset of the vomiting may have a soft, nontender abdomen.
- Stool from the rectal exam may be positive for occult blood.
- Duodenal obstruction yields air-fluid levels in the dilated stomach and duodenum with little air (doubled bubble) or no gas in the remainder of the bowel.
- Contrast studies provide conclusive diagnostic evidence. The upper gastrointestinal series is preferred.
- The findings of midgut volvulus include obstruction of the duodenum at its third portion. Intestinal obstruction of the descending duodenum, just over the right of the spine, is pathognomonic. The intestine distal to the obstruction wraps around the superior mesenteric vessels and creates a corkscrew appearance.
- Obstructed children require intestinal intubation and decompression. Volume depletion necessitates fluid resuscitation.
- Prompt laparotomy is necessary to preserve the bowel.

PYLORIC STENOSIS

- Pyloric stenosis is the most common cause of intestinal obstruction after the first month of life. The typical infant becomes symptomatic between the second and sixth week of life. Males are four times more likely to be affected than are females.
- Symptoms of gastric outlet obstruction are produced by hypertrophy of circular fibers about the pylorus. The initial symptom is intermittent nonprojectile vomiting. Within a week, nonbilious, postprandial, projectile vomiting is uniformly encountered.
- The antecedent history of a steady weight gain is replaced by weight deceleration as formula retention is compromised.

- The hydration status may be severely compromised if vomiting has been of a prolonged duration.
- A mid-abdominal peristaltic wave may be seen prior to the eventual regurgitant event. An epigastric, rounded mass, traditionally described as olive-like, is found in 80 to 90 percent of cases. In circumstances where an abdominal mass cannot be palpated, radiography or imaging may establish the diagnosis.
- An ultrasound study will reveal an elongated and hypertrophied pyloric sphincter, and thickened mucosa may be seen protruding into the gastric antrum (**antral nipple sign**).
- A barium study reveals curvature, elongation, and narrowing of the pyloric channel (**string sign**).
- Loss of both potassium and hydrogen ions from vomiting can result in a characteristic hypokalemic, hypochloremic, metabolic alkalosis.
- When infants have pyloric stenosis, a nasogastric tube should be placed and volume and electrolyte replacement initiated. Once a diagnosis is confirmed, surgical intervention with a pyloromyotomy constitutes definitive care.

INTUSSUSCEPTION

- Intussusception is an invagination of a proximal portion of the intestine into a distal adjacent part. It is the most frequent cause of intestinal obstruction between the ages of 3 months and 5 years. More than 60 percent of cases occur in the first year of life, with most of those occurring between the fifth and ninth month.
- Males are affected twice as often as females, and this difference becomes more pronounced in children over 4 years of age, rising to an 8:1 ratio.
- The classic triad of intermittent colicky pain, vomiting, and bloody stools is found in less than one third of all patients; only 85 percent of patients have classical colicky pain; 75 percent experience vomiting.
- A key diagnostic component in patients who experience pain is that it is intermittent and they look well in between episodes.
- Rectal bleeding may be found in as few as 40 percent of patients. Currant jelly stools, which are bloody, maroon-colored, and mucus laden, are typically seen late in the disease.
- Anorexia is an almost universal but nonspecific symptom. Diarrhea may be seen in about 7 to 10 percent of cases where there is complete intestinal obstruction and may be found in up to 40 percent of cases where there is an incomplete bowel obstruction.
- There is increasing appreciation that apathy or listlessness may occasionally be the dominant manifestation. This altered sensorium with intussusception may be

seen in the context of prolonged symptomatology or as the initial complaint. Mental status changes may be accompanied by pronounced pallor, mimicking shock.

- The abdomen may appear scaphoid and the right lower quadrant may seem empty (**Dance's sign**). Guarding or distension is uncommon. Bowel sounds may be normal, decreased, or absent. A sausage-shaped mass may be found. The advancing mass is typically ill-defined and variably tender on rectal examination.
- Grossly bloody stool may be found on the withdrawn examining finger, or normal-appearing stool may be positive for occult blood.
- Plain abdominal radiographs films may be normal (30 percent) or may reveal localized air–fluid levels, dilated small bowel loops, reduced intestinal air, or minimal fecal content in the colon. The intussusception itself may be visible in up to one-half of patients.
- Ultrasonography has been reported to be nearly 100 percent sensitive. Sonographic findings include a large sonographic target, bull's eye, or doughnut sign on the transverse or cross-section, and a sleeve or pseudokidney sign on the longitudinal section.
- Both an air insufflation or barium enema reduction is performed with the consent, and in the presence, of the surgeon who accepts the responsibility for operating if the reduction is unsuccessful.
- Attempted reduction with barium enema is contraindicated if there is evidence of intestinal perforation or peritonitis, due to the risk of barium peritonitis.

INCARCERATED HERNIAS

- Hernias are protrusions of tissue through an abnormal opening. In children, they occur with descending frequency at the umbilicus, inguinal and scrotal regions, midline epigastrium, and lateral border of the rectus sheath.
- When the incarcerated sac contents cannot be reduced nonoperatively into the peritoneal cavity, strangulation and necrosis of tissues may result. Male children with hernias outnumber female children by an 8:1 to 10:1 ratio.
- Both sexes have the greatest risk for incarceration during the first 6 months of life. With advancing age, incarceration becomes less likely. There is a very low incidence of incarceration after 8 years of age.
- The diagnosis of incarcerated hernia is not difficult if children are completely undressed. All children with incarceration appear uncomfortable.
- Radiographic confirmation is rarely necessary. Ultrasonography may be used in infants born prematurely to discriminate the contents of an incarcerated sac.

- Nonoperative reduction of a strangulated hernia can often be achieved by the emergency physician. Greatest success follows a period of withheld oral intake and application of ice to the hernia sac. Sedation is usually necessary.

INTRAABDOMINAL SEPSIS

ACUTE APPENDICITIS WITHOUT PERFORATION

- The late elementary school age population has the highest incidence of appendicitis in childhood. There is a gradual reduction in frequency of acute appendicitis in younger children, with a precipitous drop in children younger than 2 years of age.
- The triad of abdominal pain, vomiting, and low-grade fever is highly suggestive of appendicitis. Abdominal pain is the first manifestation of the disease. The pain is epigastric or periumbilical. At onset, the pain is described as a dull, aching sensation, later becoming more intense and constant.
- As the inflammation proceeds, the pain migrates and localizes. In most cases, the pain is maximal in the right lower quadrant.
- Pain may radiate to the flank or back with retrocecal appendicitis or the suprapubic region with a pelvic appendicitis, and to the testicle with a retroileal appendicitis.
- At least one to two episodes of nonbilious vomiting occur in over 90 percent of cases.
- Temperature elevation is a noted feature in 75 to 80 percent of patients.
- An inflamed appendix, particularly if retrocecal, may cause fecal urgency, tenesmus, and frequent passage of a small volume of stool in approximately 15 percent of children. Dysuria may be experienced by 5 to 15 percent of children with an inflamed appendix in proximity to the ureter. The latter two atypical symptoms are more often clinical features in misdiagnosed cases.
- Patients with nonperforated appendicitis will have minimal alteration of their vital signs aside from fever.
- If the appendix is in a retrocecal position or in contact with pelvic musculature, elevation and extension of the right leg against pressure of the examiner's hand causes pain (**iliopsoas sign**). Alternately, when the flexed right thigh is held at right angles to the trunk and internally rotated, hypogastric pain may result (**obturator sign**).
- Patients may voluntarily guard the entire abdomen or only the right lower quadrant. Exquisite tenderness is often noted directly over McBurney's point. Pressure applied to the descending colon may cause referred

pain at the McBurney's point (**Rovsing's sign**). A rectal examination reveals right lower quadrant tenderness but no masses.

- Ultrasonography has largely replaced the use of contrast material, with has reported sensitivity between 75 and 89 percent and specificity between 86 and 100 percent.
- Conventional computed tomography (CT) utilizing intravenous and oral contrast has a Sensitivity ranging from 87 to 100 percent and specificity from 83 to 100 percent.
- The highest accuracy has been achieved with focused appendiceal CT. For this imaging, a water-soluble contrast is administered rectally and followed by contiguous 5-mm cuts of the right lower quadrant.

ACUTE APPENDICITIS WITH PERFORATION

- Nearly 100 percent of patients in the first year of life will have perforated appendixes at the time of diagnosis, as will 94 percent of those less than 2 years of age, and 60 to 65 percent of those less than 6 years of age.
- Rapid progression with perforation has been described in preschool-age children in as little as 6 to 12 h from onset of symptoms.
- Classically, patients experience increasingly severe abdominal pain until the appendix perforates. Pain may then lessen or cease. Once the perforation has occurred, age may also influence the subsequent clinical course.
- In the first year of life, a short, thin omentum has little capacity to wall off infection. Diffuse peritonitis within hours to days is anticipated rather than focal abscess. Older children tend to isolate an expanding collection of pus.
- Children who have appendixes that have perforated may encounter vague abdominal complaints for days to weeks after the intraperitoneal event. There may be periods of remissions interspersed with exacerbations.
- Patients with perforated appendicitis appear acutely ill and their vital signs are abnormal. Tachycardia and fever are common. The temperatures tend to be higher with perforation, typically in the range of 39°C (102.2°F) to 40°C (104°F). Extreme tachycardia, hypotension, and altered tissue perfusion may be found with severe dehydration or superimposed sepsis.
- Abdominal distension may be prominent, especially in infancy. Bowel sounds are diminished or absent.
- Palpation of the abdomen in any quadrant may be painful. Rebound tenderness is most prominent in the right lower quadrant. Iliopsoas and obturator signs are variable. Rectal tenderness is noted, but a mass is an inconstant finding.
- Radiographic findings that suggest appendicitis with perforation include:

  - Focal increase in thickness of the lateral abdominal wall
  - Presence of a single gas bubble at the inferior portion of the right lower abdominal quadrant
  - Free intraperitoneal fluid
  - Pneumoperitoneum.

- Ultrasonography, in addition to revealing an enlarged, edematous appendix, may demonstrate a periappendiceal fluid collection.
- An oral, intravenous, or focused rectal contrast CT may reveal the extent and progression of an abscess.
- The preoperative management of patients with perforated appendix includes fluid resuscitation, antibiotics, and pain management.

SPONTANEOUS PERITONITIS

- In 10 to 15 percent of cases, pyoperitoneum results from a focus outside of the abdominal cavity. The bacterial access is postulated to result from bacteremia or extension of a urogenital infection.
- This spontaneous peritonitis may occur in previously healthy children, but patients with ventriculoperitoneal shunt, immunodeficiency (including splenectomy and HIV infection), and ascites from cirrhosis or nephrosis are at increased risk.
- Primary peritonitis tends to occur more often in females, with peak incidence between the ages of 5 and 10 years.
- Patients with spontaneous peritonitis have insidious onset of diffuse abdominal pain. The pain does not localize and increases in intensity over hours to days. Nonbilious vomiting, diarrhea, and fever follow the abdominal pain.
- Affected children are anxious and acutely ill and usually febrile. The abdomen is diffusely distended, and when ascites is present, evidence of free fluid will be evident. The abdomen is diffusely tender and guarded. Rebound tenderness may be generalized. Rectal examination reveals tenderness without mass.
- Plain radiographic features of peritonitis include marked gaseous distension of the large and small intestines. Multiple air–fluid levels may be present.
- Abdominal paracentesis with Gram's stain and culture of the fluid may obviate the need for exploratory laparotomy. If the diagnosis cannot be established preoperatively, laparotomy is necessary.

NECROTIZING ENTEROCOLITIS

- Diverse events in the perinatal period may lead to gastric dilatation, functional ileus, and erosive intestinal mucosal injury, all of which are characteristic of necrotizing enterocolitis (NEC). Approximately 10 percent of cases occur in term infants.

- Anorexia and gastric distension, followed by nonbilious vomiting, abdominal distension, or diarrhea are seen at the onset. Hemochezia may develop. Apnea, bradycardia, hypotension, and vascular instability may all occur. Affected infants are pale and often septic-appearing.
- Abdominal tenderness and guarding are highly variable. Bowel sounds are diminished. Rectal examination reveals grossly bloody stool or seedy stool that is guaiac positive.
- On abdominal flat plate, bowel distension is the most common finding. Intraluminal air (**pneumatosis intestinalis**) may be limited to scattered colonic segments or be generalized. Intrahepatic portal vein gas and pneumoperitoneum are ominous findings.
- Treatment includes withholding feedings, initiating parenteral nutrition, nasogastric decompression, and parenteral as well as intraluminal antibiotics.

HIRSCHSPRUNG'S DISEASE

- Hirschsprung's disease is characterized by the absence of intramural ganglion cells. The histologic deficit is usually limited to a segment of bowel in the rectosigmoid region.
- The functional abnormality with Hirschsprung's disease is an increase in muscular tone and contractility of the aganglionic segment. Relaxation needed to facilitate the onward movement of stool does not occur.
- This disease is four times more frequent in males than females.
- Newborns with aganglionosis may have delayed passage of the first meconium stool. Infants have diminished stool frequency. If undiagnosed, the clinical course in the first year of life is one of gradually increasing fecal retention, obstipation, constipation, and sporadic abdominal distention.
- Examination of affected patients may reveal mild to moderate abdominal distention. The abdomen is soft, and nontender, mobile fecal masses may be palpable in the left lower quadrant.
- Rectal examination reveals an empty vault that is not dilated. Withdraw of the examining finger may result in an explosive release of stool. If the diagnosis is not entertained, patients may precipitously develop a potentially fatal enterocolitis.
- Enterocolitis with Hirschsprung's disease is more common in the newborn period, but can occur at any age. The enterocolitis is characterized by sudden abdominal distention, generalized abdominal discomfort, and explosive diarrhea that rapidly becomes bloody.

- Temperature elevation, volume depletion, and altered mental status are typically noted. With the most severe cases, a denudation of the intestinal mucosa predisposes to colonic perforation, peritonitis, and Gram-negative septicemia.
- Progressively confirmatory steps for diagnosing Hirschsprung's disease in children with chronic constipation include plain abdominal films, barium enema, anal rectal manometry, and pathologic examination of rectal tissue.
- Barium enema confirms a normal caliber of the rectum and dilatation of the proximal colon. A cone-shaped transition zone in between is pathognomonic.
- Emergency department intervention for enterocolitis includes gastric decompression, use of a rectal tube, fluid resuscitation, parenteral antibiotics, and keeping patients NPO.

GASTROINTESTINAL FOREIGN BODIES

- The size, configuration, consistency, and chemistry of an ingested object, when coupled with children's age and personal anatomy, determines whether the children remain asymptomatic or if they develop clinical manifestations.
- Small (less than 15 to 20 mm), round, oval, and cuboid objects without sharp edges or projections cause the least difficulty. Rigid, elongated, slender objects may also traverse the intestinal tract without difficulty, but are more inclined to cause complications.
- Ingested batteries retained within the esophagus, stomach, or lodged in the appendix or a Meckel's diverticulum can lead to tragedy. Children less than 1 year of age, those most likely to inappropriately mouth objects, are at increased risk for complications due to the diminutive caliber of their digestive system.
- Complications of gastrointestinal foreign bodies include obstruction within the gastrointestinal tract and perforation. Other gastrointestinal complications include gut fistulization or hemorrhage.
- Less common, but with higher mortality, are complications of prolonged esophageal foreign bodies that include obstruction of the airway, mediastinitis, and erosion into the major vessels.
- Objects most typically become lodged at the hypopharynx, thoracic inlet, and the cardioesophageal junction.
- A metal detector is an effective diagnostic tool for locating ingested metallic bodies. If patients are found to have a metallic foreign body below the diaphragm, there is no need for radiography.
- The mainstay for locating metallic foreign bodies remains anteroposterior films of the chest and abdomen.

- Children without underlying esophageal disease who have a single coin lodged for less than 24 h in any portion of the esophagus are likely to have spontaneous passage of the coin into the stomach.
- Alternative management to watchful waiting includes balloon extraction and esophagoscopy. One of these active methods should be employed for batteries with corrosive potential, regardless of the level point of esophageal impaction. Active retrieval may also be required for objects that are pointed or elongated.

MEGACOLON

- Inflammatory bowel disease in late childhood or early adolescence may be due to ulcerative colitis, primarily a disease of the rectal and colonic mucosa, or Crohn's disease, a transmural disease primarily restricted to the distal ileum.
- Either as an exacerbation of long-standing disease or as the precipitating event of the disease, patients with either condition may develop a toxic dilatation of the colon (megacolon). The transverse colon is typically involved.
- A transmural inflammatory process occurs, and the segment of colon massively dilates. Peristalsis ceases. Significant hemorrhage and multiple areas of microperforation may be preludes to peritonitis and overwhelming sepsis.
- Patients with megacolon develop a temperature spike and experience malaise and anorexia. Abdominal pain and distension will occur over a period of a few hours to a day. Abundant, grossly bloody stools will be passed.
- The hallmark radiologic feature of toxic megacolon, seen on a supine abdominal film, is dilatation of the transverse colon greater than 6 to 7 cm in diameter.
- Initial treatment for toxic megacolon involves fluid resuscitation, with added albumin or blood as necessary.
- High-dose corticosteroids are required for patients on maintenance steroids. Pending surgical consultation, a nasogastric tube should be passed and parenteral antibiotics begun.

BIBLIOGRAPHY

D'Agostino J: Common abdominal emergencies in children. *Emerg Med Clin N Am* 20:139–153, 2002.

Daneman A, Navarro O: Intussusception part 1: A review of diagnostic approaches. *Pediatr Radiol* 33:79–85, 2003.

Heller RM, Hernanz-Schulman M: Applications of new imaging modalities in the evaluation of common pediatric conditions. *J Pediatr* 135:632–639, 1999.

Irish MS, Pearl RG, Caty MG, et al: The approach to common abdominal diagnoses in infants and children. *Pediatr Clin North Am* 45:729–772, 1998.

Kim MK, Strait RT, Sato TT, Hennes HM: A randomized clinical trial of analgesia in children with acute abdominal pain. *Acad Emerg Med* 9:281–287, 2002.

Markinson DS, Levine D, Schacht R: Primary peritonitis as a presenting feature of nephrotic syndrome: A rare case report and review of the literature. *Pediatr Emerg Care* 15:407–409, 1999.

McLario D, Rothrock SG: Understanding the varied presentation and management of children with acute abdominal disorders. *Pediatr Emerg Med Rep* 111–122, 1997.

Nance ML, Adamson WT, Hedrick HL: Appendicitis in the young child: A continuing diagnostic challenge. *Pediatr Emerg Care* 16:160–162, 2000.

Rothrock SG, Pagane J: Acute appendicitis in childhood: Emergency department diagnosis and management. *Ann Emerg Med* 36:39–51, 2000.

Seikel K, Primm PA, Elizondo BS: Handheld metal detection localization of ingested metallic foreign bodies: Accurate in any hands? *Arch Pediatr Adolesc Med* 153:853–857, 1999.

Winesett M: Inflammatory bowel disease in children and adolescents. *Pediatr Ann* 26:227–234, 1999.

QUESTIONS

1. A 1-week-old infant boy is brought to the emergency department for evaluation of persistent vomiting. Since the onset of vomiting, the parents note decreased appetite and activity. On examination, you find an ill-appearing, dehydrated infant. Abdominal examination reveals a soft, nontender abdomen without masses. You immediately begin fluid resuscitation. Which of the following signs or symptoms would be most useful in establishing the diagnosis in this infant?
   A. Decreased bowel movements
   B. Chronic abdominal distension
   C. Heme-positive stools on rectal examination
   D. Bilious vomiting
   E. Single episode of diarrhea

2. In a patient with a suspected malrotation with midgut volvulus, which of the following diagnostic studies is the **MOST** helpful in making the diagnosis?
   A. Obstructive series
   B. Upper gastrointestinal series with small bowel follow-through
   C. Barium enema
   D. Computed tomography of the abdomen
   E. Ultrasound study

3. Which of the following statements is **TRUE** regarding pyloric stenosis?

A. In early stages it is characterized by bilious vomiting.
B. It is common to see a mid-abdominal peristaltic wave following the projectile vomiting.
C. It is characterized by rapid weight loss within days of onset of vomiting.
D. Treatment involves decompression with a rectal tube.
E. The diagnosis can be made either clinically or with ultrasound study.

4. Which of the following is **NOT** a common finding in cases of intussusception?
   A. Intermittent colicky pain
   B. Listlessness
   C. Vomiting
   D. Abdominal distension
   E. Anorexia

5. The highest incidence of appendicitis is seen in which of the following age groups?
   A. Less than 2 years of age
   B. Preschool age
   C. Elementary school age
   D. Early adolescence
   E. Late adolescence

6. An 8-year-old boy is brought to the ED for evaluation of abdominal pain, vomiting, and a low-grade fever. The pain is described as a dull, aching sensation and radiates to the flank. He also reports fecal urgency. An obturator sign is positive. Based on the patient's symptoms, you would expect which of the following statements to be true?
   A. The patient has a retrocecal appendicitis.
   B. The patient has a retroileal appendicitis.
   C. The patient has a pelvic appendicitis.
   D. The patient has an ileocecal appendicitis.
   E. The patient has a perforated appendicitis.

7. A 3-day-old infant is brought to the emergency department for evaluation of nonbilious vomiting and abdominal distension. The mother notes the infant is refusing to breastfeed. On examination, you find an ill-appearing infant with diminished bowel sounds. The **MOST** useful diagnostic test is which of the following?
   A. Rectal examination
   B. Abdominal flat plate
   C. Nasogastric tube
   D. Rectal contrast study
   E. Ultrasound

8. A 6-month-old infant is brought to the emergency department by parents for constipation. The parents note diminished stool frequency. On examination, you find a well-appearing, playful infant. Which of the following findings would significantly reduce your suspicion of Hirschsprung's disease?

A. Abdominal distension
B. Presence of a mobile abdominal mass
C. Stool in rectal vault
D. Heme-positive stools
E. Abdominal pain

ANSWERS

1. D. Bilious vomiting in an infant within the first month of life is malrotation with midgut volvulus until proved otherwise. Over 75 percent of cases present within the first month of life. Other signs and symptoms include failure to thrive, chronic recurrent abdominal distension, and persistent unexplained diarrhea.

2. B. In cases of the suspected malrotation with midgut volvulus, contrast studies provide diagnostic evidence. An upper gastrointestinal series with a small bowel follow-through is preferred. In cases of duodenal obstruction, the double bubble sign may be seen on abdominal radiographs.

3. E. Pyloric stenosis is the most common cause of intestinal obstruction after the first month of life. In 80 to 90 percent of cases, an epigastric, olive-like, mass can be palpated. In cases where the mass cannot be palpated, an ultrasound or barium study can assist in establishing the diagnosis. Characteristic findings include nonbilious, postprandial, projectile vomiting. There is an antecedent history of steady weight gain followed by weight deceleration. On physical examination, often there is a midabdominal peristaltic wave preceding the projectile vomiting.

4. D. Intussusception is the most frequent cause of intestinal obstruction between the ages of 3 months and 5 years. Characteristic findings include anorexia, apathy or listlessness, intermittent colicky pain, vomiting, and bloody stools. Currant jelly stools are typically seen late in the disease. Abdominal distension and guarding are not commonly seen in intussusception.

5. C. The highest incidence of acute appendicitis is seen in the elementary school age group. There is a gradual reduction in frequency of acute appendicitis in younger children, with a precipitous drop in children younger than 2 years of age.

6. A. Based upon the clinical signs, the patient has a retrocecal appendicitis. Other signs suggestive of retrocecal appendicitis include tenesmus, frequent passage of small volumes of stool, and a positive iliopsoas sign.

7. B. The patient has necrotizing enterocolitis. Anorexia and gastric distension associated with nonbilious vomiting are characteristic findings. On abdominal flat plate, bowel distension is the most common

finding. Nasogastric decompression is a part of the treatment regimen.

8. C. In a child with a history of constipation, it is important to rule out underlying colon pathology, such as Hirschsprung's disease. A rectal examination that reveals an empty vault that is not dilated should heighten the suspicion for Hirschsprung's disease. Abdominal pain, abdominal distension, and the presence of a mass should alert the clinician to search for other causes.

ENDOCRINE AND METABOLIC EMERGENCIES

54 DISORDERS OF GLUCOSE METABOLISM

Elizabeth E. Baumann
Frank Thorp
Robert L. Rosenfield
Gary R. Strange
Valerie A. Dobiesz

DIABETIC KETOACIDOSIS (DKA)

- DKA, an endocrinologic condition caused by an absolute or relative lack of insulin, is characterized by hyperglycemia, dehydration, and metabolic acidosis. It is due to severe, uncompensated diabetes mellitus and requires immediate, careful therapeutic management.

EPIDEMIOLOGY

- The annual incidence of DKA in the United States ranges from 4.6 to 8 episodes per 1000 patients with diabetes. Recent epidemiologic studies show that hospitalizations for DKA during the past two decades have increased.

PATHOPHYSIOLOGY

- In DKA, a lack of insulin prohibits intracellular utilization of glucose by somatic cells. In response to intracellular starvation, the levels of counterregulatory hormones—glucagon, epinephrine, cortisol, and growth hormone—rise.

- Gluconeogenesis and glycogenolysis occur in the liver and proteolysis occurs in peripheral tissues. Lipolysis occurs in fatty tissues, forming the ketoacids, hydroxybutyrate and acetoacetic acid.
- Diabetic ketoacidosis is precipitated by a variety of causes. In adolescents, noncompliance with insulin is a major problem.
- Most DKA is precipitated by infection or inadequate insulin supplementation during intercurrent illness.

CLINICAL MANIFESTATIONS

- Mental status ranges from normal to lethargy and (in severe cases) coma. Virtually all patients have signs of significant dehydration, including tachycardia, dry mucous membranes, and poor skin turgor.
- Patients with severe acidosis may demonstrate Kussmaul breathing, characterized by deep, sighing respirations and fruity odor to their breath.

LABORATORY STUDIES

- In DKA, the serum glucose is almost always above 300 mg/dL. The patient's urine can also be tested at the bedside for the presence of ketones. The patient's acid–base status can be rapidly evaluated with an arterial blood gas or venous pH and bicarbonate level.
- During the resuscitation (approximately the first 12 h), serum glucose levels are monitored every h. Serum acetone is monitored every 2 h and serum electrolytes and pH every 4 h. Urine is monitored for ketones at every void.

MANAGEMENT

FLUID RESUSCITATION

- The initial fluid resuscitation is with either normal saline (NS) or Ringer's lactate at a dose of 20 mL/kg. In stable patients, the bolus is given over 1 to 2 h; patients in shock require administration as fast as possible.
- If perfusion is not adequate, a second bolus of 20 mL/kg is administered. After the initial resuscitation, rehydration is continued with 0.45 NS or 0.9 NS depending on state of hydration, serum sodium, and hemodynamic status of the patient.

INSULIN ADMINISTRATION

- An initial bolus of insulin is not necessary and can precipitate rapid fluid exchanges that may be dangerous. The starting dose is 0.1 U/kg/h.
- The goal of therapy is to decrease the serum glucose by 75 to 100 mg/dL/h. When the serum glucose reaches 250 mg/dL, 5-percent glucose is added to the infusing fluid.
- Children in mild DKA or "day after resuscitation" can be managed by providing subcutaneous insulin using their baseline or "home" dose. This typically amounts to 0.5 to 1.5 U/kg/d, depending on age and pubertal status.

POTASSIUM

- Replacement therapy is started once a normal or low serum potassium is ensured and urine output is established. The usual dose of potassium is twice-daily maintenance, or 3 to 4 mEq/kg/24h provided as 40 mEq/L in the IV fluids, with half as potassium chloride and half as potassium phosphate.

SODIUM

- For each 100-mg/dL increment in plasma glucose above a "normal" of 100 mg/dL, there is an expected decrease of 1.6 mEq/L in serum sodium.
- As the glucose falls, the reported level of serum sodium should rise.

PHOSPHATE

- The benefit of urgent replacement of phosphate during DKA is debatable; however, supplementation is indicated if the serum level is below 2 mEq/L. Phosphate can be administered in conjunction with potassium replacement as a potassium salt.

BICARBONATE

- Clinical studies have failed to demonstrate improved outcome in patients treated with supplemental bicarbonate. Its use can be considered in patients with severe acidosis (pH <7.1 or serum bicarbonate <5 mEq/L),

which is associated with insulin resistance or cardiovascular collapse.

COMPLICATIONS

- Hypoglycemia is common, especially in young diabetics, who tend to be labile. It often occurs 6 to 8 h after the initiation of therapy for DKA.
- Hypokalemia is the most common electrolyte abnormality and occurs within several hours of initiation of therapy. Since it can lead to arrhythmias, cardiac monitoring is essential until metabolic parameters have stabilized.
- Cerebral edema is the most feared and most lethal complication of DKA, accounting for at least half of DKA-related deaths. It usually occurs as the patient's metabolic parameters are improving and is often heralded clinically by complaints of headache, dizziness, changes in behavior, incontinence, and alterations in pulse and blood pressure, all of which can indicate increased intracranial pressure.
  - At present, the etiology of cerebral edema is unknown and its occurrence unpredictable. Factors implicated but not proved to be associated with cerebral edema include a rapid fall in blood glucose, hypoglycemia, fluid volume replacement, a failure of the actual serum sodium to rise during treatment, and the use of bicarbonate.
  - The treatment of cerebral edema consists of controlled ventilation, mannitol, and fluid restriction, all of which decrease intracranial pressure. Given the unpredictable nature of cerebral edema, careful attention to neurologic status, with hourly mental status checks in a critical care setting, is mandatory in the treatment of all patients with DKA.

DISPOSITION

- All patients presenting with DKA as the initial presentation of diabetes are hospitalized. Patients with severe acidosis are best treated in an intensive care unit, although criteria for this vary among institutions.
- Outpatient management of DKA has been advocated for a selected group of patients, including those with stable vital signs, the ability to tolerate oral fluids, established physician follow-up, and a competent family setting. If after 3 to 4 h of ED treatment the serum pH has risen to 7.35 or above and the serum bicarbonate is above 20 mEq/L, the patient is discharged.

HYPOGLYCEMIA

- Hypoglycemia is defined as a decrease in the plasma glucose level below 55 mg/dL in children and below

35 to 45 mg/dL in neonates. A plasma glucose level below 45 mg/dL (blood glucose <40 mg/dL) in association with symptoms requires intervention. A plasma glucose of 25 to 35 mg/dL requires intervention in an asymptomatic infant only if the infant is at risk of hypoglycemia (eg, infant of diabetic mother or fetal malnutrition) and the glucose value does not rise to 45 mg/dL or more with feeding.

SIGNS AND SYMPTOMS

- The wide variety of signs and symptoms of hypoglycemia usually results from the sympathetic stimulation driven by the insulin-antagonizing hormones that function to increase serum glucose. Newborns and young infants may be asymptomatic or may manifest nonspecific symptoms such as irritability, pallor, cyanosis, tachycardia, tremors, lethargy, apnea, or seizures.
- Older children exhibit more classic symptoms of hypoglycemia, including diaphoresis, tachycardia, tremor, anxiety, tachypnea, and weakness.

DIFFERENTIAL DIAGNOSIS

- Hypoglycemia secondary to lack of exogenous glucose is common in acutely ill infants and children, since oral intake is often decreased during an acute illness. Diarrheal diseases may cause malabsorption of substrate and result in hypoglycemia.
- Idiopathic ketotic hypoglycemia is an entity usually seen in a previously healthy, slender young child, between the ages of 2 and 7 years (typically male) with normal growth and development who presents with an episode of symptomatic fasting hypoglycemia and an appropriate degree of ketosis without hepatomegaly. It may also be associated with an intercurrent illness.
- In children seen in the ED, the most common cause of hypoglycemia is an adverse reaction to insulin therapy in a known diabetic.
- Other causes of hyperinsulinemia are not so easily recognized. These include the autosomal recessive persistent hyperinsulinemic hypoglycemia of infancy (formerly known as nesidioblastosis), infant of the diabetic mother, and the β-cell hyperplasia of Beckwith–Wiedemann syndrome. Particularly in older children, one might consider islet cell adenomas and Munchausen by proxy syndrome, that is, exogenous insulin administration by a caregiver; the earliest reported case involved an infant 2 months of age.
- Inborn errors of metabolism can result in hypoglycemia by disrupting endogenous glucose metabolism. These include a wide array of defects in amino acid metabolism, glycogen storage diseases, fatty acid oxidation (FAO) disorders, enzyme deficiencies in gluconeogenic pathways, and activating mutations of glucose transporters.
- Hormonal disorders, such as hypopituitarism and adrenal insufficiency, can also cause hypoglycemia.

DIAGNOSIS

- A rapid screen for the serum glucose level at the bedside is possible using a glucose oxidase reagent strip. More accurate confirmation is achieved by direct measurement done on an initial venous sample. This is the "critical sample" and should include not only a sample for glucose obtained in a gray top tube and placed on ice but important additional studies: insulin, C-peptide, growth hormone, cortisol, and glucagon levels.

MANAGEMENT

- Intravenous glucose is the first line of therapy. Glucose is administered to symptomatically hypoglycemic patients in a dose of 0.5 g/kg/dose. Dextrose 25 percent at a dose of 2 to 4 mL/kg is appropriate therapy. In neonates and preterm infants, dextrose 10 percent at a dose of 5 to 10 mL/kg is used to avoid sudden hyperosmolarity. In older children and adolescents, dextrose 50 percent at a dose of 1 to 2 mL/kg is used.
- If time permits prior to the administration of intravenous glucose, or in the event that intravenous access is not possible, glucagon at a dose of 0.3 mg/kg is given. A glucagon challenge is useful for both diagnosis and treatment: a negative challenge (blood glucose rise <40 mg/dL over baseline), suggests poor glycogen stores, as occurs in undernutrition, ketotic hypoglycemia, liver failure, or glycogen storage disease. A positive challenge (glycemic increment rising >40 mg/dL over baseline), suggests hyperinsulinism.
- Patients with mild hypoglycemia who are capable of eating or drinking are treated with orange juice or some other age-appropriate source of calories.
- After an episode of hypoglycemia, glucose levels are monitored every 1 to 2 h until the patient is alert and capable of eating and drinking.

DISPOSITION

- When the cause of hypoglycemia is not known, hospital admission for further evaluation is indicated.

Insulin-dependent diabetics who experience hypoglycemia can be discharged after a thorough review of the episode and when the patient and family fully understand where the care regimen deteriorated.

BIBLIOGRAPHY

DIABETIC KETOACIDOSIS

Glaser N, Barnett P, McCaslin I, et al: Risk factors for cerebral edema in children with diabetic ketoacidosis: The Pediatric Emergency Medicine Collaborative Research Committee of the American Academy of Pediatrics. *N Engl J Med* 344: 264–269, 2001.

Harris GD, Fiordalisi I: Physiologic management of DKA. *Arch Dis Child* 87:451–452, 2002.

Kaufman FR, Halvorson M: The treatment and prevention of diabetic ketoacidosis in children and adolescents with type I diabetes mellitus. *Pediatr Ann* 28:576–582, 1999.

Kitabchi AE, Umpierrez GE, Murphy MB, et al: Management of hyperglycemic crises in patients with diabetes. *Diabetes Care* 24:131–153, 2001.

White NH: Diabetic ketoacidosis in children. *Endocrinol Metab Clin North Am* 29:657–682, 2000.

Zangen D, Levitsky LL: Diabetic ketoacidosis. In: Lifshitz F, ed. *Pediatric Endocrinology.* New York: Marcel Dekker, 631–643, 1996.

HYPOGLYCEMIA

Aquilar-Bryan L, Bryan J, Nakazaki M: The focal form of persistent hyperinsulinemic hypoglycemia of infancy. *Recent Prog Horm Res* 56:47–68, 2001.

Becker DJ, Ryan CM: Hypoglycemia: A complication of diabetes therapy in children. *Trends Endocrinol Metab* 11: 198–202, 2000.

Cornblath M, Hawdon JM, Williams AF, et al: Controversies regarding definition of neonatal hypoglycemia: Suggested operational thresholds. *Pediatrics* 105:1141–1145, 2000.

Edidin DV, Farrell EE, Gould VE: Factitious hyperinsulinemic hypoglycemia in infancy: Diagnostic pitfalls. *Clin Pediatr (Phila)* 39:117–119, 2000.

Schiaffini R, Ciampalini P, Fierabracci A, et al: The continuous glucose monitoring system (CGMS) in type 1 diabetic children is the way to reduce hypoglycemic risk. *Diabetes Metab Res Rev* 18:324–329, 2002.

QUESTIONS

1. A 14-year-old female with a history of diabetes presents with complaints of a week history of fever, cough, and generalized weakness. On further questioning, she reports polyuria and polydipsia. On physical examination, the vitals are: T101°F, P120, RR 24, BP 110/70, Pulse ox 100%. Findings on examination include dry mucous membranes. Lungs are clear but she is tachypneic without wheezing or retractions. The initial accucheck is read as 600 and she is noted to have ketones in her urine. Which of the following would be the best initial approach to managing this patient?
   A. Stat CXR and initiation of antibiotics
   B. Insulin bolus of 0.1 U/kg then IV fluids
   C. A 20 mL/kg fluid bolus over 1 to 2 h
   D. Initiate potassium 40 mEq/L of IV fluids
   E. Diabetic education regarding adjusting insulin doses during illness

2. Which of the following is true regarding diabetic ketoacidosis (DKA)?
   A. Is caused by insulin resistance
   B. Is characterized by hyperglycemia, dehydration, and metabolic alkalosis
   C. Can most often be managed on an outpatient basis
   D. Most DKA is precipitated by infection
   E. Supplemental bicarbonate has been shown to improve outcome

3. A 6-year-old boy with new onset DKA is admitted to the unit. Six h after initiation of treatment, he complains of a headache and dizziness. He is noted to be drowsy and has urinary incontinence. The most likely cause of these symptoms is which of the following?
   A. Hypoglycemia
   B. Cerebral edema
   C. Hypokalemia
   D. Munchausen by proxy
   E. Hyponatremia

4. How should the patient in the previous question be managed?
   A. Hyperventilation, mannitol, and fluid restriction
   B. Consult neurosurgery for an emergent craniotomy
   C. Bilateral burr holes
   D. Order q 15-min neurologic checks
   E. Maintain the serum glucose at 150 to 200

5. Which of the following is true regarding serum sodium in cases of hyperglycemia?
   A. Serum sodium levels are accurate
   B. Must be corrected using the serum bicarbonate level
   C. Is falsely elevated
   D. Is falsely lowered
   E. Is only corrected for cases with serum glucoses above 500

6. Which of the following is the most common cause of hypoglycemia in children seen in the ED?

A. Hypopituitarism
B. Adrenal insufficiency
C. Idiopathic ketotic hypoglycemia
D. Adverse reaction to insulin therapy in a diabetic
E. Autosomal recessive persistent hyperinsulinemic hypoglycemia of infancy

7. An 8-year-old boy presents with symptoms of hypoglycemia and an accucheck of 30. A glucagon challenge is given and the blood sugar rises to 100. What is the most likely etiology of the hypoglycemia?
A. Hyperinsulinemia
B. Glycogen storage disease
C. Malnutrition
D. Ketotic hypoglycemia
E. Liver failure

ANSWERS

1. C. This patient is in DKA. The best initial therapy is fluid resuscitation with normal saline or Ringer's lactate at a dose of 20 mL/kg over 1 to 2 hours if the patient is stable. An initial bolus of insulin is not necessary and may precipitate rapid fluid exchanges. Potassium replacement is started once a normal or low serum potassium is ensured and there is a urine output. Although diabetic education is important, it is not the priority in initial management of this patient.

2. D. DKA is caused by an absolute or relative lack of insulin and is characterized by hyperglycemia, dehydration, and metabolic acidosis. Most cases are managed in the hospital and if severe acidosis in an intensive care unit. Most DKA is precipitated by infection or inadequate insulin supplementation during an illness. Clinical studies have failed to demonstrate improved outcome in patients treated with supplemental bicarbonate and is reserved for severe acidosis.

3. B. Cerebral edema is the most feared and lethal complication of DKA. Clinical complaints include headache, dizziness, changes in behavior, incontinence, and alterations in pulse and blood pressure indicative of increased intracranial pressure. The etiology is unknown.

4. A. The treatment of cerebral edema consists of hyperventilation, mannitol, and fluid restriction to decrease intracranial pressure.

5. D. The hyperglycemia causes the serum sodium to be falsely lowered. For each 100 mg/dL increment in plasma glucose above a normal, there is an expected decrease of 1.6 mg/dL in serum sodium.

6. D. All of the answers cause hypoglycemia but the most common cause of hypoglycemia in children seen in the ED is an adverse reaction to insulin therapy in a known diabetic.

7. A. A glucagon challenge is useful for both diagnosis and treatment if time permits. A positive challenge (blood glucose rising >40 mg/dL over baseline) suggests hyperinsulinism. A negative challenge (blood glucose rise <40 mg/dL over baseline) suggests poor glycogen stores such as with undernutrition, ketotic hypoglycemia, liver failure, or glycogen storage disease.

55 ADRENAL INSUFFICIENCY

Elizabeth E. Baumann
Robert L. Rosenfield
Gary R. Strange
Heather M. Prendergast

PATHOPHYSIOLOGY

- The symptoms of adrenal insufficiency (AI) result from deficiencies of two classes of hormones secreted by the adrenal cortex:
  ○ Glucocorticoid deficiency results from lack of cortisol
  ○ Mineralocorticoid deficiency results from lack of aldosterone
- Glucocorticoid deficiency impairs gluconeogenesis and glycogenolysis, resulting in fasting hypoglycemia. It also resets the "osmostat" and causes dilutional hyponatremia via the syndrome of inappropriate secretion of antidiuretic hormone (SIADH).
- Aldosterone deficiency results in decreased sodium retention by the kidney, resulting in osmotic diuresis, hyponatremia, hypovolemia, and vascular collapse. In addition, it causes a decreased distal renal tubular exchange of potassium and hydrogen ions for sodium ions, leading to hyperkalemia and acidosis.
- AI is classified as:
  ○ Primary (adrenocortical failure)
  ○ Secondary (pituitary failure)
  ○ Tertiary (hypothalamic failure)
- Primary and tertiary AI, due to withdrawal from exogenous steroid administration and suppression of cortisol synthesis, are the two most common causes of adrenal crisis.
- The most common cause of primary AI in infants is congenital adrenal hyperplasia which, in the female newborn, presents with genital ambiguity secondary to virilization in utero. Hypotension, hyponatremia, hyperkalemia, natriuresis, and shock typically do not develop until about 7 to 14 days postnatally, and may be the presenting symptoms, especially in boys.

- Acquired causes of primary AI in children are less common than congenital disorders. Acquired AI results from autoimmune, infectious, infiltrative, hemorrhagic, or ablative disorders.

CLINICAL PRESENTATION

- The onset of primary AI is usually gradual, resulting in partial corticoid deficiencies and vague symptoms of fatigue, anorexia, postural hypotension, or polyuria. However, primary AI in the presence of intercurrent illness or stress can present as shock, especially in infants.
- Signs of primary AI include hyperpigmentation, most notably in areas exposed to the sun, areas subject to friction, the buccal mucosa, areolae, and anal mucosa.
- Laboratory findings in primary AI include hypoglycemia, hyponatremia, hypochloremia, hyperkalemia, and metabolic acidosis. An increased blood urea nitrogen:creatinine ratio occurs as the result of dehydration.

MANAGEMENT

- If the patient's condition permits, synthetic ACTH (Cosyntropin) $0.15\,mg/m^2$ is administered and cortisol levels obtained 30 to 60 min later. Treatment of individuals in adrenal crisis with steroids should never be delayed inordinately to perform diagnostic tests. However, the rapid ACTH test can usually be completed in the first 30 to 60 min of treatment while fluid resuscitation is occurring. At the very least, a baseline level of cortisol and ACTH should be obtained in anyone presenting with unexplained shock.
- Fluid therapy should begin by giving a $20\,mL/kg$ bolus of 5% dextrose/normal saline IV. Specific treatment requires glucocorticoid therapy with hydrocortisone, $50\,mg/m^2/dose$ IV every 6 h. Mineralocorticoid need not be given in acute adrenal crisis, as high-dose hydrocortisone has mineralocorticoid-like action. Diagnosis and treatment of the underlying stressor, such as infection, should be addressed.

BIBLIOGRAPHY

Keffer JR: Endocrinology, In: Siberry GK, Iannone R, eds. *The Harriet Lane Handbook: A Manual for Pediatric House Officers*, 15th ed. St. Louis: Mosby, 207–228, 2000.

Muglia LJ, Mazoub JA: Disorders of the posterior pituitary. In: Sperling MA, ed. *Pediatric Endocrinology*. Philadelphia: Saunders, 195–227, 1996.

New MI, Rapaport R: The adrenal cortex. In: Sperling MA, ed. *Pediatric Endocrinology*. Philadelphia: Saunders, 195–227, 1996.

Rosenfield RL, Qin K: Adrenocortical disorders in infancy and childhood. In: Becker KL, ed. *Principles and Practice of Endocrinology and Metabolism*, 3d ed. Philadelphia: Lippincott, 806–816, 2001.

Werbel SS, Ober KP: Acute adrenal insufficiency. *Endocrinol Metab Clin North Am* 22:303, 1993.

QUESTIONS

1. Signs and symptoms of a mineralocorticoid deficiency are the result of:
   A. Lack of cortisol
   B. Excessive cortisol levels
   C. Lack of aldosterone
   D. Excessive aldosterone levels
   E. Lack of catecholamines
2. An infant with suspected primary adrenal insufficiency (AI) is brought to the emergency department for evaluation. Which of the following symptoms would heighten your index of suspicion for AI?
   A. Hyperglycemia
   B. Decreased urine output
   C. Hypernatremia
   D. Hyperkalemia
   E. Hypertension
3. Which disease state is commonly associated with a glucocorticoid deficiency?
   A. Cushing's syndrome
   B. SIADH
   C. Myxedema coma
   D. Osmotic diuresis
   E. Type I diabetes mellitus
4. Systemic manifestations of congenital adrenal hyperplasia in the newborn male are typically seen at what stage?
   A. Delivery
   B. 12 to 24 h postnatal
   C. 24 to 48 h postnatal
   D. 7 to 14 days postnatal
   E. 2 months of age
5. A management priority in a child with adrenal insufficiency during an acute adrenal crisis would include administration of which of the following?
   A. Mineralocorticoids
   B. Normal saline fluid bolus
   C. Cosyntropin
   D. Broad spectrum antibiotics
   E. Glucocorticoids

ANSWERS

1. C. Primary adrenal insufficiency results from deficiencies of both cortisol and aldosterone. However, mineral corticoid deficiency is due to a lack of aldosterone.
2. D. The onset of primary AI is often gradual; however, in the presence of intercurrent illness, it can present as shock in infants. Associated signs include hypotension, hyponatremia, hyperkalemia, and natriuresis.
3. B. Patients with a glucocorticoid deficiency experience a dilutional hyponatremia manifested via the syndrome of inappropriate secretion of antidiuretic hormone (SIADH). Addison's disease is the result of primary adrenal insufficiency secondary to the destruction of the adrenal cortex.
4. D. Presentations of congenital adrenal hyperplasia can differ between infant girls and boys. Newborn females often present with genital ambiguity secondary to virilization in utero. Infant boys tend to present in shock 7 to 14 days postnatally.
5. E. In adrenal crisis corticosteroids must be a priority, and should NEVER be delayed to perform diagnostic tests. Hydrocortisone should be given as a bolus. Fluid therapy should begin with 20 mL/kg bolus of 5% dextrose/normal saline. The rapid ACTH test (Cosyntropin) can be performed after the resuscitation has been started in patients with unexplained signs and symptoms of shock and an unclear diagnosis.

56 HYPERTHYROIDISM

Elizabeth E. Baumann
Robert L. Rosenfield
Gary R. Strange
Valerie A. Dobiesz

PATHOPHYSIOLOGY

- Thyrotoxicosis results from thyroid hormone excess due either to overproduction of thyroid hormone by the thyroid gland itself or by administration of exogenous synthetic hormone.
- Thyroid hormones activate the adrenergic system by inducing β-adrenergic receptors. Symptoms of sympathetic nervous system overactivity, including hyperthermia, may be present in thyrotoxicosis. The manifestations of thyroid hormone excess can be blocked by β-adrenergic antagonists.

- Specific conditions are known to precipitate thyroid storm in a patient with hyperthyroidism. They include thyroid surgery, withdrawal of antithyroid medications, radioiodine therapy, vigorous palpitation of a generous goiter, iodinated contrast dyes, or states in which thyroid hormone levels drastically increase, such as emotional distress, general surgery, infection, or other conditions that produce a high degree of stress.

ETIOLOGY

- The most common disorder causing thyrotoxicosis in children, as in adults, is the autoimmune disorder Graves' disease. This accounts for 10 to 15 percent of all childhood thyroid diseases.
- In 5 to 10 percent of thyrotoxicosis, the disorder is due to a variant type of chronic autoimmune thyroiditis called hashitoxicosis. Patients present with goiter without ophthalmopathy.
- In an even smaller percentage of patients, subacute thyroiditis can cause thyrotoxicosis due to destruction of thyroid tissue. This process is usually due to viral or granulomatous diseases, classically presents with a painful thyroid gland, and is self-limiting.
- Autonomously functioning thyroid nodules, typically single (toxic adenoma), are sometimes encountered in children. Multinodular goiters with thyrotoxicosis are unusual in childhood.
- Rarely, hyperthyroidism is secondary to TSH oversecretion from a pituitary tumor or to isolated pituitary resistance to negative feedback control by thyroid hormones on a genetic basis. Signs of an intracranial mass may be present with the former. Goiter is present with both.
- A less common condition is neonatal thyrotoxicosis. It is caused by transplacental passage of TSA from a mother with Graves' disease to her fetus.
- The possibility of a molar pregnancy, which may elaborate a thyroid stimulator, must be considered in adolescent females with thyrotoxicosis to guide appropriate therapy. Oversecretion of T_4 from ectopic thyroid tissue lying within a teratoma of the ovary (struma ovarii) can cause thyrotoxicosis.

CLINICAL PRESENTATION

- Children who present with thyrotoxicosis complain of nervousness, palpitations, weight loss, muscle weakness, and fatigue. A history of declining school performance, due to a decreased attention span, can usually be elicited.
- A goiter, although nonspecific, is the most common physical finding in Graves' disease. The eye signs are usually subtle in children.

- Signs of sympathetic overactivity are common and include tremor, brisk deep tendon reflexes, tachycardia, supraventricular tachycardia, flow murmur, overactive precordium, and a widened pulse pressure. Other cardiac disturbances may occur, such as atrial fibrillation, atrioventricular block, sinoatrial block, or congestive heart failure (CHF) due to the inability of cardiac function to meet metabolic demands.
- Thyroid storm is suggested by severe hyperpyrexia, atrial dysrhythmia, CHF, delirium or psychosis, severe gastrointestinal hyperactivity, and hepatic dysfunction with jaundice. A key feature in thyroid storm is a precipitating event, illness, or major stress, which should be sought and identified.

MANAGEMENT

- Complete blockade of new hormone synthesis can be accomplished by the administration of propylthiouracil (PTU) at a dosage of 175 mg/m^2 per day or 4 to 6 mg/kg per day at 6- or 8-h intervals. To block release of thyroid hormone from the gland in thyroid storm, inorganic iodine therapy (as Lugol's solution or SSKI) is started 1 h after antithyroid medication is initiated.
- Beta-adrenergic antagonists are useful in the management of severe thyrotoxicosis or thyroid storm. They are most clearly indicated for tachyarrhythmias. Propranolol, in addition to its antiadrenergic effects, modestly decreases the conversion of T$_4$ to T$_3$.
- Glucocorticoids are indicated in thyroid storm to inhibit peripheral conversion of T$_4$ to T$_3$ and for their immunosuppressive effect. Hydrocortisone should be used in stress doses of 50 mg/m^2 IV every 6 h.
- If metabolic decompensation has occurred as the result of thyroid storm, management must include a measure to reverse hyperthermia, such as acetaminophen or cooling blankets. Salicylates must be avoided because they can displace thyroid hormone from binding sites, potentially worsening the hypermetabolic state.
- Plasmapheresis has been used for the physical removal of thyroid hormone. This should be reserved for cases of thyroid storm or thyroid hormone poisoning refractory to conventional treatment.

DISPOSITION

- Patients who present in severe thyrotoxicosis or thyroid storm and those with cardiovascular compromise should immediately be transported to an intensive care unit. Patients with a milder presentation may be discharged home after baseline thyroid function studies are obtained and propranolol is initiated, as needed.

BIBLIOGRAPHY

Burch HB, Wartofsky L: Life-threatening thyrotoxicosis: Thyroid storm. *Endocrinol Metab Clin North Am* 22:263, 1993.

Dotsch J, Rascher W, Dorr HG: Graves disease in childhood: A review of the options for diagnosis and treatment. *Paediatr Drugs* 5:95–102, 2003.

Kadmon PM, Noto RB, Boney CM, et al: Thyroid storm in a child following radioactive iodine (RAI) therapy: A consequence of RAI vs withdrawal of antithyroid medication. *J Clin Endocrinol Metab* 86:1865–1867, 2001.

Keffer JR: Endocrinology. In: Siberry GK, Iannone R, eds. *The Harriet Lane Handbook*, 15th ed. St. Louis: Mosby, 207–228, 2000.

Kraiem Z, Newfield RS: Graves' disease in childhood. *J Pediatr Endocrinol Metab* 14:229–243, 2001.

Roti E, Vagenakis AG: Intrinsic and extrinsic variables; effect of excess iodide: Clinical aspects. In: Braverman LE, Utiger RD, eds. *Werner and Ingbar's, The Thyroid: A Fundamental and Clinical Text.* Philadelphia: Lippincott, 316–327, 1996.

QUESTIONS

1. Which of the following conditions would be least likely to precipitate thyroid storm in a patient with hyperthyroidism?
   A. Infection
   B. Emotional distress
   C. General surgery
   D. Radioiodine therapy
   E. Cannabinoid use
2. Which of the following is correct regarding the etiology of thyrotoxicosis in children?
   A. The most common etiology is Graves' disease.
   B. In children it is never caused by a pituitary tumor.
   C. Neonatal thyrotoxicosis is caused by a toxic adenoma.
   D. The most common etiology is hashitoxicosis.
   E. Multinodular goiters with thyrotoxicosis are common in childhood.
3. A 14-year-old female presents to the ED with the complaints of fever, palpitations, feeling nervous, muscle weakness, and weight loss. On physical examination, she has P140, BP 110/80, RR 22, T101°C. She is noted to have a goiter and her deep tendon reflexes are brisk. The cause of her symptoms is most likely due to which of the following?
   A. Parasympathetic stimulation
   B. Stimulation of the adrenergic system
   C. A toxic ingestion
   D. Adrenal insufficiency
   E. Myxedema coma

4. In the patient from the previous question, which medication should not be administered?
   A. Propylthiouracil (PTU)
   B. Inorganic iodine therapy
   C. Tylenol
   D. Salicylates
   E. Glucocorticoids
5. Which of the follow is correct in matching the treatment to its mechanism of action in the treatment of thyroid storm?
   A. Propylthiouracil – blocks the release of thyroid hormone from the gland
   B. Inorganic iodine – blocks the synthesis of hormone
   C. Glucocorticoids – inhibits peripheral conversion of T_4 to T_3
   D. Beta-adrenergic antagonists – binds to thyroid receptor sites resulting in competitive inhibition
   E. Plasmapheresis – decreases the size of the goiter

ANSWERS

1. E. Specific conditions known to precipitate thyroid storm in a patient with hyperthyroidism include thyroid surgery, withdrawal of antithyroid medications, radioiodine therapy, vigorous palpation of a generous goiter, iodinated contrast dyes, emotional distress, general surgery, infection, or other conditions that produce a high degree of stress.
2. A. The most common disorder causing thyrotoxicosis in children is the autoimmune disorder Graves' disease. Rarely, hyperthyroidism can be secondary to TSH oversecretion from a pituitary tumor. Neonatal thyrotoxicosis is caused by transplacental passage of TSA from a mother with Graves' disease to her fetus. Multinodular goiters with thyrotoxicosis are unusual in childhood.
3. B. This patient has a classic presentation for thyrotoxicosis, which causes activation of the adrenergic system by inducing beta-adrenergic receptors. The symptoms she is experiencing are related to symptoms of sympathetic nervous system overactivity.
4. D. Salicylates must be avoided because they can displace thyroid hormone from binding sites, potentially worsening the hypermetabolic state. All the other medications are appropriate in the treatment of this patient.
5. C. Glucocorticoids inhibit the peripheral conversion of T_4 to T_3 and also have an immunosuppressive effect. PTU blocks new hormone synthesis. Inorganic iodine blocks the release of thyroid hormone from the gland and must be started 1 h after antithyroid medication is initiated. Beta-adrenergic antagonists, such as propanolol, have antiadrenergic effects as well as causing modest decreases in the conversion of T_4 to

T_3. Plasmapheresis is used in refractory cases to remove thyroid hormone.

57 FLUIDS AND ELECTROLYTES

Susan A. Kecskes
Gary R. Strange
Heather M. Prendergast

FLUIDS

FLUID COMPARTMENTS

- Total body water (TBW) is divided into the intracellular and extracellular compartments, with the extracellular compartment subdivided into intravascular and extravascular compartments. The relative size of these compartments varies with age. By the time the child is 1 year of age, TBW comprises approximately 60 percent of body weight and is approaching the adult distribution of one third in the extracellular compartments and two thirds in the intracellular compartments (Table 57-1).

MOVEMENT OF FLUID

- Cellular membranes form the barrier between the extracellular and intracellular spaces. They are freely permeable to water, but impermeable to electrolytes and proteins, except by active transport. Although the specific osmoles differ in the two compartments, the osmolality is equal.
- The vascular endothelium forms the barrier between the intravascular and interstitial spaces. It is permeable to water and electrolytes, but not to protein. Two forces regulate fluid movement. Hydrostatic pressure, created by the propulsion of blood through vessels, favors movement of fluid from the intravascular space to the interstitial space. Oncotic pressure, exerted primarily by albumin found in the vascular space, favors water movement from the interstitium into the vascular space.
- Free water added to the vascular space will distribute proportionally to all three compartments. Isotonic crystalloid distributes throughout the extracellular space. Isooncotic fluid will remain in the vascular space, with the exception of a small distribution to the interstitial space because of the increase in hydrostatic pressure.

TABLE 57-1   Distribution of Body Water Between Extracellular and Intracellular Fluid as a Percent of Body Weight

AGE	TOTAL WATER, %	EXTRACELLULAR WATER, %	INTRACELLULAR WATER, %	EXTRACELLULAR WATER/ INTRACELLULAR WATER
0–1 Day	79.0	43.9	35.1	1.25
1–10 Days	74.0	39.7	34.3	1.14
1–3 Months	72.3	32.2	40.1	0.80
3–6 Months	70.1	30.1	40.0	0.75
6–12 Months	60.4	27.4	33.0	0.83
1–2 Years	58.7	25.6	33.1	0.77
2–3 Years	63.5	26.7	36.8	0.73
3–5 Years	62.2	21.4	40.8	0.52
5–10 Years	61.5	22.0	39.5	0.56
10–16 Years	58.0	18.7	39.3	0.48

SOURCE: As modified from Holiday MA: Body fluid physiology during growth, in Maxwell MH, Kleeman CR (eds): *Clinical Disorders of Fluid and Electrolyte Metabolism*, 2d ed. New York, McGraw-Hill, 1972, p 544, with permission.

FLUID REQUIREMENTS

- Fluid requirements can be divided into three categories:
  - Maintenance fluids, which replace routine daily fluid losses
  - Replacement of a fluid deficit, if needed
  - Ongoing excessive losses
- Maintenance fluids include insensible losses and routine outputs of urine and stool. These are proportional to the body surface area (BSA). Since infants and children have a higher body surface area per kilogram, they also have proportionally higher fluid requirements. There are four common methods to calculate maintenance fluids (Table 57-2).
- Many patients have fluid deficits that require replacement. In pediatrics, the most common cause is gastrointestinal disease associated with vomiting and diarrhea.
- The first priority in patients with fluid deficits is to restore circulation. To begin, the adequacy of the patient's perfusion is determined (Table 57-3).
- If the patient's perfusion is inadequate, fluid resuscitation should be initiated. An initial bolus of 20 mL/kg of isotonic crystalloid [0.9% NaCl or lactated Ringer's (LR) solution] is given intravenously over <20 min. The patient is reassessed and further boluses are given until perfusion is adequate.

TABLE 57-2   Four Methods for Maintenance Fluid Calculations

Body Surface Area Method

1500 mL/BSA (m^2)/day

100/50/20 Method

Weight	Fluid
0–10 kg	100 mL/kg/day
11–20 kg	100 mL + 50 mL/kg/day for every kg >10 kg
>20 kg	1500 mL + 20 mL/kg/day for every kg >20 kg

4/2/1 Method

Weight	Fluid
0–10 kg	4 mL/kg/h
11–20 kg	40 mL + 2 mL/kg/h for every kg >10 kg
>20 kg	60 mL + 1 mL/kg/h for every kg >20 kg

Insensible + Measured Losses Method

400–600 mL/BSA (m^2)/day + urine output (mL/mL) + L
L = other measured losses (mL/mL)

- Pediatric patients commonly require >60 mL/kg of resuscitation fluid to restore perfusion. If required, blood products may be substituted for some of the bolus fluid.
- Some patients may require replacement of ongoing fluid losses not included in normal maintenance requirements (Table 57-4).

TABLE 57-3   Signs and Symptoms of Dehydration

	MILD (5% TBW)	MODERATE (10% TBW)	SEVERE (15% TBW)
Mental status	Alert	Irritable; drowsy	Lethargic
Skin turgor	Brisk retraction	Mild delay	Prolonged retraction
Anterior fontanel	Normal	Minimally sunken	Sunken
Eyes	Moist; + tears	Dry; no tears	Sunken; no tears
Mucous membranes	Moist	Dry	Very dry
Pulses	Normal	Rapid; weak peripherally	Rapid; weak centrally
Capillary refill	<2 s	2–5 s	>5 s
Respiration	Normal	Rapid	Deep and rapid
Urine output	>1 mL/kg/h	<1 mL/kg/h	Minimal or absent
Blood pressure	Normal	Low normal	Hypotension

TABLE 57-4   Adjustments to Maintenance Fluids

Fever	Increase maintenance fluids by 10% for each degree >37.8°C.
Tachypnea (nonhumidified environment)	Increase maintenance fluids by 5–10%.
Vomiting and gastric loss	Replace with 0.45% NaCl with 10 mEq/L KCl.
Stool loss	Replace with LR with 15 mEq/L KCl or 0.45% NaCl with 20 mEq/L KCl and 20 mEq/L NaHCO$_3$.
Cerebrospinal fluid	Replace with LR or 0.9% NaCl.
Pleural fluid, peritoneal fluid, wound drainage (serous)	Replace with LR or 0.9% NaCl; may need to replace albumin periodically—base replacement on measured serum albumin levels.
Blood	≤25% TBV[a]: Replace with LR or 0.9% NaCl; assess hematocrit and physiologic status for administration of blood.
	>25% TBV[a]: Replace one-half to two-thirds of loss as whole blood and reassess. Alternatively, use "3-for-1" and replace 3 × the blood loss with LR or 0.9% NaCl.
Third-space losses	Estimate based on patient's physiologic status. Replace with LR or 0.9% NaCl.

[a]TBV = Total blood volume.

SODIUM

HYPERNATREMIA

- Hypernatremia is defined as serum sodium >150 mEq/L. It may result from intake of sodium in excess of water or, more commonly, from loss of water in excess of sodium (Table 57-5).
- Diabetes insipidus (DI) is a less common cause of hypovolemic hypernatremia. The essential feature is a functional lack of ADH, resulting in urinary water loss despite increasing osmolarity and hypovolemia. It may be caused by insufficient production and release of ADH (central DI) or end-organ unresponsiveness to ADH (nephrogenic DI).
- Clinical manifestations of hypernatremia depend on the volume status of the patient. In primary sodium excess, the skin is often described as "doughy." In hypovolemic hypernatremia, the signs and symptoms

of dehydration are manifest. In both, the central nervous system is adversely affected.

- Initial therapy of hypovolemic hypernatremia is focused on correction of circulatory failure, if present. Subsequent restoration of total body water should be gradual, over 48 h. Fatal cases of cerebral edema have occurred with correction over 24 h, as fluid enters the already volume-replete brain.
- In patients in whom DI is suspected, a trial of vasopressin may be attempted. The drug of choice is desmopressin (DDAVP). The initial dose is 0.05 to 0.1 mL (5 to 10 μg), delivered intranasally, once or twice per day.
- Primary sodium excess is treated by removal of excess sodium. First, sodium intake is curtailed. In patients with intact renal function, diuretics in combination with administration of hypotonic fluid diminish sodium concentration. Patients with renal failure require dialysis.

HYPONATREMIA

- Hyponatremia is defined as a serum sodium concentration <130 mEq/L and reflects excess body water relative to body sodium. Depending on etiology, total body sodium may be decreased, increased, or normal (Table 57-6). Hyponatremia with decreased total body sodium occurs when sodium loss exceeds water loss.
- Hyponatremia with increased total body sodium occurs when the increase in TBW exceeds sodium retention. Common etiologies include congestive heart failure (CHF) and renal failure.
- Hyponatremia with normal total body sodium is commonly associated with two etiologies in children. First, the syndrome of inappropriate antidiuretic hormone

TABLE 57-5   Causes of Hypernatremia

Sodium excess
    Inadequately diluted infant formula
    Excessive administration of sodium bicarbonate
    Excessive administration of hypertonic saline
Water deficit
    Vomiting and diarrhea
    Increased insensible water loss
    Inadequate access to water
    Diabetes mellitus (osmotic diuresis)
    Diabetes insipidus
        Central
            Brain tumors (i.e., craniopharyngioma)
            Head trauma
            Hypoxic-ischemic brain injury
        Nephrogenic
            Congenital (X-linked recessive)
            Renal disease (renal dysplasia, reflux, polycystic disease)

TABLE 57-6   Causes of Hyponatremia

DECREASED TOTAL BODY SODIUM	NORMAL TOTAL BODY SODIUM (EXCESS WATER)	INCREASED TOTAL BODY SODIUM
Extrarenal sodium loss	SIADH	Congestive heart failure
Vomiting and diarrhea	CNS disorders (ie, meningitis)	Renal failure
Burns	Pulmonary disease	
Peritonitis	Postoperative states	
Pancreatitis	Malignancies	
Renal sodium loss	Glucocorticoid deficiency	
Diuretics	Hypothyroidism	
Osmotic diuresis	Water intoxication	
Salt-losing renal disease	WIC syndrome	
Nephritis		
Obstructive uropathy		
Renal tubular acidosis		
Adrenal insufficiency		

(SIADH) leads to a dilutional hyponatremia. This syndrome is associated with diverse causes including central nervous system disorders, pulmonary disease, postoperative states, malignancies, glucocorticoid deficiency, and hypothyroidism. The most frequent etiology in the pediatric emergency room is meningitis.

- The clinical manifestations of hyponatremia depend on the volume status of the patient, the rapidity of development, and degree of hypoosmolality. In hypovolemic hyponatremia, the symptoms of dehydration and acute circulatory failure prevail. Hyponatremia produces a decrease in the osmolarity of the extracellular fluid (ECF).

- Treatment of hyponatremia begins with an assessment of the patient's volume status and correction of hypovolemic shock, if present. Correction of the hyponatremia requires a loss of water in excess of sodium. This must be undertaken with care, as aggressive correction may lead to the osmotic demyelination syndrome.

POTASSIUM

- While only 2 percent of total body potassium is in the ECF, potassium is the main cation in ICF. Normal potassium concentration in the ECF is 3.5 to 5.5 mEq/L, compared to approximately 150 mEq/L in the ICF.

- Potassium homeostasis is managed through the use of both translocation and excretion. The majority of potassium excretion occurs in the kidney.

- As only 50 percent of a potassium load is excreted in the first 4 to 6 h, translocation allows the body to maintain stable ECF potassium. In the first hours after ingestion, potassium is translocated into cells, primarily in the liver and muscle.

HYPERKALEMIA

- Hyperkalemia is defined as serum potassium >5.5 mEq/L and can result from increased potassium intake, decreased potassium loss, or from redistribution from the intracellular fluid (ICF).

- Acute renal failure is the primary cause of decreased excretion. Less commonly, adrenal insufficiency may result in hyperkalemia due to decreased mineralocorticoid activity.

- Redistribution of potassium from the ICF to the ECF may occur via cell destruction or translocation from intact cells. In patients with trauma, burns, rhabdomyolysis, massive intravascular coagulopathy, or tumor necrosis, injured cells release stores of intracellular potassium into the circulation.

- Pseudohyperkalemia is a common occurrence and must be considered in the differential diagnosis of hyperkalemia. It is associated with hemolysis from the blood draw.

- Most patients with hyperkalemia are relatively asymptomatic. Neuromuscular symptoms begin with paresthesias and progress to muscle weakness and, ultimately, flaccid paralysis.

- An ECG should always be obtained when hyperkalemia is suspected, to confirm the clinical severity. Characteristic changes include peaked T waves, prolongation of the PR interval, and progressive widening of the QRS complex. As potassium continues to rise (typically >8 mEq/L), the classic "sine wave" of hyperkalemia appears (Fig. 57-1).

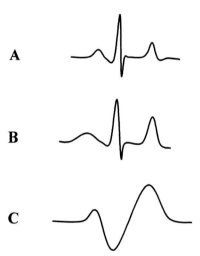

FIG. 57-1 ECG changes in hyperkalemia. *A.* Normal ECG. *B.* ECG with peaked T waves, prolonged PR interval, and widened QRS, seen in moderate hyperkalemia (potassium >7.0 mEq/L). *C.* "Sine wave" ECG seen at potassium levels >8 mEq/L.

- Treatment of hyperkalemia depends on the level of serum potassium, along with the clinical symptoms and renal status of the patient. In all cases, intake of potassium and potassium-sparing medication should be halted.
- In asymptomatic patients with intact renal function and modest (7 mEq/L) levels of serum potassium, halting intake and follow-up of serum potassium levels may be all that is required (Table 57-7).
- Those patients with serum potassium levels >7 mEq/L or who are symptomatic, require aggressive intervention to stabilize the cellular membrane, shift potassium intracellularly, and increase potassium elimination. Membrane stabilization is effected by intravenous administration of calcium. Calcium gluconate, 10 percent, in a dose of 50 to100 mg/kg, or calcium chloride, 10 percent, in a dose of 10 to 25 mg/kg, may be administered over 2 to 5 min with continuous ECG monitoring.

HYPOKALEMIA

- Hypokalemia is defined by a serum potassium level <3.5 mEq/L and can result from decreased intake, increased renal excretion, increased extrarenal losses, or a shift of potassium from the ECF to the ICF. A low-potassium diet, eating disorders such as anorexia nervosa, and prolonged administration of intravenous fluids without potassium, may all lead to hypokalemia.
- Clinical manifestations of hypokalemia are related to its rapidity of onset and degree of severity. Muscle contraction is dependent on membrane polarization and requires a rapid influx of sodium into cells and a comparable efflux of potassium.
- Hypokalemia impairs this process. The result is alteration of nerve conduction and muscle contraction. Clinical symptoms include muscle weakness, ileus,

areflexia, and autonomic instability, often manifested as orthostatic hypotension. Respiratory arrest and rhabdomyolysis can occur.

- Laboratory data should include serum electrolytes, including magnesium, serum pH, and urine potassium. Urine potassium concentration of <15 mEq/L indicates renal conservation and suggests extrarenal loss. An ECG should be done looking for flattening of the T-wave, ST segment depression, U waves, premature atrial and ventricular contractions and dysrhythmias, especially in patients who are on digitalis.

CALCIUM

- Calcium is one of the most abundant and important minerals in the body, with 99 percent of body calcium stored in bone. Of the 1 percent present in the circulation, 40 percent is bound to proteins such as albumin, 15 percent is complexed with anions such as phosphate and citrate, and 45 percent is physiologically free and ionized.
- A serum calcium level measures both ionized and protein-bound calcium. Since approximately half of serum calcium is bound to albumin, the serum calcium level may need to be adjusted for alterations in the albumin level. For every 1 g/dL decrease in serum albumin, true serum calcium may be estimated by adding 0.8 mg/dL. Alternatively, ionized calcium levels are widely available.

HYPERCALCEMIA

- Hypercalcemia is defined as a serum calcium level >10.5 mg/dL. Although often asymptomatic, complaints may include constipation, anorexia, vomiting, abdominal pain, or pancreatitis.
- The conditions in adults that are commonly associated with hypercalcemia (hyperparathyroidism and

TABLE 57-7 Treatment of Hyperkalemia

Halt potassium intake
   Eliminate high potassium food and drink
   Discontinue intravenous potassium-containing solutions
   Discontinue medications high in potassium or which cause increased potassium
Stabilize cell membranes
   Calcium chloride, 10%, 10–25 mg/kg, IV, over 2–5 min *or* calcium gluconate, 10%, 50–100 mg/kg, IV, over 2–5 min
Translocate potassium intracellularly
   Sodium bicarbonate, 1–2 mEq/kg, IV, over 5–10 min
   Regular insulin, 0.25 units/kg, with dextrose, 1 g/kg, administered as a continuous infusion over 2 h
   Albuterol, 2.5 mg for patients <25 kg and 5.0 mg for patients ≥25 kg, nebulized with 2.5 mL 0.9% NaCl
Eliminate potassium
   Sodium polystyrene sulfonate, 1–2 g/kg, PO, NG, or PR
   Diuretics
      Furosemide, 1–2 mg/kg, IV or PO
      Hydrochlorothiazide, 1 mg/kg (maximum 200 mg), PO
   Dialysis

malignancies of the breast, lung, kidney, and head and neck) are rare in children. In children, hypercalcemia with malignancy is associated with bone metastasis or tumor lysis syndrome.

- Laboratory investigation should include total or ionized serum calcium, serum albumin and total protein, electrolytes (including magnesium and phosphorus), BUN, creatinine, CBC, ECG, and urinalysis.
- In symptomatic patients or those with levels >14 mg/dL, therapy is aimed at expansion of ECF, calcium excretion, increased bone storage, and definitive treatment of the underlying cause. Volume expansion is begun with normal saline and followed by diuresis with furosemide to promote calcium excretion.

HYPOCALCEMIA

- Hypocalcemia is defined as serum calcium <9 mg/dL. Major etiologies are hypoparathyroidism and vitamin D deficiency.
- Nonspecific symptoms, including nausea, weakness, paresthesias, and irritability, are typical. Classic physical findings of neuromuscular irritability are Chvostek's and Trousseau's signs. In more severe cases, tetany, seizures, laryngospasm, and psychiatric manifestations may be seen.
- The ECG may show prolongation of the QT interval, bradycardia, and dysrhythmias.
- For significant or symptomatic hypocalcemia, intravenous calcium may be administered cautiously with continuous ECG monitoring. Calcium gluconate, 10 percent (50 to 100 mg/kg/dose), or calcium chloride, 10 percent (10 to 20 mg/kg/dose), may be administered at a maximum rate of 12 min/dose. Intravenous calcium is very irritating to tissues and veins and should be diluted prior to administration.

BIBLIOGRAPHY

Adelman RD, Solhaug MJ: Pathophysiology of body fluids and fluid therapy. In: Behrman RE, Kliegman RM, Jenson HB, eds. *Nelson Textbook of Pediatrics*, 16th ed. Philadelphia: Saunders, 197, 201, 2000.

Adrogue HJ, Madias NE: Hyponatremia. *N Engl J Med* 342:1581, 2000.

Farrar HC, Chande VT, Fitzpatrick DF, et al: Hyponatremia as the cause of seizures in infants: A retrospective analysis of incidence, severity and clinical predictors. *Ann Emerg Med* 26:42, 1995.

Gennari FJ: Current concepts: Hypokalemia. *N Engl J Med* 339:451, 1998.

Lee JH, Arcinue E, Ross BD: Brief report: Organic osmolytes in the brain of an infant with hypernatremia. *N Engl J Med* 331:439, 1994.

Taketomo CK, Hodding JH, Kraus DM: *Pediatric Dosage Handbook*, 7th ed. Hudson, Ohio: Lexi-Comp, 2000.

QUESTIONS

1. Which of the following is true regarding fluid compartments?
   A. Oncotic pressure is responsible for fluid movement from the intravascular space to the interstitial space.
   B. Most cellular membranes are impermeable to passive transport of electrolytes and proteins.
   C. The extracellular and intracellular compartments have a different overall osmolality.
   D. Hydrostatic pressure favors movement of electrolytes and proteins from the intravascular space to the interstitial space.
   E. The relative size of the intravascular and extravascular compartments is largest at birth and decreases with age.

2. A 6-year-old child presents with a history of vomiting and diarrhea for 3 days. On clinical assessment, the child is found to be dehydrated (<5%TBW). The following therapy may be indicated.
   A. An bolus of 20 ml/kg of isotonic crystalloid over 20 min.
   B. Maintenance fluids of D₅0.45 NS to replace fluid deficits and ongoing losses.
   C. A minimum of 60 ml/kg of isotonic crystalloid to restore perfusion.
   D. PO antibiotics after sample for stool culture has been obtained.
   E. Antiemetic suppositories

3. In the case of hypovolemic hypernatremia, prime considerations and management options would include which of the following?
   A. Use of diuretics in combination with hypotonic fluids
   B. Rapid restoration of TBW with successive boluses of isotonic solution within the first 24 h
   C. Prevention of osmotic demyelination syndrome by gradual correction of TBW over 48 h
   D. High index of suspicion for the syndrome of inappropriate antidiuretic hormone (SIADH)
   E. Initiating dialysis for rapid removal of excess sodium

4. Which of the following is characteristic of hypokalemia?
   A. Enhancement of nerve conduction and membrane depolarization in muscle cells

B. Shifting of potassium from the ICF to ECF

C. Symptoms include muscle weakness and areflexia

D. Is most often associated with hemolysis from blood draws

E. Impaired potassium excretion from the kidneys

5. ECG changes suggestive of hyperkalemia include which of the following?

A. Prolonged QT interval

B. Prolonged PR interval

C. T wave inversion

D. Bradycardia

E. ST depression

6. Which of the following is an accepted treatment for hyperkalemia?

A. Aggressive use of potassium-sparing medication.

B. Magnesium sulfate 2 g IV over 1 h

C. Colloid intravenous solution

D. Calcium gluconate 10% over 2 to 5 min

E. Ampule of dextrose

7. A 10-year-old boy is brought to the Emergency Department with a complaint of anorexia, vomiting, and abdominal pain. His evaluation is suggestive of pancreatitis. The patient is most likely to have which of the following associated electrolyte abnormalities?

A. Hyperkalemia

B. Hypercalcemia

C. Hypocalcemia

D. Hypokalemia

E. Hypernatremia

ANSWERS

1. B. Cellular membranes form the barrier between extracellular and intracellular spaces. While the cellular membranes are freely permeable to water, they are impermeable to electrolytes and proteins except by active transport. The overall osmolality is equal between the intracellular and extracellular compartments. The relative size of the fluid compartments varies with age; however, by the age of 1 year begins to approach adult distributions.

2. A. This patient is only mildly dehydrated. Aggressive fluid resuscitation is not warranted. In most cases, an initial bolus would be sufficient. Instituting fluids at a maintenance rate would be inappropriate for the emergency setting. Empirically starting antibiotics is not recommended.

3. A. Initial therapy should be focused on correction of circulatory failure, if present. Restoration of TBW should be done gradually over 48 h to prevent cerebral edema. In patients with intact renal function, diuretics in combination with hypotonic fluids are effective in decreasing the sodium concentration. SIADH and osmotic demyelination syndrome are typically associated with hyponatremia. Dialysis is indicated in patients with renal failure.

4. C. Potassium is the main cation in the ICF. Shifting from the ICF to ECF would lead to hyperkalemia. Hypokalemia impairs muscle contraction and nerve conduction and can lead to muscle weakness and areflexia.

5. B. Characteristic changes include peaked T waves, prolongation of the PR interval, and progressive widening of the QRS complex. Potassium levels >8 mEq/L are associated with the classic "sine wave" of hyperkalemia. Bradycardia and prolonged QT are often associated with hypocalcemia.

6. D. Treatment of hyperkalemia depends on the potassium level and patient's symptoms. Calcium gluconate IV is an effective treatment and aids in membrane stabilization. All potassium-sparing medication must be halted. Administering dextrose without insulin will be ineffective in treating hyperkalemia.

7. B. Common symptoms in hypercalcemia can include constipation, anorexia, vomiting, abdominal pain, and pancreatitis; however, most patients with hypercalcemia are asymptomatic.

58 METABOLIC ACIDOSIS

Margaret Paik
Marshall Lewis
Gary R. Strange
Patricia Lee

PATHOPHYSIOLOGY

- The normal range of pH of body fluids is between 7.35 and 7.45. Modification of two buffering systems, used by the lung and the kidney, helps restore the pH toward the normal range when a disturbance occurs in the acid–base system.

- Values for pH, P_{CO_2}, and HCO_3^- will vary during childhood (Table 58-1). These differences are attributed to the relatively higher production of acid secondary to the increased metabolic demands in children and to an inability of the developing kidney to excrete acid and resorb bicarbonate.

- In general, for every 1 mEq/L fall in the serum bicarbonate, the P_{CO_2} should decrease 1 to 1.5 mm Hg. If the P_{CO_2} is greater than expected, another acid–base disturbance, respiratory acidosis, should be considered; primary respiratory alkalosis should be considered if the P_{CO_2} is lower than expected.

TABLE 58-1 Normal Acid–Base Values for Pediatric Patients

GROUP	pH	P_{CO_2}	tCO_2
Preterm infant	7.35 ± 0.04	32 ± 3	17.9 ± 2.2
Term infant	7.34 ± 0.03	37 ± 1	20.2 ± 0.8
Children	7.41 ± 0.04	39 ± 3	25.2 ± 1.6
Male adults	7.39 ± 0.01	41 ± 2	25.2 ± 1.0

SOURCE: From Edelman CM (ed): *Pediatric Kidney Disease.* Boston: Little Brown, 217, 1992.

METABOLIC ACIDOSIS WITH ELEVATED ANION GAP

- The serum anion gap (AG) is defined as the difference between the measured serum cations and anions.
  ○ The formula for the AG is: $AG = NA^+ - (Cl^- + HCO_3^-)$.
- The normal AG is between 8 and 12 mEq/L and represents serum anions other than chloride and bicarbonate, mostly negatively charged plasma proteins. In the presence of an acid, bicarbonate decreases as it is consumed as a buffer and an unmeasured acid is generated.
- The finding of an elevated AG in the presence of a metabolic acidosis implies the presence of either an endogenously created or an exogenously ingested acid (see Table 79-4). In children, the most likely causes of acute endogenous production of acid are diabetic ketoacidosis, with the production of β-hydroxybutyric acid and acetoacetic acid, and processes that result in anaerobic metabolism and the accumulation of lactic acid.
- Another cause of elevated AG acidosis virtually unique to the pediatric patient is inborn errors of metabolism (IEM). Although these diseases are quite rare individually, as a group, their incidence approaches 1 in 5000 live births (Table 58-2).

TABLE 58-2 Inborn Errors of Metabolism Producing Acidosis

Organic acidemias
  Methylmalonic acidemia
  Propionic acidemia
  Isovaleric acidemia
Amino acidurias
  Maple syrup urine disease
Citrullinemia
Argininosuccinic aciduria
Glycogen storage disease
  Type I
  Type III
Fatty acid oxidation defects

SOURCE: From Burton B: Inborn errors of metabolism: The clinical diagnosis in early infancy. *Pediatrics* 79:359, 1987.

- The diagnosis of an IEM depends on a high degree of suspicion. The typical ED presentation is a neonate with vomiting, lethargy, poor feeding, and failure to thrive.

NONANION GAP METABOLIC ACIDOSIS

- Metabolic acidosis with a normal or near-normal AG results from loss of bicarbonate, either through the gastrointestinal tract or the kidney, or from failure of the kidney to excrete an appropriate amount of hydrogen ion. A relative or absolute compensatory increase in chloride, along with sodium, preserves a normal AG.
- In pediatric patients, acute diarrhea is the most common cause of non-AG metabolic acidosis. Intestinal fluid, high in HCO_3^- and K^+ but low in Cl^-, is lost in the diarrheal fluid.
- The different types of renal tubular acidosis (RTA) are classified as type I or distal, type II or proximal, and type IV, which is associated with hypoaldosteronism and hyperkalemia. There are primary and secondary causes of RTA.
- Distal type I RTA is a defect in the ability of the kidney to secrete H^+, with renal HCO_3^- wasting and an inability to acidify the urine in response to an acid challenge. Patients with distal type I RTA usually cannot lower their urine pH below 5.5, despite severe acidosis.
- Aside from the non-AG hyperchloremic metabolic acidosis, laboratory values in distal RTA may reveal hyponatremia and hypokalemia. Hypokalemia can be severe enough to result in severe muscle weakness.
- Proximal type II RTA can be thought of as a defect in resorbing bicarbonate. Hypokalemia is commonly seen. Unlike patients with distal type I RTA, these children retain the ability to secrete hydrogen into the distal tubule and, therefore, can acidify the urine.
- The diagnosis of RTA is unlikely to be made in the ED, but a high degree of suspicion will lead to an appropriate evaluation, which is usually made in consultation with a pediatric nephrologist.
- The fundamental treatment of all types of RTA is directed at maintaining a normal or nearly normal pH. Most patients can be managed with a supplemental alkali at a dose of 1 to 10 mEq/kg/day. Some patients may require supplemental potassium.

CLINICAL PRESENTATION

- The clinical presentation of metabolic acidosis depends on the underlying disease process and the rapidity with which it developed. Tachypnea is a universal finding in the acutely ill patient. Severe alterations in pH affect mental status, which may vary from agitation to coma.

TREATMENT

• Treatment of an elevated AG acidosis is primarily based on the treatment of the underlying disease. The role of bicarbonate and other buffering agents is somewhat controversial but, in practice, therapy with bicarbonate is rarely indicated.

BIBLIOGRAPHY

Cronan K, Mormal ME: Renal and electrolyte emergencies. In: Fleisher GR, Ludwig S, eds. *Textbook of Pediatric Emergency Medicine*, 4th ed. Philadelphia: Lippincott Williams & Wilkins, 811–858, 2000.

Jospe N, Forbes G: Fluids and electrolytes–clinical aspects. *Pediatr Rev* 17: 395, 1996.

Kartzman NA: Renal tubular acidosis syndromes. *South Med J* 93:1042–1052, 2000.

Lolekha PH, Vanavanan S, Lolekha S: Update on value of the anion gap in clinical diagnosis and laboratory evaluation. *Clin Chim Acta* 307:33, 2001.

Shapiro JI, Kaehny WD: Pathogenesis and management of metabolic acidosis and alkalosis. In: Schrier RW, ed. *Renal and Electrolyte Disorders,* 5th ed. Philadelphia: Lippincott-Raven Publishers, 130–171, 1997.

Swenson ER: Metabolic acidosis. *Respir Care* 46:342, 2001.

QUESTIONS

1. A 3-week-old presents after multiple episodes of emesis and poor feeding per mother. On examination, the neonate appears to be mildly dehydrated with minimal weight gain since birth. Electrolytes are as follows: Na 145, K 3.8, Cl 108, and bicarbonate 18. The most likely cause is:
   A. Anion gap metabolic acidosis due to inborn error of metabolism
   B. Renal tubular acidosis type I
   C. Loss of bicarbonate through the gastrointestinal tract
   D. Hypoaldosteronism
   E. Proximal type II renal tubular acidosis
2. Renal tubular acidosis is characterized by:
   A. Anion gap metabolic acidosis
   B. Failure to lower the urine pH below 5.5, despite severe acidosis
   C. Hypernatremia and hyperkalemia
   D. Hyperaldosteronism
   E. Treatment is aimed at reduction of bicarbonate.

ANSWERS

1. A. This infant presents with an anion gap metabolic acidosis. The typical ED presentation of an inborn error of metabolism is a neonate with vomiting, lethargy, poor feeding, and failure to thrive. The diagnosis of an inborn error of metabolism requires a high degree of suspicion and an anion gap metabolic acidosis is the rule. A metabolic acidosis with a normal or near-normal anion gap can result from loss of bicarbonate, either through the gastrointestinal tract or from the kidney, or from failure of the kidney to excrete an appropriate amount of hydrogen ion, EG, renal tubular acidosis (RTA). RTA is also associated with hypoaldosteronism. In pediatric patients, acute diarrhea is the most common cause of nonanion gap metabolic acidosis.
2. B. RTA is characterized by a nonanion gap acidosis. Distal type I RTA is a defect in the ability of the kidney to secrete hydrogen ions with renal bicarbonate wasting and an inability to acidify the urine in response to an acid challenge. Patients with distal type I RTA usually cannot lower their urine pH below 5.5, despite severe acidosis. Distal RTA may reveal hyponatremia and hypokalemia. Hypoaldosteronism may present with associated RTA. The fundamental treatment of all types of RTA is directed at maintaining a normal or near-normal pH. Most patients can be managed with a supplemental alkali and/or potassium.

59 MALE GENITOURINARY PROBLEMS

Marianne Gausche-Hill
Kemedy K. McQuillen
Heather M. Prendergast

TESTICULAR PAIN AND SCROTAL MASSES

- Separating the causes of scrotal swelling as painful or painless is the first step in determining its etiology (Table 59-1). In all cases of testicular pain or scrotal mass, the possibility of a surgical emergency must be considered and the evaluation and management should proceed accordingly. Additionally, a genitourinary examination should be performed on all children with abdominal or genitourinary complaints, as abdominal pain may be caused by testicular torsion, inguinal hernia, or testicular tumor.

EPIDIDYMITIS

- Epididymitis is more common in adults and adolescents than in it is in young children. It is caused by urinary

TABLE 59-1 Causes of Scrotal Swelling in Children

PAINFUL	PAINLESS
Epididymitis	Testicular tumor
Testicular torsion	Idiopathic scrotal edema
Torsion of the appendix testis	Henoch–Schönlein purpura
Incarcerated hernia	Inguinal hernia
Idiopathic scrotal edema	Hydrocele
Trauma (testicular rupture)	Varicocele
Scrotal cellulitis or inflammation	Anasarca

tract infections (*Escherichia coli, Klebsiella pneumoniae*, and *Pseudomonas aeruginosa*) in young children and by sexually transmitted disease (*Neisseria gonorrhoeae* and *Chlamydia trachomatis*) in older children and adolescents. Antibiotic selection should be based on the likelihood of each, based on age and presentation.

- During evaluation, obtain a careful history about vomiting, fever, urinary symptoms, time course for the onset of symptoms, any previous scrotal pain or surgeries, and any history of trauma or sexual activity.
  - Findings include fever, vomiting, urinary symptoms, and scrotal swelling, pain, and tenderness.
  - Symptoms in young children may be vague and nonspecific.
  - In the older child, the onset is often insidious with pain initially isolated to the hemiscrotum that then becomes diffuse.
  - Physical examination reveals an erythematous, warm, swollen epididymis, testicle, and scrotum. Epididymal tenderness is posterior and lateral to the adjacent testis and can be separated from actual testicular tenderness. Prehn's sign, or relief upon elevation of the scrotum, may be present but is not reliable in distinguishing epididymitis from testicular torsion.
- In prepubescent children, epididymitis is difficult to distinguish from testicular torsion. Although normal in 50 percent of cases of epididymitis, a urinalysis may show white blood cells (WBCs) and bacteria. If WBC and bacteria are present and a UTI is suspected, obtain a urine culture. A complete blood cell count is also usually normal but may reveal an elevated white blood cell count and left shift. In sexually active adolescents, send a urethral swab for *N. gonorrhoeae* and *Chlamydia* studies and blood for VDRL or RPR. If the cause of the scrotal pain is unclear, obtain an immediate urologic consultation and obtain a nuclear medicine testicle scan or color Doppler ultrasonography (US) to rule out a testicular torsion. With epididymitis, the

TABLE 59-2   Antibiotic Therapy for Epididymitis in Children

ANTIBIOTIC	DOSE	ROUTE
OUTPATIENT MANAGEMENT		
Nonsexually active		
Trimethoprim-sulfamethoxazole	8–10 mg/kg/24 h	PO bid for 10–14 days
or cephalexin	25–50 mg/kg/24 h	PO qid for 10 days
Sexually active		
Ceftriaxone plus (if patient ≥9 years of age)	250 mg	IM
doxycycline	100 mg	PO bid for 10 days
or tetracycline plus (if patient <9 years of age)	500 mg	PO qid for 10 days
erythromycin	50 mg/kg/24 h	PO qid for 10 days
INPATIENT MANAGEMENT		
Ampicillin	100 mg/kg/24 h	IV q 6 h
plus gentamicin	7.5 mg/kg/24 h	IV q 8 h
or cefotaxime	50–150 mg/kg/24 h	IV q 6 h
or ceftriaxone	50–100 mg/kg/24 h	IV q 12–24 h

PO, nothing by mouth; bid, twice daily; qid, 4 times daily; IM, intramuscularly.

nuclear scan and the US will reveal normal or increased flow to the affected testis.

- Management is dependent upon the age and toxicity of the child.
  - Children under 1 month of age with an associated UTI should be admitted to the hospital and receive IV antibiotics. This approach should be considered for infants up to 3 months of age.
  - Older infants and children under 2 years of age may also require admission depending on the level of toxicity and associated signs and symptoms.
  - Inpatient antibiotic therapy for infants and children with a suspected urinary source should include ampicillin and an aminoglycoside or cefotaxime (Table 59-2).
  - The majority of children can be managed as outpatients.
  - For the nonsexually active child, although drug resistance is on the rise, trimethoprim (TMP)-sulfamethoxazole orally for 10 to 14 days is the drug of choice. Cephalexin may also be used in this age group.
  - For the sexually active adolescent, especially if there is urethral discharge, antibiotic treatment should include ceftriaxone, 250 mg intramuscularly, followed by doxycycline, 100 mg orally twice a day for 10 days.
    - Patients under 9 years of age should be treated with erythromycin, 50 mg/kg/day divided 4 times a day.
  - Urologic consultation and follow-up is recommended.

TESTICULAR TORSION

- Testicular torsion may occur at any age, with the peak incidence in adolescence. Torsion of the testes is a urologic emergency and must be suspected in any child with scrotal pain or swelling. The "bell clapper" deformity is an anatomic abnormality associated with torsion. It is often bilateral and causes the testes to have a horizontal lie within the scrotal sac (Fig. 59-1). The testicular attachments to the tunica vaginalis are incomplete, allowing twisting of the testis, spermatic cord, and testicular artery. With a complete torsion, vascular compromise rapidly ensues and the testis necroses and atrophies. Intermittent torsion may spare the testes for a longer time interval. After 4 h of pain, the testis salvage rate is 96 percent, but drops to 20 percent after 12 h and to less than 10 percent at 24 h. Patients with symptoms for longer than 24 h are unlikely to have a viable testis.
- Classically, patients present with a sudden onset of unilateral scrotal or testicular pain followed by vomiting. They may also relate a history of previous symptoms on the other side. Many times, the history is less clear and 6 percent of the time includes a history of trauma. Associated symptoms of nausea, vomiting, and abdominal or flank pain are common. Unilateral lower abdominal pain may indicate an undescended testis that has torsed. Undescended testes are 10 times more likely to torse than fully descended ones.
- Physical examination often reveals a swollen, tender, and erythematous hemiscrotum. The testis may be lying horizontally or high within the scrotum. There is diffuse tenderness of the affected testis and the cremasteric reflex may be absent. Elevating the testis will cause further pain; however, this finding cannot be used reliably to include or exclude torsion as the diagnosis.
- In equivocal cases, a urinalysis should be performed looking for signs of UTI or epididymitis. Scrotal Doppler for testicular artery flow may be helpful but has

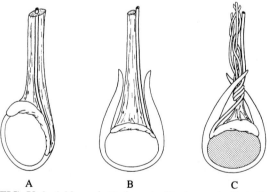

FIG. 59-1 *A.* Normal attachment of tunica vaginalis to the testis. *B.* Abnormal attachment resulting in horizontal lie of the testis. *C.* Resultant torsion of the spermatic cord.

high (20 percent) false-positive and -negative rates. Once the diagnosis of testicular torsion is considered, emergent urologic consultation should be obtained. Further diagnostic evaluation is reserved for those patients in which the diagnosis of torsion is in question and in which any delay in obtaining studies will not result in increased morbidity. Nuclear medicine scan with 99m technetium pertechnetate and color Doppler US may be helpful. With the testicle scan, a unilateral "cold" defect on the side of the testicular pain indicates lack of blood flow to the testis and indicates possible torsion. Accuracy ranges from 86 to 100 percent, but false-positive and -negative scans do occur. Color Doppler US is very accurate in adults for diagnosing testicular torsion (sensitivity: 86 to 100 percent; specificity: 100 percent; accuracy: 97 percent). There may be false-positive studies in prepubescent children because of the small testis and the low volume of arterial flow.

- Obtain rapid urologic consultation for all patients with suspected torsion. While awaiting the urologist, manual detorsion may be attempted. After sedating the patient, turn the testicle outward toward the thigh like "opening a book." Intraoperative bilateral orchiopexy to avoid recurrence is required in all patients. Orchidectomy of the affected testicle is sometimes recommended to prevent autosensitization.

TORSION OF THE APPENDIX TESTIS

- Appendices are common and may occur on the testicle, the spermatic cord, or the epididymis; the appendix testis is the most common to torse. Torsion of the appendix testis frequently occurs between 10 and 14 years of age and signs and symptoms may be indistinguishable from a torsed testicle.
- Nausea and vomiting are rare, and the physical examination may reveal focal tenderness in the upper pole of the testis or diffuse testicular enlargement and pain. A "blue dot" sign is occasionally noted in young children when the necrotic appendage casts a blue hue under the scrotal skin.
- The urinalysis is normal. Testicular scan or color Doppler US may be normal or reveal increased flow to the testicle.
- Treatment is with bed rest, urologic follow-up, and analgesia. If testicular torsion cannot be reliably excluded, surgical intervention is indicated. Patients improve within days and complications are rare.

SCROTAL AND TESTICULAR TRAUMA

- Blunt trauma is the most common cause of traumatic scrotal injury and results in a scrotal hematoma or,

rarely, a testicular rupture. Testicular rupture, which presents with a painful, swollen testis, occurs when the testis is crushed against the bony pelvis. If the injury was minor, consider the possibility of a tumor, as tumors may rupture after an insignificant trauma. Bleeding into the scrotum occurs and the scrotum may be ecchymotic or tense with blood. The testis may be difficult to palpate, ill defined, or have an irregular border. Prompt evaluation by US is essential. US can also locate a testicle that was dislocated after major trauma. Obtain immediate urologic consultation. Testicular rupture is treated by surgical exploration and repair, although salvage rates are poor.
- Scrotal hematomas and testicular contusions are treated with bed rest, scrotal support, ice packs, and analgesics.

TESTICULAR TUMORS

- Testicular tumors are rare in childhood and include teratomas, embryonal carcinomas, yolk sac, choriocarcinomas, Leydig cell, and Sertoli cell tumors. Lymphoma and leukemia can present as a testicular mass as well. The undescended testis is at increased risk for tumor, especially if it is located intraabdominally (50 times).
- Patients present with a feeling of fullness, tugging, or increased weight to the scrotum. They may have felt a mass. On physical examination, the mass is firm, smooth, or nodular and will not transilluminate. The tumor is painless but bleeding into the tumor can cause testicular, abdominal, or flank pain. Physical examination should include examination for lymphadenopathy, abdominal mass, hepatosplenomegaly, petechial rash, and gynecomastia.
- Obtain a urinalysis and complete blood cell count. Perform a rapid urine pregnancy test as human chorionic gonadotropin is often produced by germ cell tumors. Ultrasonography can confirm the presence of a tumor mass.
- Obtain urologic consultation for biopsy or removal of the mass.

INGUINAL HERNIA

- Inguinal hernia repair is the most commonly performed pediatric surgery. An inguinal hernia occurs when peritoneal or pelvic contents herniate through a patent processus vaginalis into the scrotal sac. Inguinal hernias often present in the first year of life when parents note an intermittent bulge in the scrotal sac when the infant cries or coughs. Children may note a pulling feeling or heaviness in the groin and may also note a scrotal bulge with increases in intraabdominal pressure. An inguinal hernia should transilluminate, distinguishing it from a tumor. Fever, abdominal pain, nausea, vomiting, and a firm, painful, nonreducible scrotal mass indicate an incarceration.

- An inguinal hernia can be diagnosed from history and physical examination and further diagnostic evaluation is not needed. US can be done if the diagnosis is in question.
- Reducible inguinal hernias can be referred to a surgeon for elective repair. Most incarcerated hernias can be reduced with firm finger pressure on the internal inguinal ring, analgesics, ice pack to the area, and placement of patients in the Trendelenburg position. If the hernia is reduced easily, patients can be discharged home with close surgical follow-up. Patients with hernias that do not reduce easily, but still can be reduced, should be admitted for observation and delayed surgical repair. Patients with hernias that remain incarcerated, or patients that demonstrate signs of peritonitis or bowel perforation, require immediate surgery after stabilization with fluids and antibiotics.

HENOCH–SCHÖNLEIN PURPURA

- Henoch–Schönlein purpura (HSP) is a systemic vasculitis that often results in abdominal pain, gastrointestinal bleeding, purpuric rash, nephritis, and arthritis. Patients may also complain of testicular pain, scrotal edema and swelling, or a purpuric rash on the scrotum. In some cases, it is impossible to clinically distinguish HSP from testicular torsion. Patients should be treated as if they have testicular torsion.

HYDROCELE

- A hydrocele is formed from a patent processus vaginalis that normally regresses to form the tunica vaginalis. It may be associated with an indirect inguinal hernia. Fluid is noted adjacent to the testis and may result in a swollen, bluish-appearing scrotum. Transillumination reveals that the mass is fluid filled, although it may be difficult to distinguish hydrocele from an indirect inguinal hernia. If the hydrocele becomes painful, then intraperitoneal pathology, such as a ruptured appendix, or a testicular torsion must be considered. If a painless hydrocele persists beyond the first year of life, surgical repair is indicated.

VARICOCELE

- Varicocele often presents in the adolescent male as painless scrotal swelling. Incompetent valves in the veins of the pampiniform plexus result in venous dilatation and a scrotum that feels like a "bag of worms." Approximately 85 percent of varicoceles are left-sided and benign. Fifteen percent result from a tumor obstruction at the level of the renal vein. Right-sided varicoceles may indicate obstruction at the level of the inferior vena cava (IVC). Patients should be examined in the standing position as well as in the supine position, in which findings are minimized or absent. Patients in whom the scrotal swelling persists in the supine position should be evaluated for obstruction by renal ultrasound, IVP, or angiography. Surgical repair may be necessary for cases of testicular atrophy and signs of proximal obstruction.

OTHER CAUSES OF SCROTAL PAIN OR SWELLING

- Other causes of scrotal swelling include scrotal cellulitis, idiopathic scrotal edema, and lymphadenitis.
- **Fournier's gangrene** is a rare entity of infectious origin that results in necrotizing fasciitis. It may present as cellulitis, balanitis, balanoposthitis, or scrotal pain and swelling. Patients may appear relatively nontoxic, even when obvious gangrene appears in the perineum. Although staphylococcal and streptococcal organisms are the most common organisms, management includes broad spectrum antibiotic therapy to cover anaerobic, aerobic, gram-positive, and -negative organisms. Prompt surgical consultation and operative excision of necrotic tissue is paramount. The prognosis is better in children than in adults.

PENILE EMERGENCIES

PHIMOSIS

- Phimosis occurs when the distal prepuce is unable to be retracted over the glans penis. Normally, the prepuce cannot be retracted over the glans until boys are 6 years old, at which time 90 percent will be retractable. Local irritation or infection (**balanoposthitis**) can cause a constriction of the prepuce, preventing it from retracting normally.
- Phimosis may be noted on routine examination or may be reported by parents. Pain and swelling can occur with associated infections of the glans. Urinary stream may be diverted to one side or children may

have hematuria. Physical examination establishes the diagnosis. There will be a constricted distal prepuce that is not retractable over the glans penis. Patients will sometimes have concomitant balanitis or balanoposthitis.

- Examination of the urine for UTI may be warranted in rare cases. If patients demonstrate signs of urinary tract obstruction, obtain renal function studies to assess renal function. Renal US may be obtained to better define the degree of obstruction.
- Most cases of phimosis are a result of normal growth and development and reassurance and an explanation of this condition to parents is needed. Betamethasone valerate 0.6-percent cream applied twice daily for 2 weeks may be prescribed in cases of pathologic phimosis. Patients with recurrent balanitis, balanoposthitis, UTI, or obstruction should be referred to a urologist for circumcision.

PARAPHIMOSIS

- Paraphimosis is a condition in which the prepuce is retracted over the glans and cannot be moved into normal position. This causes venous congestion that further prevents the normal placement of the prepuce.
- Patients have pain, swelling, and edema of the distal penis and prepuce.
- During the evaluation of a child with paraphimosis, establish that the child has not been circumcised and does not have a hair tourniquet.
- Treatment is manual reduction of the prepuce over the glans penis. To attempt, place ice packs over the inflammation for 10 min and then attempt manual reduction by placing the index fingers on the leading edge of the edematous foreskin with the thumbs on the glans. Direct thumb pressure inward as the prepuce is pushed back over the glans (Fig. 59-2). Once reduction is complete, the prepuce should lie over the end of the glans and the urethral opening should not be visible (see Fig. 59-2). If the retraction of the prepuce is successful and the child is able to urinate spontaneously, discharge the child with urologic follow-up. If the prepuce cannot be retracted, obtain emergent urologic consultation for circumcision. If necessary, a penile block can be done by injecting 1-percent lidocaine without epinephrine around the base of the penis.

BALANITIS AND BALANOPOSTHITIS

- Balanitis and balanoposthitis are infections of the glans and foreskin. Both are more common in the uncircumcised male. They frequently present during the preschool years and rarely prior to toilet training. Balanitis may be caused by organisms trapped under the foreskin. Gram-positive and gram-negative bacterial organisms and monilial infections may be causative (Fig. 59-3). In adolescents, syphilis may also be causative. Chronic balanitis or phimosis may result in balanitis xerotica obliterans, a sclerotic disease of the prepuce.
- Signs and symptoms include swelling, erythema, penile discharge, dysuria, bleeding, and, rarely, ulceration of the glans. Phimosis can occur, but is uncommon. Perform a careful examination for a hair tourniquet.
- Balanitis is diagnosed clinically although, in selected cases, a urinalysis or bacterial and chlamydial cultures of penile discharge may be warranted.
- Local care with Sitz baths and topical antibiotic ointment are recommended. Oral antibiotics, such as cephalexin for 5 to 7 days, should be prescribed for more severe cases. Arrange follow up within 2 days. Refer children with repeated episodes to a urologist for elective circumcision.

PRIAPISM

- Priapism is a prolonged painful erection unaccompanied by continued sexual stimulation. It is relatively uncommon in children, except in those with sickle cell disease. Polycythemia and trauma are presumed etiologies. The pathophysiology of priapism can be divided into two mechanisms: low flow or ischemic mechanism (sickle cell disease, polycythemia) or high flow or engorgement mechanism (trauma). Either mechanism results in engorgement of the corpora cavernosum with a flaccid corpora spongiosum and glans. The engorgement leads to inflammation, increased blood stasis, deoxygenation, further sludging, thrombosis, fibrosis, and impotence if unrelieved. Factors that may precipitate priapism in patients with sickle cell anemia are infection, trauma, acidosis, hypoxia, sexual intercourse, and masturbation. Other etiologies include trauma, drugs of abuse (cocaine, amphetamine, alcohol, and marijuana), leukemia, Kawasaki disease, and polycythemia.
- On physical examination, patients have an erect penis, which is firm on the dorsal surface (corpora cavernosum) and soft on the ventral surface (corpora spongiosum) and the glans. There may be associated urinary retention.
- Diagnostic evaluation may include a complete blood cell count, looking for leukemia or anemia, a hemoglobin electrophoresis, looking for possible sickle cell disease, renal function tests, and, if patients have

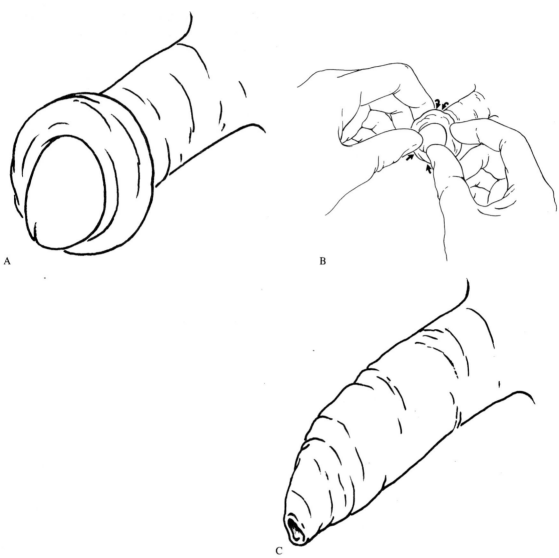

FIG. 59-2 *A.* Paraphimosis. *B.* Manual retraction of the prepuce over the glans. *C.* Normal position of the prepuce.

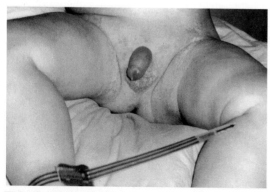

FIG. 59-3 Balanoposthitis in an infant with monilial diaper rash.

suffered perineal trauma, a retrograde cystourethrogram. Color Doppler US can determine if the priapism is due to a low- or high-flow state.

- Treatment is based on the etiology.
  - Provide oxygen, hydration, and analgesics to patients with sickle cell disease and perform an exchange transfusion with 30 mL/kg of packed cells to get the patient's hemoglobin above 10 g/dL.
  - Hydrate and treat pain in patients with leukemia.
  - Place a urinary catheter to relieve bladder distension.
  - Obtain urologic consultation and admit all patients for observation.
  - If medical management is not successful within 24 h, intracavernous injection of a vasoconstrictor (epinephrine, ephedrine, or phenylephrine) should be done.

○ If that is unsuccessful, surgical shunting of blood from the cavernosum to the spongiosum or the glans is recommended. Intravenous ketamine and parenteral vasodilators, including hydralazine or terbutaline, have been used to treat priapism with varying success.

BIBLIOGRAPHY

Cornel EB, Karthaus HF: Manual derotation of the twisted spermatic cord. *Br J Urol* 83:672–674, 1999.

Gahukamble DE, Khamage AS: Early versus delayed repair of reduced incarcerated inguinal hernias in the pediatric population. *J Pediatr Surg* 31:1218, 1996.

Herberner TE: Ultrasound in the assessment of the acute scrotum. *J Clin Ultrasound* 24:405–421, 1996.

Kadish H, Bolte R: A retrospective review of pediatric patients with epididymitis, testicular torsion, and torsion of testicular appendages. *Pediatrics* 102:73–76, 1998.

Klein BL, Ochsenschlager DW: Scrotal masses in children and adolescents: A review for the emergency physician. *Pediatr Emerg Care* 9:351–361, 1993.

Langer J, Coplen D: Circumcision and pediatric disorders of the penis. *Pediatr Clin North Am* 45:801–812, 1998.

Mulhall JP, Honig SC: Priapism: diagnosis and management. *Acad Emerg Med* 3:810–816, 1996.

Niedzielski J, Paduch D, Racynski P: Assessment of adolescent varicocele. *Pediatr Surg Int* 12:410–413, 1997.

Paltiel HJ: Acute scrotal symptoms in boys with an indeterminate clinical presentation: Comparison of color Doppler sonography and scintigraphy. *Radiology* 207:223–231, 1998.

Van Howe R: Cost-effective treatment of phimosis. *Pediatrics* 102:1–4, 1998.

QUESTIONS

1. A 14-year-old boy presents to the emergency department for evaluation of dysuria and lower abdominal pain. He reports mild scrotal swelling and tenderness. He is not sexually active. Physical examination reveals an erythematous, warm, swollen epididymis, testicle, and scrotum. There is tenderness posterior and lateral to the adjacent testis. There is relief upon elevation of the scrotum. A color Doppler ultrasonography (US) reveals increased flow to the affected testis. What is the **MOST** likely diagnosis in this patient?
   A. Testicular torsion
   B. Torsion of the appendix testis
   C. Epididymitis
   D. Inguinal hernia
   E. Testicular tumor

2. A 12-year-old boy is brought by his parents for evaluation of the sudden onset of unilateral right scrotal pain followed by vomiting. The parents report a similar previous episode following minor trauma involving the left scrotal area. Physical examination reveals a swollen, tender, and erythematous hemiscrotum. There is diffuse tenderness of the right testis and you are unable to elicit the cremasteric reflex. Elevation of the testis causes further pain. Which of the following is the **MOST** appropriate management for this patient?
   A. Obtain a stat scrotal Doppler for testicular artery flow
   B. Emergent urologic consultation and comfort measures for patient
   C. Obtain a urinalysis to look for signs of UTI or epididymitis
   D. Obtain a stat color Doppler ultrasound
   E. Emergent urologic consultation and attempt manual detorsion

3. Which of the following is **NOT** true regarding torsion of the appendix testis?
   A. Occurs most frequently between 10 and 14 years of age
   B. A "blue dot" sign is pathognomonic when present
   C. Urinalysis is normal.
   D. Surgical intervention is the preferred treatment.
   E. Signs and symptoms may be indistinguishable from a torsed testicle.

4. A 4-year-old boy is brought by his parents for evaluation of "heaviness" in his groin. On physical examination, you note a scrotal bulge that transilluminates. The mass reduces with firm finger pressure. The **MOST** appropriate course of action would be which of the following?
   A. Admit for 23-h observation
   B. Discharge home with close surgical follow-up
   C. Begin oral antibiotics
   D. Obtain a surgical consultation in the ED
   E. Admit for observation and delayed surgical repair

5. A patient presents for evaluation of a scrotal mass. Transillumination reveals that the mass is fluid filled. What is the **MOST** likely diagnosis?
   A. Hydrocele
   B. Varicocele
   C. Testicular tumor
   D. Epididymitis
   E. Lymphadenitis

6. Which of the following is **NOT** considered a risk factor for priapism?
   A. Sickle cell disease
   B. Trauma

C. Drugs of abuse
D. Leukemia
E. Wilms' tumor

ANSWERS

1. **C.** Epididymitis is more common in adults and adolescents than in younger children. It is caused by urinary tract infections in young children and by sexually transmitted disease in older children and adolescents. Prehn's sign, or relief upon elevation of the scrotum, may be present but is not reliable in distinguishing epididymitis from testicular torsion. Management is dependent upon the age and toxicity of the child.

2. **E.** Testicular torsion may occur at any age, with the peak incidence in adolescence. Torsion of the testes is a urologic emergency and must be suspected in any child with scrotal pain or swelling. Once the diagnosis of testicular torsion is considered, emergent urologic consultation is paramount. Further diagnostic testing is reserved for those patients in which the diagnosis of torsion is in question and in which delay will not cause increased morbidity to the patient. While awaiting the urologist, manual detorsion may be attempted.

3. **D.** Appendices are common and may occur on the testicle, the spermatic cord, or the epididymis. The appendix testis is the most common to torse. Treatment is with bed rest, urologic follow-up, and analgesia. Surgical intervention is indicated when testicular torsion cannot reliably be excluded.

4. **B.** Inguinal hernia repair is the most commonly performed pediatric surgery. An inguinal hernia should transilluminate, distinguishing it from a tumor. Reducible inguinal hernias can be referred to a surgeon for elective repair. Patients with hernias that do not reduce easily, but still can be reduced, should be admitted for observation and delayed surgical repair. Patients with incarcerated hernias require immediate surgery after stabilization with fluids and antibiotics.

5. **A.** A hydrocele is formed from a patent processus vaginalis that normal regresses to form the tunica vaginalis. Fluid is noted adjacent to the testis and may result in a swollen, bluish–appearing scrotum. Transillumination reveals that the mass is fluid filled.

6. **E.** Priapism is a prolonged painful erection unaccompanied by continued sexual stimulation. It can commonly occur in children with sickle cell anemia, polycythemia, and trauma. Risk factors that may precipitate priapism include, drugs of abuse, leukemia, Kawasaki disease, and polycythemia.

60 URINARY TRACT DISEASES

Marianne Gausche-Hill
Kemedy K. McQuillen
Heather M. Prendergast

URINARY TRACT INFECTION

- Urinary tract infection (UTI) affect approximately 5 to 7 percent of infants and children and is a frequent cause of fever. Girls are affected more frequently than boys and uncircumcised boys more frequently than circumcised boys.
- UTIs are caused by bacteria (*Escherichia coli, Proteus* spp., *Klebsiella* spp., *Staphylococcus epidermidis, Pseudomonas aeurginosa,* and *Enterococcus* spp.) that enter the urinary tract from the bowel, the urethra or, in infants less than 3 months old, the bloodstream. Approximately 75 percent of children under 5 years of age with a UTI and fever have pyelonephritis.
- In the infant, signs and symptoms may be nonspecific and include fever, vomiting, and irritability. Older children may have frequency, urgency, dysuria, and hematuria. Patients may also have abdominal or flank pain and vomiting.
- Urine culture is the most important diagnostic test to establish the diagnosis of UTI.
- Urinalysis results may be helpful but can be misleading: approximately 20 percent of young children with a documented UTI have a normal urinalysis for leukocytes and nitrites.
- Bagging the perineum is the least reliable method of obtaining urine with false-positive rates between 85 to 99 percent but they can be used in low-risk patients such as circumcised boys under 1 year of age.
  - If the urine is then positive, obtain urine by catheterization or suprapubic aspiration for culture.
- In infants under 1 year of age and girls or uncircumcised boys under 2 years of age, a catheterized urine specimen should be used.
- If infants require immediate antibiotic administration and are less than 2 years old, the specimen may be collected by suprapubic aspiration.
  - To perform a suprapubic aspiration, prep the infraumbilical abdomen with povidone solution and inject a small wheal of 1-percent lidocaine subcutaneously in the midline, one fingerbreadth above the symphysis pubis. Then, while pulling back on the plunger, insert a 22-gauge, 1½" needle, with a 10-mL syringe at a 60- to 90-degree angle cephalad until urine is obtained. Withdraw the needle, clean the abdomen of

the povidone solution, and apply a bandage over the aspiration site.

○ Complications include hematuria, bowel perforation, cystitis, and abdominal wall hematoma or infection.

- With adequate instruction and supervision, older children may be able to provide a clean catch specimen.
- Electrolyte and renal function tests should be obtained in infants, males, patients with signs of upper tract disease, and those with signs of dehydration or toxicity.
- Neonates, females with pyelonephritis or recurrent UTI, and males of any age should undergo radiologic evaluation for urinary tract abnormalities: up to 50 percent of these patients will have anatomic abnormalities.

○ The most common anatomic abnormality of the urinary tract is vesicoureteral reflux (VUR). It is usually diagnosed in the first decade of life and, in most cases, resolves spontaneously.

○ Voiding cystourethrogram (VCUG) is the diagnostic test for boys and girls. Girls can also be evaluated with isotope cystography (IC).

○ Table 60-1 summarizes the types of diagnostic tests and their indications.

○ Renal cortical scintigraphy (RCS) is displacing intravenous urography (IVU) as the test of choice for upper tract infection evaluation because it is not obscured by bowel contents, does not use highly osmotic agents, rarely causes allergic reactions, is more sensitive in patients with poor renal function, and delivers a lower radiation dose to the gonads. Renal cortical scintigraphy should be performed on patients with fever and UTI to determine upper tract involvement. An algorithm for the radiologic evaluation of children with their first UTI is summarized in Fig. 60-1.

- Empiric antibiotic against likely organisms should be used until urine culture results are available. Almost 80 percent of causative organisms are resistant to ampicillin and amoxicillin, and many are resistant to trimethoprim-sulfamethoxazole (TMP-SMX). While TMP-SMX remains the drug of choice for outpatient UTI treatment, other options include sulfisoxazole (Gantrisin), 120 to 150 mg/kg per 24 h orally every 6 h, or cephalexin (Keflex), 50 to 100 mg/kg per 24 h orally every 6 h (Table 60-2). Children over 6 years of age may benefit from the addition of phenazopyridine (Pyridium), 10 mg/kg/day in 3 divided doses for 2 to 3 days. Admission criteria are listed in Table 60-3. Intravenous antibiotic therapy that includes an aminoglycoside, such as gentamicin, 7.5 mg/kg per 24 h divided every 8 h, continues until the sensitivity of the organism is known and patient's clinical status is improved. Patients may be discharged on an oral antibiotic and treated for a total of 14 days. Rapid

TABLE 60-1 Diagnostic Tests and Their Indications

DIAGNOSTIC TEST	INDICATION(S)
Renal cortical scan	Pyelonephritis; UTI; fever
Voiding cystourethrogram	Vesicoureteric reflux: *Initial* evaluation of boys with UTI; initial evaluation of girls with UTI (in some centers)
Isotope cystography	Vesicoureteric reflux: *Initial* evaluation of girls with UTI without suspected urethral pathology
Renal ultrasonography	Hydronephrosis; nephrolithiasis
Diuretic renography	Obstructive uropathies
Intravenous pyelogram	Nephrolithiasis; isolated renal or ureteral trauma
Computed tomography	Nephrolithiasis; renal and abdominal trauma

UTI, urinary tract infection.

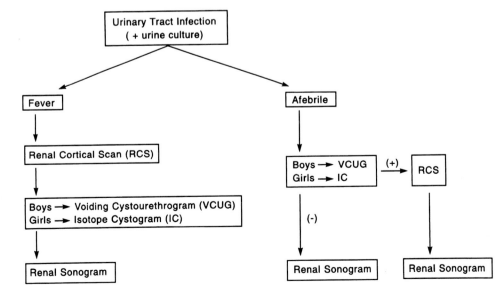

FIG. 60-1 Algorithm for the radiographic evaluation of children with their first UTI. (Adapted from Andrich MP, Majd M: Diagnostic imaging in the evaluation of the first urinary tract infection in infants and young children. *Pediatrics* 90:436, 1992.)

TABLE 60-2   Antibiotic Therapy for Treatment of Urinary Tract Infections in Children

OUTPATIENT MANAGEMENT	
Cotrimoxazole (trimethoprim in combination with sulfisoxazole)	8 to 10 mg/kg/24 h divided bid
or cefixime	8 mg/kg/24 h divided bid
or cephalexin	50 to 100 mg/kg/24 h divided qid
or cefpodixime	10 mg/kg/24 h divided bid
INPATIENT MANAGEMENT	
Ampicillin *plus*	100 mg/kg/24 h divided qid
Cefotaxime	150 mg/kg/24 h divided qid
or cetriaxone	75 mg/kg/24 h
or ceftazidime	150 mg/kg/24 h divided qid
or gentamicin	1.5 mg/kg/24 h divided tid
or tobramycin	5 mg/kg/24 h divided tid

bid, twice daily; qid, 4 times daily; tid, three times daily.

diagnosis and appropriate antibiotic therapy reduces the risk of complications, including renal scarring, hypertension, nephrolithiasis, and renal failure.

UROLITHIASIS

- Urolithiasis refers to stone formation in the bladder, ureter, or kidney and is rare in children. Its incidence varies geographically, with the southeastern and western United States having the highest incidence of stones (1/1380 hospital admissions). In the United States, most urinary calculi are calcium oxalate or calcium phosphate (58 percent).
- Urinary stasis from anomalies of the urinary tract, concentration of solute (calcium, oxalate, uric acid, and cystine) in the urine, presence of urinary infection (struvite), and concentrated urine promote stone formation. The most common causes are listed in Table 60-4.
- Patients may present with abdominal or flank pain (44 percent), hematuria (38 percent), fever (15 percent), and other urinary complaints (18 percent). Historical clues include a history of recurrent UTIs, frequent bouts of abdominal pain, microscopic or gross hematuria, passage of stones or gravel in the urine, intake of vitamins C and D, hydration status, recent trauma,

TABLE 60-3   Admission Criteria for Children with Urinary Tract Infection

Neonate
Pyelonephritis (Infants)
Known urinary tract abnormality
Urinary tract obstruction (stone)
Ureteral stents or other urinary tract foreign bodies
Immunocompromised state
Intractable vomiting and dehydration
Renal insufficiency
Toxic-appearing infant or child

TABLE 60-4   Causes of Urolithiasis in North American Children

CAUSE	NUMBER (%)
Metabolic	162 (32.9)
Idiopathic hypercalciuria	
Cystinuria	
Myeloproliferative disorders	
Hyperoxaluria	
Renal tubular acidosis	
Primary hyperparathyroidism	
Hypercortisolism	
Other	
Endemic (urate)	10 (2.2)
Developmental anomalies of the genitourinary tract	160 (32.5)
Infection	21 (4.3)
Idiopathic	139 (28.3)

genitourinary surgery, and a family history of stones. Routine physical examination, including blood pressure and growth parameters, should be performed.

- Urinalysis, urine culture, and renal function studies should be obtained. Urinalysis may be normal or reveal gross or microscopic hematuria. A complete blood cell count, renal function tests, electrolytes, uric acid, total protein, and albumin may also be obtained.
- Computed tomography (CT) scan of the abdomen without contrast is the test of choice for the evaluation of children with renal stones. Although approximately 90 percent of renal stones are radiopaque and visible on plain radiographs, CT delineates underlying congenital abnormalities and degree of obstruction. Renal ultrasound or an intravenous pyelogram (IVP) may be performed if CT is not available. Renal ultrasound may be useful in those patients who are pregnant; however, it cannot distinguish obstructive from nonobstructive causes of hydronephrosis.
- Assess patients for signs of infection and dehydration. Give NSAIDs and morphine sulfate, or another narcotic, to control pain. Patients with complete urinary obstruction, intractable pain, dehydration, a solitary kidney, renal insufficiency, or inability to keep fluids down may need to be admitted. If stones cannot pass spontaneously, extracorporeal shock wave lithotripsy or surgical removal may be necessary. Sixteen percent of patients will have a recurrence of stones, so close follow-up and outpatient dietary management are critical.

BIBLIOGRAPHY

American Academy of Pediatrics: Practice parameter: The diagnosis, treatment, and evaluation of the initial urinary tract infection in febrile infants and young children. *Pediatrics* 103:843–852, 1999.

Hoberman A, Chao HP, Keller DM, et al: Prevalence of urinary tract infection in febrile infants. *J Pediatr* 123:17–23, 1993.

Hoberman A, Charron M, Hickey RW: Imaging studies after a first febrile urinary tract infection in young children. *N Engl J Med* 348:195–202, 2003.

Jakobsson B, Esbjorner E, Hansson S: Minimum incidence and diagnostic rate of first urinary tract infection. *Pediatrics* 104:222–225, 1999.

Nelson DS, Gurr MB, Schunk JE: Management of febrile children with urinary tract infections. *Am J Emerg Med* 16: 643–647, 1998.

Shaw KN, Gorelick MH: Urinary tract infection in the pediatric patient. *Pediatr Clin North Am* 46:1111–1124, 1999.

QUESTIONS

1. Parents bring an 8-year-old girl for evaluation of frequency, urgency, and dysuria. Parents report low-grade fevers at home. On examination, you note a well-appearing child. Abdominal examination demonstrates suprapubic tenderness without rebound or guarding. You suspect a urinary tract infection. You have excluded other diagnoses through history and physical; however, a urine dipstick is negative. Which of the following would be the **MOST** appropriate in managing this patient?
   A. Obtain a catheterized urine specimen, if negative no further intervention is necessary
   B. Obtain a catheterized urine specimen, a urine culture, and begin empiric antibiotics
   C. Begin empiric antibiotics
   D. Send a formal urinalysis, if negative no further intervention is necessary
   E. No further intervention is necessary

2. Parents bring a 1-year-old child for evaluation of fevers, vomiting, and irritability. A bagged urine specimen is positive. Which of the following would **NOT** be recommended in management of this patient?
   A. Obtain a catheterized urine specimen
   B. Suprapubic aspiration prior to starting antibiotics
   C. Urine culture
   D. Voiding cystourethrogram
   E. Intravenous pyelogram

3. A 15-year-old girl presents for evaluation of flank pain radiating to her abdomen. On arrival to the emergency department, the patient appears very uncomfortable. A urinalysis demonstrates microscopic hematuria. A urine pregnancy test is negative. You learn that the patient has a strong family history of kidney stones. Which of the following would be the **MOST** helpful in establishing the diagnosis of urolithiasis?
   A. Urinalysis
   B. Intravenous pyelogram
   C. Renal cortical scintigraphy

D. Computed tomography of the abdomen without contrast
E. Plain radiographs

ANSWERS

1. B. Urine culture is the most diagnostic test to establish the diagnosis of UTI. Approximately 20 percent of young children with a documented UTI have a normal urinalysis for leukocytes and nitrites. Empiric antibiotics against likely organisms should be used until urine cultures results are available. While TMP-SMX remains the drug of choice for outpatient UTI treatment, sulfisoxazole and cephalexin are options.

2. E. Bagging the perineum is the least reliable method of obtaining urine with false-positive rates between 85 to 99 percent. If the urine is positive, obtain urine by catheterization or suprapubic aspiration for culture. Intravenous pyelogram is useful when evaluation the urinary system for stones.

3. D. Urolithiasis refers to stone formation in the bladder, ureter, or kidney. Patients may present with abdominal or flank pain (44 percent), hematuria (38 percent), and fever (15 percent). Historical clues include recurrent UTIs, microscopic or gross hematuria, genitourinary surgery, recent trauma, and a family history of stones. Computed tomography (CT) scan of the abdomen without contrast is the test of choice for evaluation of children with renal stones. Although approximately 90 percent of renal stones are radiopaque and visible on plain radiographs, CT delineates underlying congenital abnormalities and degree of obstruction.

61 SPECIFIC RENAL SYNDROMES

Roger Barkin
Kemedy K. McQuillen
Heather M. Prendergast

ACUTE GLOMERULONEPHRITIS

- Glomerulonephritis is a histopathologic diagnosis associated with hematuria, edema, and hypertension. It commonly occurs 1 to 2 weeks after a group A beta-hemolytic streptococcus infection in children between 3 and 7 years of age. Patients under 2 years old are rarely affected. It results from the deposition of circulating immune complexes in the basement membrane of the kidney, causing reduced glomerular filtration.

- The physical findings reflect the duration of illness; initially, there may be mild facial or extremity edema with a minimal rise in blood pressure but over time, patients develop fluid retention and edema and commonly have hematuria (90 percent), hypertension (60 to 70 percent), and oliguria (80 percent). Fever, malaise, and abdominal pain are frequently reported and circulatory congestion and hypertensive encephalopathy may be noted. Anuria and renal failure occur in 2 percent of children.
- Microscopic or gross hematuria is noted on urinalysis. Erythrocyte casts tend to be present and proteinuria is generally under $2\,g/m^2$ per 24 h. Hematuria (Fig. 61-1) and proteinuria (Fig. 61-2) may present independently and require a specific evaluation. Leukocyturia and hyaline and granular casts are common. The fractional excretion of sodium may be reduced (Table 61-1). The blood urea nitrogen (BUN) level is elevated disproportionately to the creatinine level. Total serum complement and C3 is reduced in most children during the first 2 weeks of the illness. The antistreptolysin (ASO) level is elevated and anemia, hyponatremia, and hyperkalemia may be present.
- Treatment includes fluid and salt restriction and, occasionally, diuretics. Hypertension, congestive heart failure, renal failure, and hyperkalemia must be anticipated and treated.
- Over 80 percent of patients recover without residua. Children without hypertension, congestive heart failure, or azotemia may be followed as outpatients. Nephrology consultation is recommended.

NEPHROTIC SYNDROME

- Nephrotic syndrome is associated with increased glomerular permeability producing massive proteinuria. Hypoalbuminemia results, producing a decrease in the plasma osmotic pressure and shifting fluids from the vascular to interstitial spaces. This shrinks plasma volume, thereby activating the renin-angiotensin system and enhancing sodium reabsorption. Edema develops. Serum cholesterol is elevated and remains high after resolution of urinary protein loss. The etiology of nephritic syndrome is usually idiopathic, but it has been associated with glomerular lesions, intoxications, allergic reactions, infections, and other entities (Table 61-2).
- Patients have edema, often with a preceding flu-like syndrome. Edema is periorbital and then becomes generalized and is associated with weight gain. Edema of the intestinal wall may result in abdominal pain, nausea, vomiting, and ascites. Pleural effusion, pulmonary edema, and malnutrition from protein loss may occur. Blood pressure may be decreased if the

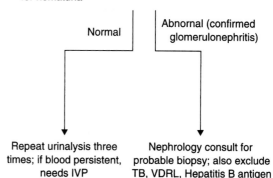

History: illness, rashes, arthralgia, growth pattern, etc., urinary stream; family history of renal failure, deafness, hematuria; check for previous TB testing

↓

Physical examination: blood pressure, cardiac and pulmonary examination, palpate bladder and kidneys

↓

Urinalysis: microscopic (look for free RBCs and RBC casts); dipstick (if proteinuria and hematuria, needs complete work-up); specific gravity (in chronic renal disease, poor concentrating ability present)

↓

Urine culture

↓

Basic labs: BUN, creatinine, Ca^{2+}, urine calcium for Ca^{2+}/Cr ratio; 24 h urine creatinine clearance and total protein; streptozyme, ANA, immunoglobulins; complement (CH_{50}, C_3, C_4); check family for hematuria

Normal — Abnornal (confirmed glomerulonephritis)

Repeat urinalysis three times; if blood persistent, needs IVP

Nephrology consult for probable biopsy; also exclude TB, VDRL, Hepatitis B antigen

FIG. 61-1 Evaluation for hematuria. TB, tuberculosis; RBC, red blood cell; BUN, blood urea nitrogen; Ca, calcium; Cr, creatinine; ANA, antinuclear antibody; CH; IVP, intravenous pyelogram; VDRL. [From Barkin RM, Rosen P (eds): *Emergency Pediatrics: A Guide to Ambulatory Care*, 5th ed. St. Louis, MO: Mosby-Year Book, p 266, 1999, with permission.]

intravascular volume is depleted or increased in the presence of significant renal disease. Renal failure may develop. Due to chronic steroid use and low immune protein levels from urinary losses, children with nephrotic syndrome are considered immunocompromised and are at risk for life-threatening infections and peritonitis. Other complications include hypercoagulability (leading to an increased risk of thromboembolism), hypoalbuminemia, proteinuria, and hyperlipidemia. Renal vein thrombosis should be

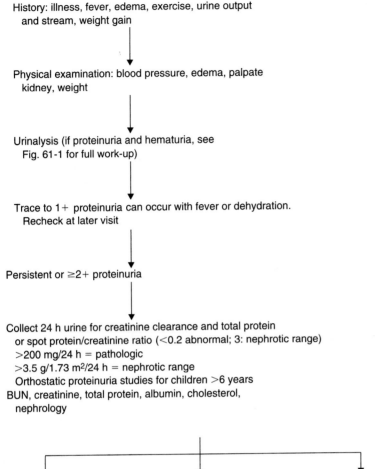

History: illness, fever, edema, exercise, urine output and stream, weight gain

↓

Physical examination: blood pressure, edema, palpate kidney, weight

↓

Urinalysis (if proteinuria and hematuria, see Fig. 61-1 for full work-up)

↓

Trace to 1+ proteinuria can occur with fever or dehydration. Recheck at later visit

↓

Persistent or ≥2+ proteinuria

↓

Collect 24 h urine for creatinine clearance and total protein or spot protein/creatinine ratio (<0.2 abnormal; 3: nephrotic range)
>200 mg/24 h = pathologic
>3.5 g/1.73 m²/24 h = nephrotic range
Orthostatic proteinuria studies for children >6 years
BUN, creatinine, total protein, albumin, cholesterol, nephrology

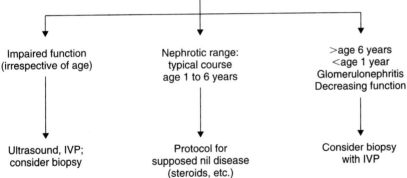

Impaired function (irrespective of age)	Nephrotic range: typical course age 1 to 6 years	>age 6 years <age 1 year Glomerulonephritis Decreasing function
↓	↓	↓
Ultrasound, IVP; consider biopsy	Protocol for supposed nil disease (steroids, etc.)	Consider biopsy with IVP

FIG. 61-2 Evaluation for proteinuria. BUN, blood urea nitrogen; IVP, intravenous pyelogram. [From Barkin RM, Rosen P (eds): *Emergency Pediatrics: A Guide to Ambulatory Care*, 5th ed. St. Louis, MO: Mosby-Year Book, p 267, 1999, with permission.]

suspected if hematuria, flank pain, and decreased renal function occur. Avoid deep vein punctures to prevent triggering a deep vein thrombosis.

o A 24-h urine collection reveals a protein excretion of >3.5 g/1.73 m² per 24 h. A spot protein:creatinine ratio of >3.0 is noted, and BUN and creatinine levels are elevated in 25 percent of children. Serum complement is decreased. Plasma cholesterol carriers (low-density lipoprotein and very low-density lipoprotein) are increased. Elevated lipids result from increased synthesis and catabolism of phospholipid. Imaging studies show normal renal structure. A renal biopsy should be considered if the patient is over 10 years old or if there is azotemia, decreased complement, hematuria, persistent hypertension, or no response to steroids.

• Other causes of edema should be excluded. These include congestive heart failure, vasculitis, hypothyroidism, starvation, cystic fibrosis, protein-losing enteropathy, and drug ingestions (i.e., glucocorticoids).

• During treatment, assure hemodynamic stability, balance intake and output, and restrict salt and water. Treat hypovolemia with albumin and fluids. Treat hypertension if it occurs. Subsequent evaluation is described in Fig. 61-3. Most patients require hospitalization and nephrology consultation. Patients under 10

TABLE 61-1 Evaluation of Renal Failure

PRERENAL	INTRARENAL	POSTRENAL
Ultrasound: normal	Ultrasound: Can have increased renal density or slight swelling	Ultrasound: Dilated bladder or kidney
Serum BUN:creatinine ratio >15:1		History and examination may be diagnostic
Urine Na$^+$ <15 mEq/L	Urine Na$^+$ >20 mEq/L	Indexes not helpful
Urine osmolality >500 mOsm/kg H$_2$O	Urine osmolality <350 mOsm/kg H$_2$O	
Urine:plasma creatinine ratio >40:1	Urine:plasma creatinine ratio <20:1 (often <5:1)	
Fractional excretion of Na$^+$ <1 (<2.5 in neonates)	Fractional excretion of Na$^+$ >2 (>2.5 in neonates)	

$$\text{Fractional excretion of Na}^+ = \frac{\text{Urine Na}^+ \text{ (mEq/L)}}{\text{Plasma Na}^+ \text{ (mEq/L)}} \times \frac{\text{Plasma creatinine (mg/dL)}}{\text{Urine creatinine (mg/dL)}}$$

SOURCE: From Barkin RM, Rosen P (eds): *Emergency Pediatrics: A Guide to Ambulatory Care*, 5th ed. St. Louis, MO: Mosby-Year Book, p 811, 1999, with permission.

TABLE 61-2 Nephrotic Syndrome: Etiology

Primary renal disorders	Nil or minimal change disease
	Focal glomerulosclerosis
	Membranoproliferative glomerulonephritis
	Membranous glomerulonephritis
Intoxication	Heroin
	Mercury
	Probenecid
	Silver
Allergic reaction	Poison ivy or oak, pollens
	Bee sting
	Snake venom
Infection	Bacterial
	Viral: hepatitis B, cytomegalovirus, Epstein–Barr virus
	Protozoa: malaria, toxoplasmosis
Neoplasm	Hodgkin's disease, Wilms' tumor, etc.
Autoimmune disorder	Systemic lupus erythematosus
Metabolic disorder	Diabetes mellitus
Cardiac disorders	Congenital heart disease
	Congestive heart failure
	Pericarditis
Vasculitis	Henoch–Schönlein purpura
	Wegener's granulomatosis

years old without gross hematuria and large protein losses who have normal complement levels, are treated with prednisone (2 mg/kg per 24 h up to 80 mg) and tapered once a response is noted. Most patients respond within 14 days. Treatment continues for about 2 months but is reinstituted if relapse occurs. Diuretics may be used judiciously for pulmonary edema.

HEMOLYTIC-UREMIC SYNDROME

• Patients with hemolytic uremic syndrome (HUS) have nephropathy, microangiopathic hemolytic anemia, and thrombocytopenia. It occurs when endothelial damage of the renal microvasculature causes a mechanically induced microangiopathic hemolytic anemia. Subsequent platelet aggregation produces renal microthrombi and hypoxia and decreased C3 results from complement deposition in the glomeruli. HUS progresses rapidly and occurs most commonly in children under 5 years of age. It may follow an episode of gastroenteritis or respiratory infection or may occur in siblings due to a familial genetic component. *Escherichia coli* serotype 0157:H7 is the most common agent associated with HUS. *Shigella, Salmonella*, group A streptococcus, coxsackievirus, influenza, and respiratory syncytial virus (RSV) are also associated with HUS.

• On presentation, patients usually have a history of vomiting, bloody diarrhea, and crampy abdominal pain within the 2 weeks preceding the onset of HUS. Children who present without this prodrome have a poor prognosis. Findings include low-grade fever, pallor, hematuria, oliguria, gastrointestinal bleeding, and central nervous system symptoms that range from irritability to seizures or coma. Disease severity ranges from a mild elevation of BUN with anemia to acute nephropathy and anuria with severe anemia and thrombocytopenia. Patients may develop hypertension, petechiae, easy bruising, hepatosplenomegaly, edema, hyponatremia, and hypocalcemia. Additionally, acute abdominal conditions (intussusception, bowel perforation, and toxic megacolon), hepatic and pancreatic injury, cardiomyopathy, myocarditis, or high-output failure may develop. Recurrences may occur and have a high mortality rate.

• Laboratory evaluation includes electrolyte, BUN, and creatinine levels, and a urinalysis. A complete blood count will demonstrate thrombocytopenia and low hemoglobin with a microangiopathic, hemolytic anemia. Burr cells are common. Coagulation studies are usually normal.

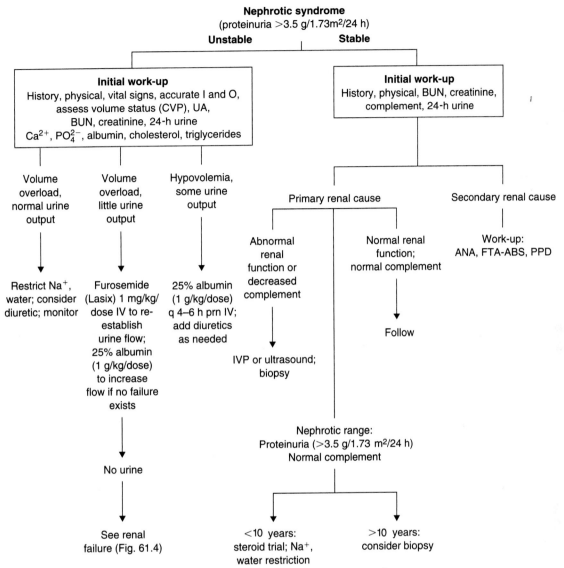

FIG. 61-3 Management of nephrotic syndrome. I, input; O, output; CVP, central venous pressure; UA, urine analysis; BUN, blood urea nitrogen; Ca, calcium; PO, by mouth; Na, sodium; IV, intravenous; ANA, antinuclear antibody; FTA-ABS = Fluorescent treponema antigen-antibody; PPD = purified protein derivative for T.B.; IVP, intravenous pyelogram. [From Barkin RM, Rosen P (eds): *Emergency Pediatrics: A Guide to Ambulatory Care*, 4th ed. St. Louis, MO: Mosby-Year Book, p 735, 1994, with permission.]

• Stabilize and admit all patients with HUS. Treat hypertension if the diastolic pressure is above 120 mm Hg: nifedipine, labetalol, captopril, and hydralazine may be used. Carefully balance intake and output and treat hyperkalemia, acidosis, hypocalcemia, hyperphosphatemia, and other metabolic abnormalities. Peritoneal dialysis may be required if the BUN is over 100 or if the patient has congestive heart failure, hyperkalemia or encephalopathy, or if anuria has been present for 24 h. Transfuse packed red blood cells for a serum hemoglobin <5g/dL or a hematocrit <15 percent.

Infuse platelets if there is active bleeding. Treat seizures (usually caused by hypertension or uremia) with anticonvulsants, antihypertensives, and dialysis. There is no role for streptokinase or heparin.

ACUTE RENAL FAILURE

• The etiology of acute renal failure is categorized by the type of renal injury: prerenal with decreased kidney perfusion, intrarenal with nephron damage, or postrenal from downstream obstruction of the urinary tract (see Table 61-1). Prerenal patients usually have dehydration from vomiting, diarrhea, diabetic ketoacidosis, or decreased intravascular volumes associated with nephrotic syndrome, burns, or shock. Nephron damage is caused by glomerulonephritis (hematuria, proteinuria, edema, and hypertension), HUS, nephrotoxic exposures, crush injuries, sepsis, or disseminated intravascular coagulation. Obstructive postrenal failure may be insidious and asymptomatic or may present with abdominal pain and an abdominal mass. Causes include posterior urethral valves, ureteropelvic junction abnormalities, renal stones, and trauma.

• The history and physical examination may suggest the mechanism of renal failure, the degree of hypovolemia, volume overload, and hypertension, and the amount of urine output. Patients in renal failure may be oliguric (urine output <1 mL/kg/h) or nonoliguric.
  ○ Laboratory evaluation includes electrolytes, BUN, creatinine, and a search for the underlying pathology. The creatinine clearance is a good measure of GFR and is useful in initial assessment and ongoing monitoring.

Creatinine clearance (mL/min/1.73 m^2) =
$$\frac{UV}{P} \times \frac{1.73}{SA}$$

[U = urinary concentration of creatinine (mg/dL); V = volume of urine divided by the number of min in collection period (mL/min); P = plasma concentration of creatinine (mg/dL); SA = surface area (m^2).]
A rapid approximation can be made using the formula:

Creatinine clearance
$$(mL/min/1.73\,m^2) = [0.55 \times ht\,(cm)]/P$$

Normal values vary by age:
  ○ Newborn and premature infants: 40 to 65 mL/min/1.73 m^2
  ○ Female child: 109 mL/min/1.73 m^2
  ○ Male child: 124 mL/min/1.73 m^2
  ○ Adult female 95 mL/min/1.73 m^2
  ○ Adult male 105 mL/min/1.73 m^2

In adult patients with stable renal function, a spot protein:creatinine ratio of >3.0 represents nephrotic range proteinuria (<0.2 is normal). An ultrasound should also be obtained. Combining data helps differentiate

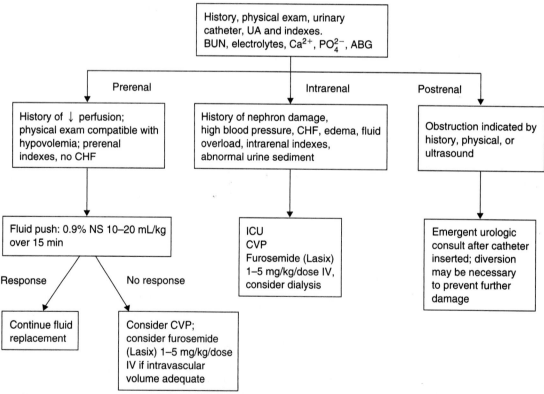

FIG. 61-4 Acute renal failure: initial assessment and treatment. UA, urine analysis; BUN, blood urea nitrogen; Ca, calcium; PO, by mouth; ABG, arterial blood gas; CHF, congestive heart failure; NS, normal saline; ICU, intensive care unit; CVP, central venous pressure; IV, intravenous. [From Barkin RM, Rosen P (eds): *Emergency Pediatrics: A Guide to Ambulatory Care,* 5th ed. St. Louis, MO: Mosby-Year Book, p 812, 1999, with permission.]

among prerenal, intrarenal, and postrenal failure (see Table 61-1).

- Initial treatment includes stabilization and correction of fluid imbalance (Fig. 61-4). Give furosemide (1 mg/kg increased as needed up to 6 mg/kg/dose) to enhance urine output if the intravascular volume is adequate or overloaded and there is no evidence of obstruction. Give mannitol (0.5 to 0.75 mg/kg/dose IV) if there is no response to furosemide. In oliguric or anuric patients with decreased intravascular volume, administer fluid slowly: central venous pressure monitoring can help guide therapy. Consider low-dose dopamine to increase renal blood flow and GFR. In patients with high output renal failure, administer sufficient fluid to avoid hypovolemia. Hypertension may be caused by fluid overload or high renin secretion. Treat hypertensive patients who have a diastolic pressure over 100 mm Hg with parenteral nitroprusside or nifedipine. Treat potassium levels above 7.0 mEq/L with calcium chloride (20 to 30 mg/kg slowly), sodium bicarbonate (1 to 2 mEq/kg/dose), a glucose and insulin infusion (1 mL/kg of D50W followed by 1 mL/kg of D25W and 0.5 U/kg of regular insulin per h to keep serum glucose between 120 to 300 mg/dL), or Kayexalate (1 g/kg/dose every 4 to 6 h orally or rectally). Treat anemia, metabolic acidosis, hyponatremia, and hyperphosphatemia as needed. Consider dialysis for fluid overload, hyperkalemia, hyponatremia, hypernatremia, or metabolic acidosis refractory to medical management, BUN >100 mg/ dL, or an altered mental status secondary to uremia.

BIBLIOGRAPHY

ACUTE GLOMERULONEPHRITIS

Roy S, Stapleton FB: Changing perspective in children hospitalized with post streptococcal acute glomerulonephritis. *Pediatr Nephrol* 4:585, 1990.

Wingo CS, Clapp WL: Proteinuria: Potential causes and approach to evaluation. *Am J Med Sci* 320:188–94, 2000.

NEPHROTIC SYNDROME

Hudson EM, Knight JF, Willis NS, Craig JC: Corticosteroid therapy for nephrotic syndrome in children (Cochrane Review). *Cochrane Database Syst Rev* (1):CD001533, 2003.

Warshaw BL: Nephrotic syndrome in children. *Pediatr Ann* 23:495, 1994.

HEMOLYTIC-UREMIC SYNDROME

Brandt JR, Fouser LS, Watkins SL, et al: *E. coli* 0157:H7–associated hemolytic-uremic syndrome after ingestion of contaminated hamburgers. *J Pediatr* 125:519, 1994.

Kelles A, Van Dyck M, Proeshan W: Childhood haemolytic uraemic syndrome: Long-term outcome and prognostic features. *Eur J Pediatr* 153:38, 1994.

Siegler RC, Milligan MK, Burningham TH, et al: Long-term outcome and prognostic indicators in the hemolytic uremic syndrome. *J Pediatr* 118:195, 1991.

ACUTE RENAL FAILURE

Sehic A, Chesney RW: Acute renal failure: Diagnosis, therapy. *Pediatr Rev* 16:101, 137, 1995.

Thadhani R, Pascual M, Bonventre JV: Acute renal flow. *N Engl J Med* 334:1448, 1996.

QUESTIONS

1. A 5-year-old girl is brought to the emergency department for evaluation of hematuria and swollen legs. You also learn that the child was recently treated for a "strep throat." On examination, you note a slightly elevated blood pressure and mild extremity edema. Urinalysis reveals microscopic hematuria. Which of the following, if present, would increase your suspicion of acute glomerulonephritis?
   A. Proteinuria
   B. Decreased antistreptolysin (ASO) level
   C. Hypernatremia
   D. Hypokalemia
   E. Leukocyturia

2. A 10-year-old child is brought for evaluation of generalized body edema. While obtaining a history, you learn that 2 weeks ago, the child was treated for a "flu-like" syndrome with antibiotics and subsequently developed an allergic reaction. The mother states the child appeared to be doing well until 3 days ago when he began having nausea, vomiting, and body swelling. Physical examination reveals marked periorbital edema. You suspect nephrotic syndrome. Which of the follow would **NOT** be consistent with a diagnosis or complication of nephrotic syndrome?
   A. Cardiomegaly on chest radiograph
   B. Pleural effusion
   C. Pulmonary edema
   D. Hypotension
   E. Renal failure

3. Paramedics bring a 3-year-old child in for recurrence of vomiting, blood diarrhea, and abdominal pain. Parents report that the child was previously evaluated

for gastroenteritis 2 weeks prior to this episode and had fully recovered. On evaluation, you note a low-grade fever, pallor, and hematuria. You suspect hemolytic-uremic syndrome. Additional findings that you would expect in a patient with hemolytic-uremic syndrome would include all of the following **EXCEPT**:

A. Hypertension
B. Petechiae
C. Prolonged prothrombin time
D. Hypocalcemia
E. Thrombocytopenia

4. Which of the following is **NOT** typically associated with hemolytic-uremic syndrome?

A. Intussusception
B. Toxic megacolon
C. Acute cholecystitis
D. Bowel perforation
E. Pancreatic injury

ANSWERS

1. E. Glomerulonephritis is a histopathologic diagnosis associated with hematuria, edema, and hypertension. It commonly occurs 1 to 2 weeks after a group A beta-hemolytic streptococcus infection in children between 3 and 7 years of age. Microscopic or gross hematuria is noted on urinalysis. Other findings include leukocyturia, hyaline and granular casts, elevated ASO levels, hyponatremia, hyperkalemia, and anemia.

2. A. Nephrotic syndrome is associated with increased glomerular permeability producing massive proteinuria. The etiology of nephrotic syndrome is usually idiopathic, but it has been associated with glomerular lesions, allergic reactions, infections, and other entities. Patients have edema, often with a preceding flu-like syndrome. Edema is periorbital and then becomes generalized and is associated with weight gain. Other causes of edema should be excluded. These include congestive heart failure, vasculitis, hypothyroidism, starvation, and drug ingestions.

3. C. Patients with hemolytic uremic syndrome (HUS) have nephropathy, microangiopathic hemolytic anemia, and thrombocytopenia. HUS progresses rapidly and occurs most commonly in children under 5 years of age. Patients may develop hypertension, petechiae, easy bruising, hepatosplenomegaly, edema, hyponatremia, and hypocalcemia. Coagulation studies are usually normal.

4. C. Acute abdominal conditions associated with hemolytic-uremic syndrome (HUS) include intussusception, bowel perforation, toxic megacolon, and hepatic and pancreatic injury.

62 PETECHIAE AND PURPURA

Julia A. Rosekrans
Kemedy K. McQuillen
William R. Ahrens

INTRODUCTION

- Petechiae and purpura develop when small blood vessels in the skin rupture and bleed. They can occur because of increased capillary fragility, decreased ability to clot, or due to traumatic injury (Table 62-1). Petechiae may signify a life-threatening illness or a benign viral syndrome.

PETECHIAE DUE TO SEPSIS

- Septic illnesses cause petechiae through local vasculitis and consumption of coagulation factors. Petechial rashes in acute infections range from scattered small petechiae to widespread purpura and shock (purpura fulminans). Causes of **purpura fulminans** include *Neisseria meningitides*, gonococcus, *Salmonella typhi*, and *Escherichia coli*. Patients with rickettsial (Rocky Mountain spotted fever) and viral illnesses may also have petechiae.
- Children with septic illnesses may appear toxic with high fever, delirium, and, hypotension or they may look well and present only with fever. On physical examination, petechiae and purpura do not blanch. Small fresh lesions are red, while large lesions are blue to purple. Lesions darken and change color over several days as hemoglobin degrades. Petechiae above the nipple line suggest increased intravenous pressure in the superior vena cava and may result from vomiting or coughing. Petechiae in an acral distribution suggest infectious vasculitis.

TABLE 62-1   Differential Diagnosis of Purpura

A.	Infectious:	
	Acute:	Meningococcemia
		Rocky Mountain spotted fever
		Escherichia coli sepsis
		Gonococcemia
		Subacute bacterial endocarditis
		Atypical measles
		Echovirus 9, 4, 7
		Epstein–Barr virus
		Coxsackie A9
	Neonatal:	Rubella
		Toxoplasma
		Cytomegalovirus
		Syphilis
B.	Thrombocytopenic	
	Idiopathic thrombocytopenic purpura	
	Leukemia	
	Systemic lupus erythematosus	
	Hemangioma with platelet trapping	
C.	Nonseptic normal platelet count	
	Henoch–Schönlein purpura (anaphylactoid purpura)	
	Coagulation disorders	
	Trauma, including child abuse	

- Laboratory evaluation includes a complete blood cell count to evaluate total white blood cell and platelet counts. Blood cultures will identify bacterial causes. A lumbar puncture should be done if meningitis is suspected.
- Complications of purpura fulminans include vascular compromise with loss of digits and sloughing of skin. Meningitis can complicate sepsis and bacteremia.

HENOCH–SCHÖNLEIN PURPURA

- **Anaphylactoid purpura** is a systemic vasculitis that involves the skin, viscera, and joints. Infectious illnesses have been implicated as instigators of an immune complex response that reacts with blood vessel walls causing capillary leaking and Henoch–Schönlein purpura (HSP) symptoms. Skin biopsies show perivascular extravasation of blood.

- Children present variably with findings that may include rash, abdominal pain, joint pain, or seizures. The rash can develop before or after any systemic symptoms or it may be the only manifestation of the disease. It can begin with 1- or 2-mm palpable purpura or urticaria that progresses to palpable purpura over 24 h. Characteristically, the rash is acral, symmetric, and most prominent on the buttocks and thighs, although it can also be seen on hands, arms, and genitalia. Most skin changes last for about 4 to 6 weeks. Very rarely, skin ulcerations may occur. Abdominal pain may resemble appendicitis and some children may develop intussusception. Many children have microscopic intestinal bleeding and guaiac-positive stools. Arthralgia or arthritis is present about 80 percent of the time; it is usually mild and transient. Renal involvement is common and most children have microscopic hematuria at some point during the illness. A minority of children develop nephrotic syndrome that can progress to chronic renal failure. Rarely, children with vasculitis of the cerebral vessels may have seizures, coma, or paralysis.
- The diagnosis of HSP is clinical. Obtain a complete blood cell count to evaluate the white blood cell and platelet counts and check a urinalysis for hematuria and proteinuria.
- Most children can be discharged with mild analgesics and close follow-up. Inpatient treatment should be considered for children with significant joint pain or abdominal pain that precludes eating. Prednisone, 2 mg/kg/day, has been used to treat abdominal pain, although the efficacy is unproven. Corticosteroid therapy does not prevent nephritis.

IDIOPATHIC THROMBOCYTOPENIC PURPURA

- Idiopathic thrombocytopenic purpura is a common cause of an acute low platelet count and is heralded by petechiae and ecchymosis in no particular distribution over the body. Thrombocytopenia is due to IgG antiplatelet antibodies that develop in response to a preceding viral infection. The antibodies fix to normal platelets that are then destroyed by reticuloendothelial phagocytic cells. The antibody titer is inversely related to the platelet count. Most children have mild, self-limited illnesses, although bleeding into vital organs, including intracranial hemorrhage, may occur.
- Children present with bruises on areas of the body that are not usually bruised with or without bleeding of the oral cavity and the gastrointestinal and genitourinary tracts. The physical examination is otherwise normal without lymphadenopathy or splenomegaly.
- Obtain a complete blood count to identify the low platelet count and to assess the white blood cell count and hemoglobin. Antiplatelet antibody titers are not required.
- The differential diagnosis of thrombocytopenia includes autoimmune collagen vascular disease (especially lupus), drugs (thiazides, quinidine, and sulfa antibiotics), leukemia, lymphoma, and myeloma.
- Most cases of ITP are mild and self-limited and require only close follow-up. When cases are more severe, anti-D or intravenous immunoglobulin or prednisone may be given to interrupt platelet destruction. Splenectomy may be needed for patients whose illness does not remit spontaneously. Children with platelet counts below 50,000 require inpatient management.

CHILD ABUSE

- See Chapter 118 for a comprehensive discussion of child abuse.
- Child abuse should be considered if bruising is noted on nonbony prominences and the history does not match the physical findings. The pattern of injury and correlation of the pattern with the history of the injury are the best clues. In many fatal cases due to abuse, bruises had been seen on the child in previous encounters but were not recognized as unaccidental.
- Physical examination reveals bruising in areas that are not easily and commonly bruised: abdomen, trunk, cheeks, and buttocks. Bruises of different ages are frequently noted. All bruises should be evaluated for patterns such as bite marks, cord marks from being tied up, or belt shapes from a beating. During the physical examination look for bruises that are not consistent with the reported cause.
- Order a complete blood cell count to identify platelet abnormalities. In some cases, clotting studies may be needed. A skeletal survey may be helpful for infants under 18 months to identify subtle unsuspected fractures.
- Children with unexplainable bruises may have a problem with platelet number or activity, such as idiopathic thrombocytopenic purpura, leukemia, medication allergy, clotting disorders such as Wiskott-Aldrich syndrome, or Henoch-Schönlein purpura.
- Physician reporting of suspicious cases is mandated by law. If the diagnosis of child abuse is not clear, consult with social workers or physicians with experience in abuse. Consider emergency placement or hospital admission for children whose safety cannot be assured.

BIBLIOGRAPHY

Adams JR, Nathan DP, Bennett CL: Pharmacoeconomics of therapy for ITP: steroids, i.v.Ig, anti-D, and splenectomy. *Blood Rev* 16:65–7, 2002.

Cohen B: *Pediatric Dermatology*, 2d ed. St. Louis, Mosby Year Book, 1999.

Edwards L: *Dermatology in Emergency Care*. New York, Saunders, 1997.

Lilleyman J: *Pediatric Hematology*. New York, Churchill Livingstone, 1999.

Monteleone J: *Child Maltreatment*, 2d ed. Elk Grove Village, IL, GW Medical Publishers, 1998.

Schachner LA, Hansen RC (eds): *Pediatric Dermatology* 2d ed. New York, Saunders, 1995.

Weston WL, Lane AT: *Color Textbook of Pediatric Dermatology*. St. Louis, Mosby Year Book, 1996.

QUESTIONS

1. Petechiae in an acral (hands and feet) distribution suggest which of the following?
   A. Child abuse
   B. Idiopathic thrombocytopenic purpura
   C. Acute leukemia
   D. Infectious vasculitis
   E. Cardiac disease
2. The purpuric rash of Henoch-Schönlein purpura is often associated with which of the following?
   A. Severe headache
   B. Pneumonitis
   C. Conjunctivitis
   D. Meningismus
   E. Arthralgias or arthritis
3. The petechial/purpuric rash associated with idiopathic thrombocytopenic purpura (ITP):
   A. is usually associated with intracranial bleeding.
   B. has no particular distribution.
   C. is associated with severe neutropenia.
   D. usually occurs in combination with joint pains.
   E. occurs mostly on the hands and feet.
4. Management of ITP includes which of the following?
   A. Immediate platelet transfusion
   B. Transfusion of fresh frozen plasma
   C. Transfusion of cryoprecipitate
   D. Therapy with steroids or immunoglobulin
   E. Broad spectrum antibiotics

ANSWERS

1. D. Infectious vasculitis results from direct bacterial invasion of capillary endothelial cells.
2. E. Arthralgias or arthritis are associated with 80 percent of cases of HSP; they are usually transient and respond to analgesics.
3. B. The rash of ITP has no particular distribution. Intracranial bleeding is an uncommon but potentially devastating complication of ITP.
4. D. Platelet transfusion is avoided in patients with ITP; therapy with steroids or immunoglobulin is effective in raising platelet counts, but should be initiated in consultation with a pediatric hematologist.

63 PRURITIC RASHES

Julia A. Rosekrans
Kemedy K. McQuillen
William R. Ahrens

INTRODUCTION

- Some rashes that present with itching are acute problems that can be diagnosed and rapidly treated; others are chronic problems that can be controlled but not cured (Table 63-1).

ATOPIC DERMATITIS

- Atopic dermatitis is a chronic relapsing condition that appears in children who have a tendency to produce specific IgE when exposed to environmental antigens. It is associated with other atopic conditions, including allergic rhinitis and asthma. Atopic dermatitis appears to be an inherited disorder; if one parent has atopy, there is a 60 percent chance that a child will be atopic and if both parents are atopic, the child's risk is 80 percent. In comparison, the likelihood that a child whose parents are not atopic will develop atopy is about 20 percent. Environmental pollutants may also play a role in causing atopy. Atopic dermatitis is more common in children than it is in adults and usually begins in infancy. Most children improve over time.
- On skin biopsy, there is an inflammatory exudate in the epidermis with excessive numbers of lymphocytes and monocytes. There is no convincing data as to

TABLE 63-1   Pruritic Rashes

CHRONIC	ACUTE
Atopic dermatitis	Urticaria
Seborrhea	Scabies
	Insect bites
	Head lice
	Contact dermatitis

what triggers atopic dermatitis, although food and house dust mite allergies, cellular immunodeficiency, and abnormal beta-adrenergic receptors have been implicated.

- Infants tend to present with involvement of the cheeks and extensor surfaces of the legs. Later in childhood, the antecubital and popliteal fossae are most affected.
- Children with extensive involvement are more likely to have problems as adults. The rash may range from dry itchy skin to weeping open fissures. The most consistent symptom is itchiness, which may be severe enough to interfere with sleep. Associated physical findings include signs of scratching, rubbing, and other atopic problems. Some children have shiny buffed fingernails from constant rubbing. Denny's lines on the lower eyelid and allergic shiners are commonly seen. There may also be hypopigmented skin patches.
- Atopic dermatitis is a clinical diagnosis. The definitive features of the diagnosis are pruritus, flexural lichenification, and a chronic relapsing condition.
- The differential diagnosis includes seborrheic dermatitis, scabies, contact dermatitis, tinea corporis, Hurler's syndrome, phenylketonuria, and histiocytosis X.
- The most common acute complication is bacterial superinfection with *Staphylococcus aureus*, which can cause abscesses, cellulitis, and lymphangitis. Cataract formation and **keratoconus**, an abnormally shaped cornea, may be late complications.
- There is no cure for atopic dermatitis, so treatment is aimed at relieving dryness, inflammation, and itching. Baths should be limited and should not be with hot water. Mild, nonperfumed soap and bath oil should be recommended. Topical moisturizers and skin lotions should be used after a bath and daily. Treat inflammation with topical corticosteroid ointments, although take care to avoid fluorinated steroids, which are systemically absorbed and can cause permanent thinning of the skin. Strong potency steroids can be used to quell a severe flare; however, a rapid change to less powerful ointments is important. H_1 antihistamines, such as diphenhydramine (5 mg/kg per 24 h, not to exceed 300 mg divided into 4 doses daily) and hydroxyzine (2 to 4 mg/kg per 24 h divided into 2 or 3 doses), are commonly used to relieve the itch.

CONTACT DERMATITIS

- Allergic contact dermatitis is a type IV lymphocyte-mediated reaction to a particular allergen.
- Common allergens include nickel, chemicals from rubber in elastic or latex gloves, and chemicals used for tanning leather or dying fabric. The most common cause of contact dermatitis in the United States is the *Rhus* group of plants: poison ivy, poison oak, and poison sumac. Mango rind and cashew nut oil also contain a similar chemical material.
- A reaction usually occurs after the skin is sensitized, which can occur within 7 to 10 days after exposure. On subsequent exposures, a reaction can occur within 24 h.
- Patients present with erythema and a papulovesicular eruption. The rash may be linear when the reaction is from contact with plant leaves and stems or discrete and under jewelry when caused by nickel. In general, there are few complications from contact dermatitis; infrequently, scarring may occur.
- The diagnosis of contact dermatitis is made by recognizing the sudden development of a vesicular weeping eruption in a pattern suggestive of contact with an allergen. If necessary, patch testing can be done to delineate the cause. Other pruritic vesicular rashes include atopic dermatitis, ichthyoses, and scabies.
- Treat contact dermatitis by removing the inciting agent. With *Rhus* dermatitis, wash the skin, clothes, and under the nails to remove *Rhus* oleoresin. Fluid from the blisters does not spread the reaction so, if new lesions appear over several days, the child is probably being reexposed. Use topical corticosteroids to relieve the inflammation. In severe cases, use systemic steroids such as prednisone (1 to 2 mg/kg per 24 h over 10 to 14 days). Taper the steroids gradually to prevent rebound. Systemic H_1 antihistamines, such as hydroxyzine, can help relieve itching. Use cool compresses with tap water or Burow's solution to relieve discomfort. The rash can last for several weeks.

PEDICULOSIS

- *Pediculus humanus capitus*, the common head louse, is a wingless insect about 2- to 4-mm long, which feeds on human blood and is spread by direct contact or through fomites. The female louse attaches to a hair shaft and lays eggs along the hair. The eggs hatch in about 10 days.
- Head lice are most common in school age children and prefer to attach to fine straight hair. The presence of head lice is not related to poor hygiene.
- Scratching the scalp may be the first sign of head lice. Nits are commonly found close to the scalp, especially behind the ears and at the nape of the neck, and are firmly stuck to the hair shaft. Dandruff, seborrhea, and neurotic excoriation of the scalp can all be confused with head lice. Bacterial superinfection may develop as a result of scratching.
- Treatment includes eradication of the infestation and education to prevent reinfection. Several shampoos

and cream rinses effectively kill adult lice and nits: permethrin 1-percent cream rinse (Nix) has an excellent safety record. Treat all members of the household at the same time and apply a second treatment 7 days later. Although insecticides usually kill the larva inside the egg case, it may be difficult to dislodge the nit. Diluted vinegar can be used with a fine-tooth comb to remove the nits. In addition to treating the household members, wash and dry clothing and bedding using a hot air dryer. Clothing or hats that cannot be heat-treated can be disinfected if sealed in a plastic bag for 4 weeks. Warn parents that pruritus can last for several weeks after successful treatment. Some lice have become resistant to insecticides and barrier methods to suffocate the lice may be used; examples include Vaseline or mayonnaise applied thickly to the hair and left in place under a shower cap for at least 12 h. Treat itching with oral antihistamines and topical hydrocortisone cream.

SCABIES

- Scabies, a very pruritic skin infestation, is caused by a mite, *Sarcoptes scabiei*. It is quite contagious and easily spreads from one person to the next. Mites are very small, white transparent insects less than a half a millimeter in length with four pairs of legs. They are host-species specific and transmission generally requires close human contact. Adult mites can survive for several days off the human body so it is possible for scabies to be transmitted without skin-to-skin contact. The female mite burrows into the stratum corneum and lays two to three eggs per day for about a month. Larvae hatch in 3 to 4 days and crawl off to make a new burrow, either on the same person or someone in close contact.
- Patients present with burrows, papules, and itching. Itching may be the only manifestation of infestation. Infants may develop papules and vesicles all over their body, including palms, soles, face, and scalp. Older children and adults tend to develop papules on the hands, wrists, elbows, and belt line, and in the gluteal cleft and interdigital webs. Atopic dermatitis, papular urticaria, and simple insect bites can be confused with scabies. The existence of multiple family members with pruritic papules is an important diagnostic feature. Scraping papules and fresh vesicles may yield the mite or its stool pellets.
- Secondary infection with streptococcus or staphylococcus is the most common complication of scabies.
- Treat the affected child and close personal contacts with permethrin cream (Elimite): apply to the body overnight and rinse it off in the morning. Retreat after

7 days. Wash and dry clothing and bed linens with ordinary soap at usual temperatures to eliminate mites. Use oral antihistamines to control itching.

PAPULAR URTICARIA

- Papular urticaria is an intense hypersensitivity reaction to insect bites that may progress to a hard papule and persist for several days. It is seen in preschool children and infants in the second summer season when they are exposed to insect bites.
- The papules represent a delayed-type hypersensitivity reaction and as time goes by, and the child is repeatedly exposed to the offending antigen, hyposensitization and resolution of the reaction develop.
- Children present with dome-shaped papules on areas of the body that are exposed to insect bites; there may also be vesicles and bullae. Papules may last for 2 weeks. Papular urticaria can be confused with simple insect bites, viral exanthems, and sun sensitivity reactions. Complications include bacterial superinfection.
- Treat papular urticaria by protecting children from insect bites: pants and long sleeves with insect repellent applied to the clothes should be recommended. De-flea pets if bites are coming from fleas. Topical hydrocortisone cream and oral antihistamines may be helpful.

URTICARIA

- While urticaria may develop in response to a specific allergen, most cases of urticaria are idiopathic. Common causes include medications, seafood, strawberries, peanuts, tomatoes, viruses, and group A beta-hemolytic streptococci. Insect stings can cause local urticaria or progress to a systemic anaphylactic reaction. Hives are a result of a specific IgE mediated antibody reaction that causes histamine release with subsequent vasodilatation and enhanced vascular permeability. Prior sensitization is required to produce this reaction and hives do not develop on exposure to a new substance. Some urticarial reactions, especially those related to bee stings and food allergies, signal the potential for future anaphylactic reaction.
- Hives occur on all parts of the body and are very pruritic. They are more prominent on areas of skin that are warm or under pressure and they last from minutes to hours. Hives are accentuated by heat and often develop after a bath or when children are wrapped in warm clothing.
- Erythema multiforme is frequently confused with urticaria. They can be differentiated because erythema

multiforme is a fixed skin reaction with individual lesions that last for several days. Subcutaneous epinephrine clears urticaria but does not change erythema multiforme.

- For short-term relief, treat severe urticaria with subcutaneous epinephrine (1:1000) at a dose of 0.01 mL/kg (maximum 0.3 mL). For longer relief, use H_1 antihistamines. There is no role for topical steroids or antihistamines. In most cases, systemic corticosteroids are not needed

ERYTHEMA MULTIFORME

- Erythema multiforme (EM) is a hypersensitivity reaction that includes a variety of skin problems from minor itching and urticaria-like lesions to severe blistering and desquamation. It is most commonly caused by infections and drug exposures; sulfa, phenytoin, penicillin, cephalosporins, recurrent herpes simplex, and *Mycoplasma pneumoniae* have all been implicated. In 50 percent of cases, no inciting agent is identified. Skin biopsies show epidermal damage with perivascular lymphatic infiltration and edema below the epidermis.
- Patients with EM minor present with pruritic, non-blistering urticaria-like lesions with little systemic reaction. The lesions are different from urticaria because they are fixed in the skin and fade slowly over a week's time. They do not clear when subcutaneous epinephrine is given. The lesions may develop a characteristic target shape or they may remain as round-topped papules. They last for about 1 week and become darker as they start to resolve.
- **Stevens–Johnson syndrome**, or EM major, is a more severe illness with fever, general malaise, and blistering of mucous membranes. The mucous membranes of the mouth can become deeply eroded and crusted. Conjunctivae and urogenital mucous membranes also become inflamed.
- **Toxic epidermal necrolysis (TEN)** is the most severe variant of EM. Dramatic blisters develop rapidly over all areas of the body. High fever and severe mucous membrane involvement is common. EM can be confused with urticaria, varicella, and staphylococcal scalded-skin syndrome.
- Mild cases of EM resolve completely. Problems with hydration and nutrition may develop in cases with oral blistering. Severely blistered lesions may produce scarring. There is a serious risk of mortality for patients with TEN.
- Mild cases need symptomatic care with oral antihistamines. When mucous membranes are involved, consider intravenous fluids and hyperalimentation. Steroids are not required for mild cases of EM. For patients with TEN, the risk of complications, such as gastrointestinal hemorrhage and sepsis, outweigh the potential value of decreasing blistering and steroids should not be used. In moderate cases, blistering may be diminished if steroids are initiated within the first 2 weeks of an eruption.

BIBLIOGRAPHY

American Academy of Pediatrics 2003 Red Book: *Report of the Committee on Infectious Diseases*, 26th ed. American Academy of Pediatrics, Elk Grove Village, IL.

Cohen B: *Pediatric Dermatology*, 2d ed. St. Louis, Mosby Year Book, 1999.

Edwards L: *Dermatology in Emergency Care.* New York, Saunders, 1997.

Schachner LA, Hansen RC (eds): *Pediatric Dermatology*, 2d ed. New York, Saunders, 1995.

Weston WL, Lane AT: *Color Textbook of Pediatric Dermatology*, St. Louis, Mosby Year Book, 1996.

QUESTIONS

1. Which of the following is true regarding infants with atopic dermatitis?
   A. Most commonly have involvement of the cheeks and extensor surfaces of the legs
   B. Usually have no family history of atopy
   C. Most commonly present with fever
   D. Are almost always breast fed
   E. Even children with extensive skin involvement are likely to clear in later childhood and are not likely to have skin problems as adults
2. Treatment of atopic dermatitis includes which of the following?
   A. The use of astringents
   B. Topical steroids
   C. Increasing the use of soaps
   D. Chronic suppressive therapy with antibiotics
   E. Isopropyl alcohol rubs
3. Which of the following is the most common cause of contact dermatitis in the United States?
   A. The Rhus group of plants
   B. Plastic material
   C. Denim
   D. Silk products
   E. Laundry adjuncts
4. Treatment for head lice (pediculosis) includes which of the following?
   A. Bactrim
   B. Chloramphenicol

C. Washing the hair in alcohol
D. Mayonnaise
E. Mustard
5. Concerning urticaria and erythema multiforme, which of the following is correct?
 A. Neither are caused by allergies
 B. Subcutaneous epinephrine will at least transiently clear urticaria but not erythema multiforme.
 C. Neither is associated with infection
 D. Neither will resolve spontaneously
 E. Erythema multiforme is a macular-type lesion while urticaria is raised.

ANSWERS

1. A. In infants, atopic dermatitis commonly involves the cheeks and extensor surfaces of the legs; in older children, the antecubital and popliteal fossae are commonly affected.
2. B. Topical medium-potency steroids are used to control acute exacerbations of inflammation; the mainstay of therapy for atopic dermatitis is maintaining moisture in the skin.
3. A. The most common cause of contact dermatitis in the United States is the Rhus family of plants, which includes poison ivy, poison oak, and poison sumac.
4. D. Some lice are resistant to treatment with permethrin shampoo; believe it or not, suffocating the lice by applying mayonnaise or Vaseline to the hair and covering it with a shower cap may be effective.
5. B. Erythema multiforme is a "fixed" lesion, while urticaria will usually at least temporarily clear following the administration of subcutaneous epinephrine. Lesions in erythema multiforme may vary from urticarial-like lesion to severe blistering.

64 SUPERFICIAL SKIN INFECTIONS

Julia A. Rosekrans
Kemedy K. McQuillen
William R. Ahrens

IMPETIGO AND ECTHYMA

- Impetigo is the most common skin infection in children. It develops when the protective barrier of the skin is broken and colonizing skin bacteria invade deeper epidermal tissues. Impetigo is superficial while ecthyma involves the entire thickness of the epidermis. Skin biopsy shows tiny vesicles within the epidermis

containing polymorphonuclear infiltrates and bacteria. Bullous impetigo is caused by *Staphylococcus aureus* and nonbullous impetigo and ecthyma are caused by *S. aureus* and group A beta-hemolytic streptococci (GABHS). Superficial skin infections are more common during warm seasons and in tropical climates and spread easily from child to child. If left untreated, a single lesion may heal spontaneously; however, new lesions crop up so that a single episode of impetigo may last for many weeks.

- Children with bullous impetigo present with small papules that develop into 1- to 2-cm bullae that rupture easily, exposing the shiny, wet, red base of the blister. The lesions can occur anywhere on the body but are found most often on the buttocks, perineum, or the face. Children with nonbullous impetigo present with a pustular reaction that has a serous honey-colored crust. Unless they complicate an insect bite or pruritic dermatitis, the lesions are not pruritic. Sometimes, the lesions spread, leaving a central clear, healed area. Regional lymph nodes may be enlarged if the infection is deep or has been present for a long period. Ecthyma, because it is deeper, is often painful and may include cellulitis or lymphangitis. Impetigo rarely causes any scarring. Ecthyma does tend to scar. Poststreptococcal glomerulonephritis is possible when nephrogenic strains of streptococci are involved.

- Herpes simplex lesions may resemble impetigo and a viral culture or Tzank prep can differentiate the two. Varicella and contact dermatitis may resemble the vesicle stage of impetigo. Tinea capitus that has progressed to kerion formation looks as if it is impetiginized; however, the reaction is a response to the fungal infection.

- In widespread cases, treat impetigo with oral antibiotics active against staphylococci: dicloxacillin, 20 to 50 mg/kg per 24 h divided in four doses, or cefadroxil, 30 mg/kg per 24 h in two doses, work well. Use mupirocin (Bactroban) 2-percent ointment if the infection is localized.

STAPHYLOCOCCAL SCALDED-SKIN SYNDROME

- Staphylococcal scalded-skin syndrome (SSSS) is a superficial skin infection characterized by erythema and generalized blistering and peeling of the skin. It is a serious systemic illness that is caused by an infection with a strain of *S. aureus* that produces an epidermolytic toxin. The infecting bacteria may be located in the nose, conjunctivae, or umbilical stump. SSSS is most often seen in children under 5 years old.
- Children present with fever and painful skin. Initially, the rash looks like sunburn with generalized erythema

but progresses to large bullae with desquamation of large sheets of skin. Serous crusts may be seen around the nose and mouth. In the initial erythematous phase, scarlet fever, toxic shock syndrome, severe erythema multiforme, and even sunburn may be considered.

- Cultures of the skin or bullae are often sterile; however, *S. aureus* may be cultured from the nose, sores, or wounds.
- With early recognition and management, patients recover fully without permanent sequelae or scarring. Manage fluid loss, electrolyte imbalance, heat loss, and pain. Give antibiotics to eradicate staphylococci: cefazolin or nafcillin are effective. Mild lubricant creams may reduce skin discomfort in the healing stages.

FUNGAL INFECTIONS

- Superficial fungal infections of the epidermis, hair, or nails are caused by dermatophytes.

TINEA CAPITIS

- Fungal infections of the scalp are most common in children between 2 and 10 years old. Most cases in the United States are caused by *Trichophyton tonsurans* (90 percent) and *Microsporum audouinii* (10 percent). *M. canis* can also cause infection, but is usually transmitted from an infected cat rather than a dog. Infections are very contagious, persist for years if untreated, and are more frequent in hot, humid climates and in crowded living conditions.
- The most common pattern of fungal infections in the United States is endothrix. Fungal spores develop entirely within the hair shaft leading to fragile hairs that break easily. A kerion, which is a tender boggy crusted pustular mass caused by an immune response to the fungal antigen, develops in about one third of cases.
- Children present with 1- to 5-cm round or oval areas of alopecia with stubby hair shafts broken off at the level of the scalp, causing a "black dot" appearance that differentiates it from alopecia areata. Tinea capitis can also resemble flaky dandruff without any clear patches of alopecia, although close examination will still show black dots. If a kerion occurs, there may be occipital and cervical lymphadenopathy and a low-grade fever. Tinia capitis can be mistaken for alopecia areata, trichotillomanis, traction alopecia, seborrhea, dandruff, or psoriasis. Kerions are frequently confused with bacterial skin infections but are differentiated by the sterile exudate. Complete destruction of the hair follicle with scarring and permanent baldness can result if tinea capitis is untreated.

- Hairs infected by *Microsporum species* will fluoresce yellow–green under a Wood's lamp. Unfortunately, this organism causes the minority of infections.
- Other fungi are diagnosed with a potassium hydroxide (KOH) preparation of hair and scalp scrapings. Spores and hyphae, either along side or within the hair shaft will be seen.
- Fungal cultures should be obtained because the course of therapy is very long.
- Treat tinea capitis with oral griseofulvin (15 mg/kg/day) for at least 6 weeks. Oral prednisone may be helpful in reducing the kerion. Instruct families to wash barrettes, combs, and brushes to kill fungal spores that can remain viable for a long period. Check family members for infection. Children can return to school after 1 week of griseofulvin therapy.

TINEA CORPORIS

- Dermatophyte infections of the epidermis can be found on any part of the body and are less problematic than tinea capitis. Any organism that can cause tinea capitis can also cause tinea corporis. Tinea corporis is most common in children and more prevalent in warm climates. Domestic and farm animals are a common source of infection. The dermatophyte invades the stratum corneum and does not extend to deeper epidermal layers. Hair follicles may be invaded and act as a reservoir for recurrent disease.
- Infection may present with papules, vesicles, eczematous plaques, or the classic oval ringworm shape with a scaly inflammatory border and a clear center. The rash is often pruritic and regional lymph nodes are usually not involved. Pityriasis rosea, granuloma annulare, and atopic dermatitis can be confused with tinea corporis.
- To diagnose, do a potassium hydroxide (KOH) prep of border scrapings looking for spores or hyphae. Cultures are not needed because topical treatment is usually effective. Infections usually clear without scarring.
- Treat tinea corporis with topical antifungal agents twice a day for a minimum of 2 to 3 weeks after initial clearing. Effective medications include tolnaftate (Tinactin), miconazole (Micatin), haloprogin (Halotex), and clotrimazole (Lotrimin). Failure to improve after 3 weeks should prompt further evaluation.

BIBLIOGRAPHY

American Academy of Pediatrics 2003 Red Book: *Report of the Committee on Infectious Diseases*, 26th ed. American Academy of Pediatrics, Elk Grove Village, IL.

Cohen B: *Pediatric Dermatology*, 2d ed. St. Louis, Mosby Year Book, 1999.

Edwards L: *Dermatology in Emergency Care.* New York. Saunders, 1997.

Schachner LA, Hansen RC (eds): *Pediatric Dermatology*, 2d ed. New York, Saunders, 1995.

Weston WL, Lane AT: *Color Textbook of Pediatric Dermatology*, St. Louis, Mosby Year Book, 1996.

QUESTIONS

1. Which of the following is true regarding nonbullous impetigo?
   A. It is caused exclusively by group a beta-hemolytic streptococcus.
   B. It is most common during the winter months.
   C. It is a manifestation of a contact allergy.
   D. It can be associated with glomerulonephritis.
   E. It is associated with a papular reaction with white purulent drainage and crusting.
2. Which of the following is true regarding staphylococcal scalded-skin syndrome?
   A. It is not associated with systemic manifestations.
   B. It does not cause painful skin.
   C. It is usually associated with blisters that are culture positive for *Staphylococcus aureus.*
   D. It is a toxin-mediated phenomenon.
   E. It has low morbidity and mortality.
3. Which of the following is true with regard to tinea capitis?
   A. Kerion formation is rare.
   B. Aspiration of the exudate of a kerion usually reveals gram-negative rods.
   C. Alopecia is rare.
   D. Scarring and permanent hair loss can result if treatment is not instituted.
   E. It occurs more commonly in girls.

ANSWERS

1. D. Nonbullous impetigo can be caused by *Staphylococcus aureus* and group A beta-hemolytic streptococcus. Nephritogenic strains of streptococci associated with impetigo can cause glomerulonephritis. Lesions are pustular and associated with honey-colored crusts.
2. D. The blistering in staphylococcal scalded-skin syndrome (SSSS) results from an epidermolytic toxin. The patient often complains of painful skin; there is some risk of mortality.
3. D. Kerion formation occurs in about 30 percent of cases of tinea capitis. If untreated, permanent scarring and hair loss can result. Tinea capitis occurs equally in girls and boys.

65 EXANTHEMS

Julia A. Rosekrans
Kemedy K. McQuillen
William R. Ahrens

INTRODUCTION

- In addition to diagnosing a rash, the physician needs to educate the family about the course of the illness, risk to others, incubation period, and potential complications.

RUBEOLA (MEASLES)

- The incidence of measles has dropped precipitously since a live attenuated virus vaccine was introduced in 1963. Most cases now occur as community epidemics in inadequately immunized children. Measles virus is a single-stranded ribonucleic acid (RNA) paramyxovirus that is spread by droplets and is highly contagious. It has an incubation period of 9 to 12 days. Patients are most contagious during the prodromal period, from about 3 days before until 4 days after the onset of the rash. The virus enters the body through the respiratory tract and, by the time symptoms appear, is distributed throughout the body. Multinucleated giant cells can be recovered from urine, sputum, and nasal secretions.
- Typical measles begin with a prodrome of respiratory symptoms. Cough, conjunctivitis, and coryza (nasal congestion) are usually present. **Koplik's spots**, tiny white spots on erythematous buccal mucosa opposite the lower molars, appear during the prodrome and last for about 24 hours. They are usually present when the rash begins. The erythematous, maculopapular exanthem appears about 14 days after exposure, starting at the hairline behind the ears and spreading from head to feet in about 3 days. Individual spots become confluent over time. Patients look most ill on the second or third day with high fever, brassy cough, and photophobia. The illness lasts for about 7 days.
- Complications include otitis media (most common), croup, laryngitis, pneumonia, and encephalitis with neurologic sequelae.
- There are no specific laboratory tests that identify the disease acutely. Serologic testing may be helpful for community surveillance.
- Treatment for measles is supportive. Live attenuated measles vaccine given within 72 h of exposure can provide some protection by stimulating active antibody production. Immune serum globulin [0.25 mL/kg

intramuscularly (IM), maximum 15 mL] will prevent or modify the disease if given within 6 days of exposure. Documented cases of measles should be reported to local public health authorities.

RUBELLA (GERMAN MEASLES)

• Rubella is a single-stranded RNA virus. The incidence of the disease has fallen since introduction of a live attenuated virus vaccine in 1969. It is spread by respiratory droplets and highly contagious. The incubation period is 14 to 23 days and patients are contagious from 1 week before to about 5 days after the rash appears. Infants with congenital rubella syndrome shed the virus for months after birth. There is a high rate of subclinical infection.

• Rubella is a very mild disease that causes fussiness, slight fever, and prominent postauricular and suboccipital nodes that occur with the rash. The rash is a nonspecific, diffuse, erythematous maculopapular eruption. Older children have transient joint pain. Complications include thrombocytopenia, encephalitis, and arthritis or arthralgias that may begin during the prodrome or following the appearance of the rash. The most significant complication is fetal malformation following a maternal rubella infection during the first or second trimester of pregnancy. The infection affects the organ system that is undergoing the most rapid development of the time of the viremia.

• Serologic tests can be done if the diagnosis is in question.

• Treatment is symptomatic. NSAIDs may be needed to control arthritis symptoms.

ROSEOLA (EXANTHEM SUBITUM)

• Roseola is caused by human herpes virus C. Roseola is a common illness that rarely occurs before 6 months or after 2 years of age. It is spread by respiratory droplets, has an incubation period of 5 to 15 days, and occurs most frequently in the spring and fall. Subclinical infection is common.

• Most children with roseola look well despite a high fever. The fever starts suddenly and persists for 3 to 4 days. The rash appears when the fever vanishes and resolves within 48 h. Some infants have a bulging fontanel without other meningeal symptoms and lumbar punctures are unremarkable.

• Roseola is a clinical diagnosis and there are no laboratory tests that are diagnostic.

• There are no known complications of roseola and care is supportive.

FIFTH DISEASE (ERYTHEMA INFECTIOSUM)

• Fifth disease is caused by parvovirus B19, a single-stranded DNA virus. It occurs in school age children in the spring and winter, is probably droplet spread, but is only mildly contagious.

• Viremia occurs about 1 week after exposure and lasts for 3 to 5 days, resolving prior to the onset of the rash. The rash develops abruptly with bright red cheeks giving the "slapped cheek" appearance. A maculopapular faintly pink rash develops on the trunk and extremities and then clears in a lacy pattern. The rash fades over several days but can reappear intermittently for weeks. Children may have a low-grade fever but generally appear well. Transient arthritis may complicate fifth disease in adults, although this is rare in children. Patients with sickle cell disease who contract parvovirus may develop bone marrow suppression and aplastic crisis. Parvovirus infection during pregnancy can result in fetal death or red blood cell aplasia with fetal hydrops.

• Fifth disease is a clinical diagnosis. Serologic testing is suggested for pregnant women who develop the disease or who are in close contact with children who have the illness.

• Treatment is symptomatic.

SCARLET FEVER

• Scarlet fever, caused by erythrogenic strains of GABHS, can develop in association with throat or skin infections. There are three different toxins and several different strains of erythrogenic GABHS so it is possible to have scarlet fever more than once.

• Children present with a sandpaper rash that begins in the skin folds, spares the area around the mouth and nose, and goes on to desquamate. The exanthem develops 12 to 48 h after the onset of fever and chills. Generalized lymphadenopathy is common. Viral illnesses may cause a similar rash. Complications of scarlet fever include rheumatic fever and glomerulonephritis; both of which occur at the same rate as in GABHS infection without a rash.

• Diagnose scarlet fever with a culture looking for GABHS.

• Treat scarlet fever with oral penicillin VK (15 to 50 mg/kg per 24 h divided in 3 doses) or erythromycin (20 to 50 mg/kg per 24 h in 3 to 4 divided doses). Children can return to school 24 h after starting antibiotics.

CHICKENPOX

- Chickenpox is caused by varicella zoster, a herpes-type virus that can remain latent in the body for years after a primary infection, only to reactivate and cause herpes zoster years later. The incubation period is 14 to 21 days. It is spread by direct contact and airborne droplets.
- Chickenpox begins with a mild 1- or 2-day prodrome of respiratory symptoms and low-grade fever.
- The rash appears on the trunk as small, red papules that progress to tiny vesicles giving the "dew drop on a rose petal" appearance. Crops of vesicles develop for 3 to 5 days, making all stages of the lesions present at the same time on any part of the body. When the vesicles dry and crust, they are no longer infectious. Subclinical infections are common.
- Although varicella usually gives life-long immunity with the first infection, second attacks can occur. With a family epidemic, subsequent children develop more severe illnesses.
- Papular urticaria, hand-foot-and-mouth, and disseminated herpes simplex can be confused with varicella.
- Complications of varicella include scarring, bacterial superinfection of the skin, otitis media, pneumonia, arthritis, hepatitis, Reyes's syndrome, and encephalitis. Adolescents are more at risk for complications than are young children.
- Chickenpox is a clinical diagnosis. If in doubt, a Tzanck preparation demonstrating multinucleated giant cells confirms the diagnosis. A viral culture can be used to differentiate chickenpox from disseminated herpes simplex.
- For children with uncomplicated illnesses, treatment is symptomatic and supportive. Antihistamines, such as diphenhydramine, may help control itching. Oatmeal and tea baths are also quite soothing. Consider intravenous acyclovir for immunocompromised children or those with significant complications. If a child presents within 24 h of the appearance of the rash, consider oral acyclovir to decrease the duration of the illness. Children who are at high risk for severe or complicated infections should be given varicella zoster immune globulin (125 U per 10 kg of body weight with a maximum dose of 625 U) within 48 h of exposure.
- Routine vaccination with a live attenuated varicella vaccine began in the United States in 1995. It offers close to 100 percent protection from severe chickenpox and 90 percent protection from illness.

HERPES ZOSTER

- Herpes zoster is the reactivation of the varicella zoster virus that has remained latent in a spinal-sensory nerve-root ganglia. It can erupt years after the initial infection. The incidence of zoster increases with age and is more common in people with immune suppression.
- Virus is present within the vesicles and can be spread by direct contact.
- Tingling pain usually precedes the appearance of vesicles that occur in two or three crops within one or more dermatomes.
- The most commonly involved areas are the thoracic and lumbosacral areas. In children, the least commonly involved areas are the cranial nerves; however, a trigeminal nerve eruption can involve the cornea causing significant morbidity.
- For most people, herpes zoster is painful but self-limited. Serious complications, however, may occur, especially in immunosuppressed patients. Postherpetic neuralgia is rare in children.
- Herpes zoster can be treated with acyclovir, or other antivirals, and varicella zoster immune globulin (VZIg).

HERPES SIMPLEX

- HSV-1 (type 1) and HSV-2 (type 2) cause infection in humans; HSV-1 is more common in oral infections and HSV-2 is more common in genital infections. Both viruses can cause subclinical infection and both remain latent within the body after the initial infection. Herpes simplex virus is species-specific and affects only humans. It is passed by direct contact with another person or with droplets on fomites. Even if lesions are not present, virus can still be shed. The incubation period ranges from 1 day to 4 weeks. At the time of an initial infection, the virus enters the epithelium and travels to regional nerve ganglia where it remains for the host's lifetime. Because it is intracellular, normal immune protection mechanisms do not work against these latent viruses and current antiviral agents do not eradicate the latent state.
- Clinically, herpes simplex infection can manifest with symptoms that range from recurrent cold sores to encephalitis.
  ○ **Herpes gingivostomatitis** is a primary infection usually caused by HSV-1.
    ▪ The peak incidence is in children less than 5 years of age.
    ▪ Patients appear quite ill with high fever, painful vesicles on the tongue and mucous membranes, and regional lymphadenopathy. They frequently drool and refuse to eat. The fever may last for 1 week, with sores persisting for up to 2 weeks.
  ○ **Herpetic whitlow** is a painful inoculation of herpes virus onto a finger. This occurs in children who

suck their fingers and in medical personnel from direct contact or through a needle stick. A primary infection with fever, local pain, regional lymphadenopathy, and general malaise may develop.

- ○ **Genital herpes** results from sexual contact with an infected partner or from self-inoculation from an oral infection with virus spread from the patient's hands or fomites. Primary infections include painful localized vesicles, regional lymphadenopathy, and fever. Many primary infections are subclinical. With recurrence, the pain is less severe and there is no fever or lymphadenopathy. Itching and burning may be present for a day before vesicles appear and pain can last for up to a week. Recurrences can be triggered by spicy foods, stress, or trauma, although many patients cannot determine a specific trigger. Most cutaneous herpes infections resolve without scarring.
- ○ **Neonatal herpes simplex infection**, usually caused by HSV-2, results from intrauterine, intrapartum, or postpartum exposure. Symptoms can develop up to 6 weeks after birth. Infants may develop disseminated systemic illness, an infection limited to the skin, or encephalitis without any skin lesions. Infants with herpes encephalitis usually develop permanent long-term neurologic sequelae. Other rashes that can be confused with oral herpes infections include hand-foot-and-mouth disease, herpangina, or impetigo. Herpetic whitlow is often confused with bacterial cellulites. Genital herpes infections can be mistaken for other venereal problems and may coexist with gonorrhea or syphilis.
- A Tzanck smear with multinucleated giant cells identifies herpes simplex infections. Confirmation with viral culture or rapid assay may be necessary.
- Acyclovir (15 mg/kg, 5 times daily for 5 to 7 days) will shorten the course of a primary herpes infection if started early in the illness. Local acyclovir 5-percent ointment applied 6 times a day may provide relief and shorten viral shedding for localized perioral or genital infections. If no treatment is given, up to 70 percent of infants will develop disseminated infection and there is a 50 percent chance of mortality with systemic illness. Intravenous acyclovir is recommended for neonatal herpes infections when systemic illness or encephalitis is present. Because infants with skin lesions may develop encephalitis as a late complication, some authorities recommend oral acyclovir during the first few months of life. Local symptomatic care includes analgesics, cool compresses, ice packs, and forcing of fluids. Consider intravenous fluids if patients refuse to drink. While local eruptions do shed virus, this virus is so common that isolation to prevent contagion is not practical.

ENTEROVIRUSES

- Nonspecific viral rashes may be maculopapular, scarlatiniform, vesicular, or urticarial. Many infections are subclinical and isolation from day care is impractical. A few clinical syndromes can be differentiated.
- **Hand-foot-and-mouth syndrome** is caused by coxsackievirus. It has a variable incubation period, usually a few days, and is most common in summer and fall. There may be a prodrome of low fever, malaise, and abdominal pain. Children may complain of a sore mouth or painful hands and feet. Vesicles about 5 mm in diameter are found on palms, soles of feet, buttocks, and sometimes on the trunk. Oral lesions usually appear later on the soft palate, gingivae, and tongue. The illness lasts about 3 to 6 days. Cases may recur for several weeks. Infrequent complications include myocarditis, pneumonia, and meningoencephalitis.
- **Herpangina** is caused by several enteroviruses and herpes simplex virus, and causes an enanthem of tiny vesicles on the soft palate, uvula, and tonsils. Findings include sore throat, dysphagia, fever, headache, myalgias, and vomiting.
- Treatment is symptomatic: soft diet, bed rest if needed, and analgesics for pain. Hand washing may reduce viral spread.

PITYRIASIS ROSEA

- Pityriasis rosea is a self-limited disorder of unclear etiology. It is most common in adolescents and young adults. Most cases begin with a single, large, oval scaly patch about 2 to 5 cm in diameter. This "herald patch" is followed by crops of small, oval, scaly patches that appear on the trunk and run parallel to skin cleavage lines. They create a "Christmas tree" pattern. The herald patch fades quickly. The secondary patches take several weeks to fade. There may be mild itching, pharyngitis, and malaise. The distribution of the rash is diagnostic. Differential considerations include tinea corporis and secondary syphilis. An RPR and VDRL should be ordered in all sexually active teenagers. Pityriasis rosea resolves without sequelae.
- Most patients require only reassurance and education. Exposure to sunlight may hasten disappearance of the rash and moisturizers may stop itching. There is no role for topical steroids.

BIBLIOGRAPHY

American Academy of Pediatrics 2003 Red Book: *Report of the Committee on Infectious Diseases*, 26th ed. American Academy of Pediatrics, Elk Grove Village, IL.

Amir J: Clinical aspects and antiviral therapy in primary herpetic gingivostomatitis. *Paediatr Drugs* 3:593–597, 2001.

Cohen B: *Pediatric Dermatology*, 2d ed. St. Louis, Mosby Year Book, 1999.

Edwards L: *Dermatology in Emergency Care.* New York, Saunders, 1997.

Gershon AA: Live-attenuated varicella vaccine. *Infect Dis Clin North Am* 15:65–81, 2001.

Schachner LA, Hansen RC (eds): *Pediatric Dermatology*, 2d ed. New York, Saunders, 1995.

Skull SA, Wang EE: Varicella vaccination—A critical review of the evidence. *Arch Dis Child* 85:83–90, 2001.

Weston WL, Lane AT: *Color Textbook of Pediatric Dermatology.* St. Louis, Mosby Year Book, 1996.

QUESTIONS

1. Which of the following is true of rubeoloa (measles)?
   A. It is associated with cough, coryza, and conjunctivitis.
   B. It is associated with a rash that travels from the feet upward.
   C. It is not highly contagious.
   D. The most common associated problem requiring hospitalization is encephalitis.
   E. The most common means of spread is by hand-to-hand contact.

2. Which of the following is true for rubella (German measles)?
   A. It is associated with a severe flu-like illness in children.
   B. It rarely causes adenopathy.
   C. It is not an illness associated with teratogenicity.
   D. It is often complicated by pneumonia.
   E. It can be associated with joint pain.

3. Which of the following is true for roseola (exanthem subitum)?
   A. It is caused by herpes simplex virus.
   B. It is associated with a low-grade fever.
   C. It can be associated with a bulging fontanelle.
   D. It usually requires hospitalization.
   E. The rash precedes the fever.

4. Which of the following is true of fifth disease (erythema infectiosum)?
   A. It is caused by an enterovirus.
   B. It is associated with glomerulonephritis.
   C. It can cause aplastic crisis in patients with sickle cell disease.
   D. It causes a diffuse vesicular rash.
   E. It is associated with children who appear ill.

5. The management of chickenpox includes which of the following?
   A. Hospitalization of virtually every patient
   B. Empiric antibiotics in all patients to prevent secondary skin infection
   C. Intravenous acyclovir in all patients with chickenpox less than 2 years old
   D. Varicella zoster immune globulin in immunocompromised patients exposed to chickenpox
   E. Systemic steroids

6. Which of the following is true regarding herpes simplex virus?
   A. It does not cause gingivostomatitis in children.
   B. It rarely causes subclinical infection.
   C. It can cause serious systemic disease in neonates.
   D. It often causes liver failure in previously healthy patients.
   E. The peak incidence is in adolescents.

ANSWERS

1. A. Cough, coryza, and conjunctivitis are characteristic of measles; the most common problem for which children with measles require hospitalization is pneumonia. It is spread by the respiratory route.

2. E. Rubella is a mild, self-limited illness, mostly significant for its teratogenic potential in women infected in the first or second trimester of pregnancy. It can be associated with arthralgias in older children.

3. B. Roseola is associated with a well-appearing child with a high fever; occasionally, the fontanelle can be bulging, but lumbar puncture is normal. The rash appears as the fever vanishes.

4. C. Fifth disease is associated with the "slapped cheek" appearance in well-appearing children. It is caused by parvovirus, which can cause aplastic crisis in patients with sickle cell disease.

5. D. Certain immunosuppressed patients, especially leukemics, are at high risk for severe illness from varicella, and should receive varicella zoster immunoglobulin within 48 h of exposure to a patient with chickenpox.

6. C. Herpes simplex can cause devastating disease in neonates; it usually presents as a vesicular rash; treatment includes hospitalization and intravenous acyclovir. The peak incidence is in children under 5 years of age.

66 INFANT RASHES

Julia A. Rosekrans
Kemedy K. McQuillen
William R. Ahrens

SEBORRHEIC DERMATITIS

- Seborrheic dermatitis occurs in young infants and adolescents and is characterized by greasy, scaly skin. It is caused by an overproduction of sebum that leads to accumulation of scaly exfoliated skin on the scalp, eyebrows, behind the ears, and in the axillae. Lipophilic yeasts of the Malassezia genus, as well as genetic, environmental, and general health factors, contribute to this disorder. Seborrhea is more common in warm weather. It is a chronic, relapsing condition that usually resolves before 1 year of age. Infantile seborrhea does not increase the risk of seborrhea or acne in adolescence. The differential diagnosis includes dandruff, psoriasis, yeast infections, atopic dermatitis, and Letterer-Siwe disease.
- Use low-potency topical corticosteroids to treat inflamed weeping areas. Using a soft brush, soften scalp scales with mineral oil, and wash the scalp with a mild selenium sulfide, pyrithione zinc, or ketoconazole-containing shampoo. Diaper area seborrhea requires treatment with antifungal medication to eradicate superinfection with *Candida*.

DIAPER DERMATITIS

- The biggest factor that contributes to diaper rash is chronically wet skin. Wet skin is vulnerable to injury, and any condition that irritates the skin will be accentuated in a moist environment. Ammonia, although easy to smell, probably does not contribute to diaper area irritation.
- *Candida albicans* frequently causes a secondary infection of damaged skin, although it is not a primary cause of diaper rash.
- Infants with atopic dermatitis or seborrhea frequently have trouble with nonspecific diaper rash and may be more prone to *Candida* infection.
- Diaper rash due to **chafing** occurs mainly on the thighs and around the waist where skin folds rub together. The skin is mildly erythematous, dry, and may be lichenified. It tends to appear and resolve quickly. **Irritant diaper rash** occurs on the lower abdomen, buttocks, and inner thighs and spares intertriginous folds. The skin is reddened with papules, vesicles, and scaly lesions. *Candida* **diaper dermatitis** appears as reddened skin involving the intertriginous areas with sharply demarcated margins and pustular or vesicular "satellite lesions." A perianal **GABH streptococcal infection** is characterized by a painful, bright, glistening red eruption around the anus. Psoriasis may be confused with a nonspecific diaper rash. It can be differentiated by the presence of plaques on other areas of the body and a strong family history.

- The mainstay of diaper dermatitis treatment is keeping the skin dry. Frequent diaper changes and the use of cornstarch powder to reduce friction may help to reduce development of diaper rash. When an inflamed rash is present, avoid rubbing the skin: it may be necessary to rinse the baby in warm water to circumvent the need for cleaning with a washcloth or premoistened wipe. Use emollients containing zinc oxide to provide barrier protection and decrease friction. Use hydrocortisone cream (1 percent) two or three times a day to reduce inflammation. Avoid fluorinated steroids since they are absorbed excessively from the diaper area. Treat *Candida* diaper rash with topical imidazole or nystatin with or without a 1 percent hydrocortisone cream. Tell parents to avoid cornstarch powder until the *Candida* rash is resolved. Treat perianal streptococcal infections with oral penicillin or erythromycin. Parents should be instructed to follow up in one week if the diaper rash is not improved.

BIBLIOGRAPHY

Cohen B: *Pediatric Dermatology*, 2d ed. St. Louis, Mosby Year Book, 1999.

Edwards L: *Dermatology in Emergency Care.* New York, Saunders, 1997.

Johnson BA, Nunley JR: Treatment of seborrheic dermatitis. *Am Fam Physician* 61:2703–2714, 2000.

Schachner LA, Hansen RC (eds): *Pediatric Dermatology*, 2d ed. New York, Saunders, 1995.

Weston WL, Lane AT: *Color Textbook of Pediatric Dermatology*, St. Louis, Mosby Year Book, 1996.

QUESTION

1. Which of the following is correct regarding diaper dermatitis?

A. It is caused by local irritation due to ammonia
B. It is almost always caused by chronically wet skin
C. It is best prevented by keeping the perineal skin moist
D. It is often a manifestation of an allergic reaction
E. The primary cause is *Candida albicans*

ANSWER

1. B. Diaper dermatitis usually results from chronically wet skin. Candida albicans is a common secondary infection; it appears as reddened skin with sharply demarcated margins.

67 EAR AND NOSE EMERGENCIES

Thomas J. Abrunzo
John P. Santamaria
Kemedy K. McQuillen
Gary R. Strange

ACUTE OTITIS EXTERNA

- Acute otitis externa is a common childhood illness that refers to any inflammatory condition of the external ear.
- The external ear extends from the pinna to the tympanic membrane.
  - The lateral third, or cartilaginous portion, has hair follicles, glands that produce bacteriostatic cerumen, and tightly applied skin.
  - The medial two-thirds, or osseous portion, does not contain glands that produce cerumen.
  - Additionally, the avascular cartilage of the pinna and external acoustic meatus limits host resources in wound healing and infection control.
- The development of acute otitis externa is dependent upon the presence of microorganisms in a moist, warm environment: the bony end of the canal supports bacterial growth since it lacks cerumen, traps moisture, and approximates body temperature. Anything that interrupts the integrity of the epithelial lining can predispose to infection.
- *Pseudomonas, Staphylococcus, Streptococcus*, gram-negative organisms and diphtheroids cause acute otitis externa.
- *Aspergillus,* which causes approximately 90 percent of fungal cases, is more common in immunosuppressed or hyperglycemic patients.

- Itching and mild pain are early symptoms of otitis externa. As bacterial invasion progresses, worsening edema and tissue tension cause worsening pain. Pain is exacerbated by traction to the pinna, pressure on the tragus, or movement of the jaw from side to side. If untreated, swelling of the ear canal will occur and an exudate may develop. For patients with a fungal etiology, white, yellow-green, or dark-pigmented masses composed of hyphae are seen. Acute otitis externa is characterized by local symptoms and systemic toxicity suggests another diagnosis.
- Stains and cultures of ear discharge are necessary when disease is unresponsive to usual treatment or when unusual microorganisms are suspected.
- Differential considerations include a retained foreign body, a furuncle or localized pyogenic infection, atopic dermatitis, seborrheic dermatitis, dyshidrosis, contact dermatitis, and otitis media with perforation. Furuncles are frequently caused by *Staphylococcus aureus*, and if not fluctuant, are treated with warm compresses and systemic antibiotics.
- The first step of treatment is cleaning out the ear canal with suction, dry mopping, curetting, or irrigation. This improves examination, removes inflammatory exudates, and allows better contact between topical medications and the diseased area. When treating, instill enough topical medication to fill the canal. If there is significant edema, use a wick to facilitate medication transport to the end of the canal. Wicks should be removed within 2 days. In mild cases, antiseptic drops, such as boric acid or aluminum acetate, can be used. With more severe inflammation, antibiotic-steroid topical preparations should be used. They are effective against *Pseudomonas*, other gram-negative bacteria, and staphylococci and they also have anti-inflammatory and antipruritic effects. If fungal infection is suspected, consult an

otolaryngologist. Several weeks of topical tolnaftate therapy are usually required.

- **Malignant otitis externa**, a deeper infection with necrosis, thrombosis and vasculitis, is almost always caused by *P. aeroginosa*. It is refractory to conventional treatment, has a high mortality rate, and rarely occurs in children, primarily affecting diabetic adolescents and those who are immunosuppressed. Contiguous structures such as cartilage, bone, the mastoid air spaces, lymph glands, and the parotid gland may be involved. Sequelae include facial nerve paresis, stenosis of the external canal, and hearing loss. Malignant otitis externa requires an otolaryngologist, prolonged intravenous antibiotic therapy, and possible surgical debridement.

OTITIS MEDIA AND MASTOIDITIS

- Otitis media includes acute suppurative otitis media and otitis media with effusion. The incidence peaks between 6 and 13 months and mastoiditis is an uncommon complication.
- Eustachian tube dysfunction is important in the pathogenesis of otitis media. The eustachian tube has three major functions: equilibration of the middle ear and atmospheric air pressures, protection from secretions of the nasopharynx, and clearance of middle ear secretions into the nasopharynx. Allergy, infection, or anatomic predisposition causes congestion of the eustachian tube, blocking the clearance of middle ear secretions. Accumulated secretions serve as a culture medium and suppuration and rupture of the tympanic membrane may result. Supine positioning and shorter eustachian tubes in young children enhance reflux of nasopharyngeal pathogens into the middle ear, while a more horizontal orientation hampers drainage, all of which predispose to otitis media. Hematogenous spread of bacteria into the middle ear is possible in newborns, but uncommon.
- The posterior wall of the middle ear communicates with the mastoid antrum and air cells via the aditus. The mucous membrane lining the tympanic cavity and mastoid structures is continuous.
- Otitis media and mastoiditis are caused by *Streptococcus pneumoniae*, nontypeable *Haemophilus influenzae*, *Branhamella catarrhalis*, group A streptococcus, and *S. aureus*. *Chlamydia trachomatis* can cause otitis media in infants less than 6 months old, and *S. aureus*, group B streptococcus, and gram-negative enteric bacteria can cause otitis media in neonates. *Mycoplasma pneumoniae* should be considered in cases unresponsive to initial therapy or when tympanic bullae are present. The role of viruses is poorly understood.

- Historic findings include ear pain, discharge, hearing loss, fever, headache, malaise, gastrointestinal irritation, altered behavior, and anorexia. As part of the physical exam, inspect the pinna, postauricular area, and external auditory canal for inflammation. Use a pneumatic otoscope with a well-fitting speculum to evaluate the color, lucency, light reflex, bony landmarks, and mobility of the tympanic membrane. Findings in otitis media include redness, opacity, absence of landmarks, alteration of the light reflex, and lack of mobility. Tympanic membrane immobility is the only reliable sign of otitis media in crying children. Cerumen must be removed for an adequate exam: curettage, suction, and irrigation are commonly used. In mastoiditis, redness and swelling over the mastoid area may be seen. Outward, downward protrusion of the pinna is suggestive of subperiosteal abscess.
- Laboratory evaluation is not required for uncomplicated otitis media. In mastoiditis, blood cultures should be done even though the yield is low. Culture of material from the mastoid mucosa or subperiosteal abscess cavity may also provide a microbiologic diagnosis. Computed tomography or magnetic resonance imaging may be helpful in the diagnosis of mastoiditis, brain abscess, or lateral sinus thrombosis.
- Otitis media can be confused with dysbaric injury and otitis externa. Crying, otherwise normal children can also have physical findings consistent with acute otitis media.
- Complications of acute otitis media include bacteremia, tympanic perforation, mastoiditis, cholesteatoma, facial paralysis, labyrinthitis, and infectious eczemoid dermatitis. Intracranial complications such as meningitis, brain abscess, encephalitis, and lateral sinus thrombosis may be heralded by worsening ear pain while on antibiotics, persistent headache, intractable emesis, or behavior change. Meningismus, visual changes, papilledema, seizure, and focal neurologic findings may not be present, especially when patients are "partially treated" with oral antibiotics.
- An antimicrobial effective against *S. pneumoniae*, *H. influenzae*, and *B. catarrhalis* is indicated.
  - Amoxicillin is the first-line agent.
    - For children over 2 years old who attend day care with recent antibiotic exposure, higher-dose amoxicillin is recommended.
    - If there are frequent treatment failures on amoxicillin, or if there is a large proportion of beta-lactamase–producing strains, other drugs should be considered as first-line therapy.
  - For children with treatment failures after 3 days (persistent ear pain, otorrhea, or red, bulging tympanic membranes), second-line antimicrobial treatment is recommended. Second-line agents include high-dose

amoxicillin-clavulanate, cefuroxime, and intramuscular ceftriaxone.

- Observation without initial antibiotic use, while predominant in other countries, remains controversial in the United States.
- Recommend analgesics, topical anesthetic otic drops, antipyretics, and local heat for pain. Oral narcotics may be necessary.
- In neonates, the possibility of hematogenously spread disease requires a complete septic workup, admission, and intravenous broad-spectrum antibiotics pending culture results.
- Some authorities recommend that in otherwise well neonates over 2 weeks old, otitis media without systemic toxicity can be treated on an outpatient basis with oral antibiotics.
- There is no conclusive evidence supporting the use of topical or systemic steroids, decongestants, or antihistamines.
- Patients with otitis media should be rechecked if symptoms worsen or if there is no improvement in 3 days. Otherwise, reevaluation in 2 weeks is appropriate.
- Children with concomitant systemic bacterial infection or toxic appearance may require hospitalization and intravenous antibiotics.
- In cases of mastoiditis, admit all patients, consult an otolaryngologist, and start a broad-spectrum intravenous antibiotic; ceftriaxone or a penicillinase-resistant penicillin with an aminoglycoside can be used. Breakdown of bony septae between mastoid air cells (mastoid osteitis) and subperiosteal abscess are indications for mastoidectomy. Tympanostomy tubes are placed if concurrent otitis media is present.

FOREIGN BODY OF THE NOSE AND EAR

- Foreign bodies are most commonly self-inserted, either in play or as a response to an itch or irritation. Animal foreign bodies, such as insects, worms, and larvae, can be deposited as eggs or enter as adults. The position, movement, size, and antigenicity of the foreign body influence bleeding and tissue reaction, and anatomic characteristics of the ear and nose predispose to foreign body retention. The external acoustic meatus is oval in transverse section, with a constriction near the medial end of the cartilaginous part and another in the osseous portion; while in the nose, the turbinates impede visualization and removal of foreign bodies.
- Excessive cerumen, while not a foreign body, is the most common cause of aural obstruction. It may present with a headache, hearing loss, or a painful, itchy, or draining ear. Its production and clearance are influenced by ethnic, familial, and individual factors. Cerumen retention is also exacerbated by the use of cotton swabs that pack the cerumen into the canal, sometimes adding cotton fibers to the wax mixture. Small, tortuous external ear canals associated with syndromes such as trisomy 21 can also impede cerumen clearance.
- Historical clues to the presence of a foreign body include bleeding from the ear or nose, pain, fever, discharge, and alterations in smell or hearing. Foreign bodies can masquerade as chronic infections, tumors, recurrent epistaxis, and generalized body odor (bromidrosis). Both sides of the nose and both ears must be examined.
- Plain radiographs generally are not helpful unless a rhinolith, or a mineralized nasal foreign body, is present. Gradually increasing in size, it is usually discovered as an incidental finding on plain radiograph. More sensitive radiographic techniques or direct visualization with an endoscope can demonstrate the presence of a foreign body in the posterior portion of the nose that is not readily visualized on examination. In difficult cases, radiographic studies can be used prior to removal to demonstrate the size and position of a retained foreign body.
- Complications can occur due to the foreign body, the examination, or the removal and include blockage and infection. Infection can occur locally or in the sinus if the ostia is blocked or in the middle ear if the eustachian tube is blocked. Nasal foreign bodies may present with recurrent epistaxis due to mucosal erosion and local irritation. Aspiration is a risk if foreign bodies are pushed into the nasopharynx. A case of meningitis and death secondary to a foreign body is reported in the literature.
- Adequate restraint and sedation of the child before instrumentation will minimize potential complications.
- The first attempt at removal is the most likely to be successful, because removal attempts may stimulate bleeding, mucosal edema, and movement of the object to a less accessible area. Therefore, any case with a low probability of successful removal in the emergency department should be referred to an otolaryngologist.
- Before attempting foreign body removal, it is prudent to be prepared for complications (Table 67-1).
- After explanation of the procedure to children and family, adequate immobilization should be ensured.
- Do not attempt removal without a good light source: for most foreign bodies of the nose and ear, direct visualization and instrumentation through an otoscope is adequate, although a nasal speculum and headlight may be better for nasal foreign bodies.

TABLE 67-1   Equipment for Examination and Removal of a Nasal or Aural Foreign Body

Immobilization device (sheet or papoose board)
Sedative medications (see Chap. 24)
Otoscope for instrumentation under direct visualization
Nasal speculum
Headlight (optional)
Topical vasoconstrictor (phenylephrine 0.125%–0.5%, cocaine 4%, or epinephrine 1:1000)
Alligator or Hartman forceps
Wire loop or curette
Suction apparatus, including catheters of various sizes
Foley or Fogarty catheter no. 8 (optional)

- Foreign body shape, location, and composition influence the removal technique. Insects are usually easier to remove when they are not moving: they can be killed with alcohol, viscous lidocaine, or mineral oil before removal is attempted. Wood and other vegetable matter swell when wet and are best removed before irrigating the ear canal. Mineral-based foreign bodies, such as round plastic beads, are difficult to grasp. When the object cannot be grasped with forceps, a wire loop curette may be slipped behind the foreign body or a cotton-tipped applicator with superglue on it can be applied, held in place until the glue dries, and removed with the foreign body attached. Some practitioners remove foreign bodies with suction or small Foley catheters.

- To avoid damaging the ear canal or tympanic membrane while using an otoscope, curette, or other instrument, anchor part of that hand against the child's head. If the child's head moves suddenly, the examining hand and instrument will then move with it. Use a curette or irrigation to remove impacted cerumen. Small aural foreign bodies close to the tympanic membrane may be removed with tap water irrigation. A 30 to 60-mL syringe attached to a plastic infusion catheter, or a butterfly needle with the tubing cut off 3 cm from the hub, will deliver adequate volumes for irrigation at adequate pressures. If the canal is traumatized during cerumen or foreign body removal, consider prophylactic therapy for acute otitis externa.

- When removing a nasal foreign body, apply a topical vasoconstrictor to reduce tissue edema and aid removal; additionally, opening the nasal speculum vertically will help avoid septal damage. Nasal foreign bodies may also be removed by occluding the unaffected nares and blowing air into the mouth and out through the nose using an ambu bag.

- Since children may pack a nose or ear with several objects at once, a thorough recheck for other objects is advisable after a foreign body is removed.

- If emergency department removal is not possible and immediate removal is not necessary, start the child on oral antibiotics to cover normal upper respiratory flora and refer them to an otolaryngologist for outpatient treatment.

EPISTAXIS

- Nosebleeds tend to occur in the preteenage population and are almost exclusively anterior in location, either at the nasal vestibule or the plexus of vessels on the anterior, inferior portion of the nasal septum (Little's area, Kiesselbach's plexus). Less commonly, occult bleeding from the respiratory and gastrointestinal tracts can present as epistaxis. Epistaxis digitorum, or "nose picking," is the most frequent cause of nosebleed in children. Dry air, forceful nose blowing, increased vascularity associated with local infection, systemic bleeding disorders, drug use, barotrauma, tumors, postsurgical changes and deviated nasal septum are also predisposing factors to nosebleed. No association with hypertension has been demonstrated. Careful examination is important to exclude nasal foreign bodies and septal hematomas.

- Historically there may be recent trauma, upper respiratory infection, allergy, or exposure to dry air. Prolonged bleeding or easy bruising in patients or family members is an important clue to systemic disorders. In bilateral epistaxis, the history of which side bled first usually reveals the bleeding site. Ask how much bleeding occurred, but expect an overestimation. History of behavior change, pallor, or orthostatic dizziness suggests significant blood loss: altered mental status, delayed capillary refill, tachycardia, and tachypnea may be noted. Hypotension is a late finding. Blood under the nails may be evidence of nose picking. Associated lymphadenopathy or evidence of other bleeding suggests systemic disease.

- Supplies, including suction apparatus for emesis and blood, should be readied before attempting evaluation of epistaxis, so that treatment can accompany examination. The head down position will lessen the risk of aspiration from swallowed blood. Careful physical examination, facilitated by the use of a headlamp and nasal speculum, usually reveals the bleeding point. Open the speculum in a rostrocaudal direction to avoid damaging the nasal septum. Removal of blood with a Fraser suction tip aids localization of the bleeding point. Positioning small children in their parent's lap with manual restraint is often helpful.

- Hemoglobin and type and cross-match are indicated if there is evidence of hypovolemia. Epistaxis alone is usually self-limited and does not warrant evaluation for a coagulation defect.

- Number of recurrences, general health of patients, and hydration status should be considered when deciding whether or not to treat a nosebleed.
- No treatment is required for patients whose bleeding resolves spontaneously or with direct pressure.
- For persistent bleeding, remove as much blood and clot as possible, fill the anterior nasal cavity with topical thrombin and have the patient or parent apply 10 min of firm, constant pressure: this is more effective and better tolerated than using silver nitrate cautery.
- Alternatively, place a cotton pledget soaked in Neo-Synephrine (0.125 to 0.5 percent), epinephrine (1:1000), or cocaine (4 percent) into the nose for 10 min.
- If bleeding persists, use cautery judiciously: children's have a thin nasal septum that may be perforated.
- Epistaxis can also be treated with local injection of 1 to 2 mL of lidocaine with epinephrine (1:100,000): it has tamponading and vasoconstrictive effects but systemic effects should be anticipated.
- Rarely, nasal packing may be required and should be done in consultation with an otolaryngologist. Use nasal sponges instead of packing with petrolatum gauze; they are easily inserted when dry, can be cut to size, and expand when moistened. Prescribe antibiotics (cephalosporins, amoxicillin/clavulanate, or macrolides) and arrange for packing removal within 2 days.
- Complications include syncope during packing, sinusitis, bacteremia, local infection, toxic shock syndrome, and iatrogenic sleep apnea if bilateral sponges are placed.
- Suspect a posterior bleed if a bleeding site cannot be visualized and anterior packs are ineffective. With posterior bleeds, admission and an otolaryngology consult is needed. Temporize bleeding with Foley catheters or pneumatic nasal catheters: eustachian tube obstruction and subsequent otitis media can occur. A posteriorly placed pack, arterial ligation, pterygopalatine fossa block, and embolization are rarely needed in a child.
- Pediatric epistaxis is likely to recur. Recommend humidifiers, petroleum jelly rubbed onto the anterior nasal septum and the skin at the nasal orifice, and short fingernails. Habitual nose-pickers may benefit from covering their hands with socks during sleep.

RHINITIS

- Rhinitis is the most frequent cause of nasal discharge, with children suffering 6 to 21 episodes per year.
  - Rhinovirus, influenza, parainfluenza, respiratory syncytial virus (RSV), and adenovirus are common causes.
  - Bacterial rhinitis may complicate viral rhinitis and is usually heralded by the development of a purulent discharge and persistence of symptoms. Sinusitis often coexists. Pathogens include *H. influenzae*, *Staphylococcus* spp., *B. catarrhalis*, and *S. pneumoniae*.
    - Children under 3 years of age may develop, streptococcosis, a subacute condition characterized by rhinitis, prolonged course, low-grade fever, and adenopathy.
  - Rhinitis can also result from pertussis, diphtheria, congenital syphilis, *Chlamydia trachomatis, Ureaplasma urealyticum, Pneumocystis carinii*, or cytomegalovirus.
  - IgE-mediated allergic rhinitis peaks in late adolescence.
  - Topical toxin exposure (eg, vasoconstrictor drops or cocaine) or systemic absorption (eg, aspirin or estrogens) may cause rhinitis. Prolonged topical vasoconstrictor use can cause rhinitis medicamentosa, characterized by inflammation and chronic nasal congestion, which further encourages the use of the offending agent.
- Ask about known precipitants; discharge quality, quantity, and timing; factors that improve or worsen the discharge; and associated symptoms. Solicit history of previous episodes, known sensitivities, medications, prior therapy, and topical decongestant use. Examine the nasal mucous membrane with a good light source and nasal speculum: a large-caliber otoscope speculum can also be used. Swelling, erythema, and secretions are evidence of inflammation. Laboratory and radiographic evaluation are not needed in the acute management of infectious or allergic rhinitis.
- Rhinitis therapy is disease specific (Table 67-2). Recommend oral or topical decongestants (vasoconstrictors); however, limit topical therapy to 5 days to minimize rebound phenomena. Some authors advocate the use of unilateral decongestant nasal spray: the unsprayed side improves in approximately 3 days. Bacterial rhinitis should be treated with antibiotics effective against *S. pneumoniae* and *H. influenzae*: amoxicillin, trimethoprim-sulfamethoxazole, and cefaclor are first-line agents. When avoidance, decongestants, and

TABLE 67-2 Response to Treatment of Infectious and Allergic Rhinitis

	INFECTIOUS	ALLERGIC
Decongestants	Fair	Fair
Antihistamines	Poor	Good
Steroids	None	Excellent
Immunotherapy	None	Variable
Cromolyn	None	Fair
Antibiotics and antivirals	Disease specific	None

antihistamines fail, steroids, cromolyn sodium, and immunotherapy may be tried. Inhaled steroids cause less adrenal suppression and are preferred to oral preparations.

SINUSITIS

- Sinusitis is a bacterial inflammation of the paranasal sinuses associated with nasal mucosal inflammation and obstruction of the sinus ostia. The condition is most often manifested as a prolongation or complication of a viral upper respiratory tract infection. Children average six to eight upper respiratory infections per year and 0.5 to 5 percent are complicated by sinusitis. Symptoms range from the more common, persistent, purulent rhinorrhea and cough to the less common fever, headache, facial pain, and swelling. It is classified as acute (less than 4 weeks duration), subacute (4 to 12 weeks duration), or chronic (over 12 weeks duration). Further, symptoms lasting under 10 days, without recent antibiotic use, tend to be viral upper respiratory infections and do not require antibiotic therapy.
- The paranasal sinuses are four paired structures: maxillary, ethmoid, sphenoid, and frontal. Maxillary and ethmoid sinuses are aerated soon after birth, while the frontal sinuses do not appear radiographically until the seventh year and the sphenoids until the ninth year of life. Sinusitis can occur at any age and the maxillary and ethmoids are involved most frequently. The sinuses drain beneath two of the three shelf-like turbinates of the lateral nasal wall. The sphenoids and posterior ethmoids drain into the superior meatus and the maxillary, frontal, and anterior ethmoids drain into the middle meatus, which can sometimes be directly visualized. Normal paranasal sinuses function depends on patency of the sinus ostia, function of the ciliary apparatus, and the nature of sinus secretions. An abnormality of any of these will predispose to bacterial infection. Predisposing factors include allergies, rhinitis, foreign bodies, choanal atresia, cleft palate, neoplasm, septal deviation, adenoidal hypertrophy, polyps (allergic, cystic fibrosis), dental infection, immunodeficiency, and immotile cilia syndromes (such as Kartagener's syndrome). Swimming, trauma, and rhinitis medicamentosa may also cause mucosal swelling and sinus ostium obstruction. Bacterial sinusitis pathogens are similar to those of acute otitis media.
- The key to differentiating upper respiratory infections from sinusitis is the unusual severity or protraction of symptoms found in the latter. Severe signs and symptoms include fever over 39.0°C (102.2°F), purulent nasal discharge, and periorbital swelling. Protracted (>10 days) findings are more common and may include nasal discharge (clear or purulent), cough that is frequently worse at night, bad breath, facial pain, and periorbital edema that is worse in the morning. Fatigue, malaise, decreased appetite, and weight loss are sometimes noted. Headache, dental pain, and facial tenderness are uncommon. Sphenoid sinusitis, although rare in children, often occurs without respiratory complaints and is associated with frontal, temporal, or retroorbital pain: it can result in severe intracranial complications and is an important consideration in the differential diagnosis of headache. Physical exam may include purulent drainage from the middle meatus, boggy nasal mucosa, postnasal drip, and cobblestoning of the posterior pharynx. Transillumination is of limited value: in older children, it is useful if it is normal or absent.
- The white blood cell count and blood cultures are occasionally useful in toxic patients. If a sinus puncture is done, the material should be sent for Gram's stain and culture for aerobes and anaerobes. Radiographs have variable reliability. Normal sinus films are helpful while abnormal sinus films are difficult to interpret: beyond 6 years of age the interpretation can be more definitive. Abnormal radiographic findings include clouding, mucoperiosteal thickening of more than 4 mm, and air fluid levels, with the last being most helpful in defining acute infection. Sinus films should include the occipitomental or Water's view (maxillary sinus), the anteroposterior or Caldwell view (frontal and ethmoidal sinuses), the submentovertex view (sphenoid sinus), and lateral view (sphenoid sinus). If maxillary sinusitis is suspected, a single Water's view may suffice. With equivocal plain radiographs, computed tomography scan is indicated if children are seriously ill, have had recurrent episodes, have chronic disease, or have suspected suppurative complications.
- The differential diagnosis of sinusitis includes acute viral upper respiratory tract infection, allergy, foreign body, neoplasm, or polyp. Functional and organic causes of headache should also be excluded.
- Sinusitis can seed the systemic circulation resulting in bacteremia or septicemia. Local extension can result in facial cellulitis, facial abscess, periorbital and orbital cellulitis, osteomyelitis of the skull (Pott's puffy tumor), cavernous sinus thrombosis, epidural abscess, subdural empyema, meningitis, and brain abscess.
- Although sinusitis resolves spontaneously in 40 percent of cases, antibiotic therapy is indicated to hasten resolution of symptoms and to prevent complications.

- ○ Antibiotics should be continued for one week beyond the resolution of symptoms; generally 14 days.
- ○ The choice of antibiotic therapy depends on duration of symptoms and local drug-resistance patterns.
  - ▪ Initial treatment includes amoxicillin (40 mg/kg per day divided bid) or, in the penicillin sensitive, a macrolide such as clarithromycin (15 mg/kg per day divided bid), or azithromycin (10 mg/kg per day on day 1, and 5 mg/kg per day on days 2 through 5).
  - ▪ For nonresponsive cases and suspected resistant organisms, amoxicillin doses of 80 to 90 mg/kg per day divided bid; cefuroxime axetil 30 mg/kg per day divided bid; amoxicillin clavulanate at 40 mg/kg per day divided bid; or a combination of amoxicillin and amoxicillin clavulanate each at 40 mg/kg per day are recommended.
  - ▪ With known penicillin-resistant *S. pneumoniae*, clindamycin is also used.
  - ▪ Nonresponders should be referred for otolaryngologist consultation.
- ○ Needle or surgical drainage is necessary for patients unresponsive to antibiotics.
  - ▪ Antral puncture by an otolaryngologist is indicated if there is severe pain unresponsive to medical management; sinusitis in a seriously ill, toxic child; an unsatisfactory response; suppurative complications; or if patients are immunocompromised.
  - ▪ Recurrent or refractory sinusitis may be further evaluated by antral lavage.
  - ▪ Persistent infection, unresponsive to multiple antibiotics, is treated surgically with an antral window or endoscopic enlargement of the osteomeatal unit.
- ○ Degree of toxicity, ability to tolerate oral fluids, complicated or serious disease, age, and reliability of follow-up will dictate whether inpatient management is necessary.
  - ▪ Immunocompromised hosts, toxic children, and those with sphenoid sinusitis require inpatient therapy for parenteral antibiotics.
- ○ Antihistamines, decongestants, steroids, and cromolyn sodium are variably (in)effective in pediatric sinusitis.

BIBLIOGRAPHY

Barnett ED, Teele DW, Klein JO, et al: Comparison of ceftriaxone and trimethoprim-sulfamethoxazole for acute otitis media. *Pediatrics* 99:23, 1997.

Bluestone CD, Stool SE, Kenna MA: *Pediatric Otolaryngology.* New York, Saunders, 1996.

Dowell SF, Butler JC, Giebink GS, et al: Acute otitis media: management and surveillance in an era of pneumococcal resistance—A report from the drug-resistant *Streptococcus pneumoniae* Therapeutic Working Group. *Pediatr Infect Dis J* 18:1, 1999.

Green SM, Rothrock SG: Single-dose intramuscular ceftriaxone for acute otitis media in children. *Pediatrics* 91:23, 1993.

Kadish, HA, Cornell, HM: Removal of nasal foreign bodies in the pediatric population. *Am J Emerg Med* 15(1):54, 1997.

McCracken GH: Diagnosis and management of acute otitis media in the urgent care setting. *Ann Emerg Med* 39:413–421, 2002.

Van Zuijlen DA, Schilder AG, Van Balen FA, et al: National differences in incidence of acute mastoiditis: Relationship to prescribing patterns of antibiotics for acute otitis media? *Pediatr Infect Dis J* 20:140–144, 2001.

QUESTIONS

1. Malignant otitis externa is almost always caused by:
   A. *Streptococcus* spp.
   B. *Aspergillus*
   C. *Staphylococcus aureus*
   D. *Pseudomonas*
   E. Numerous gram negative bacteria
2. A 3-year-old child is brought to the ED with ear pain. He is crying loudly and resists examination. Which of the following is an essential component of the diagnosis of acute otitis media in this patient?
   A. Fever.
   B. Erythema of the tympanic membrane.
   C. Opacification of the tympanic membrane.
   D. Immobility of the tympanic membrane.
   E. Alteration of the light reflex.
3. Bullous myringitis is typically associated with infection due to:
   A. *Pseudomonas*
   B. *Mycoplasma pneumoniae.*
   C. *Streptococcus spp.*
   D. *Aspergillus*
   E. *Hemophilus influenzae* type b
4. In removing a foreign body from the nose, which of the following tips is correct?
   A. Explain the procedure to the child and continue to talk to her in a calm reassuring manner during the procedure. Physical restraint is rarely required.
   B. Most nasal foreign bodies are easily visualized and removable with the use of only a penlight.
   C. When using a nasal speculum, it is best to open it in a vertical manner in the nostril.
   D. Topical vasoconstrictors should not be used.
   E. Nasal foreign bodies composed of organic material are very difficult to remove and should be referred directly to an otolaryngologist.

5. A 15-year-old girl presents to the ED with persistent epistaxis for several hours. She has moderate flow of blood from the right nostril. With suction and a headlight, you are able to visualize a bleeding site on the anterior septum. Which management option is most appropriate?
   A. Digital pressure for 10 min.
   B. Fill the anterior nasal cavity with topical thrombin and then apply digital pressure for 10 min.
   C. Silver nitrate cautery of the bleeding site.
   D. Electrical cautery of the bleeding site.
   E. Pack the right nasal cavity with nasal sponges.

ANSWERS

1. D. Malignant otitis externa is almost always due to *Pseudomonas* infection and is resistant to conventional treatment. It is seen primarily in diabetic or immunosuppressed adolescents. It requires intravenous anti-pseudomonal antibiotics.

2. D. Tympanic membrane immobility is the only reliable sign of otitis media in crying children, since abnormalities of the color, lucency, light reflex, and landmarks can be false-positive findings.

3. B. Myringitis with bullae is an infection of the tympanic membrane caused by various bacteria and viruses but it is most commonly associated with infection caused by *Mycoplasma pneumoniae.*

4. C. Opening the nasal speculum in a vertical orientation avoids pressure and possible damage to the septum. Physical restraint is essentially always required for nasal foreign body removal in a child. Failure to restrain can lead to injury. No attempts at removal should be made without a good light source. An otoscope may be sufficient if the foreign body is easily visualized and accessed, but a headlight is preferable. Topical vasoconstrictors can be very helpful. Foreign bodies that are composed of organic material are notorious for absorbing water and swelling. They also may shred when they are grasped. However, there is no contraindication to attempting removal in the ED.

5. B. Filling the anterior nasal cavity with topical thrombin followed by 10 minutes of firm, constant pressure is safe, effective, technically simpler, and better tolerated than is using silver nitrate cautery. Children's thin nasal septum must be considered at risk for perforation when cautery is done. It is uncommon for childhood epistaxis to require nasal packing and it should only be done in consultation with an otolaryngologist.

68 EMERGENCIES OF THE ORAL CAVITY AND NECK

Thomas J. Abrunzo
John P. Santamaria
Kemedy K. McQuillen
Gary R. Strange

DENTOALVEOLAR INFECTIONS

- Infections originating from dental structures begin in the dental pulp or, less commonly, the periodontium, the tissue investing and supporting the tooth. Periodontal infections tend to localize to intraoral soft tissue and seldom extend to deeper structures of the face and neck. These infections include gingivitis, periodontitis, or periodontal abscess and pericoronitis. Periodontitis is a chronic inflammation and infection of the dental-gingival interface usually seen in adults, but also occurring in immunosuppressed children. Pericoronitis is an acute, localized infection caused by food particles and microorganisms that have become trapped under the gum flaps (opercula) of partially erupted or impacted teeth.

- Dental pulp infections are usually the result of caries that occur secondary to bacteria-facilitated disintegration of enamel, dentin, and cementum. These infections can erode the periodontal membrane and extend into the mandible and maxilla. Infection of the pulp can also result from a fracture or a defect in the apical foramen or lateral canals. Hematogenous seeding with bacteria may also occur. Once infected, pus may exit the pulp canal apically, forming a periapical or alveolar abscess or it may track laterally, through the alveolar bone and gingiva to form a parulis ("gum boil"). Dental infections can extend locally to involve deep fascial spaces of the mandible (Ludwig's angina). *Bacteroides, Peptostreptococcus, Actinomyces*, and *Streptococcus* are common pathogens.

- A history of recent restoration or extraction; sensation of a change in the surface; and thermal, percussion, or chemical sensitivity suggest failed dental therapy, dental fracture, or new caries as a cause of pain. Pain, fever, gingival swelling, and purulent gingival discharge suggest periodontal abscess, periapical abscess, pulpitis, pericoronitis, or gingivitis. Dental examination includes a search for discoloration, fractures, swelling, fluctuance, and percussion tenderness. Palpation may disclose tenderness or purulent discharge. Anterior cervical adenopathy may be present.

- A panoramic radiograph (panorex) may reveal dental disease or maxilla or mandible involvement. A computed tomography (CT) scan may be necessary to diagnose deep fascial space infection. A complete blood cell count and cultures of the site and blood may be useful in toxic patients.

- Treat caries with analgesics and a dental referral. Pulpitis and periapical abscess require analgesia and systemic antibiotics against oral flora. Incision and drainage may be necessary. Pericoronitis and periodontitis are treated similarly; incision and drainage may be avoided with irrigation and gentle debridement of opercula, with removal of retained debris. Treat patients with uncomplicated dental infections as outpatients and admit those with deep fascial space infections.

GINGIVOSTOMATITIS

- Gingivitis presents as tender, swollen, edematous, and sometimes friable gum tissue with or without vesiculation or ulceration. It may be accompanied by stomatitis, which presents as either diffuse erythema or vesicoulceration (Table 68-1).
- Poor oral hygiene, neutropenia, and mouth breathing predispose to gingivitis. Gingivitis may accompany prepubertal and pubertal maturation.
- Phenytoin causes a painless, extensive, firm, lobulated, hypertrophic gingivitis.
- Hypovitaminosis C (scurvy) causes gingivitis with bone pain, irritability, petechial hemorrhage, poor wound healing, and the sicca syndrome of Sjögren.
- Primary dental disease can cause localized gingivitis.
- Histiocytosis X can cause gingivitis, swelling of the palate, and loss of teeth. It is associated with dermatitis, proctitis, vaginitis, and hepatosplenomegaly.

TABLE 68-1   Oral Ulcers: Diagnostic Considerations

Acute necrotizing gingivostomatitis
  (trench mouth: Vincent's angina)
Aphthous stomatitis
Autoimmune
Candidiasis (oral thrush)
Chemical (antineoplastic)
Drugs (phenytoin)
Epstein-Barr virus
Erythema multiforme and Stevens-Johnson syndrome
Hand-foot-and-mouth disease
Herpangina
Herpes simplex
Herpetic gingivostomatitis
Malignancy (leukemia)
Radiation-induced
Syphilis (primary and secondary)
Traumatic
Varicella zoster
Vitamin deficiency (scurvy)

- Exposure history frequently assists in diagnosis. Fever is common, except with *Candida.* Posterior pharyngeal ulcers likely represent coxsackie virus: buccal and lingual vesicles and maculovesicles on the hands and feet (hand-foot-and-mouth disease) may be present. Gingivitis from a primary herpes simplex infection is usually accompanied by high fever and swollen, red, friable gums with diffuse oropharyngeal mucosal lesions that may become confluent. It is differentiated from trench mouth (Vincent's angina) by the latter's isolated gingival involvement. Syphilis may present in its primary stage as oral, lingual, and tonsillar chancres and, in its secondary stage, as superficial, excoriated, weeping, exudative lesions found anywhere in the oropharynx. Mucosal blistering occurs in the Stevens-Johnson form of erythema multiforme. *Candida* stomatitis presents with white, flocculent, confluent patches found diffusely over the tongue and oropharyngeal mucosa.
- Laboratory evaluation is not helpful in most cases of gingivostomatitis. A complete blood cell count can diagnose leukemia and Epstein-Barr virus (EBV) infection. A "monospot" may also diagnose an EBV infection. Syphilis is diagnosed with serologic studies and dark-field microscopy.
- Treat uncomplicated gingivitis with good oral hygiene. Children with painful lesions may benefit from gargling or oral administration of kaopectate and diphenhydramine with or without viscous lidocaine. Use lidocaine cautiously as overuse may cause seizures. Systemic analgesics are sometimes necessary. With secondary gingivitis, treat the underlying cause. Use nystatin for a *Candida* infection and penicillin for trench mouth (ANUG). Syphilitic ulcers require benzathine penicillin, tetracycline, or erythromycin with serologic follow-up at specified intervals. Patients with Stevens-Johnson syndrome have significant morbidity and mortality and should be admitted. Use acyclovir for herpes simplex virus infections.

PHARYNGITIS

- The pharynx is the musculomembranous sac adjacent to the mouth, nares, and esophagus and includes tonsillar and adenoidal lymphoid tissue. Infectious, allergic, mechanical, and chemical processes can cause pharyngeal inflammation. Viruses, bacteria, spirochetes, *Chlamydia, Mycoplasma*, mycobacteria, fungi, and parasites can all cause pharyngitis; viruses are the most common infectious cause. Common viral pathogens include adenovirus, parainfluenza virus, rhinovirus, herpes simplex, respiratory syncytial virus, Epstein-Barr virus, influenza virus, enterovirus (coxsackie virus and echo virus), coronavirus, and cytomegalovirus. Group A beta-hemolytic streptococcus is the most common bacterial cause of pharyngitis in children under 3 years of age. One must also consider groups C and G streptococci, *Neisseria gonorrhoeae*, and *Corynebacterium diphtheriae*. *Corynebacterium hemolyticum* causes pharyngitis with a scarletiniform rash. Pneumococcus, *Staphylococcus aureus, N. meningitides*, and *Haemophilus influenzae* can cause pharyngitis, usually after a viral upper respiratory infection. Syphilis may present with diffuse pharyngeal inflammation and focal chancres primarily; gray mucous patches are noted secondarily. *Chlamydia trachomatis* and *Mycoplasma pneumoniae* can be responsible for pharyngitis in adolescence. *Candida* may cause a diffuse oropharyngeal erythema with thick white exudate in immunosuppressed patients and in those taking antibiotics. A "scratchy" throat may be due to sinusitis, posterior nasal drip, or respiratory irritants. Caustic ingestions can present with pharyngeal pain. Agranulocytosis, lymphoma, and lymphocytic leukemia may present with pharyngeal inflammation. Uvula inflammation results from bacterial infection (group A hemolytic streptococcus, *H. influenzae* type B, *Streptococcus pneumoniae*), trauma, and allergy. It is most worrisome when associated with epiglottitis or angioneurotic edema, both potentially life-threatening conditions.

- Infants and toddlers with pharyngitis may have nonspecific irritability, poor feeding, anorexia, drooling, or oral lesions. Older children can localize pain to the throat. Clear rhinorrhea, cough, hoarseness, or mucosal ulcers suggest a viral etiology. Epstein-Barr virus and cytomegalovirus infection often have pharyngeal inflammation, diffuse lymphadenopathy, and hepatosplenomegaly. Herpangina causes small vesicular lesions and punched-out ulcers in the posterior pharynx. Hand-foot-and-mouth disease causes vesicles and ulcers in the areas noted. Low-grade fever, follicular conjunctivitis, sore throat, and cervical lymphadenopathy characterize pharyngoconjunctival fever. Streptococcal pharyngitis tends to have an acute onset and may include fever, throat pain, dysphagia, headache, vomiting, abdominal pain, and scarletiniform rash (fine, erythematous, sandpaper-like). It most often occurs in late winter and early spring. Diphtheria presents with an adherent, grayish pharyngeal membrane, bull neck, and toxic appearance. Tularemia follows exposure to small animals. Pharyngitis accompanied by rash, joint pain, and urethral or vaginal discharge, may indicate gonorrhea. Urticaria, wheezing, or stridor may indicate an allergic etiology.
- Rapid streptococcus detection by latex agglutination or enzyme immunoassay is useful when positive. A negative rapid screening test should be confirmed with a culture. Local suppurative complications, manifested by severe dysphagia, stridor, dysphonia, and odynophagia, may require soft tissue radiographs of the lateral neck or CT of the neck. Incision and drainage may be necessary. CBC, EBV titers, monospot, syphilis screening tests, and cultures for *N. gonorrhoeae* are indicated for atypical presentations. Nonsuppurative complications of streptococcal infection may require urinalysis, antistreptolysin-O (ASO), "Streptozyme," renal function tests, and electrocardiogram.
- Suppuration can spread to contiguous tissue, causing:
  ○ Peritonsillar abscess (quinsy).
  ○ Life-threatening Lemierre's postanginal sepsis (aerobic or anaerobic bacteremia from septic thrombophlebitis of the tonsillar vein).
  ○ Ludwig's angina (submandibular abscess).
- Hematologic spread may result in mesenteric adenitis, meningitis, brain abscess, cavernous sinus thrombosis, suppurative arthritis, endocarditis, osteomyelitis, sepsis, and septic embolization to the lung.
- Nonsuppurative complications of streptococcal infection include scarlet fever, rheumatic fever, and glomerulonephritis.
- Gonococcus and syphilis can disseminate systemically. Untreated diphtheria may progress to seizures or respiratory failure.
- Streptococcal pharyngitis requires antibiotics. Treatment includes oral penicillin, 250 mg twice a day for children under 12 years of age and 500 mg twice a day for children older than 12; each for 10 days. If compliance and follow-up are in doubt, give intramuscular benzathine penicillin, 600,000 U for children weighing less than 60 lb and 1,200,000 U for children who weigh more than 60 lb. Treat penicillin-allergic patients with erythromycin ethylsuccinate, 40 mg/kg per day in 2 to 4 doses daily for 10 days. If diphtheria is suspected, give diphtheria antitoxin and penicillin or erythromycin. Treat tularemia with streptomycin or gentamicin. Allergic entities may require epinephrine, 1:1000, 0.01 mL/kg per dose, subcutaneously. Antihistamines, such as diphenhydramine, (1.25 mg/kg per dose) and corticosteroids, such as prednisone, (2 mg/kg per dose orally) are also used.

PERITONSILLAR ABSCESS

- Peritonsillar abscess (quinsy) is the most common deep infection of the head and neck. Usually a complication of bacterial tonsillitis, it can also occur with EBV infection and can extend to the peripharyngeal space and tissues. They are rare in children under 12 years old. Most peritonsillar abscesses are polymicrobial: Group A streptococci predominates but *Peptostreptococcus,*

Peptococcus, Fusobacterium, anaerobes, *H. influenzae, S. pneumoniae*, and *S. aureus* may also be detected.

- Historically, there is gradually increasing pharyngeal discomfort and ipsilateral otalgia, followed by drooling, trismus, dysarthria, dysphagia and odynophagia. The voice has a muffled, "hot potato" quality and patients are often toxic.

- The oropharynx examination may show cellulitis (diffuse peritonsillar swelling and edema) or an abscess (trismus, peritonsillar mass, soft palate and uvula displacement contralaterally, fluctuance, and ipsilateral cervical adenopathy). Spiking fevers, chills, neck stiffness and pain, torticollis toward the opposite side (from sternocleidomastoid spasm), and swelling around the parotid gland may herald peripharyngeal extension.

- The white blood cell count may be elevated and the throat culture will often document a streptococcal infection. Blood and tonsillar aspirate cultures are helpful. If patients are not responding to standard antibiotic therapy, a CT of the head and neck can delineate the extent of the disease.

- Peritonsillar abscess may be confused with peripharyngeal space infections, cervical adenitis and abscess, foreign bodies, dental infections, tetanus, salivary gland infections, tumors, tonsillitis or peritonsillar cellulitis.

- Complications include peripharyngeal extension, necrotizing fasciitis, airway obstruction, aspiration pneumonia, mediastinitis, lung abscess, thrombophlebitis, and sepsis.

- Most patients with a peritonsillar abscess require admission for hydration, intravenous antibiotics, analgesia, and, possibly, surgical drainage. Appropriate antibiotics include a third generation cephalosporin, such as ceftriaxone (100 mg/kg per day q 12 h IV), cefotaxime (150 mg/kg/day q 8 hours IV), or clindamycin (40 mg/kg per day q 6-8 h IV). If resolution is slow, nafcillin, 100 to 150 mg/kg per day q 4 h IV is started. Needle aspiration is sometimes used diagnostically to differentiate between cellulitis and peritonsillar abscess and can be employed for definitive treatment instead of incision and drainage in cooperative patients. Tonsillectomy may be necessary in children with recurrent problems or slow resolution of symptoms.

RETROPHARYNGEAL ABSCESS

- A retropharyngeal abscess is an accumulation of pus in the prevertebral soft tissue of the upper airway. Fifty percent of cases occur between 6 and 12 months of age, and 96 percent occur in children under 6 years old. Infections in the nasopharynx, middle ear, adenoids, and posterior paranasal sinuses drain into the retropharyngeal lymphoid tissue and can result in suppuration of the nodes and abscess formation. Less commonly, retropharyngeal abscess is the result of extension of infection from penetrating injuries or vertebral osteomyelitis Causative organisms include *S. aureus*, group A hemolytic streptococci, *H. influenzae*, and anaerobes (*Bacteroides, Peptostreptococcus*, and *Fusobacterium* spp).

- Diagnostically, there is usually a prodromal nasopharyngitis or pharyngitis followed by the abrupt onset of high fever, dysphagia, refusal to eat, severe throat pain, hyperextension of head, and noisy respirations. Patients may complain of a pain in the back or shoulders with swallowing. There may be labored respirations, drooling, and stridor. A bulge in the retropharynx is frequently visible and meningismus may result from irritation of the paravertebral ligaments.

- An elevated white blood cell count with a shift to the left is present but is not needed for a therapeutic decision. Gram stain and culture of purulent material obtained from incision and drainage is essential. A soft tissue lateral neck radiograph with proper hyperextension will usually demonstrate the retropharyngeal mass: the prevertebral space is normally less than 7 mm anterior to C2 and less than 5 mm anterior to C3 and C4 or less than 40 percent of the anteroposterior diameter of the C3 or C4 vertebral bodies.

- Differential considerations include epiglottitis, croup, mononucleosis, peritonsillar abscess, cystic hygroma, hemangioma, and primary neurogenic neoplasms. Trauma to the retropharynx from foreign body ingestion, instrumentation, and cervical spine injury can also cause swelling.

- Retropharyngeal abscess complications include airway obstruction, aspiration, and rupture into the esophagus, mediastinum, or lungs with subsequent empyema and pneumonia. Blood vessels may erode and hemorrhage can occur. Inadequate drainage can allow abscess reformation.

- Airway maintenance is vital since airway obstruction and aspiration can occur at any time. Admit patients for hydration, intravenous antibiotics, analgesia, and surgical drainage. Antibiotics include penicillin G 25 to 50 mg (40,000 to 80,000 U)/kg per 24 hours q 4 h IV or nafcillin 100 to 150 mg/kg per 24 hours q 4 h IV. A third-generation cephalosporin such as ceftriaxone (100 mg/kg per 24 hours q 12 h IV) or cefotaxime (150 mg/kg per 24 hours q 8 h IV) may also be added.

CERVICAL LYMPHADENOPATHY

- Lymphadenopathy is enlargement of one or more lymph nodes. Benign lymph node enlargement and lymphadenitis account for most childhood neck masses.

- Bacterial, viral, mycobacterial, fungal, and parasitic infections, Kawasaki's disease, cat-scratch disease, Kikuchi's lymphadenitis, sarcoidosis, and antigenic stimulation by drugs, bites, or stings can stimulate node inflammation and enlargement.
- *S. aureus* accounts for 60 percent and group A streptococcus accounts for 85 percent of primary lymphadenitis in children. Less common agents include *Mycobacterium tuberculosis*, nontuberculous mycobacteria, anaerobic bacteria, *Francisella tularensis* (tularemia), *Yersinia pestis* (plague), *Brucella melitensis* (brucellosis), *Chlamydia* spp., *Mycoplasma* spp., *Treponema pallidum* (syphilis), *Actinomyces israelii*, *Streptococcus pyogenes*, *H. influenzae*, *Pseudomonas aeruginosa*, and *Toxoplasma gondii*.
- Viral causes include rhinovirus, adenovirus, enterovirus, EBV, mumps, rubella, rubeola, chickenpox, and herpes simplex.
- Kikuchi's disease (necrotizing lymphadenitis) is a benign condition of concern primarily for its variable association with fever and leukopenia, which can be confused with lymphoma.
- Cat-scratch disease causes regional lymphadenitis, is usually diagnosed after a recent kitten scratch, and can be confirmed with an antigenic skin test (Hanger-Rose test) or by biopsy.
- Noninfectious causes of lymphadenopathy include traumatic soft tissue swelling, malignancy, congenital muscular torticollis, branchial cleft cyst, thyroglossal duct cyst, cystic hygroma, lymphangioma, sarcoidosis, and vascular abnormalities.
- History should include time of symptom onset and clinical course, upper respiratory infection, concurrent sore throat, duration of symptoms, skin lesions of the scalp or face, fever, dental problems, pets, and exposure to tuberculosis or other infections. The most useful differentiating finding on examination of an enlarged lymph node is the presence or absence of inflammation. A hot node presents with erythema, warmth, tenderness, and sometimes fluctuance. "Cold" or uninflammed nodes require a thorough search for associated disease such as cat-scratch disease, tuberculosis, nontuberculous mycobacterial infections, and malignancy. A painless, firm neck mass should be considered malignant until proven otherwise.
- If malignancy is suspected, a CBC with manual differential may reveal anemia, thrombocytopenia, or abnormal white blood cell count with immature cells. If tuberculosis is suspected, place a 5TU purified protein derivative (PPD) skin test: if anergy is suspected, also place a control skin test. Nontuberculous mycobacteria may weakly react to PPD. Specific antigenic skin tests are available for some of the non-tuberculous mycobacteria, but culture is the only reliable means of confirming the diagnosis. Culture spontaneously draining nodes. In immunocompromised patients, neonates, or when antibiotic therapy has failed, the abscess material should be cultured for aerobic and anaerobic bacteria, mycobacteria, and fungi.
- Treatment is directed against the primary cause of the adenopathy: tuberculosis is treated by medical means, but non-tuberculous mycobacterial infections usually require complete node excision. If the cause is cat-scratch disease, then patients should be treated with rifampin or trimethoprim-sulphamethoxazole. Hot or suppurative nodes are most commonly caused by beta-hemolytic group A streptococci (*S. pyogenes*) and penicillin-resistant *S. aureus* and can be treated with cephalexin, amoxicillin/clavulanic acid, or erythromycin. Arrange follow-up in 2 to 3 days to reevaluate, read skin tests if placed, and examine for fluctuance. Toxic appearance, advanced disease, young age, unreliable follow-up, unresponsiveness to oral therapy, immunocompromised host, or inability to tolerate oral medications mandate inpatient therapy. Inpatient management should include semisynthetic penicillin, such as intravenous oxacillin. If fluctuance occurs or if patients are unresponsive to medical management, obtain surgical consultation. Emergency physician incision and drainage of the nodes should be avoided because a persistent draining sinus can result. Total surgical excision of the node is curative, prevents a draining sinus, and allows a clear etiologic diagnosis. The disease process determines the therapy of cold lymphadenopathy. An otolaryngologist should follow children with suspected malignancy.

BIBLIOGRAPHY

Alvarez A, Schreiber JR: Lemierre's syndrome in adolescent children—anaerobic sepsis with internal jugular vein thrombophlebitis following pharyngitis. *Pediatrics* 96:354–359, 1995.

Amsterdam JT: Dental emergencies: Part I—Pain and trauma. *Emer Med* 26:21–39, 1994.

Kureishi A, Chow AW: The tender tooth: Dentoalveolar, pericoronal and periodontal infections. *Infect Dis Clin North Am* 2:163, 1988.

Pickering LK (ed): Red Book 2000. Report of the Committee on Infectious Disease. *American Academy of Pediatrics*, 213, 2000.

QUESTIONS

1. Children with stomatitis, ulcers, or severe sore throat may safely benefit symptomatically from gargling or careful administration of:

A. A saline solution made by adding 2 tablespoons of salt to an 8-ounce glass of warm water.
B. 2 percent lidocaine solution
C. Over-the-counter mouthwashes
D. A combination of kaopectate, diphenhydramine and viscous lidocaine
E. Steroid solutions

2. Suppurative pharyngitis can spread to cause all of the following EXCEPT:
A. Peritonsillar abscess (quinsy)
B. Septic thrombophlebitis of the tonsillar vein (Lemierre's postanginal sepsis)
C. Kawasaki disease
D. Meningitis
E. Submandibular abscess (Ludwig's angina)

3. A 9-month-old child presents to the ED with upper respiratory and pharyngeal symptoms for several days. He has been previously healthy and his immunizations are up-to-date. On the day of presentation, a fever spiked to 104°F, the child refused feedings and water. He appears to experience pain on attempting to swallow and there is some increased drooling. He maintains the head in a hyperextended position. Respirations are stridorous. What is the most likely cause of this child's problem?
A. Epiglottitis
B. Viral croup
C. Peritonsillar abscess
D. Retropharyngeal abscess
E. Foreign body

ANSWERS

1. D. This combination is safe and effective. Saline solutions may be used but should not be concentrated; 1 teaspoon in 8 ounces of warm water is a common recommendation. Concentrated lidocaine solutions can lead to seizures. Mouthwashes may be irritating to inflamed tissues. Systemic steroids have been shown to be useful in severe sore throat patients but there is no evidence to support their topical oropharyngeal use.

2. C. Suppuration can spread to contiguous tissue causing peritonsillar or submandibular abscess, as well as septic thrombophlebitis of the tonsillar vein. Hematologic spread can result in serious bacterial illness including meningitis. Kawasaki disease is of unknown etiology and is associated with pharyngeal injection but not suppuration.

3. D. Many of this child's symptoms are suggestive of epiglottitis but the long prodrome, young age and up-to-date immunization status make this diagnosis less likely. Viral croup would not usually present with such a toxic appearance. Peritonsillar abscess is a disease of older children and adolescents and generally does not cause this degree of airway involvement. Foreign body is possible but the acute onset of high fever suggests an infectious etiology. This presentation is very typical for retropharyngeal abscess which tends to present between the ages of 6 months and 2 years, with abrupt onset of fever following an upper respiratory prodrome, and with dysphagia, drooling and stridor.

69 EYE EMERGENCIES

Katherine M. Konzen
Ghazala Q. Sharieff
Kemedy K. McQuillen
Gary R. Strange

INTRODUCTION

- The visual acuity in both eyes must always be checked. Information about the unaffected eye can help guide in the assessment of the affected eye.
- If the possibility of a globe perforation exists, manipulation of the eye should not be performed. A metal shield should be used to protect the eye; a pressure patch is contraindicated.

PHYSICAL EXAMINATION OF THE EYE AND DIFFERENTIAL CONSIDERATIONS

VISION

- Some method of testing visual acuity must be available for both preverbal and verbal children.
  - For very young children, the ability to focus on an object such as a toy may give a rough assessment of visual acuity. A newborn can fixate on a close object, and a 1-month-old should be able to follow a moving object.
  - For older children, Snellen letters or Allen figures are useful to check visual acuity in both eyes.
- Normal visual acuity is:
  - 20/40 in a 3 year old
  - 20/30 in a 4 year old
  - 20/20 in a 5 to 6 year old

LIDS AND ORBIT

- Children with periorbital cellulitis will often have significant edema and erythema of both the upper and lower eyelids.
- The upper lid must be everted to rule out the presence of a foreign body by firmly grasping the lashes at the lid margin and everting the lid against countertraction at the superior tarsal margin using a cotton-tip applicator.
- Lacerations involving the medial canthus may result in a lacrimal duct injury and should be repaired by an ophthalmologist.
- Examination of the orbit includes palpation for defects in the orbital bony structure or for subcutaneous emphysema. Orbital fractures are often accompanied by ecchymosis, lid swelling, proptosis, and limitation in extraocular movements.
- Herniation and entrapment of the inferior rectus muscle within the orbital floor fracture results in paralysis of upward gaze.

ANTERIOR SEGMENT

- Conjunctival infections often begin unilaterally but may spread to the other eye within a few days. Crusting and exudate are usually present.
- In North America, the most common corneal infection causing permanent visual impairment is herpes simplex. Throughout the rest of the world, the most common agent is trachoma.
- Traumatic injuries to the cornea should be considered in even the youngest of children and can be the cause of a crying infant. Fluorescein examination for a corneal abrasion may be appropriate during the initial examination.

- Acute iritis (anterior uveitis) is rare in children and may be associated with juvenile rheumatoid arthritis or sarcoidosis. One should consider the possibility of iritis in children who have unilateral, sudden onset of pain, photophobia, and redness. Physical examination reveals a miotic pupil, perilimbal injection, and aqueous flare and cells on slit lamp examination.
  - Treatment includes early ophthalmologic consultation, cycloplegics, and steroid drops if recommended by the specialist.
- A hyphema occurs when there is hemorrhage in the anterior chamber. Complications of hyphemas include rebleeding, increased intraocular pressure, glaucoma, and corneal bloodstaining.
- Under penlight or direct ophthalmoscopic examination, the lens should be clear. If opacification is present, cataracts should be considered.

PUPILS AND EXTRAOCULAR MOVEMENTS

- Pupils should be black, round, symmetric, and equally reactive to light.
- Assess extraocular movements in all visual fields and clearly document all deficits.
- Pupillary assessment includes evaluation for an afferent pupillary defect known as a Marcus Gunn pupil in which pupillary constriction is delayed and diminished in both eyes when light is shone in the affected eye as compared to the normal eye. A Marcus Gunn pupil is evidence of injury to the anterior visual system and is a poor prognostic sign.

POSTERIOR SEGMENT

- The direct ophthalmoscope can be used to examine for papilledema, hemorrhages, retinal detachment, and intraocular foreign bodies.
- Blunt or penetrating trauma to the eye can lead to a vitreous hemorrhage. Other causes of hemorrhage include diabetes mellitus, hypertension, sickle cell disease, leukemia, retinal tears, central retinal vein occlusion, and tumor. Presentation of these patients is usually due to sudden loss of vision.
- Retinal artery occlusion is a true ocular emergency and can be due to emboli in patients with endocarditis and systemic lupus erythematosus or result from hypercoagulability in patients with sickle cell disease. When central retinal artery occlusion occurs, there is sudden, painless loss of vision in one eye. Ophthalmoscopic examination reveals the cherry-red spot of the fovea, a pale optic nerve and markedly narrowed arteries. A Marcus Gunn pupil may be present.
  - Ophthalmology consultation should be immediately obtained for possible paracentesis of the anterior chamber to decompress the globe.
  - Temporizing measures include ocular digital massage, topical beta-blocker (Timoptic 0.5 percent), acetazolamide, and CO_2 rebreathing by having patients blow into a paper bag for 5 to 10 min.
- Retinal vein obstruction also leads to sudden painless loss of vision that varies depending on the extent of the obstruction. Retinal hemorrhages and a blurred, reddened optic disk may be seen. These findings are often described as a "blood and thunder" fundus.
  - Aspirin therapy may be initiated to inhibit further thrombosis.
- Retinal detachment may take years to develop after a tear. As the detachment progresses, patients may have a visual field deficit or may complain of flashing lights or a "curtain" draping over the affected eye. Ophthalmoscopic examination will reveal a light-appearing retina in the area of detachment.
- Optic neuritis is usually due to inflammation or demyelination. It is characterized by an abrupt, rapid, unilateral loss of vision while pain is variable. Rarely does optic neuritis present as a separate entity in children.

INTRAOCULAR PRESSURE

- Pain and blurred vision should alert one to the possibility of glaucoma. Findings include a pupil that is nonreactive and dilated, and the appearance of halos around objects.
- Accurate measurement is accomplished by slit lamp tonometry or with a handheld tonometer. This should not be undertaken, however, if the possibility of a ruptured globe exists. Normal eye pressure in children ranges from 10 to 22 mm Hg.
  - An ophthalmologist must be immediately involved in the care and treatment of children with suspected glaucoma.
  - Immediate medical management includes:
    - Topical pilocarpine 1 to 2 percent once the intraocular pressure is below 40 mm Hg
    - Adrenergic agents
    - Mannitol 1 to 2 g/kg IV
    - Carbonic anhydrase agents
      - Acetazolamide is most often used at an oral dose of 15 mg/kg per day

COMMON ERRORS

- In managing eye emergencies, physicians should avoid some common mistakes:
  - Forgetting to examine the unaffected eye
  - Not thoroughly examining the injured eye
  - Failing to consider and recognize globe perforation
  - Prescribing topical anesthetics and steroids
  - Using eye drops or ointment when a perforation exists
  - Failure to ensure proper follow-up for patients

COMMON EYE COMPLAINTS

RED EYE

- Although conjunctivitis is common in childhood, other etiologies must be thoroughly considered prior to arriving at the diagnosis.
- All of the following are important in the consideration of the differential diagnosis (Table 69-1):
  - Time of onset
  - Exposure to chemicals or noxious stimuli
  - Exposure to other children with similar problems
  - Presence of systemic illness
  - History of trauma
  - Photophobia
  - Excessive tearing

TABLE 69-1   Differential Diagnosis of Red Eye

Conjunctivitis
   Bacterial
   Viral
   Herpes simplex
   Chemical
   Allergic or seasonal
   Neonatal ophthalmia
Corneal abrasion and corneal ulcer
Foreign bodies
Glaucoma
Hordeolum or chalazion
Iritis
Keratitis, episcleritis, scleritis
Periorbital or orbital cellulitis
Systemic disorders
   Ataxia-telangiectasia
   Collagen vascular disease
   Infectious disease—mumps, measles, otitis media
   Inflammatory bowel disease
   Juvenile rheumatoid arthritis
   Kawasaki disease
   Lyme disease
   Leukemia
   Stevens–Johnson syndrome
Trauma
   Chemical burns and thermal burns
   Ruptured globe
   Subconjunctival hemorrhage
   Hyphema

EYE PAIN

- Two fiber systems are involved in the transmission of eye pain.
  - Myelinated fibers transmit the sharp transient pain
  - Unmyelinated fibers transmit the dull aching sensations
- Pain fibers innervating the eye and periorbital structures arise from the trigeminal or fifth cranial nerve. The first (ophthalmic) division is the most important one responsible for eye pain.
- Eye pain in children results from a variety of causes including foreign bodies, corneal abrasions, conjunctivitis, episcleritis, acute dacryocystitis, congenital glaucoma, uveitis, optic neuritis, hordeolum, herpes zoster, and a wide array of trauma. Physicians should attempt to characterize the pain and then thoroughly search for the underlying etiology.

EXCESSIVE TEARING

- Usually noted in infants, excessive tearing can be due to nasolacrimal obstruction (dacryostenosis) or may be secondary to bacterial, viral, or allergic conjunctivitis. Sometimes infants with a corneal abrasion or glaucoma will have tearing.

EYE DISCHARGE

- Purulent eye discharge is most often associated with bacterial conjunctivitis while viral and allergic conjunctivitis are more often associated with mucoid discharge.
- Patients with blepharitis have crusting in addition to the discharge.

NONTRAUMATIC EYE DISORDERS

EYELID INFECTIONS

- Eyelid infections (blepharitis) often involve one of two glands.
  - Glands of Zeis: sebaceous glands attached directly to the hair follicles.
  - Meibomian glands: sebaceous glands that extend through the tarsal plate.
- The most common infections of the eyelid include chalazion, hordeolum, impetigo contagiosa, and herpes simplex.

CLINICAL FINDINGS

- An external hordeolum or stye is a suppurative infection of the glands of Zeis, whereas an internal hordeolum or chalazion is an acute infection of a Meibomian gland.
  - A chalazion presents as a painless, hard nodule and is often located in the midportion of the tarsus, away from the lid border caused from obstruction of the gland duct.
- Impetigo contagiosa is a pyoderma usually presenting with vesicles; it then develops a yellowish crust, which occurs due to local invasion by staphylococci or streptococci.
- Herpes simplex can present on the eyelids of children and can lead to latent infection, which may persist throughout life and be reactivated. Recurrent infection often involves the cornea.

MANAGEMENT

- The management of a hordeolum includes warm compresses and eyelid hygiene using baby shampoo on a washcloth. Twice-daily application of an antistaphylococcal antibiotic ointment (erythromycin ophthalmic ointment or polymyxin B sulfate) or ophthalmic drops should also be initiated.
- A chalazion is initially managed in the same manner, and antibiotic treatment should be continued for several days after rupture of the chalazion to prevent recurrence. If there is a lack of response to medical treatment, surgical incision and drainage under general anesthesia is recommended for young children.
- Impetigo contagiosa should be treated with removal of crusts and topical antistaphylococcal and streptococcal antibiotics. A cotton-tip applicator soaked in baby shampoo can be used to clean the lid margins.
  - Bacitracin ophthalmic ointment, topical erythromycin or gentamicin can be used.
- Herpes simplex blepharitis should be treated with vidarabine ophthalmic ointment and trifluorothymidine topical drops. Topical and oral acyclovir should be considered but may be of limited value.

CELLULITIS OF THE PERIORBITAL AND ORBITAL REGION

- The following classification has been described for orbital infections:
  - Class I: Periorbital or preseptal cellulitis. Cellulitis is confined to the anterior lamella tissue due to a lack of flow through the drainage ethmoid vessels. Lid edema and erythema may be mild or severe.

The globe ordinarily is not involved so that vision and function remain normal.
  - Class II: Orbital cellulitis. Orbital tissue is infiltrated with bacteria and cells, which extend through the septum into the orbital fat and other tissues. Manifestations usually include proptosis, impaired or painful movement, and periocular pain. Visual acuity may be impaired and septicemia may be present.
  - Class III: Subperiosteal abscess. Purulent material collects between the periosteum and the orbital wall. Medial wall involvement causes the globe to be displaced inferiorly or laterally. Symptoms include edema, chemosis, and tenderness with ocular movement, while vision loss and proptosis vary in severity.
  - Class IV: Orbital abscess. When pus accumulates within the orbital fat inside or outside the muscle cone, an orbital abscess has developed. The infectious process becomes localized and encapsulated, unlike orbital cellulitis, which tends to be more diffuse. Exophthalmos, chemosis, ophthalmoplegia, and visual impairment are generally severe; systemic toxicity may be impressive.
  - Class V: Cavernous sinus thrombosis. Thrombosis results from extension of an orbital infection into the cavernous sinus. Nausea, vomiting, headache, fever, pupillary dilation, and other systemic signs may be present. There is marked lid edema and early onset of third, fourth, and sixth cranial nerve palsies.
- In the newborn period and up to the age of 5 years, *Haemophilus influenzae* and *Streptococcus pneumoniae* are predominant, particularly in children with upper respiratory tract infections, conjunctivitis, sinusitis, or otitis media. In patients with a history of skin infections or trauma, *Staphylococcus aureus* and streptococcal species are the main offending agents.

MANAGEMENT

- Mild cases of preseptal cellulitis due to local trauma or conjunctivitis can be treated with oral antibiotics such as amoxicillin-clavulanate (20 to 40 mg/kg per day), to cover against *S. aureus*. Close follow-up is mandatory.
- For patients requiring hospitalization, a complete blood cell count, blood cultures, lumbar puncture, and CT of the head may be warranted. A lumbar puncture should be considered to rule out meningitis if patients appear toxic and are less than 2 years of age.
- The following management scheme has been recommended by several authors:
  - All patients hospitalized for orbital inflammation should receive ophthalmologic and otolaryngology consultation.

- Broad-spectrum antimicrobial therapy should be instituted at once while awaiting blood or intraoperative culture results.
  - Children under 5 years of age, without a history of trauma, should be placed on appropriate coverage against *H. influenzae* type B, *S. pneumoniae*, and group A streptococcus. A suggested initial regimen consists of ceftriaxone, 100 mg/kg per day, with the addition of vancomycin, 40 mg/kg per day in severe cases.
  - Children over 5 years of age or those fully immunized with the *Haemophilus influenzae* vaccine, do not generally require coverage for *Haemophilus*; appropriate antimicrobials are similar to those used for treatment of severe sinusitis.
- Attempts must be made to delineate the extent of the cellulitis. Computed tomography of the head is a helpful diagnostic aid but may not differentiate between subperiosteal abscess and reactive periosteal edema.
- Surgical indications include diminishing visual acuity, lack of improvement despite adequate antibiotics, or spiking fevers suggesting possible development of an orbital abscess or cavernous venous thrombosis.
- Orbital cellulitis secondary to sinusitis should be managed with the consultation of ophthalmology and otolaryngology. Intravenous antibiotics should consist of a third-generation cephalosporin and a penicillinase-resistant penicillin.

SCLERITIS AND EPISCLERITIS

- Scleritis is uncommon but can be associated with juvenile rheumatoid arthritis or various infectious processes.
- The thin vascular membrane between the sclera and conjunctiva is called the episclera. Inflammation of this area produces some irritation but not the severe pain associated with scleritis.

CONJUNCTIVITIS

OPHTHALMIA NEONATORUM

- Conjunctivitis in the newborn period (first 28 days of life) is not uncommon (Table 69-2). Because of the potential complications from ocular infections in infancy, neonates with symptoms mandate a thorough evaluation.
- Important guidelines for evaluation include:
  - Obtaining a detailed maternal history including prenatal care, history or exposure to venereal disease, duration of rupture of membranes, type of delivery, agent used for ocular prophylaxis at birth, recent exposure to conjunctivitis, and timing of onset of symptoms. History should also include a description of excessive tearing, type and amount of exudate, and elucidation of systemic signs of illness in the baby, such as fever, vomiting, irritability, or lethargy.
  - Physical examination must be thorough including a comprehensive eye examination searching for evidence of eyelid erythema, edema, discharge, corneal ulceration, globe perforation, or foreign body. In addition, general physical examination must be complete; special attention must focus on the skin, respiratory, and genitourinary system for evidence of concomitant systemic involvement.
  - Conjunctival scrapings should be obtained for Gram's stain, Giemsa's stain, and viral and bacterial cultures including *Neisseria*. A rapid antigen test is sensitive and specific for *Chlamydia* and can be obtained easily from the conjunctiva. Culture is usually not necessary.

DIFFERENTIAL DIAGNOSIS

Chemical Conjunctivitis

- Chemical conjunctivitis caused from silver nitrate drops in the immediate newborn period occurs in almost 10 percent of newborns.
- Signs of this type of conjunctivitis include bilateral conjunctival hyperemia and mild discharge that begin in the first 24 hours of life and usually subside within 48 hours.
- Gram's stain reveals no organisms and only a few white blood cells.
- The inflammation is typically quite mild and does not require intervention.

Chlamydia Trachomatis

- Typically, the conjunctiva becomes hyperemic and edematous with the palpebral conjunctiva more involved than is the bulbar conjunctiva. Unilateral, purulent involvement is characteristic.
- The diagnosis is confirmed by identification of chlamydial antigen, detection of intracellular inclusions from Giemsa's stain, or isolation of the organism. Antigen detection tests are rapid, sensitive, and specific and are the most efficient means of confirming the diagnosis. Gram's stain is not helpful in confirming the diagnosis.
- Systemic therapy is absolutely essential in the treatment of this condition. The treatment of choice is oral erythromycin (40 to 50 mg/kg per day) for a 2 to 3-week course to eliminate both conjunctival and nasopharyngeal colonization.
- Administration of a topical agent is unnecessary.

TABLE 69-2   Ophthalmia Neonatorum

	CHEMICAL CONJUNCTIVITIS	CHLAMYDIA	BACTERIAL	NEISSERIA	HERPES SIMPLEX	VIRAL
Onset	0–2 days	1–2 weeks	1–4 weeks	0–30 days	2–14 days	0–30 days
Discharge	–	+	+	+++	+	+
Unilateral/ bilateral hyperemia	B	U	U/B	B	U/B	U/B
Fever	–	±	–	±	±	–
Diagnosis	Negative Gram's stain, few WBCs	Rapid antigen, Giemsa's stain, or culture	Gram's stain, culture	Gram's stain, culture	Fluorescein staining, multinucleated giant cells, intranuclear inclusion cells, fluorescent antigen tests	History of contact exposure, negative Gram's stain, and viral culture
Treatment	None	Systemic oral erythromycin, 2–3 weeks	Topical antimicrobial	Intravenous third-generation cephalosporin	Intravenous acyclovir, topical trifluorothymidine	Topical antimicrobial
Associated findings	None	Pneumonia, otitis media	None	Rhinitis, anorectal infection, arthritis, meningitis	Skin lesions, septicemia	Upper respiratory tract infection
Long-term complications	None	Conjunctival scarring, micropannus formation	None	Blindness	Keratitis, cataracts, chorioretinitis, optic neuritis, others	None

WBC, white blood cells; – = absent; ± = may or may not be present; + = mild; + + = moderate; + + + = severe.

NEISSERIA GONORRHOEAE

- Gonococcal ophthalmia neonatorum classically presents as a purulent, bilateral conjunctivitis. Conjunctival hyperemia, chemosis, eyelid edema, and erythema may also be seen.
- This entity is diagnosed by Gram's stain, revealing gram-negative intracellular diplococci. Cultures should be sent immediately on blood and chocolate agar, because the organisms die rapidly at room temperature.
- Treatment must be systemic; there is no role for oral or topical antibiotics. Neonates without meningitis should be treated for 7 days with either ceftriaxone or cefotaxime. If meningitis is present, treatment continues for 10 to 14 days.

HERPES SIMPLEX

- The onset is generally 2 to 14 days after birth.
- Characteristics are not clinically distinctive; however, unilateral or bilateral epithelial dendrites are virtually diagnostic. Fluorescein staining reveals these defects.
- Treatment should consist of intravenous acyclovir for 10 days and topical trifluorothymidine.

- Parents must be aware of the high risk of recurrence of keratitis later in life; an ophthalmologist ought to follow these children closely.

OBSTRUCTED NASOLACRIMAL DUCT

- Congenital nasolacrimal duct obstruction, or dacryostenosis, is often only recognized when infants have a history of recurrent ocular infections. The blockage is frequently caused by failure to canalize a membrane called the *valve of Hasner*, which is located at the lower end of the nasolacrimal duct.
- Conservative treatment consists of massaging the lacrimal sac, suppressive topical antimicrobials, and warm compresses.
- Probing of the nasolacrimal system is not recommended until after 1 year of age because 95 percent of children younger than 13 months will experience spontaneous opening of the lacrimal duct.

NONINFECTIOUS ETIOLOGIES

- Corneal abrasions can be detected in infants and may often be secondary to a scratch from their fingernail. Conjunctival hyperemia may be present; fluorescein staining is diagnostic. Linear abrasions on the superior aspect of the cornea should alert the physician to an upper eyelid foreign body.

CONJUNCTIVITIS BEYOND THE NEONATAL PERIOD

- Conjunctivitis is a frequently encountered entity in children (Table 69-3).
- Conjunctivitis in older children is characterized by normal vision, a gritty sensation in the eye, diffuse injection, and exudate. Photophobia and lacrimation are not usually associated with conjunctivitis.
- Keratitis and iritis typically are associated with impaired vision, true pain, photophobia, and lacrimation.
- Clinically, viral conjunctivitis is difficult to distinguish from bacterial conjunctivitis. Marked exudate, severe injection, and lid matting is more typical of bacterial or chlamydial infections.

BACTERIAL CONJUNCTIVITIS

- Outbreaks of acute catarrhal conjunctivitis, also known as "pink eye," may occur in day care or among school-aged children. The offending organisms are most frequently *S. pneumoniae* or *Haemophilus aegyptius*.
- Although most types of acute bacterial conjunctivitis are self-limited, the use of topical antibiotic therapy is thought to shorten the clinical course and more quickly eradicate the organism, thereby decreasing the amount of time patients are contagious.
- Routine Gram's stain and culture usually is unnecessary unless there is a history of copious mucopurulent exudate (*Neisseria*) or a chronic history of conjunctivitis.
- Treatment is empiric with topical antimicrobial ointments or ophthalmic drops. Specific drugs include polymyxin B sulfate (Polysporin) ointment, which has a broad spectrum of activity including coverage for *H. influenzae*, erythromycin ointment or sodium sulfacetamide (Sulamyd), trimethoprim-polymixin (Polytrim), or gentamicin drops.
- Contact lenses can cause conjunctivitis and corneal abrasions.
  - Lens wear should be discontinued; storage and cleaning solutions must be replaced to prevent further contamination.
  - Although patching is no longer recommended in these patients, topical antibiotics to avoid *Pseudomonas* or secondary bacterial infection may be initiated.
    - An aminoglycoside such as tobramycin (Tobrex) drops or a fluoroquinolone such as ciprofloxacin (Ciloxan) or ofloxacin (Ocuflox) should be administered 4 times a day for 5 to 7 days.
  - Corneal ulcers should always be considered in patients who wear contact lenses and have a red eye.

TABLE 69-3 Conjunctivitis in Childhood

	BACTERIAL	PHARYNGO CONJUNCTIVAL	ACUTE HEMORRHAGIC	HERPES SIMPLEX	GONOCOCCAL	ALLERGIC
Organism	See text	Adenovirus	Enterovirus 70, coxsackie A24	Herpes simplex	*Neissera gonorrhoeae*	None
Discharge	++	+	+++	±	+++	−
Unilateral/ bilateral hyperemia	U/B	U/B	B	U	U/B	B
Fever	−	+	+	++	±	−
Diagnosis	History and Gram's stain, culture if necessary	History and associated symptoms, viral culture if necessary	Subconjunctival hemorrhages and viral culture	Antifluorescent test Gram's stain, culture	Gram's stain, culture	History, physical examination
Treatment	Topical antimicrobial	Topical antimicrobial to prevent secondary infection	Topical antimicrobial to prevent secondary infection	Topical vidarabine, trifluorothymidine	Intramuscular ceftriaxone	Topical antihistamine, vasoconstrictors, and/or glucocorticoids
Associated findings	Otitis media with *Haemophilus*	Upper respiratory infection, regional adenopathy	Malaise, myalgias, upper respiratory infection	Eyelid vesicles, preauricular adenopathy	Periorbital inflammation	Atopy
Long-term complications	None	None	None	Corneal ulcerations, cataracts	Blindness, septicemia	None

Key: − = absent; ± = may or may not be present; + = mild; + + = moderate; + + + = severe.

These patients should be referred to an ophthalmologist.

- Gonococcal conjunctivitis can occur in sexually active children and adolescents; the mode of transmission is similar to adults. Treatment may consist of ceftriaxone, 1 g IM plus saline irrigation.

VIRAL CONJUNCTIVITIS

- Adenoviruses are the most common cause of viral conjunctivitis in children. Pharyngoconjunctival fever is most common in children and is associated with an upper respiratory tract infection, regional lymphadenopathy, and fever.
- Epidemic keratoconjunctivitis is more common in the second to fourth decades of life and causes preauricular lymphadenopathy with diffuse superficial keratitis.
  - Treatment is symptomatic with cool compresses. Many physicians prescribe a topical antimicrobial to prevent secondary bacterial infection, but this practice has not been proven.

HERPES SIMPLEX AND VARICELLA ZOSTER

- Vesicular lesions on the eyelid can be due to herpes simplex, varicella-zoster, impetigo, or contact dermatitis.
- Infections are characterized by unilateral, follicular conjunctivitis with vesicles localized to the eyelids. Preauricular lymphadenopathy is commonly present.
- Ocular involvement with varicella is relatively uncommon, occurring in fewer than 5 percent of cases.
- Zoster is uncommon in children, with only 5 percent of all cases occurring in children under 5 years of age. Zoster infections of the eye notably follow the distribution of the first division of the trigeminal nerve. Lesions are usually located on the forehead and upper eyelid and can be located on the tip of the nose.
  - Trifluorothymidine is the preferred agent for treatment of herpes simplex because of its increased solubility, diminished toxicity, and lack of viral resistance. For herpetic eye lesions, systemic acyclovir is not recommended because the drug does not penetrate the avascular cornea.

ALLERGIC CONJUNCTIVITIS

Seasonal and Perennial Allergic Conjunctivitis

- Itching is frequently the hallmark of allergic conjunctivitis. The conjunctiva is mildly inflamed with varying degrees of edema.
  - Treatment consists of a combination of topical vasoconstrictors (naphazoline-antazoline and naphazoline pheniramine), antihistamines (levocabastine 0.05 percent and olopatadine 0.1 percent), steroids, and anti-inflammatory agents (ketorolac 0.5 percent). Systemic antihistamines may be of some benefit.
  - Cromolyn sodium 4 percent and Iodoxamide tromethamine 0.1 percent eyedrops have also been shown to be effective when used as a prophylactic agent.

VERNAL CONJUNCTIVITIS

- Vernal keratoconjunctivitis is a rare condition mainly affecting children under the age of 10. It is common in warm, dry climates, and males have a 2:1 ratio of being affected. Often there is a significant history of atopy. Patients usually have a history of bilateral itching, foreign-body sensation, clear mucoid discharge, photophobia, and injection. The giant papillae involve the upper tarsal conjunctiva and consist of large "cobblestone" papillae.

SPECIAL FORMS OF CONJUNCTIVITIS

- Patients with Stevens-Johnson syndrome may have severe conjunctival involvement. In the acute phase of the disease, the palpebral and ocular conjunctiva can scar together.
- Kawasaki disease is associated with a bilateral bulbar, non-exudative conjunctivitis. This diagnosis should be suspected in patients who have fever for more than 5 days and have conjunctivitis, strawberry tongue, cervical adenopathy, fissuring of the lips, diffuse oral injection, erythema and induration of the hands and feet, and desquamation of the fingers and toes.
- A chronic blepharoconjunctivitis can be caused by *Pthirus pubis* when the eyelashes are infected by nits or by the bug itself. The only recognized lice to infect the eyelashes are pubic lice. Family members should be screened.
  - Systemic treatment of the organism is necessary for successful eradication.
  - Eye ointments have been used for treatment because they are thought to paralyze and smother the lice. A cotton-tip applicator should be used for debridement prior to the placement of the ointment.
- *Molluscum contagiosum* can cause conjunctivitis when the virus is shed into the eye. Typically, it causes a chronic conjunctivitis that does not respond to topical antimicrobials. Eradication of the virus requires that the lesions be opened with a needle and the central core of the umbilicated region be removed.
- Other viral syndromes can be associated with nonspecific conjunctivitis. These include:
  - Rubella
  - Influenza
  - Mumps
  - Measles
  - Infectious mononucleosis
  - Cytomegalovirus

BIBLIOGRAPHY

Ambati B, Ambati J, Azar N, et al: Periorbital and orbital cellulitis before and after the advent of *Haemophilus influenzae* type B vaccination. *Ophthalmology* 107:1450–1453, 2000.

Hart A: The management of corneal abrasions in accident and emergency. *Injury* 28:527–529, 1997.

Herpetic Eye Disease Study Group: Oral acyclovir for herpes simplex virus eye disease. *Arch Ophthalmol* 118:1030–1036, 2000.

Kaufman H, Varnell E, Thompson H: Trifluridine, cidofovir, and penciclovir in the treatment of experimental herpetic keratitis. *Arch Ophthalmol* 116:777–780, l998.

Laskowitz D, Liu G, Galetta S: Acute visual loss and other disorders of the eyes. *Neurol Clin North Am* 16:323–353, 1998.

Mitchell J: Ocular emergencies. In: Tintinalli J, Kelen G, Stapczynski, eds. *Emergency Medicine: A Comprehensive Study Guide.* New York: McGraw-Hill, 1501–1518, 1999.

Wallace D, Steinkuller P: Ocular medications in children. *Clin Pediatr* 37:645–652, 1998.

Wright K: *Textbook of Ophthalmology.* Baltimore: Williams & Wilkins, 1997.

QUESTIONS

1. A 5-year-old boy presents to the ED with complaints of sudden onset of right eye pain associated with photophobia. On examination, he has a miotic pupil and perilimbal injection. With the slit lamp, you detect an aqueous flare and cells. You arrange for ophthalmologic follow-up the next morning and plan to discharge him on steroid and cycloplegic drops. What further action is essential in the management of this case?
   A. Patch the right eye
   B. Add antibiotic drops to the treatment plan.
   C. Institute oral acyclovir.
   D. Examine the eye after fluorescein staining.
   E. Add oral non-steroidal anti-inflammatory agent to the treatment plan

2. A 1-week-old baby that was born at home is brought to the ED due to bilateral eye swelling. On examination, you find marked erythema and purulent drainage from both eyes. There is chemosis and associated eyelid edema and erythema. On Gram's stain, you identify gram-negative intracellular diplococci. Which of the following is appropriate management for this case?
   A. Gentamicin eyedrops and follow-up in 24 hours with ophthalmology
   B. Ceftriaxone, 50 mg/kg IM and 24-hour follow-up with pediatrician
   C. Full sepsis workup with lumbar puncture and CSF analysis
   D. Hospitalize and treat with intravenous acyclovir for 10 days.
   E. Oral erythromycin, 50 mg/kg per day for 2 to 3 weeks.

3. A 10-year-old girl has received a splash of Drano to the left eye. This occurred 5 to 10 minutes ago and the mother has carried the child to your ED, which is near her home. Which of the following approaches is most appropriate?
   A. Rinse the eye with saline drops, instill fluorescein and do a complete slit lamp examination.
   B. Instill a mildly acidic eye drop to assist in neutralizing the alkaline drain cleaner.
   C. Irrigate with normal saline, 1 to 2 liters
   D. Irrigate continuously until the pH of the tears is 6 to 8 as measured by litmus paper; then instill fluorescein and proceed with examination.
   E. Fluorescein is contraindicated but complete examination is otherwise indicated after copious irrigation

ANSWERS

1. D. Prior to initiating the use of steroid drops for this case of iritis, you MUST rule out herpes keratoconjunctivitis by examining the eye after fluorescein staining. Herpetic keratitis is associated with corneal ulceration in a characteristic dendritic pattern.

2. C. This child has ophthalmia neonatorum due to *Neisseria gonorrhoeae*. It is rarely seen now due to the common use of postnatal prophylaxis. Neonates with suspected gonococcal conjunctivitis or any neonate with fever and conjunctivitis should have a sepsis evaluation, including a lumbar puncture.

3. D. Irrigation should be continued until the pH is neutral as tested with litmus paper. Then fluorescein examination should be performed.

GYNECOLOGIC AND OBSTETRIC EMERGENCIES

70 PEDIATRIC AND ADOLESCENT GYNECOLOGY

Geetha Gurrala
Michael Van Rooyen
William R. Ahrens
Heather M. Prendergast

EVALUATION OF PREMENARCHEAL PATIENTS

- The evaluation of prepubescent patients requires particular sensitivity to the emotional concerns of the patient and family. Continuous reassurance during the examination is necessary to address the concerns and fears of the child, particularly in cases of sexual assault.
- A standard speculum examination is not indicated in most children; it is necessary only in patients who are sexually active and those with suspected vaginal foreign bodies or bleeding from trauma.
- Children are best examined by placing them in either the frog-leg position or the prone knee-chest position, usually with the assistance of the parent. The child may be positioned on the mother's lap. If necessary, an otoscope may be used as an adjunct to check for vaginal lacerations or foreign bodies.
- Vaginal cultures are obtained by gently swabbing the vaginal introitus or by using a soft dropper with a small amount of saline to lavage the introitus and obtain a specimen.

GYNECOLOGIC DISORDERS OF INFANCY AND CHILDHOOD

CONGENITAL VAGINAL OBSTRUCTION

- The most common etiology of vaginal obstruction is imperforate hymen. Less commonly seen is vaginal atresia, also called transverse vaginal septum. If the disorder is not detected on the initial physical examination of the infant, vaginal obstruction and uterine distension, termed hydrocolpos, can develop.
- If congenital vaginal obstruction remains undiagnosed until puberty, the patient may present with the complaint of noncyclic lower abdominal pain and amenorrhea.
- The obstructed flow of menstrual blood, termed hematocolpos, often presents with abdominal distension, urinary complaints, and a dark-blue, bulging introitus.
- Congential renal anomalies are associated with vaginal atresia.
- The treatment of imperforate hymen or vaginal atresia is surgical intervention.

LABIAL ADHESIONS

- Labial adhesions, also called labial agglutination, represent an acquired and potentially recurrent condition than occurs in 3 to 7 percent of all prepubescent females, mostly between the ages of 1 and 6 years.
- The child is usually brought to the physician by the parents with the concern that the vagina is "closing." Upon examination, this disorder may resemble congenital absence of the vagina or ambiguous genitalia. Adhesions may be differentiated by the presence of a vertical connecting line that forms a central seam or raphe.
- The treatment of labial adhesions in asymptomatic girls is expectant; no specific therapy is required since

the condition is usually self-limiting. In children who appear to have local recurrent irritation and adhesions, estrogen cream applied to the adhesions at bedtime for 3 to 4 weeks will usually be sufficient to facilitate labial opening.

PREPUBERTAL VAGINAL BLEEDING

- The most common cause of genital trauma in childhood is accidental injury due to a fall. Vaginal hematomas are commonly seen in blunt injuries to the perineum.
- Penetrating trauma to the perineum from falling on a sharp object requires careful evaluation to exclude injury to the urethra, rectum, and peritoneum.
- Vaginal hematomas from trauma rarely require surgical intervention and are most appropriately treated conservatively with cool packs and sitz baths.
- Early gynecologic or surgical consultation should be considered in cases of vaginal laceration, or when there is a suspicion of pelvic penetration. General anesthesia may be required to fully explore the extent of a vaginal laceration.

URETHRAL PROLAPSE

- Urethral prolapse is the protrusion of the urethral mucosa outward through its meatus, producing red or purplish edematous mucosa at the meatus, which is soft and doughnut shaped; the central dimple indicates the urethral lumen.
- Most cases of urethral prolapse are found in African American children between the ages of 2 and 10 years. If left untreated, urethral prolapse may progress to mucosal thrombosis and necrosis.
- In most cases, warm compresses or sitz baths, combined with a 2-week course of topical estrogen cream, can be used to shrink the swelling of urethral tissue.
- Surgical management to excise redundant tissue may be required if the urethral tissue has become gangrenous.

PRECOCIOUS PUBERTY

- Precocious puberty is defined as the appearance of secondary sex characteristics before the age of 8 years or the appearance of menarche before the age of 9 years.
- True precocious puberty is premature maturation of the pituitary and it results in both menstruation and ovulation. Pseudoprecocious puberty is not secondary to pituitary control, and menses may occur without ovulation.
- In up to 74 percent of cases, precocious puberty is idiopathic and simply represents early sexual development.

TABLE 70-1   Tanner Stages

Stage 1 (prepubertal): Elevation of breast papilla; no pubic hair
Stage 2 (age 9.8–10.5 years): Elevation of papilla; areolar diameter enlarged; sparse hair on labia majora
Stage 3 (age 11.2–11.4 years): Enlargement without separation of breast and areola; dark, coarse, curled hair over mons
Stage 4 (age 12.0–12.1 years): Secondary mound of areola and papilla above the breast; adult-type hair, abundant, covers mons and extends about halfway out to inguinal regions
Stage 5 (age 13.7–14.6 years): Mature, with projection of papilla only because of recession of areola to contour of the breast; adult-type hair in quality and distribution

Familiarity with the Tanner staging criteria may be helpful to the emergency physician (Table 70-1).
- The most appropriate management of patients with suspected precocious puberty is referral to a pediatric gynecologist or endocrinologist for evaluation.

GENITAL TRACT INFECTIONS IN CHILDREN

VULVOVAGINITIS
- Vulvovaginitis, or inflammation of the vaginal and vulvar region, is the most common gynecologic problem in childhood and adolescence.
- Historical considerations include an overview of nutritional and hygienic practices (irritating soaps, constrictive clothing), underlying medical disorders (diabetes, immunocompromised state), and the potential for sexual abuse.
- Most childhood vulvovaginitis is due to irritation of the vulva and secondary involvement of the lower third of the vaginal canal. In the young child, inadequate local hygiene is the most common predisposing factor in nonspecific vulvovaginitis.
- Vaginal cultures yield mixed bacterial flora unrelated to a specific disease.
- Treatment includes antimicrobial therapy, when indicated, and encouraging proper hygiene and preventive measures (Table 70-2).

NEONATAL LEUKORRHEA
- Neonatal leukorrhea is a physiologic vaginal discharge seen in female newborns. The discharge occurs in response to high levels of circulating maternal estrogens.
- This transient condition usually subsides within a few weeks as the influence of maternal estrogen subsides.

VAGINAL FOREIGN BODIES
- Vaginal foreign bodies may cause local irritation and secondary infection of the vagina. Discharge may be purulent and bloody.

TABLE 70-2 Nonspecific Vulvovaginitis in Children

Causes
  Poor toilet hygiene following bowel evacuation
  Tight-fitting underclothing
  Lack of proper bathing
  Irritative agents: bubble baths, harsh soaps
  Vaginal foreign bodies
  Upper respiratory infections
Treatment
  Elimination of the irritative agents
  Improved local hygiene
  Sitz baths (2 tbsp baking soda and lukewarm bathwater)
  Aveeno oatmeal baths
  Loose-fitting underclothing
  Hydroxyzine or diphenhydramine for pruritus
  Antibiotics directed by culture and sensitivity

VAGINITIS DUE TO UPPER RESPIRATORY INFECTIONS

- Bacterial upper respiratory infections can precede a vaginal infection by 3 to 5 days. Organisms can be transmitted from the nose or mouth to the genitalia
- Cultures can confirm the presence of respiratory flora, including *Haemophilus influenzae*, hemolytic streptococci, or *Staphylococcus aureus.*
- Most cases of vaginitis related to upper respiratory infection involve instructing the patient to use proper hygiene.

CANDIDAL VAGINITIS

- Vulvovaginitis due to *Candida albicans* is uncommon during infancy and childhood. This may be the first manifestation of occult diabetes in older children.
- Diagnosis is made by preparing a wet mount with potassium hydroxide (KOH) preparation, which reveals branching spores and pseudohyphae.
- Effective treatment can be accomplished by a variety of antifungal agents.

SHIGELLA VAGINITIS

- Chronic cases of vulvovaginitis may be caused by organisms from the intestinal tract. *Shigella* vaginitis presents with whitish to yellow discharge in three quarters of cases and is unresponsive to antifungal agents.
- Cultures will reveal growth of *Shigella flexnerni*, which can be treated with trimethoprim-sulfamethoxazole for 5 days.

PARASITIC VULVOVAGINITIS

- Parasites, which can cause vulvar pruritus, irritation, and discharge, include pinworms (*Enterobius vermicularis*), roundworms (*Ascaris lumbricoides*), or whipworms (*Trichuris trichiura*).
- Diagnosis is best made by pressing a piece of cellophane adhesive tape against the perianal area in the early morning to recover the parasitic.
- The treatment of pinworms is albendazole.

GYNECOLOGIC DISORDERS OF ADOLESCENCE

DYSMENORRHEA

- Primary dysmenorrhea is pain with menstruation that is not associated with recognized pelvic pathology. It is due to uterine contractions induced by increased prostaglandin production.
- Secondary dysmenorrhea is pain occurring during menstruation that is caused by underlying pelvic pathology.
- Primary dysmenorrhea is much more common than secondary dysmenorrhea, particularly in adolescents.
- Symptoms typically last for the first 24 to 48 h of the menstrual period. Associated symptoms may include headaches, backache, thigh pain, nausea, and vomiting.
- Initial treatment of mild dysmenorrhea includes the use of aspirin, ibuprofen, mefenamic acid, or naproxen to inhibit prostaglandin synthesis, which is effective in 80 to 90 percent of cases.

DYSFUNCTIONAL UTERINE BLEEDING

- Dysfunctional uterine bleeding (DUB) is defined as vaginal bleeding that is irregular (metrorrhagia), excessive in duration and amount (menorrhagia), or both (menometrorrhagia).
- Dysfunctional uterine bleeding results from the absence of progesterone release during the luteal phase.
- Other causes of vaginal bleeding must be excluded in the evaluation of the patient with suspected DUB, including ectopic pregnancy, spontaneous abortion, pelvic inflammatory disease, and uterine pathology, such as endometriosis and carcinoma.
- Since DUB occurs most commonly in the anovulatory state, accompanying dysmenorrhea is absent.
- Laboratory testing includes pregnancy testing, hemoglobin, and a coagulation profile if the suspicion of coagulopathy exists.
- Patients with minimal bleeding may be reassured and observed
- Patients with moderate bleeding may be treated with medroxyprogesterone 10 mg/day orally for 5 days. If bleeding persists, this regimen may be repeated for a total of three cycles, after which normal menses should occur.
- Patients with severe vaginal bleeding and unstable vital signs are treated aggressively. After the patient is stabilized, treatment is begun with high-dose estrogens, such as Premarin, 20 to 25 mg, every 4 h until bleeding stops, with a maximum of 6 doses.

MITTELSCHMERZ

- Mittelschmerz is pain on ovulation caused by peritoneal irritation from minor ovarian bleeding.
- This disorder, which presents with right or left lower abdominal pain in midcycle, is benign and resolves spontaneously.

OVARIAN CYSTS

- Ovarian cysts are most commonly painless and are usually discovered on routine pelvic examination.
- Cysts can rupture and cause lower abdominal pain and hemoperitoneum; they may, therefore, be confused with appendicitis or ectopic pregnancy.

OVARIAN TORSION

- Ovarian torsion, or twisting of the ovary and adnexa may present with intermittent unilateral abdominal pain, low-grade fever, and a tender mass on pelvic examination.
- Predisposing factors include ovarian enlargement from pregnancy, ovarian cysts, and polycystic ovary disease.
- Although Doppler ultrasound may be helpful in excluding this diagnosis, laparoscopy is the most reliable diagnostic procedure.

GENITAL TRACT INFECTIONS

Candidal Vaginitis
- Vulvovaginitis due to *Candida albicans* is common in adolescence and adulthood. Most commonly, patients present with thick vulvovaginal discharge associated with intense pruritus and inflammation.
- A KOH preparation will reveal pseudohyphae and branching spores.
- Treatment may be accomplished by a variety of antifungal agents, including miconazole nitrate (vaginal suppository, 200 mg) intravaginally at bedtime for 3 days or 2-percent cream intravaginally at bedtime for 7 days.

Trichomonas Vaginitis
- *Trichomonas* is typically sexually transmitted and is a common cause of vaginitis in sexually active adolescents.
- Patients may complain of pruritus, a frothy yellowish or greenish discharge that smells foul. The vaginal mucosa and the cervix may have a spotted "strawberry" appearance.
- The diagnosis can be confirmed by a wet mount, which may demonstrate motile, flagellated trichomonads.
- Treatment is most commonly accomplished with metronidazole.

Gardnerella Vaginitis
- *Gardnerella* vaginitis, which is also known as nonspecific vaginitis or bacterial vaginosis, results from overgrowth of an organism that may be found in the normal vaginal flora.
- Patients often complain of white or grayish discharge with a "fishy" odor.
- KOH prep may reveal characteristic "clue" cells, which are vaginal epithelial cells that have been invaded by bacteria.
- Effective treatments include metronidazole 500 mg twice daily for 7 days or clindamycin 300 mg twice daily for 7 days.

Herpetic Vulvovaginitis
- Herpetic vulvovaginitis is a sexually transmitted disease usually caused by the herpes simplex II virus.
- Genital herpes most commonly presents with labial or perianal vesicles, which rupture and progress to painful ulcerations. Ulcerations may be surrounded by a variable inflammatory reaction, and inguinal lymphadenopathy may be present.
- Genital herpes infections are self-limiting but recurrent. The course of the disease may be shortened by administration of acyclovir, 200 mg every 4 h for 10 days.

Bartholin Cyst
- A Bartholin cyst is an enlargement of the Bartholin gland, located at 4 and 8 o'clock positions in the vestibule.
- Treatment requires incision and drainage. After incision and drainage, iodoform gauze or a balloon catheter should be inserted to promote healing.

Gonorrhea
- Gonorrhea is a sexually transmitted disease that can present as pelvic inflammatory disease (30 percent), cervicitis (40 percent), or as an asymptomatic infection (30 percent).
- During the last few years, nucleic acid amplification techniques using the polymerase chain reaction (PCR) and ligase chain reaction (LCR) have been developed that are highly sensitive and specific for *Neisseria gonorrhoeae* when used on urethral and cervicovaginal swabs and on first-void urine specimens.
- The diagnosis can also be made by endocervical cultures on Thayer-Martin media.

- Positive DNA probe test results should be verified by culture in cases where a false positive result will have adverse medical, social, or legal consequences.
- Patients are most appropriately treated with single-dose therapy, to ensure compliance, by either a single dose of ceftriaxone 125 mg intramuscularly or cefixime given as a single oral dose of 400-mg tablets.

CHLAMYDIAL INFECTIONS

- Infections due to *Chlamydia trachomatis* have become the most common sexually transmitted diseases in the United States. *Chlamydia trachomatis* can cause acute cervicitis, lymphogranuloma venereum, and pelvic inflammatory disease.
- The polymerase chain reaction (PCR) and ligase chain reaction (LCR) are useful for evaluating urine specimens from either sex.
- Patients with suspected cervicitis or pelvic inflammatory disease are treated presumptively with doxycycline, 100 mg twice daily for 7 days, or with azithromycin, 1 g as a single dose.

CONDYLOMA ACUMINATA

- Condyloma acuminata, or "venereal warts," are found in both pre-menarcheal patients and adolescents. The causative agent is the human papillomavirus.
- In adolescents with condyloma, the infection is usually sexually transmitted.
- Cryotherapy is the most effective treatment for young children, and podophyllin 25-percent ointment used once weekly for 3 to 4 weeks is effective in adolescents and adults. Laser fulguration may be used on larger lesions.

PELVIC INFLAMMATORY DISEASE

ETIOLOGY

- Pelvic inflammatory disease (PID) is an acute infection of the endometrium and the fallopian tubes. It is usually a sexually transmitted disease caused most frequently by *N. gonorrhoeae, C. trachomatis*, and a variety of anaerobic pathogens.
- The consequences of untreated or inadequately treated PID include recurrent infections, tubo-ovarian abscesses, infertility, and subsequent ectopic pregnancies.

CLINICAL PRESENTATION

- Patients may present with a wide variety of symptoms, including dull, generalized lower abdominal pain beginning 2 to 5 days after menstruation. Associated complaints may include dyspareunia, vaginal discharge, and pain on ambulation. Fever may also be present.

- Physical examination may reveal tenderness of the uterine fundus, adnexal fullness and pain to bimanual manipulation, and marked cervical motion tenderness.

MANAGEMENT

- Indications for hospitalization include a toxic appearance, marked peritoneal findings, repeated vomiting, a failed course of outpatient therapy, and pregnancy.
- Outpatient treatment should consist of antibiotic coverage for both gonorrhea and chlamydial infections, which consists of ceftriaxone, 250 mg IM or cefoxitin, 2 g IM with probenecid, 1 g PO, and doxycycline 100 mg twice daily for 14 days.
- Inpatient treatment may include clindamycin and gentamicin intravenously for 4 to 7 days and subsequent 14-day outpatient therapy with doxycycline and clindamycin.

DISORDERS OF PREGNANCY

HYPERTENSION IN PREGNANCY

- All pregnant patients presenting to the emergency department are screened for hypertension because of the high maternal and fetal mortality associated with preeclampsia.

PREECLAMPSIA AND ECLAMPSIA

- Preeclampsia, also called toxemia of pregnancy, occurs in patients who are greater than 20 weeks of gestation. It is a leading cause of maternal death in the United States.
- Preeclampsia can be classified into mild or severe forms.
- Mild preeclampsia is defined as:
  - Systolic BP greater than 140 mm Hg or greater than 30 mm Hg above baseline
  - Diastolic BP greater than 90 mm Hg or greater than 15 mm Hg above baseline
  - Urine protein greater than 300 mg or greater than 2+ on dipstick
- Severe preeclampsia is defined as:
  - Systolic BP greater than 160 mm Hg
  - Diastolic BP greater than 110 mm Hg
  - Urine protein greater than 2 g/24 h
  - Serum creatinine greater than 1.2 mg/dL, unless known to be previously elevated
  - Platelets less than 100,000/mm^3
  - Elevated ALT and AST
  - Increased LDH
  - Persistent headache or other cerebral or visual disturbance
  - Persistent epigastric pain

CLINICAL PRESENTATION

- Patients with mild preeclampsia may be asymptomatic or may complain of progressive edema and headache.
- Twenty percent of women with severe preeclampsia or eclampsia develop hemolysis, elevated liver enzymes, and low platelets (**HELLP syndrome**).
- Neurologic irritability may herald this onset of seizures. Cerebrovascular accidents can occur.

MANAGEMENT

- If mild preeclampsia is suspected, the patient is admitted for fetal monitoring. The most widely used antihypertensive agent in pregnancy is methyldopa.
- In all patients who meet criteria for severe preeclampsia, 4 g of magnesium sulfate is given intravenously as a loading dose, followed by 1 to 2 g/h to prevent seizures. If respiratory depression occurs with magnesium administration, 1 g of calcium gluconate may be given over 3 min.
- Hypertension is controlled emergently and is reduced to a diastolic blood pressure of 90 to 100 mm Hg. Hydralazine, 5 mg/30 min IV, is the drug of choice for control of hypertension. Alternatively, intravenous labetalol, 20 to 50 mg, may be used.
- The ultimate treatment for preeclampsia is delivery of the fetus.

ECLAMPSIA

- Eclampsia is defined as preeclampsia with associated tonic-clonic seizures. There is a high risk of maternal and fetal mortality, as well as DIC and placental abruption.
- Magnesium sulfate is the anticonvulsant of choice and may be given as a bolus dose of 6.0 g intravenously. The maximum dose should not exceed 8 g.
- Benzodiazepines are not routinely used. After seizures are controlled, arterial blood gas analysis and fetal and maternal monitoring is performed.
- Laboratory testing includes CBC, electrolytes (including calcium and magnesium), coagulation profile, and liver function studies.
- Patients should be admitted for induction of labor or cesarean section.

VAGINAL BLEEDING IN PREGNANCY

THREATENED ABORTION ETIOLOGY

- Threatened abortion occurs in approximately 20 percent of all pregnancies. Of all patients diagnosed with threatened abortion, 40 to 50 percent progress to a complete spontaneous abortion.

- Patients commonly present to the emergency department with the complaint of vaginal bleeding with or without lower abdominal pain. Bleeding is usually mild, but in some cases, is severe. The lower abdominal pain is usually cramping in character.
- A complete spontaneous abortion may be diagnosed if the conceptus is expelled, the cervical os closes, and the uterus returns to normal size.
- Septic abortions carry the risk of septic shock and disseminated intravascular coagulation and should be suspected in patients with a nonviable pregnancy and fever.
- Spontaneous abortion carries a 2 percent risk of Rh isoimmunization. It is mandatory for the Rh-negative woman who aborts to be given Rh prophylaxis.

ECTOPIC PREGNANCY

ETIOLOGY

- An ectopic pregnancy results when a fertilized ovum implants outside of the uterus. The most common site of an ectopic pregnancy is the fallopian tube (95 percent).
- The most common predisposing factor for ectopic pregnancy is chronic salpingitis or PID. This leads to fibrosis and scarring of the fallopian tube.

CLINICAL PRESENTATION

- The most common symptom of ectopic pregnancy is vaginal bleeding, which occurs in 60 percent of patients. Unilateral lower abdominal pain is a relatively common finding.
- Few patients actually present to the emergency department with the classic findings of acute abdominal pain, vaginal bleeding, and hypotension.
- Life-threatening hemorrhage is possible in any patient with an ectopic pregnancy.
- Urine pregnancy tests are very reliable in excluding pregnancy (98 percent sensitivity).
- In normal pregnancy, serum quantitative β-hCG levels should double approximately every 2 days.
- An intrauterine pregnancy is generally detectable by 6 weeks of gestation by transabdominal ultrasound, and as early as 5 weeks of gestation by transvaginal ultrasound.
- The correlation of serum β-hCG with accurate visualization of an intrauterine pregnancy on vaginal probe ultrasound is probably not static.

MANAGEMENT

- The most common surgical treatment is salpingectomy, although the unruptured ectopic pregnancy may be resected from the tube (salpingostomy) or milked from the fimbriated end of the tube while preserving the normal tubal anatomy.

- Low-dose methotrexate with a single IM dose of 50 mg/m2, is a viable nonsurgical option for treating stable patients with ectopic pregnancy.

HYDATIDIFORM MOLE

- Hydatidiform mole is a proliferative abnormality of trophoblastic tissue. Nausea and vomiting are common, and the uterus is often larger than expected.
- Preeclampsia in the first trimester is uncommon in normal pregnancy and is very suggestive of a molar pregnancy. The diagnosis should be considered if the serum β-hCG is greater than expected.
- Patients with molar pregnancies are most commonly managed by dilatation and suction curettage.

ABRUPTIO PLACENTAE

ETIOLOGY
- Placental abruption is defined as the detachment of the placenta from the uterus prior to delivery of the fetus. Premature detachment can occur in varying degrees.

CLINICAL PRESENTATION
- Placental abruption must be suspected in patients who present to the emergency department with third-trimester vaginal bleeding and lower abdominal pain. Bleeding may be minimal.
- The uterus is firm and tender, and fetal heart tones may be absent because of fetal demise.

MANAGEMENT
- Laboratory studies include a coagulation profile to exclude potential coagulopathy.
- Pelvic examination must be delayed until the patient is in the operating room because of the potential for massive hemorrhage and fetal demise.

PLACENTA PREVIA

ETIOLOGY
- Placenta previa is the implantation of the placenta in the lower pole of the uterus over or near the internal os.
- Vaginal bleeding may occur because of tearing of the placental attachments due to cervical effacement and dilatation.

CLINICAL PRESENTATION
- Placenta previa can be distinguished from abruption by the absence of abdominal pain, a contracted uterus,

and the presence of bright red blood instead of dark, clotted blood, as found in placental abruption.
- Placenta previa must be suspected in any patient presenting with third-trimester vaginal bleeding.

MANAGEMENT
- The most important principle in the management of possible placenta previa is avoidance of vaginal examination.
- Pelvic examination may precipitate massive hemorrhage and fetal demise. Ultrasonic examination is necessary and immediate obstetric consultation is indicated.

EMERGENCY CONTRACEPTION

- Emergency treatment is indicated for the prevention of pregnancy in women after unprotected sex or suspected contraceptive failure.
- The Preven Emergency Contraceptive kit contains a pregnancy test and four oral contraceptive tablets, each containing 50 micrograms of ethinyl estradiol and 0.25 mg of levonorgestrel. Two tablets are taken within 72 h of intercourse followed, 12 h later, by the second dose.
- Best results are seen if the pills are taken within 72 h of intercourse. The efficacy rate is 75 percent.

BIBLIOGRAPHY

American Academy of Pediatrics: Diagnostic tests, in Pickering LK (ed): *2003 Red Book: Report of the Committee on Infectious Diseases*, 26th ed. Elk Grove Village, Il: American Academy of Pediatrics, 2003.

Centers for Disease Control and Prevention: 1998 guidelines for treatment of sexually transmitted diseases. *MMWR* 47(No. RR–1):57–62, 79–84, 1998.

Dart RG: Role of pelvic ultrasonography in evaluation of symptomatic first-trimester pregnancy. *Ann Emerg Med* 33:310–320, 1999.

Embling ML, Monroe KW, Oh MK, et al. Opportunistic urine ligase chain reaction screening for sexually transmitted diseases in adolescents seeking care in an urban emergency department. *Ann Emerg Med* 36:28–32, 2000.

Molitch ME: Endocrine problems of adolescent pregnancy. *Endocrinol Metab Clin North Am* 22:649, 1993.

Smith YR, Berman DR, Quint EH: Premenarchal vaginal discharge. Findings of procedures to rule out foreign bodies. *J Pediatr Adolesc Gynecol* 15:227–230, 2002.

Tay JI, Moore J, Walker JJ: Ectopic pregnancy. *BMJ* 320:916–919, 2000.

QUESTIONS

1. A 6-year-old girl is brought to the emergency department by parents with the concern that the child's vagina is "closing." There is no history of similar symptoms in the past and no history of recurrent irritation. Upon examination, you note the presence of a vertical connecting line that forms a central seam. Which of the following is the **MOST** appropriate management plan?
   A. Gynecologic consultation
   B. Outpatient surgical consultation
   C. Estrogen cream at bedtime
   D. ED manipulation
   E. No specific therapy is necessary.

2. A 7-year-old girl is brought to the emergency department following a fall from her bike. On arrival, she complains of abdominal pain, but is otherwise stable. On examination, the abdomen is relatively benign; however you note the presence of a vaginal hematoma. There is no evidence of a vaginal laceration. Which of the following is the **MOST** appropriate intervention?
   A. Admit for 23-h observation
   B. Evacuate the hematoma in the ED
   C. Obtain a gynecologic consultation
   D. Obtain a surgical consultation
   E. Treat conservatively with cool packs

3. A 7-year-old girl is brought to the ED for evaluation of "vaginal irritation." The mother states the child frequently complains about discomfort while bathing. You suspect vulvovaginitis secondary to hygienic practices. Which of the following **HISTORICAL** considerations would be **MOST** useful in making this diagnosis?
   A. History of vaginal foreign body
   B. Regular use of perfumed soaps
   C. Parent suspicion of sexual abuse
   D. Precocious puberty
   E. History of Type I Diabetes

4. Neonatal leukorrhea is a physiologic vaginal discharge seen in female newborns. Which of the following is responsible for the discharge?
   A. Low levels of neonatal estrogen
   B. Low levels of maternal estrogen
   C. High levels of maternal estrogen
   D. High levels of maternal progesterone
   E. Low levels of maternal progesterone

5. A 13-year-old girl is brought to the ED for evaluation of pain with menstruation, nausea, and vomiting. A previous gynecologic evaluation was unremarkable for pelvic pathology. A urine pregnancy test is negative. Which of the following would be the **MOST** appropriate in management of this patient?
   A. Obtain a pelvic ultrasound
   B. Obtain a gynecologic consultation in ED
   C. Outpatient gynecologic follow-up
   D. Begin oral contraceptives
   E. Recommend ibuprofen and reassurance

6. An adolescent girl presents with complaints of unilateral intermittent abdominal pain, low-grade fever, and nausea. On examination, you find an ill-appearing girl with otherwise normal vitals. Physical examination reveals no abdominal tenderness; however, you note a tender mass on pelvic examination. A urine pregnancy test is negative. Which of the following is the **MOST** likely diagnosis?
   A. Vaginal foreign body
   B. Ovarian cyst
   C. Ovarian torsion
   D. Bartholin Cyst
   E. Ectopic pregnancy

7. Gonorrhea, a sexually transmitted disease, presents as asymptomatic infection in what percentage of patients?
   A. 10 percent
   B. 20 percent
   C. 30 percent
   D. 40 percent
   E. 50 percent

8. A sexually active teenage presents with a complaint of dull, generalized lower abdominal pain beginning 3 days after the start of her menstruation. She also complains of pain on ambulation, and a vaginal discharge. On physical examination, the patient has a low-grade fever and appears dehydrated. Abdominal examination reveals a mild lower abdominal tenderness without rebound or guarding. Pelvic examination demonstrates uterine tenderness, and marked cervical motion tenderness. Which of the following would **NOT** be an appropriate part of a management plan?
   A. Urine pregnancy test
   B. Single dose therapy covering both *Chlamydia* and gonorrhea
   C. Inpatient hospitalization for intravenous antibiotics
   D. Pelvic ultrasound
   E. Gynecologic consultation

9. A 14-year-old girl is brought by paramedics after a syncopal episode while playing basketball. You learn that the patient has no medical problems and has been previously healthy. Which of the following would **NOT** increase your suspicion of an ectopic pregnancy in this patient?
   A. History of amenorrhea
   B. History of pelvic inflammatory disease

C. Previous ectopic pregnancy

D. Multiple ovarian cysts palpated on pelvic examination

E. History of tuboovarian abscess

10. Which of the following would **NOT** be classified as mild preeclampsia?

A. Urine protein >2 g/24 h

B. Diastolic BP >90 mm Hg or >15 mm Hg above baseline

C. Systolic BP >140 mm Hg or >30 mm Hg above baseline

D. Headache without neurologic findings or visual disturbances

E. Progressive edema

ANSWERS

1. E. Labial adhesions represent an acquired and often recurrent condition that occurs in 3 to 7 percent of all prepubescent females between the ages of 1 and 6 years. The treatment of labial adhesions in asymptomatic girls is expectant. No specific therapy is required since the condition is usually self-limiting. In children who appear to have local recurrent irritation and adhesions, estrogen cream applied to the adhesions at bedtime for 3 to 4 weeks is usually sufficient.

2. E. Vaginal hematomas are commonly seen in blunt injuries to the perineum. Vaginal hematomas from trauma rarely require surgical intervention and are most appropriately treated conservatively with cool packs and sitz baths. Early gynecologic and surgical intervention should be considered in cases of vaginal lacerations.

3. B. Vulvovaginitis is the most common gynecologic problem in childhood and adolescence. Historical considerations include an overview of nutritional and hygienic practices, ie: irritating soaps, and constrictive clothing.

4. C. Neonatal leukorrhea occurs in response to high levels of circulating maternal estrogens. This transient condition usually subsides within a few weeks as the influence of maternal estrogen subsides.

5. E. Primary dysmenorrhea is pain with menstruation that is not associated with recognized pelvic pathology. Symptoms typically last for the first 24 to 48 h of the menstrual period. Associated symptoms may include headaches, backache, thigh pain, nausea, and vomiting. Initial treatment of mild dysmenorrhea includes aspirin, ibuprofen, or naproxen.

6. C. Ovarian torsion may present with intermittent unilateral abdominal pain, low-grade fever, and a tender mass on pelvic examination. Predisposing factors include ovarian enlargement from pregnancy and ovarian cysts.

7. C. Gonorrhea is a sexually transmitted disease that can present as an asymptomatic infection in 30 percent of patients.

8. B. The patient presents with signs and symptoms consistent of pelvic inflammatory disease (PID). Indications for hospitalization include a toxic appearance, marked peritoneal findings, repeated vomiting, a failed course of outpatient therapy, and pregnancy. Single-dose therapy is **NOT** appropriate treatment for PID. Outpatient treatment should consist of antibiotic coverage for both gonorrhea and chlamydial infections, which consists of ceftriaxone, 250 mg IM or cefoxitin, 2 g IM with probenecid, 1 g PO, and doxycycline 100 mg twice daily for 14 days.

9. D. An ectopic pregnancy results when a fertilized ovum implants outside the uterus. The most common predisposing factor for ectopic pregnancy is chronic salpingitis or PID. This leads to fibrosis and scarring of the fallopian tube. Few patients actually present to the emergency department with the classic findings of acute abdominal pain, vaginal bleeding, and hypotension.

10. A. Preeclampsia occurs in patients who are greater than 20 weeks of gestation. It is a leading cause of maternal death in the United States. Preeclampsia can be classified into mild or severe forms. A urine protein greater than 2 g/24 h is consistent with severe preeclampsia.

71 ANEMIAS

David F. Soglin
Jane E. Kramer
William R. Ahrens
Valerie A. Dobiesz

INTRODUCTION

- Anemia is defined as a hemoglobin concentration more than 2 standard deviations below the mean for a comparable population.
- Infants reach a nadir in hemoglobin concentration at 2 to 3 months of life, with anemia defined as a hemoglobin level below 9 g/dL. This nadir is deeper and occurs at a younger age in premature infants.
- Patients with mild to moderate anemia are usually asymptomatic, and the anemia is most commonly discovered on a routine complete blood count (CBC).
- When the hemoglobin becomes low enough to produce symptoms, patients may present with fatigue, irritability, or shortness of breath on exertion.
- Physicians are not able to predict hemoglobin levels based on the appearance of pallor.
- Anemias are most easily classified based on red blood cell (RBC) size and degree of bone marrow activity.
- The size of RBCs is measured as mean corpuscular volume (MCV), the normal values of which vary with age.
- Bone marrow activity is reflected by the reticulocyte count. Correcting the measured reticulocyte count for the degree of anemia allows an accurate determination of marrow activity.
- The appearance of the RBCs on the peripheral smear, the total number of RBCs, and the red cell distribution width (RDW), which measures the variability in RBC size, are also helpful in determining the etiology of anemia.

MICROCYTIC ANEMIA

- Microcytic anemia is defined by an MCV lower than 2 standard deviations below the population mean. The vast majority of microcytic anemia in young patients is caused by iron deficiency, but thalassemia is also an important cause (Table 71-1).

IRON DEFICIENCY

- Risk factors for iron deficiency anemia include age between 6 months and 2 years, decreased prevalence or duration of breast-feeding, lack of use of iron-fortified formulas, early introduction of whole cow's milk into the diet, and low socioeconomic status.
- Fetuses absorb most of their total body iron during the last trimester, so premature infants are at greater risk for iron-deficiency anemia.
- Iron deficiency anemia develops slowly, and patients rarely present with acute symptoms. Even with drastically reduced hemoglobin levels, patients are usually well compensated.

TABLE 71-1 Differentiating Microcytic Anemia

PARAMETER	IRON DEFICIENCY	THALASSEMIA TRAIT
History	Prematurity or high milk intake	None or family history
Reticulocyte count		
MCV	Low	Normal
RDW	Low	Very low
Mentzer's index (MCV/RBC)	High >13	Low <11

MCV, mean corpuscular volume; RDW, red cell distribution width; RBC, red blood cell.

- The diagnosis is usually made on the basis of the history and CBC results showing anemia, microcytosis, and a high RDW. The reticulocyte count is not elevated.
- In the usual setting, a trial of iron therapy is both diagnostic and therapeutic. An increase in the reticulocyte count is typically seen in a matter of days, and the hemoglobin level increases in 1 to 2 weeks.

THALASSEMIA

- Thalassemias are inherited defects resulting in the inability to synthesize sufficient quantities of various globin chains of the hemoglobin molecule. The production of beta chains is generally the most affected.
- The defect is most common in people of Mediterranean ancestry and is present in a small percentage of African Americans.
- In general, the disease is classified as thalassemia minor or major, corresponding to heterozygous and homozygous states, respectively. The heterozygous form of thalassemia is often referred to as thalassemia trait.
- Thalassemia trait produces marked microcytosis out of proportion to the degree of anemia. There is typically a high total RBC count and narrow RDW, which helps differentiate thalassemia trait from iron deficiency anemia.
- Unlike iron deficiency, the reticulocyte count in thalassemia trait should be normal or slightly elevated.
- Beta-thalassemia major produces severe hemolytic anemia with marked microcytosis and reticulocytosis. It usually presents within the first year of life. Pallor, jaundice, and hepatosplenomegaly are present.
- Because patients require life-long transfusion therapy, the use of uncrossmatched blood is avoided except in the direct circumstances.
- The major side effect of long-term transfusion therapy is iron overload, which adversely affects multiple organs, especially the pancreas, liver, and heart.

LEAD POISONING

- Lead poisoning must be considered in the child with microcytic anemia. High levels of lead can interfere with hemoglobin production.
- Much of the anemia seen with lead poisoning is actually due to concomitant iron deficiency.

NORMOCYTIC ANEMIA

- Although normocytic anemia is less common than microcytic anemia, the differential diagnosis in childhood is extensive (Table 71-2).

TABLE 71-2 Differential Diagnosis for Normocytic Anemia

Blood loss (high reticulocyte count)
Hemolytic anemia (high reticulocyte count)
   Immune
      Autoimmune hemolytic anemia
      Neonatal-maternal blood group incompatibility
   Nonimmune
      Microangiopathic
         Disseminated intravascular coagulation (DIC)
         Hemolytic uremic syndrome (HUS)
      Macroangiopathic
         Artificial cardiac valve
      Membrane abnormalities
         Spherocytosis
         Elliptocytosis
         Stomacytosis
      Metabolic abnormalities
         G6PD deficiency
         Pyruvate kinase deficiency
         Hemoglobinopathies
Nonhemolytic anemia (low or normal reticulocyte count)
   Abnormality isolated to red cell line
      Chronic hemolytic anemia with concurrent aplastic crisis
      Transient erythroblastopenia of childhood (TEC)
      Chronic disease
         Renal insufficiency
         Diamond–Blackfan anemia
   Abnormality affecting other cell lines
      Bone marrow infiltration
         Leukemia
         Lymphoma
         Tumor metastasis
      Acquired aplastic anemia

- It is important to establish whether the anemia is due to decreased production (low reticulocyte count) or increased blood loss or destruction (high reticulocyte count).

NORMOCYTIC ANEMIA WITH HIGH RETICULOCYTE COUNT

- If there is no evidence of blood loss, a hemolytic anemia is likely.
- The workup for a patient with hemolytic anemia includes a Coombs' test to determine whether the hemolytic anemia is immunologic in nature. Immune hemolytic anemia may be the result of a drug reaction, infection, collagen vascular disorder, or malignancy, but commonly no etiology is determined.
- The differential diagnosis for nonimmune hemolytic anemia includes micro- and macroangiopathic destruction, membrane disorders, metabolic abnormalities, and hemoglobinopathies. Sickle cell anemia is discussed in detail in Chapter 72.
- Microangiopathic RBC destruction can occur with disseminated intravascular coagulation and hemolytic

uremic syndrome. The peripheral smear will demonstrate schistocytes, burr cells, and other RBC fragments.

- Hereditary spherocytosis results in a hemolytic anemia due to splenic destruction of red blood cells. The diagnosis is confirmed by osmotic fragility studies. Splenectomy is curative. The major hematologic crisis is aplastic anemia, which is usually secondary to a parvovirus infection.
- Pyruvate kinase deficiency may present because of an increase in hemolysis or an aplastic crisis.
- There are multiple variants of glucose 6 phosphate dehydrogenase deficiency (G6PD). The A variant is seen in approximately 10 percent of African American males and becomes symptomatic only after a significant challenge from a drug or infection.

NORMOCYTIC ANEMIA WITH LOW RETICULOCYTE COUNTS

- A low reticulocyte count in the face of significant anemia indicates bone marrow underproduction.
- An acquired red cell aplasia, TEC spares the white blood cells (WBCs) and platelets and, as the name implies, resolves after a number of weeks. It typically affects children between 1 and 4 years of age. Supportive therapy is usually sufficient. Steroids have not been shown to speed recovery.
- Diamond–Blackfan anemia is a congenital RBC aplasia that usually presents in the first year of life with severe anemia.
- Thrombocytopenia or WBC abnormalities associated with normocytic anemia and poor reticulocyte response suggests marrow infiltration or acquired aplastic anemia.
- Marrow infiltration is most commonly due to leukemia, with acute lymphoblastic leukemia being the most frequent type.
- Acquired aplastic anemia in the absence of an underlying hemolytic anemia has been associated with drugs and infections. Often no etiology is determined. The prognosis is quite poor, and bone marrow transplantation is often required. Blood transfusion is performed judiciously for patients who are candidates for bone marrow transplantation.

MACROCYTIC ANEMIA

- Macrocytic anemia is quite uncommon in pediatric patients.
- Folate and vitamin B_{12} deficiencies can result in megaloblastic anemia. These are rare in otherwise healthy children.

BIBLIOGRAPHY

Farhi DC, Luebbers EL, Rosenthal NS: Bone marrow biopsy findings in childhood anemia: Prevalence of transient erythroblastopenia of childhood. *Arch Pathol Lab Med* 122:638–641, 1998.

Hung OL, Kwon NS, Cole AE, et al: Evaluation of the physician's ability to recognize the presence or absence of anemia, fever and jaundice. *Acad Emerg Med* 7:146–156, 2000.

Sherry B, Bister D, Yip R: Continuation of decline in prevalence of anemia in low income children: The Vermont experience. *Arch Pediatr Adolesc Med* 151:928–930, 1997.

QUESTIONS

1. Which of the following is true regarding anemia in children?
   A. Physicians are able to accurately predict hemoglobin levels by the appearance of pallor.
   B. Bone marrow activity is reflected by the reticulocyte count.
   C. Anemia is defined as a hemoglobin concentration less than 12.
   D. Premature infants have no nadir in hemoglobin levels after birth as do full term infants.
   E. Patients with mild anemia are always symptomatic.

2. A 5-year-old female is discovered on routine CBC to have a microcytic anemia. What is the most likely etiology?
   A. Iron deficiency
   B. Thalassemias
   C. Lead poisoning
   D. Blood loss
   E. Sideroblastic anemia

3. Which of the following is true regarding iron deficiency anemia?
   A. Patients typically present with acute symptoms.
   B. The treatment is transfusion of pRBCs.
   C. Premature infants are at increased the risk of developing it.
   D. The CBC will show anemia and macrocytosis.
   E. Typically develops over a short period of time.

4. A 3-year-old patient is diagnosed with a thalassemia during a work up for anemia. Which of the following is correct regarding this disorder?
   A. It is secondary to radiation injury.
   B. It is most common in African Americans.
   C. The heterozygous form of thalassemia is a more severe form of the disease.
   D. The reticulocyte count will be normal or slightly elevated.
   E. It is typically treated with bone marrow transplant.

5. Which of the following is true regarding hereditary spherocytosis?
   A. Causes a hemolytic anemia
   B. Transfusion of pRBCs is curative
   C. Is a common etiology of childhood anemias
   D. Is secondary to an enzyme deficiency in hemoglobin production
   E. The reticulocyte count will be suppressed.

6. Which of the following is true regarding a decreased reticulocyte count in a patient with a normocytic anemia?
   A. There is increased RBC destruction.
   B. May be due to increased blood loss
   C. Is caused by congenital disorders only
   D. May be caused by marrow stem cell failure
   E. Lead poisoning is the most common cause.

ANSWERS

1. B. Physicians are not able to predict hemoglobin levels based on the appearance of pallor. Bone marrow activity is reflected by the reticulocyte count. Anemia is defined as a hemoglobin concentration of more than 2 standard deviations below the mean for a comparable population. Premature infants reach a deeper nadir and this occurs at a younger age than full term infants. Patients with mild to moderate anemia are usually asymptomatic.

2. A. The majority of microcytic anemia in young patients is caused by iron deficiency.

3. C. Iron deficiency anemia develops slowly and patients rarely present with acute symptoms. The treatment is with iron therapy. Fetuses absorb most of their total body iron during the last trimester so premature infants are at greater risk. The CBC will show anemia, microcytosis, and a high RDW.

4. D. Thalassemias are inherited defects resulting in the inability to synthesize sufficient quantities of various globin chains of the hemoglobin molecule. It is most common in people of Mediterranean ancestry. The heterozygous form is referred to as thalassemia trait or thalassemia minor and is a less severe form of the disease. The reticulocyte count should be normal or slightly elevated. Patients will require life-long transfusion therapy.

5. A. Hereditary spherocytosis results in a hemolytic anemia due to splenic destruction of red blood cells. It will cause a normocytic anemia with high reticulocyte counts. Splenectomy is curative.

6. D. A low reticulocyte count in the face of anemia indicates bone marrow underproduction or marrow stem cell failure. These may be congenital or acquired such as in acquired aplastic anemia. Lead poisoning may cause microcytic anemia as lead interferes with hemoglobin production.

72 SICKLE CELL DISEASE

David F. Soglin
Jane E. Kramer
William R. Ahrens
Valerie A. Dobiesz

INTRODUCTION

- Sickle cell anemia (SCA) is a chronic hemolytic anemia that is most common among African Americans. It is secondary to a hemoglobinopathy that occurs when valine is substituted for glutamic acid in the 6 position of the beta-chain.
- The diagnosis of SCA is applied to patients who are heterozygous for HbS and heterozygous for another abnormal hemoglobin such as HbC or beta-thalassemia.
- Patients with a single abnormal gene for HbS have sickle cell trait. The concentration of HbS is typically 40 percent, and the large percentage of normal hemoglobin allows the patients to remain asymptomatic except under the most severe hypoxic stress.

VASOOCCLUSIVE CRISIS

- The most common of the sickle cell crises, vaso-occlusive pain, presumably occurs when sickled red blood cells (RBCs) obstruct blood flow and cause tissue ischemia.
- Dactylitis, or hand-foot syndrome, is vaso-occlusion in the metacarpal or metatarsal bones. This is often the earliest presentation of SCA. It is common in infants, who present with hand and foot swelling and tenderness, refusal to walk, and irritability.
- Older patients typically experience vaso-occlusive pain crises in the long bones, back, joints, and abdomen.
- Patients with high levels of fetal Hb typically suffer less severe and less common crises, as do patients with HbSC and HbSB thalassemia.
- A complete blood count and reticulocyte count is indicated.
- Typically, patients remain at baseline levels of Hb during a painful event.
- Oxygen has not been shown to be beneficial in the management of pain crises unless hypoxemia is a complicating factor.

- Oral agents such as acetaminophen, nonsteroidal anti-inflammatory drugs (NSAIDs), and codeine used separately or in combination are the mainstays of treatment for mild to moderate pain.
- Ketorolac tromethamine is an NSAID that can be given intramuscularly or intravenously for acute pain. Its use should not be extended beyond 3 to 5 days.
- Parenteral agents such as morphine are often necessary in the ED setting.
- Although meperidine has commonly been used in the past, the availability of other potent analgesics has reduced its use for SCA vaso-occlusive pain.
- If adequate pain relief is not achieved with the oral agent, the patient is admitted for parenteral analgesia. Patient-controlled analgesia (PCA) with a morphine drip allows baseline levels of pain relief.

ACUTE CHEST SYNDROME

- Patients with SCA presenting with chest pain, hypoxemia, and infiltrates on chest radiograph are said to have *acute chest syndrome* (ACS). Fever may be present. ACS can result from pneumonia or pulmonary infarction due to vaso-occlusion.
- In most patients with ACS, no infectious etiology is isolated. When the etiology is bacterial pneumonia, *Pneumococcus* is the most common organism. *Mycoplasma* and *Chlamydia* are frequent causes, as are viral pneumonias.
- Because the etiology of ACS is often elusive, most patients receive antibiotic therapy directed at *Streptococcus pneumoniae* or *Mycoplasma*.
- The mainstay of therapy for pulmonary infarction in patients with SCA is early blood transfusion, with consideration of exchange transfusion.
- Bronchodilation has been demonstrated to be helpful in a significant minority of patients.

INFECTION

- Patients with SCA are at high risk for infection with encapsulated bacteria, especially *Pneumococcus*.
- Pneumococcal sepsis is a common cause of mortality. Children younger than 3 years are particularly susceptible to pneumococcal bacteremia.
- Children younger than 5 years with SCA who present to the ED with fever are at high risk for bacteremia. After obtaining a complete blood count and blood culture, children with SCA are treated with parenteral antibiotics effective against *Streptococcus pneumonia*.
- Although hospital admission is generally recommended, some institutions use outpatient ceftriaxone along with close follow-up to reduce the number of hospitalizations for these children.
- Older children can be managed on an individual basis.
- Unlike the general population, the most common organism identified as the cause of osteomyelitis in patients with SCA is *Salmonella*.

CEREBROVASCULAR ACCIDENTS

- Cerebrovascular accidents (CVAs) are common in children with SCA and are thought to be due to intimal damage and RBC sickling.
- These patients are at high risk for subsequent CVAs and are usually managed with long-term blood transfusions to maintain their percentage of HbS below 30 percent. Exchange transfusion is unnecessary in the chronic phase of transfusion therapy.
- Problems with iron overload may develop with chronic transfusions.

SPLENIC SEQUESTRATION

- Splenic sequestration crisis occurs when RBCs become entrapped in the spleen, resulting in a rapidly enlarging spleen and a sudden drop in Hb and hematocrit.
- Affected patients present with a history of decreased exercise tolerance.
- Among patients with SS hemoglobinopathy, splenic sequestration occurs almost exclusively in young children, because as the SCA patients age, they undergo "autosplenectomy."
- The mainstay of therapy is rapid blood transfusion. Fluid resuscitation is performed carefully to avoid volume overload.
- Sequestration can recur, and occasionally splenectomy is necessary.

APLASTIC CRISIS

- Viral infections, especially with parvovirus, can result in marrow suppression in children with SCA.
- Patients may present in a decompensated state, complaining of fatigue and shortness of breath.
- There will be a significant drop in Hb from baseline and little or no reticulocytosis.
- Symptomatic patients may require a transfusion of packed RBCs.
- Folate deficiency is common in patients with SCA and may be responsible for a small percentage of aplastic crises.

BIBLIOGRAPHY

Hargrave DR, Wade A, Evans JP, et al: Nocturnal oxygen saturation and painful sickle cell crises in children. *Blood* 101:846–848, 2003.

Steinberg MH: Drug therapy: Management of sickle cell disease. *N Engl J Med* 340:1021–1030, 1999.

Vichinsky EP, Neumayr LD, Earles AN, et al: Causes and outcomes in acute chest syndrome in sickle cell disease. *N Engl J Med* 342:1855–1865, 2000.

Yaster M, Kost-Byerly S, Maxwell LG: The management of pain in sickle cell disease. *Pediatr Clin North Am* 47:699–710, 2000.

QUESTIONS

1. What is the most common organism causing osteomyelitis in sickle cell patients?
   A. *Staphylococcus aureus*
   B. *Streptococcus pneumoniae*
   C. *Salmonella*
   D. *Bacteroides*
   E. *Mycoplasma*
2. A 4-year-old male presents with the complaint of abdominal pain. He has a history of sickle cell disease. He is noted to be hypotensive, pale, and has splenomegaly on examination. Which of the following is true regarding his condition?
   A. Typically seen in adolescence
   B. Is usually precipitated by infection
   C. He will have a sudden rise in hemoglobin and hematocrit
   D. May need a blood transfusion
   E. Splenectomy is contraindicated
3. Which of the following is true regarding aplastic crisis?
   A. Is usually precipitated by an infection especially with parvovirus
   B. Most commonly caused by folate deficiency
   C. Is diagnosed by an elevated reticulocyte count and a low hemoglobin
   D. Treatment is oxygen and antibiotics
   E. Patients typically present with fever, chest pain, and dyspnea
4. A 15-year-old female with a history of sickle cell anemia presents with a complaint of chest pain, shortness of breath, fever, and cough. She has an infiltrate on CXR. Which of the following is true regarding her condition?
   A. The cause is related solely to infection
   B. The cause is related solely to pulmonary infarction
   C. The treatment consists of supplemental oxygen, hydration, antibiotics and early blood transfusion or exchange transfusion
   D. Viral pneumonias are the most common cause
   E. Bronchodilation is contraindicated
5. Which of the following is true regarding sickle cell anemia in children?
   A. Dactylitis is an osteomyelitis of the hands
   B. Patients with HbSC and HbSB thalassemia have more severe crises than patients with HbS
   C. The most common crises is hemolytic crises
   D. Patients with sickle cell anemia are at high risk for infection with encapsulated bacteria
   E. Young children with sickle cell disease are less susceptible to bacteremia than children without the disease

ANSWERS

1. C. Unlike the general population, the most common organism causing osteomyelitis in sickle cell disease is Salmonella.
2. D. This patient has splenic sequestration, which is seen in young children (6 months to 6 years old). Splenic sequestration crises occur when RBCs become entrapped in the spleen causing a rapidly enlarging spleen and a sudden drop in hemoglobin and hematocrit. The mainstay of therapy is rapid blood transfusion. Sequestration can recur, and occasionally splenectomy is necessary.
3. A. Aplastic crisis is usually precipitated by an infection, most often human B19 parvovirus. Folate deficiency is rarely the underlying cause. The diagnosis is made by noting a very low hemoglobin and little or no reticulocytosis secondary to severe bone marrow depression. Treatment is supportive and possible transfusion with packed RBCs. Patients may present pale, lethargic and in shock.
4. C. This patient has an acute chest syndrome, which may result from pneumonia or pulmonary infarction and is multifactorial. The treatment consists of supplemental oxygen, hydration, antibiotics, early blood transfusion and possible exchange transfusion. In most patients with ACS, no infectious etiology is isolated. Bronchodilation has been demonstrated to be helpful in a significant minority of patients.
5. D. Dactylitis is vasoocclusion in the metacarpal or metatarsal bones and is common in infants. Patients with HbS have more severe and more common crises than do patients with HbSC or HbSB thalassemia. The most common crises are vasoocclusive crises. Patients with sickle cell anemia are at high risk for infection with encapsulated bacteria, especially

Pneumococcus. Young children with sickle cell anemia with fever are at higher risk for bacteremia.

73 BLEEDING DISORDERS

David F. Soglin
Jane E. Kramer
William R. Ahrens
Valerie A. Dobiesz

HEMOPHILIA

- Hemophilia is an X-linked recessive disorder of coagulation caused by deficiency of factor VIII (hemophilia A) or factor IX (hemophilia B or Christmas disease).
- Two thirds of American hemophiliacs have severe disease.
- In both hemophilia A and B, prothrombin time (PT) and bleeding time are normal and partial thromboplastin time (PTT) is prolonged. The same types of bleeding occur in both diseases.

ACUTE HEMARTHROSIS

- Knees, elbows, and ankles are the most commonly affected joints.
- It is generally agreed that even if joint bleeding cannot be confirmed, treatment is indicated. This philosophy is based on the potentially crippling sequelae of hemarthrosis.
- Joint swelling that is persistent and associated with fever may indicate a septic joint.
- A single factor infusion to raise levels to 25 to 30 percent is usually sufficient to terminate bleeding. A joint that has bled repeatedly may require several doses of factor.
- Hip bleeds are especially worrisome, because pressure within the joint can lead to aseptic necrosis of the femoral head.

INTRAMUSCULAR BLEEDS

- Such hemorrhage is usually identifiable by pain, tenderness, and swelling in the muscle and is treated with factor replacement to 30 percent levels.
- Forearm, calf, and hand bleeding can result in a compartment syndrome.
- Iliopsoas hemorrhage, which can be massive, presents with flexion of the thigh, groin and abdominal pain, and paresthesias. Ultrasound or computed tomography (CT) can confirm the diagnosis.

INTRACRANIAL HEMORRHAGE

- A potentially devastating complication, intracranial bleeding may be traumatic or spontaneous. Minor trauma may present with neurologic changes days after the event.
- Symptomatic children need immediate factor replacement to 100 percent levels even before imaging results are available.

OTHER BLEEDING MANIFESTATIONS

- Subcutaneous hemorrhage, abrasions, and lacerations that do not require sutures do not require factor replacement.
- Painless gross hematuria can occur. An anatomic source of the bleeding is usually not found. Treatment with factor may not be necessary if the bleeding is spontaneous.
- Factor replacement is necessary before laceration repair, lumbar puncture, surgery, and dental extractions.

MANAGEMENT ISSUES

- Factor replacement for hemophilia A is accomplished by transfusion with a variety of factor VIII concentrates. These products are made from either plasma-derived or recombinant proteins. Product selection is based on cost and purity.
- Hemophilia B is treated with factor IX complex concentrates, the older, and least pure of which contain significant amounts of factors VII and X and prothrombin. These carry the risk of disseminated intravascular coagulation (DIC) or thrombosis.
- More recently, monoclonal and recombinant factor IX became available.
- The amount of factor to be delivered will be dependent on the nature and severity of the bleeding episode. For life- or limb-threatening bleeds, treatment with factor replacement is generally required every 12 hours or by continuous infusion until healing occurs.
- Some 10 to 20 percent of severe hemophiliacs form factor inhibitors that are capable of neutralizing infused factor VIII. Alternatives for treating patients with high titers of inhibitor include highly purified porcine factor VIII, prothrombin complexes, and plasmapheresis followed by factor replacement.

- The rare patient with factor IX inhibitor can be managed with prothrombin complex concentrates or by exchange transfusion followed by factor IX infusion, if hemorrhage is life threatening.
- No cases of HIV-1 transmission from clotting factor concentrates have been documented since 1986.

VON WILLEBRAND DISEASE

- Von Willebrand disease exists when there is decreased or defective vWf, which is necessary for platelet adhesion to blood vessel walls.
- Clinical manifestations include epistaxis, easy bruising, menorrhagia, and bleeding after dental extraction. Posttraumatic and postsurgical hemorrhage can occur, but hemarthroses are uncommon.
- Typical laboratory findings include a normal PT and platelet count, with a prolonged bleeding time and a PTT that may be normal or prolonged.
- Type I von Willebrand disease is often amenable to DDAVP therapy, which stimulates the endogenous release of vWf. This corrects the bleeding time for 3 to 4 hours.
- The treatment for hemorrhage in these patients may include the administration of cryoprecipitate, which contains intact vWf, or of intermediate or high-purity factor VIII concentrate.

ACQUIRED COAGULOPATHIES

- Vitamin K deficiency leads to decreases in the vitamin K–dependent factors (II, VII, IX, and X) and prolongation of the PT. It can be seen in malabsorption syndromes, such as cystic fibrosis and celiac disease, biliary obstruction, and prolonged diarrhea.
- Vitamin K deficiency can also be caused by drugs such as diphenylhydantoin, phenobarbital, isoniazid, and coumadin.
- Administration of vitamin K is safest by the subcutaneous route. Severe anaphylactoid reactions are described with intravenous infusion.

IDIOPATHIC THROMBOCYTOPENIC PURPURA

- Idiopathic thrombocytopenic purpura (ITP) is the most common cause of thrombocytopenia in a well-appearing young child.
- The platelet surface is covered with increased amounts of IgG and the spleen removes the affected platelets from the circulation.

- Platelet production is increased in the bone marrow, but not enough to offset the rapid destruction.
- Patients present with the acute onset of bruising, petechiae, and purpura; they have normal physical examinations other than for skin findings.
- The most serious complication, intracranial hemorrhage, occurs in less than 0.1 to 0.5 percent of patients and almost exclusively with platelet counts under 20,000/μL.
- The diagnosis of ITP is likely when the complete blood count reveals thrombocytopenia in association with normal red and white blood cell numbers and morphology.
- The natural history of the condition is that 80 percent of children make a full recovery within 6 months.
- High-dose steroids can hasten the rate at which patients recover but are not necessary in most patients, who have only skin manifestations and platelet counts above 30,000/μL.
- Intravenous gamma globulin has been shown to promptly increase counts in patients with profound thrombocytopenia even more predictably than steroids and may be useful during active bleeding or intracranial hemorrhage.
- Transfused platelets will be rapidly destroyed due to the immune response and have no role in the management of these patients except in the circumstance of life-threatening hemorrhage, which most commonly occurs intracranially.
- Intravenous anti-Rh(D) immunoglobulin (Winrho-SD) is another technique to increase platelet counts. Anti-D appears to be as safe and effective as IVIG in Rh-positive patients. The cost is much less, and infusion takes minutes as opposed to hours for IVIG.

BIBLIOGRAPHY

Blanchette V, Imback P, Andrew M, et al: Randomized trial of intravenous immunoglobulin G, intravenous anti-D, and oral prednisone in childhood acute immune thrombocytopenic purpura. *Lancet* 344:703, 1994.

DiMichele D, Neufeld EJ: Hemophilia: A new approach to an old disease. *Hematol Oncol Clin North Am* 12:1315, 1998.

Holt D, Brown J, Terrill K, et al: Response to intravenous immunoglobulin predicts splenectomy response in children with immune thrombocytopenic purpura. *Pediatrics* 111: 87–90, 2003.

Mannucci PM, Tuddenham EGD: Medical progress: The hemophilias—From royal genes to gene therapy. *N Engl J Med* 344:1773–1779, 2001.

Scaradavou A, Woo B, Woloski BMR, et al: Intravenous anti-D treatment of immune thrombocytopenic purpura: Experience in 272 patients. *Blood* 89:2689, 1997.

QUESTIONS

1. Which of the following is true regarding the bleeding disorder hemophilia?
   A. It is an autosomal dominant disorder
   B. Factor IX deficiency is also known as hemophilia B
   C. In hemophilia A, prothrombin times and bleeding times are abnormal
   D. Only one third of American hemophiliacs have severe disease
   E. HIV transmission is common in hemophiliacs

2. An 8-year-old male with a history of hemophilia A presents with the complaint of left elbow swelling and pain for several hours. He has a decreased range of motion of the elbow. He has been afebrile and denies trauma or injury. He has had similar symptoms in the past. Which of the following would be the most appropriate management of this patient?
   A. Arthrocentesis to rule out infection
   B. If radiographs are negative immobilize in a splint, ice, elevation
   C. A single factor infusion to raise levels to 25 to 30 percent
   D. Immediate factor replacement to 100 percent levels
   E. Admission for serial examinations and continuous factor infusion until swelling resolves

3. Which of the following is true regarding hemophiliacs?
   A. Acute hemarthrosis most commonly affects the small joints of the hands
   B. Asymptomatic intracranial bleeds need no factor replacement
   C. Laceration repairs requiring suturing need no factor replacement
   D. Forearm, calf and hand intramuscular bleeding can result in a compartment syndrome
   E. Symptomatic intracranial bleeds should have an immediate CT scan prior to factor replacement

4. Which of the following is correct regarding Von Willebrand's disease?
   A. Von Willebrand's factor (vWF) is necessary for platelet adhesion to blood vessel walls
   B. Clinical manifestations are most commonly hemarthroses
   C. Laboratory findings include a prolonged prothrombin time, decreased platelet count and a normal PTT
   D. DDAVP therapy contains von Willebrand factor and is used in treatment
   E. The treatment of hemorrhage is with packed RBCs

5. A 5-year-old girl presents with the complaint of multiple bruises, petechiae and purpura on her skin. She has noticed them over the past 3 to 4 days. She is afebrile and is well appearing. She has no past medical history and has a completely normal physical examination except for the skin findings. She has a history of a recent viral illness. Her CBC reveals normal red and white blood cell numbers and morphology but her platelet count is 30,000/μL. Which of the following is true regarding the treatment of this patient?
   A. Platelet transfusion is recommended
   B. Intracranial hemorrhage is a common complication
   C. She will most likely develop chronic ITP
   D. High dose steroids and IV gammaglobulin may be used if she develops active bleeding or intracranial hemorrhage
   E. Renal disease and altered mental status are common findings

ANSWERS

1. B. Hemophilia is an X-linked recessive disorder of coagulation caused by a deficiency of factor VIII (hemophilia A) or factor IX (hemophilia B or Christmas disease). In hemophilia A and B, prothrombin time (PT) and bleeding time are normal and PTT is prolonged. Two-thirds of American hemophiliacs have severe disease. No cases of HIV transmission from clotting factor concentrates have been documented since 1986.

2. C. This patient has an acute hemarthrosis. Treatment is indicated with a single factor infusion to raise levels to 25 to 30 percent. This is usually sufficient to terminate bleeding.

3. D. Knees, elbows, and ankles are the most commonly affected joints in acute hemarthrosis. Intracranial bleeding whether symptomatic or asymptomatic require immediate factor replacement to 100 percent levels even before imaging results are available as this is a potentially devastating complication. Factor replacement is necessary before laceration repair, lumbar puncture, surgery, and dental extractions. Intramuscular bleeds in the forearm, calf, and hand bleeding can result in a compartment syndrome.

4. A. Von Willebrand's disease is due to decreased or defective vWf, which is necessary for platelet adhesion to blood vessel walls. Clinical manifestations include epistaxis, easy bruising, menorrhagia, and bleeding after dental extraction. Hemarthroses are uncommon. Laboratory findings include a normal PT and platelet count, with a prolonged bleeding time and a PTT that may be normal or prolonged. DDAVP therapy stimulates endogenous release of vWf. The treatment of hemorrhage may include cryoprecipitate, or factor VIII concentrate.

5. D. This patient has idiopathic thrombocytopenic purpura which most often affects children 2 to 6 years of age and frequently follows a viral infection.

It is a self-limited disorder and 89 percent of children make a full recovery within 6 months. Platelet transfusion is limited for life-threatening hemorrhage. Intracranial hemorrhage is a rare complication. High dose steroids and IV gammaglobulin are reserved for patients with active bleeding or intracranial bleeding. Renal disease and altered mental status are seen in TTP and not ITP.

74   BLOOD COMPONENTS

David F. Soglin
Jane E. Kramer
William R. Ahrens
Valerie A. Dobiesz

WHOLE BLOOD

- Transfusion of whole blood is rarely performed but may be indicated for prompt restoration of red cells and volume after trauma or surgery.
- The risk of transfusion reactions is doubled when transfusing whole blood.

PACKED RED BLOOD CELLS

- PRBC units have a hematocrit ranging from 60 to 80 percent.
- There are no functional platelets or granulocytes in this preparation.
- Patients with recurrent or severe allergic reactions to transfusions should receive PRBCs that have been saline washed.

PLATELET CONCENTRATE

- Platelets should be ABO and Rh-compatible, but crossmatching is not necessary.
- Platelet transfusions are indicated for patients with thrombocytopenia or platelet dysfunction who are actively bleeding.
- Patients with immune thrombocytopenia rarely benefit from platelet transfusions.

FRESH FROZEN PLASMA

- Fresh frozen plasma contains all clotting factors.
- ABO compatibility is important, but crossmatching is not necessary.
- Allergic reactions are possible.

- Fresh frozen plasma is not indicated for volume expansion.

CRYOPRECIPITATE

- Cryoprecipitate is prepared by slow thawing of FFP at 4°C and subsequent refreezing of the protein precipitate.
- Cryoprecipitate does not require crossmatching.
- It is indicated for treatment of hypo- or a-fibrinogenemia and of von Willebrand's disease.

FACTORS VIII AND IX

- Highly purified concentrates of factors VIII and IX are now produced by monoclonal antibody techniques and by recombinant DNA technology.
- These products avoid or greatly diminish the risk of infectious disease transmission.

ALBUMIN

- Available in both 5 and 25 percent solutions, albumin is most frequently used for blood volume expansion in shock, trauma, burns, and surgery.
- It contains no blood group antibodies.
- Only the 5 percent solution is isosmotic with plasma, and the 25 percent solution is never used to treat shock without other fluids.

INDICATIONS FOR TRANSFUSION

- Transfusion of blood in the emergency department is usually performed because of shock secondary to acute blood loss.
- Blood typing (for ABO and Rh) takes about 5 minutes, and screening for antibodies and crossmatching takes 30 minutes or more.
- The use of O-negative (universal donor) blood is reserved for life-threatening hemorrhage.
- The use of group- and Rh type-specific blood is preferred over O-negative transfusions when time precludes complete cross-matching.

COMPLICATIONS

ACUTE HEMOLYTIC TRANSFUSION REACTIONS

- Acute hemolytic transfusion reactions (AHTR) occur when a patient's anti-A or anti-B antibodies bind to incompatible transfused red cells.

- Symptoms include fever, chills, back or chest pain, nausea and vomiting, dyspnea, flushing, tachycardia, and hypotension.
- Disseminated intravascular coagulation, shock, renal failure, and death may ensue.

DELAYED HEMOLYTIC TRANSFUSION REACTIONS

- Delayed hemolytic transfusion reactions (DHTR) are caused by sensitization to non-ABO antigens from a previous transfusion.
- The reaction is delayed for 3 to 10 days.
- Signs and symptoms include fever, back pain, anemia, jaundice, and, rarely, hemoglobinuria.
- No treatment is usually required.

FEBRILE NONHEMOLYTIC TRANSFUSION REACTIONS

- Febrile or nonhemolytic transfusion reactions (FNHTR) are benign and self-limiting.
- They account for the majority of transfusion reactions and occur most commonly in the multiply transfused patient.
- Symptoms include fever and chills.
- If the patient is very uncomfortable, the transfusion should be stopped. Antipyretics may be given.

ALLERGIC TRANSFUSION REACTION

- Urticarial reactions may involve cytokines or histamine in stored blood products.
- The transfusion must be interrupted and the patient watched closely for signs and symptoms of anaphylaxis.
- An antihistamine such as diphenhydramine, 1 mg/kg per dose, should be administered. When the urticaria fades, transfusion can be resumed.
- Anaphylactic reactions occur in patients with congenital IgA deficiency who have high-titer IgG anti-IgA antibodies.
- Activation of a complement and chemical mediator cascade precipitates increased vascular permeability, resulting in angioedema, respiratory distress, urticaria, and shock.
- The transfusion is stopped, epinephrine is administered, and blood pressure is stabilized with crystalloid and vasopressive agents if necessary.

COMPLICATIONS OF MASSIVE TRANSFUSIONS

- This generally refers to the transfusion of greater than 1 entire blood volume within 24 hours.
- Complications include hypothermia, hyperkalemia, hypocalcemia, and coagulation disorders from the dilution of platelets and clotting factors.

INFECTIOUS COMPLICATIONS

- Donated blood is routinely screened for HIV-1 and -2, HTLV, hepatitis B surface antigen, hepatitis B core antibody (a surrogate marker for non-A, non-B hepatitis), hepatitis C virus, and syphilis.
- The current estimated risk of transmitting HIV through a blood transfusion is 1 in 493,000; hepatitis B, 1 in 63,000; and hepatitis C, 1 in 103,000.

BIBLIOGRAPHY

Goodnough LT, Shander A, Brecker ME: Transfusion medicine: Looking to the future. *Lancet* 361:161–169, 2003.
Manno C: What's new in transfusion medicine? *Pediatr Clin North Am* 43:793, 1996.
Schreiber GB, Busch MP, Kleinman SH et al: The risk of transfusion-transmitted viral infections. *N Engl J Med* 334: 1685–1690, 1996.

QUESTIONS

1. Which of the following is true regarding the transfusion of whole blood?
   A. Commonly ordered in patients needing routine transfusions
   B. Is readily available
   C. Has an increased risk of transfusion reactions
   D. Does not replete volume
   E. Refrigerated storage does not alter clotting factors
2. A 10-year-old boy has sustained significant blood loss and is determined to need a blood transfusion. He is stable after fluid resuscitation. Which of the following is correct regarding his transfusion?
   A. Type O negative is considered the universal donor
   B. When transfusing pRBCs, ABO compatibility is important but crossmatching is not necessary
   C. Transfusing pRBCs will also provide platelets and granulocytes

   D. O-negative transfusions are preferred over type-specific blood
   E. Blood typing for ABO and Rh compatibility usually takes about two hours

3. A 6-year-old female is found to have severe thrombocytopenia <20,000/μL and is bleeding actively. Which of the following is true regarding the management of this patient?
   A. Cross-matching is necessary when ordering platelets
   B. There is no risk of infectious disease transmission when transfusing platelets
   C. There is no indication for transfusion of platelets in this patient
   D. A platelet pack increases the platelet count by 10,000
   E. Patients with immune thrombocytopenia often benefit from platelet transfusions

4. A 15-year-old male who has a history of protein C deficiency and is on warfarin therapy presents after a head injury. He is found to have an intracranial bleed and needs to go to the operating room. His PT is elevated and his INR is 3. What is the most appropriate treatment of this patient?
   A. Transfusion of type specific pRBCs
   B. Transfusion of 10 units of platelets
   C. Transfusion of fresh frozen plasma
   D. Transfusion of cryoprecipitate
   E. Transfusion of 5 percent albumin solution

5. Which of the following is not known to be a complication of massive transfusions?
   A. Hypothermia
   B Hyperkalemia
   C. Hypocalcemia
   D. Coagulopathies
   E. Acute renal failure

6. Which of the following is the most common transfusion reaction?
   A. Acute hemolytic reaction
   B. Delayed hemolytic reaction
   C. Febrile nonhemolytic reaction
   D. Allergic reaction
   E. Extravascular hemolysis

7. A 2-year-old female is receiving a transfusion of pRBCs and subsequently develops an urticarial rash. Which of the following is indicated in this patient?
   A. Continue the transfusion and give antipyretics
   B. Continue the transfusion and give diphenhydramine

   C. Stop the transfusion and give no medications
   D. Stop the transfusion and give diphenhydramine
   E. Stop the transfusion and send the blood to the blood bank for ABO testing

ANSWERS

1. C. Whole blood is rarely used today and is not readily available. It is reserved for acute massive blood loss after trauma or surgery. The risk of transfusion reactions is doubled when using whole blood. It restores red cells and volume. Refrigerated storage causes a reduction in clotting factors.

2. A. Type O negative blood is the universal donor and is reserved for life-threatening hemorrhage. When transfusing pRBCs, ABO compatibility and cross-matching are important and will take about 30 minutes or more. There are no functional platelets or granulocytes in this preparation. The use of type specific blood is preferred over O negative transfusions when time precludes complete crossmatching and takes about 5 minutes.

3. D. When ordering platelets crossmatching is not necessary. There is an associated risk of infectious disease transmission. A platelet pack increases the platelet count by 10,000. Patients with immune thrombocytopenia rarely benefit from platelet transfusions.

4. C. Fresh frozen plasma contains all the coagulation factors except platelets and is indicated in the correction of clinically significant depletion of clotting factors and correction of coagulopathies prior to surgery.

5. E. Massive transfusion refers to the transfusion of greater than one entire blood volume within 24 hours. Complications include hypothermia, hyperkalemia, hypocalcemia, and coagulopathies from the dilution of platelets and clotting factors.

6. C. Febrile nonhemolytic transfusion reactions account for the great majority of transfusion reactions and are benign and self-limited. Symptoms include fever, chills, and malaise.

7. D. This patient has developed an allergic transfusion reaction. The urticaria may involve cytokines or histamine in stored blood products. The transfusion must be stopped and the patient watched closely for signs and symptoms of anaphylaxis. An antihistamine such as diphenhydramine 1mg/kg per dose should be given.

75 ONCOLOGIC EMERGENCIES

Brenda N. Hayakawa
William R. Ahrens
Heather M. Prendergast

INTRODUCTION

- Approximately 10 percent of childhood deaths are related to cancer. The leukemias, central nervous system (CNS) tumors, and lymphomas account for more than one-half of all childhood malignancies (Table 75-1).

COMMON PEDIATRIC MALIGNANCIES

ACUTE LEUKEMIAS

- Leukemia is a condition in which there is uncontrolled growth of immature white blood cells within

TABLE 75-1   Cancer Incidence Rates in Children Aged 0 to 14 Years: SEER[a] 1974–1991

CANCER	RATE[b]
Leukemia	41
Central nervous system tumors	29
Lymphoma	15
Neuroblastoma	9
Rhabdomyosarcoma	8
Wilms' tumor	8
Bone	6
Retinoblastoma	4

[a] SEER: Surveillance, Epidemiology and End Results program of the National Cancer Institute.
[b] Annual incidence rates per million children aged 0 to 14.
SOURCE: Adapted from Ries LAG, Gurney JG, Linet M, et al: Cancer incidence and survival among children and adolescents: United States SEER Program 1975–1995, National Cancer Institute, NIH Publication No. 99-4649; Bethesda, MD, 1999.

the bone marrow, with subsequent suppression of normal hematopoiesis.
- Acute leukemia is the most common childhood malignancy, representing approximately 30 percent of newly diagnosed cancers; 75 percent of these are of acute lymphoblastic leukemia (ALL).
- Overall, about 60 to 70 percent of patients survive more than 5 years beyond diagnosis. Although the exact cause of leukemia is unknown, certain genetic, environmental, viral, and immunologic risk factors have been implicated.
- Common presentations include pallor, fatigue, petechiae, purpura, bleeding, and fever. Lymphadenopathy, hepatomegaly, and splenomegaly reflect extramedullary involvement. Bone pain results from leukemic involvement of the periosteum and bone, causing patients to limp or even refuse to walk.
- The leukocyte count is greater than 10,000/mm^3 in approximately one half of patients with ALL. Most patients will be anemic and thrombocytopenic.
- Treatment consists of combination chemotherapy for induction of remission, CNS preventative therapy, consolidation, and maintenance therapy.

COMPLICATIONS OF LEUKEMIA

- Complications of leukemia include CNS involvement, which may be present at the time of initial diagnosis or can occur with relapse. Patients may have headache, nausea, vomiting, irritability, papilledema, or other signs of raised ICP. Diagnosis is confirmed through the demonstration of leukemic blasts in the cerebrospinal fluid.
- Leukemia may relapse in the testes, where it causes painless, usually unilateral, testicular enlargement.
- Hematologic complications include anemia, hemorrhage, and hyperleukocytosis.

- Blood product irradiation helps minimize the occurrence of posttransfusion graft-versus-host disease by inhibiting the mitotic activity of lymphocytes in donor blood products.
- Hemorrhage is a complication of leukemia and is most often due to thrombocytopenia.
- Most cases of spontaneous intracranial hemorrhage are associated with a platelet count less than $5000/mm^3$. Platelet transfusions are warranted for patients who have a platelet count in the range of 20,000 to $50,000/mm^3$ and who have significant bleeding.
- Hyperleukocytosis, with an initial white blood cell (WBC) count greater than $100,000/mm^3$, may be seen with acute leukemias and chronic myelocytic leukemia. Patients may be asymptomatic but are more often dyspneic, confused, or agitated or experience blurred vision.
- Patients with hyperleukocytosis are at risk for tumor lysis syndrome and are treated with intravenous hydration, alkalinization measures, and allopurinol; they are admitted for antileukemic therapy.
- Although hypercalcemia, with a serum calcium greater than 10.5 mg/dL, is more commonly associated with adult malignancies, it may occur with ALL, non-Hodgkin's lymphoma (NHL), neuroblastoma, and Ewing's sarcoma.
- Clinically, patients may experience nausea, vomiting, constipation, polyuria, and polydipsia, which may progress to dehydration, lethargy, seizures, and coma.
- Treatment begins with intravenous hydration with normal saline, followed by furosemide to promote calcium excretion.

HODGKIN'S DISEASE

- Hodgkin's disease is a malignancy of the lymph nodes, which may spread to other local nodes and lymphatic channels. The malignant cell is the Reed-Sternberg cell. The first peak in incidence occurs from ages 13 to 35 years, with a late peak at 50 to 75 years.
- The majority of pediatric patients have painless supraclavicular or cervical lymphadenopathy. A lymph node is considered enlarged if it is more than 10 mm at its greatest diameter, with the exception of an epitrochlear node, which is considered enlarged at 5 mm, and an inguinal node, at 15 mm.
- Splenomegaly, which indicates more advanced disease.
- Systemic symptoms occur in one third of the patients and include unexplained fever, weight loss, and night sweats.

- A screening CBC and chest radiograph are indicated, as well as a tuberculin skin test. Patients are referred for lymph node biopsy if the node is enlarging after 2 to 3 weeks, remains enlarged, and has not returned to normal size by 5 to 6 weeks, or is associated with an abnormal chest radiograph finding such as mediastinal enlargement.
- Once the diagnosis of Hodgkin's disease is confirmed and histologically classified, patients undergo further workup for staging, which may involve exploratory laparotomy and splenectomy. Treatment regimens include multidrug chemotherapy and/or radiation, with a cure rate of over 80 percent.

NON-HODGKIN'S LYMPHOMAS

- Non-Hodgkin's lymphomas are a heterogeneous group of malignancies of lymphatic tissue. They account for 10 percent of all childhood cancer and usually occur in children over 5 years of age.
- Although the etiology of NHL is unknown, Epstein-Barr virus and immunodeficiency diseases have been linked to this malignancy.
- Bone, bone marrow, and the CNS are common sites of metastasis.
- Chest radiograph may reveal a mediastinal mass. Other mediastinal tumors in children are listed in Table 75-2.
- Multiagent chemotherapy is the mainstay of treatment, with up to 80 percent long-term disease-free survival.

TABLE 75-2 Mediastinal Tumors in Children

	MALIGNANT	BENIGN
Anterior mediastinum	Non-Hodgkin's lymphoma Hodgkin's disease Teratocarcinoma Thymoma Sarcoma	Teratoma Cystic hygroma Thymic cyst Hemangioma Bronchogenic cyst Lipoma
Middle mediastinum	Non-Hodgkin's lymphoma Hodgkin's disease Rhabdomyosarcoma Teratocarcinoma Other Sarcoma	Bronchogenic cyst Granuloma Teratoma Esophageal cyst Diaphragmatic hernia
Posterior mediastinum	Neuroblastoma Ganglioneuroblastoma Ewing's sarcoma Pheochromocytoma Lymphoma	Ganglioneuroma Neurolemmoma Neurofibroma Enterogenous cyst

SOURCE: Adapted from King RM, Telander RL, Smithson WA, et al: Primary mediastinal tumors in children. *J Pediatr Surg* 17:512–520, 1982. Used with permission.

CENTRAL NERVOUS SYSTEM TUMORS

- The second most common group of pediatric malignancies is those of the CNS, accounting for 20 percent of all pediatric cancers. Two incidence peaks occur, one in the first decade and the other beyond the fourth decade of life.
- Tumors arising in the supratentorial region include cerebral astrocytoma, optic glioma, and craniopharyngioma.
- Infratentorial tumors such as cerebellar astrocytoma, medulloblastoma, ependymoma, and brain stem glioma are more commonly seen after 2 years of age. Cerebellar astrocytomas account for 40 percent of CNS tumors in childhood.
- Supratentorial tumors may cause headache, seizures, or visual impairment.
- Truncal ataxia or incoordination is typical of infratentorial tumors. Raised ICP in infants and toddlers may manifest as vomiting, anorexia, irritability, developmental regression, or impaired upward gaze ("sunsetting" sign).
- Tumors of the CNS may be diagnosed by CT, which is relatively accessible and can detect up to 95 percent of CNS lesions. Magnetic resonance imaging (MRI) is more sensitive than CT in detecting tumors.
- Treatment is multimodal, utilizing surgical resection, chemotherapy, and radiation therapy. Newer therapies include immunotherapy and gene therapy.

WILMS' TUMOR

- Wilms' tumor (nephroblastoma), the most common pediatric abdominal malignancy, arises from embryonal renal cells.
- Most Wilms' tumors occur in children less than 6 years of age and present with a nontender or tender abdominal mass. If present, hematuria is usually microscopic.
- Ultrasound is a noninvasive means of evaluating a renal mass.
- Management includes surgical resection and chemotherapy or radiation.

NEUROBLASTOMA

- Neuroblastoma is a malignant tumor arising from sympathetic neuroblasts in the adrenal medulla and sympathetic chain. It is the most common extracranial solid tumor in childhood.
- Two-thirds of neuroblastomas arise in the abdomen and pelvis. Impingement of renal vasculature may lead to renin-mediated hypertension. Other sites of origin include the posterior mediastinum and neck.
- Tumors of the paraspinal ganglia may grow around and through the intervertebral foramina, causing spinal cord or nerve root compression.
- At the time of diagnosis, more than one-half of patients with neuroblastoma will have metastases involving the lymph nodes, bone marrow, cortical bone, liver, or skin.
- Massive hepatomegaly due to liver involvement, more common in infants, can cause respiratory compromise or liver failure. Skin manifestations appear as bluish, nontender subcutaneous nodules. They rarely occur outside of infancy.
- Paraneoplastic syndromes seen with neuroblastoma include opsoclonus, myoclonus, and cerebellar ataxia.
- A CBC may reveal neutropenia or pancytopenia due to marrow involvement. Chest radiography may show a posterior mediastinal mass.
- All patients are referred to a pediatric oncologist.

PRIMARY BONE TUMORS

- Common primary pediatric malignancies of the bone include osteosarcoma and Ewing's sarcoma. Osteosarcoma has a predilection for the metaphysis of long bones, particularly around the knee. Ewing's sarcoma may also arise in extraosseous tissues.
- Local pain, the most common symptom, may be exacerbated with activity and may cause a limp. The pain may be intermittent, remit for several weeks, and later return with increasing severity.
- Other presentations include a palpable mass, fever, and pathologic fracture.
- Plain radiographs of the affected bone reveal bony destruction and soft tissue swelling.
- Osteosarcoma may metastasize to the lung, causing pulmonary hemorrhage, pneumothorax or, rarely, SVC obstruction.

RHABDOMYOSARCOMA

- Rhabdomyosarcoma is a malignant solid tumor from mesenchymal tissue that normally forms striated muscle.
- It most often presents as a painless mass. The most common site of origin is the head and neck region.
- Rhabdomyosarcoma of the extremities or trunk usually presents as an enlarging soft tissue mass. Common sites of metastasis include lymph nodes, lungs, bones, bone marrow, brain, spinal cord, and heart.

- CT scan is used to evaluate suspected head or neck lesions. Ultrasound is a useful initial tool to define a pelvic mass.
- Treatment of rhabdomyosarcoma is multimodal, utilizing surgery, chemotherapy, and radiation.

RETINOBLASTOMA

- Retinoblastoma is the most common intraocular tumor of childhood. In 30 percent of cases, the disease is bilateral. Infants and young children are most commonly affected.
- Retinoblastoma most commonly presents with leukocoria or strabismus. Other rare findings include vitreous hemorrhage, microphthalmos, and orbital cellulites.
- A CT scan or MRI is needed to determine the presence of choroidal or optic nerve spread and orbital, subarachnoid, or intracranial involvement.
- Unilateral disease is predominantly treated with enucleation. With bilateral or more extensive disease, other modalities include radiation, chemotherapy, thermotherapy, and cryotherapy.

COMMON COMPLICATIONS OF CHILDHOOD CANCER

INFECTIOUS COMPLICATIONS

- Infection is the leading cause of death in children with cancer. The single most important factor is the development of neutropenia due to replacement of healthy bone marrow by malignant cells or from myelosuppressive chemotherapy
- The best estimate of production of neutrophils is the absolute neutrophil count (ANC), calculated as the total WBC count multiplied by the sum of the percentages of band cells plus polymorphonuclear neutrophils. Patients are defined as being neutropenic if their ANC is less than 500/mm^3.
- Splenectomized patients are at greatly increased risk for sepsis with encapsulated bacteria such as pneumococcus and *Haemophilus influenzae.*
- Patients are at risk of infection from their own endogenous flora, as well as nosocomial pathogens from previous recent hospitalizations.
- About 75 percent of neutropenic cancer patients with fever have an infection, most commonly bacterial. Of the nonneutropenic cancer patients with fever, approximately 17 percent have associated infection. The common pathogens are listed in Table 75-3.

TABLE 75-3   Common Pathogens in Children With Cancer

Bacteria:
Gram-positive aerobes:
   Staphylococcus aureus
   Coagulase-negative staphylococci
   Alpha-hemolytic streptococci
   Enterococci

Gram-negative aerobes:
   Enterobacteriaceae (*Escherichia coli, Klebsiella pneumoniae*)
   Enterobacter, Citrobacter, Serratia
   Anaerobes

Fungi:
   Candida species
   Aspergillus species
   Cryptococcus

Parasites:
   Pneumocystis carinii
   Cryptosporidium species
   Strongyloides stercoralis

Viruses:
   Herpes simplex virus
   Varicella-zoster virus
   Cytomegalovirus

SOURCE: Adapted from Pizzo PA, Rubin M, Freifeld A, et al: The child with cancer and infection. I. Empiric therapy for fever and neutropenia and preventative strategies. *J Pediatr* 119:674–694, 1991.

- Initial investigations include a chest radiograph, urinalysis and urine culture, and CBC; in addition, two sets of blood cultures, obtained from different sites, are sent for bacterial and fungal cultures. If an indwelling catheter is present, one blood specimen is obtained from the line and one from a peripheral vein.
- Prompt initiation of empiric antibiotic therapy in febrile neutropenic children has been associated with a reduction in morbidity and mortality. Traditionally, all patients are admitted to the hospital for intravenous antibiotics.
- The choice of antibiotic regimen must consider the microbial sensitivity patterns in the institution. Combination therapy has been the usual approach to provide broad-spectrum antibiotic coverage (Table 75-4).
- For febrile neutropenic patients with an indwelling catheter, vancomycin should be included in the initial therapy.
- The presence of a pulmonary infiltrate may represent a bacterial, viral, fungal, or parasitic infection.
- Patients with diffuse or interstitial infiltrates receive trimethoprim-sulfamethoxazole (TMP-SMX) for possible *Pneumocystis carinii* infection, as well as erythromycin for *Legionella* and *Mycoplasma* coverage.
- Cancer patients who are febrile and neutropenic are at risk for fungal infections, particularly *Candida* species.

TABLE 75-4   Empiric Antibiotic Therapy for Febrile Neutropenic Patients

REGIMEN	DRUG	DOSE	NOTES
Monotherapy	Ceftazidime	150 mg/kg/day IV, divided q 8 h	Poor coverage for coagulase-negative staphylococci, methicillin-resistant *Staphylococcus aureus*, eneterococci, some strains of penicillin-resistant *Streptococcus pneumoniae* and *viridans* streptococci; meropenem and cefipime have enhanced gram-positive and gram-negative coverage
	Or Imipenem/cilastin	40–60 mg/kg/day IV divided q 6 h (max 2 g/day)	
	Or Meropenem	60–120 mg/kg/day IV divided q 8 h	
	Or Cefipime	150 mg/kg/day IV divided q 8 h	
Duotherapy (without vancomycin): Aminoglycoside			Avoid if patients are receiving nephrotoxic, ototoxic, or neuromuscular blocking agents or have renal dysfunction, severe electrolyte disturbance, or suspected meningitis (poor blood–brain barrier)
	Gentamicin	5–7.5 mg/kg/day IV divided q 8 h	
	Or Tobramycin	5–7.5 mg/kg/day IV divided q 8 h	
	Or Amikacin	30 mg/kg/day IV divided q 8 h	
PLUS Antipseudomonal penicillin	Ticarcillin	300 mg/kg/day IV divided q 6 h	
	Or Ticarcillin/ clavulanate	300 mg/kg/day IV divided q 6 h	
	Or Mezlocillin	300 mg/kg/day IV divided q 6 h	
	Or Piperacillin	300 mg/kg/day IV divided q 6 h	
OR Aminoglycoside PLUS Antipseudomonal cephalosporin	As above Ceftazidime OR Cefipime	As above As above As above	
If immediate-type penicillin allergy	Aztreonam	75–150 mg/kg/day IV divided q 4–6 h	
	Plus aminoglycoside	As above	
Regimen with vancomycin for additional gram-positive coverage (*viridans* streptococci, enterococci)	Vancomycin	40–60 mg/kg/day IV divided q 6 h	Indications: Obvious catheter-related infection Severe mucositis Quinolone prophylaxis prior to fever Colonization with methicillin-resistant *S. aureus* or penicillin/cephalosporin-resistant *S. pneumoniae* Hypotension
PLUS Antipseudomonal cephalosporin	Ceftazidime	As above	
Is suspect *Pneumocystis carinii*	Add trimethoprim/ sulfamethoxazole	15–20 mg/kg/day IV divided q 6 h (based on trimethoprim component)	

SOURCE: Adapted from Hughes WT, Armstrong D, Bodey GP, et al: 1997 guidelines for the use of antimicrobial agents in neutropenic patients with unexplained fever. *Clin Infect Dis* 25:551, 1997. Used with permission.

- In pediatric patients, the oral cavity is the most common site for fungal infection. Any patient with difficulty breathing, hoarseness, or stridor should be considered to have epiglottic or laryngeal candidiasis.
- Herpes simplex virus (HSV) infections tend to be localized, even in the immunocompromised patient, and commonly involve the mouth, nares, esophagus, genitals, and perianal region.

- Varicella-zoster virus (VZV) infections in immunocompromised patients are associated with significant morbidity and mortality, including potential dissemination to the lung, CNS, and liver.
- Cancer patients with VZV infection are usually admitted for intravenous acyclovir. Varicella-zoster seronegative patients who are seen within 96 hours of virus exposure receive varicella-zoster immune globulin at a

dose of 125 U per 10 kg body weight IM with a maximum dose of 625 U.

- *P. carinii* is the most common parasitic infection in immunocompromised patients. Children with hematologic malignancies are most at risk.
- Typically, patients will have fever, dry cough, tachypnea, and intercostal retractions without detectable rales. The chest radiograph may be normal in early disease, but later progresses to bilateral alveolar infiltrates. Immunocompromised patients should be started on empiric therapy with TMP-SMX pending definitive diagnosis, as well as erythromycin for empiric *Legionella* coverage.

TUMOR LYSIS SYNDROME

- Tumor lysis syndrome results from the rapid degradation of tumor cells and release of the intracellular metabolites, uric acid, phosphate, and potassium in excess of their renal clearance.
- The syndrome occurs prior to or within several days after the initiation of cancer therapy. It is more commonly seen in patients with a large tumor cell load or rapidly growing tumors.
- Signs and symptoms of tumor lysis syndrome include nausea, vomiting, lethargy, abdominal or back pain, and change in urine color and amount.
- Hypocalcemia may manifest as muscle weakness, spasms, tetany, convulsions, altered level of consciousness, photophobia, or abdominal pain.
- Therapy is directed at treatment of hyperuricemia and hyperphosphatemia and prevention of renal failure. Hydration is important in facilitating uric acid and phosphate excretion. Intravenous fluid is administered at a minimum of twice the patient's maintenance rate, aiming at a urine specific gravity less than 1.010.
- To treat hyperuricemia, uric acid production may be reduced with allopurinol.
- In addition to hydration therapy, alkalinization of the urine increases uric acid solubility and excretion.
- Calcium supplementation for hypocalcemia is indicated only in patients who are severely symptomatic with a normal serum phosphate. Giving calcium in the face of hyperphosphatemia may increase the precipitation of calcium phosphate.

SUPERIOR VENA CAVA SYNDROME

- SVC syndrome refers to the signs and symptoms resulting from obstruction of the SVC. In children, compression of the narrow, more compliant trachea poses an additional complication.
- The presence of central venous catheters predisposes to vascular thrombosis and SVC syndrome.
- In children and adolescents, symptoms of SVC syndrome may progress rapidly over several days, unlike adults where the onset is more insidious.
- Patients have edema and plethora of the face, conjunctivae, neck, and upper torso. Tortuous collateral veins appear on the chest and upper abdomen. Headache, papilledema, seizures, coma, cerebral hemorrhage, and engorgement of retinal veins are a result of cerebral venous hypertension.
- Fatalities from SVC syndrome are related to airway obstruction, cerebral edema, or cardiac compromise.
- Computed tomography or MRI allows for identification of the lesion causing obstruction and the anatomic level of obstruction.
- The first priority in management is to protect and secure the airway.
- Radiation has been the traditional mode of therapy for tumor-induced SVC syndrome. More recently, treatment of SVC syndrome utilizes a combination of endovascular techniques, including thrombolysis, angioplasty, stent therapy and surgical bypass.

SPINAL CORD COMPRESSION

- Spinal cord compression due to a tumor occurs in approximately 4 percent of pediatric cancer patients. Extradural metastatic tumors such as soft tissue sarcomas, neuroblastoma, germ cell tumors, and Hodgkin's disease account for the majority of cases.
- Pain is the most common and usual initial presenting symptom. The pain is usually worse when supine and localized in the thoracic region; it is tender with percussion.
- Muscle weakness, which is usually symmetric, is a later finding.
- Sensory deficits are less common than is weakness and present with ascending numbness and paraesthesias.
- Changes in bladder or bowel function are also a common but late finding. Most patients will usually have objective neurologic deficits at the time of presentation.
- Plain spine radiographs will show an abnormality in less than 50 percent of patients with spinal cord compression.
- Contrast myelography or MRI provides a more definitive study.
- Epidural masses require immediate decompression with corticosteroids or radiation therapy. Chemotherapy is an option for chemotherapy-sensitive diseases such as Hodgkin's disease, NHL, neuroblastoma, or germ cell tumors.

BIBLIOGRAPHY

Abramson DH, Frank CM, Susman M, et al: Presenting signs of retinoblastoma. *J Pediatr* 132:505, 1998.

Barri YM, Knochel JP: Hypercalcemia and electrolyte disturbances in malignancy. *Hematol Oncol Clin North Am* 10:775, 1996.

Cairo MS, Sposto R, Perkins SL, et al: Burkitt's and Burkitt-like lymphoma in children and adolescents: A review of the Children's Cancer Group experience. *Br J Haematol* 120:660–670, 2003.

Fisman DN, Kaye KM: Once-daily dosing of aminoglycoside antibiotics. *Infect Dis Clin North Am* 14:475, 2000.

Freifeld AG, Pizzo PA: The outpatient management of febrile neutropenia in cancer patients. *Oncology* 10:599, 1996.

Hughes WT, Armstrong D, Bodey GP, et al: 1997 Guidelines for the use of antimicrobial agents in neutropenic patients with unexplained fever. *Clin Infect Dis* 25:551, 1997.

Klaassen RJ, Goodman TR, Doyle JJ: "Low-risk" prediction rule for pediatric oncology patients presenting with fever and neutropenia. *J Clin Oncol* 18:1012, 2000.

Mullen CA, Petropoulos D, Roberts WM, et al: Outpatient treatment of fever and neutropenia for low risk pediatric cancer patients. *Cancer* 86:126, 1999.

Schiff D, Butchelor T, Wen PY: Neurologic emergencies in cancer patients. *Neurol Clin* 16:449, 1998.

Schinder N, Vogelzang RL: Superior vena cava syndrome: Experience with endovascular stents and surgical therapy. *Surg Clin North Am* 79:684, 1999.

QUESTIONS

1. An 8-year-old is brought to the emergency department for evaluation of generalized fatigue. The parents state that the child was previously very active playing both soccer and softball. On examination, you note the child to have pallor, a low grade fever and marked lymphadenopathy. The remainder of the examination is essentially normal. You have a suspicion of leukemia. If your suspicion is correct, which of the following abnormalities would you expect to see on a complete blood count (CBC)?
   A. Pancytopenia
   B. Thrombocytopenia
   C. Neutropenia
   D. Thrombocytosis
   E. Elevated hematocrit

2. Which of the following is NOT a common complication of leukemia?
   A. CNS involvement
   B. Testicular enlargement in males
   C. Thrombocytopenia-induced hemorrhage
   D. Hypocalcemia
   E. Tumor lysis syndrome

3. A child is brought to the ED for evaluation of isolated cervical lymphadenopathy. Parents report that the lymph nodes have continued to increase in size over the last several weeks. Based on the history obtained and your physical examination, you suspect Hodgkin's disease. You obtain a screening CBC, and a chest radiograph. Which of the following lymph node measurements, if present, would increase your suspicion?
   A. Inguinal node of 10 mm
   B. Epitrochlear node of 5 mm
   C. Supraclavicular node of 7 mm
   D. Submandibular node of 4 mm
   E. Postauricular node of 8 mm

4. A 5-year-old boy is brought by parents for evaluation of a non-tender abdominal mass. Parents state the mass has increased in size over the last several months. The parents have noticed increased fatigue in the child. A screening urinalysis demonstrates microscopic hematuria. An ultrasound reveals in renal mass. Which of the following is the MOST likely diagnosis in this patient?
   A. Wilm's tumor
   B. Neuroblastoma
   C. Rhabdomyosarcoma
   D. Hodgkin's lymphoma
   E. Leukemia

5. A 4-year-old girl with leukemia is brought to the ED for evaluation of fever. Which of the following is NOT mandatory in the management of this patient?
   A Complete blood cell count
   B. Two sets of blood cultures
   C. Chest radiograph
   D. Empiric antibiotics
   E. Urine culture

ANSWERS

1. B. Acute leukemia is the most common childhood malignancy. Common presentations include pallor, fatigue, petechiae, purpura, bleeding and fever. The CBC often demonstrates leukocyte count greater than 10,000/mm^3, anemia, and thrombocytopenia.

2. D. Complications of leukemia can include CNS involvement, unilateral testicular enlargement in males, anemia, hemorrhage, hyper-leukocytosis, and hypercalcemia. Hypercalcemia is treated with intravenous hydration with normal saline, followed by furosemide to promote calcium excretion.

3. B. Hodgkin's Disease is a malignancy of the lymph nodes. The majority of pediatric patients have

painless supraclavicular or cervical lymphadenopathy. A lymph node is considered enlarged if it is more than 10 mm at its greatest diameter, with the exception of an epitrochlear node, which is considered enlarged at 5 mm, and an inguinal node, at 15 mm.

4. A. Wilm's tumor (nephroblastoma), the most common pediatric abdominal malignancy, arises from embryonal renal cells. Most Wilm's tumors occur in children less than 6 years of age and present with an abdominal mass and microscopic hematuria. Management includes surgical resection and chemotherapy or radiation.

5. D. Infection is the leading causes of death in children with cancer. The single most important factor is the development of neutropenia. The best parameter to assess is the absolute neutrophil count (ANC). Initial investigations include a chest radiograph, urinalysis and urine culture, CBC, and blood cultures. Prompt initiation of empiric antibiotic therapy is indicated in febrile neutropenic children.

76 INFECTIOUS MUSCULOSKELETAL DISORDERS

Gary R. Strange
Diana Mayer
Heather M. Prendergast

SEPTIC ARTHRITIS

- Septic arthritis occurs more commonly in children than in adults, and the frequency is greater in infants and toddlers than in older children. Half of all cases occur in the first 2 years of life, and three fourths of all cases are in children younger than 5 years.

ETIOLOGY

- Seeding of the joint with bacteria occurs either by hematogenous spread, direct inoculation of infected material into the joint capsule, or spread from an adjacent site of infection.
- Spread from a contiguous focus is uncommon, but in neonates and small infants, metaphyseal osteomyelitis can spread to the joint via blood vessels that bridge the epiphysis. In otherwise healthy children, most cases of septic arthritis are thought to be of hematogenous origin.
- The bacterial pathogen in septic arthritis depends largely on the age of the patient. In the first 2 months of life, *Staphylococcus aureus* and group B *Streptococcus* are the most common pathogens.
- *Staphylococcus aureus* predominates as the cause of septic arthritis until adolescence, when *Neisseria gonorrhoeae* becomes a frequent pathogen.
- Immunosuppressed patients are particularly vulnerable to infection with gram-negative organisms, including *Pseudomonas*.

CLINICAL PRESENTATION

- Neonates and young infants are particularly vulnerable to infection of the hip. The first manifestation of disease may be nonspecific irritability. Parents may note that the baby appears to be in pain when its diaper is changed.
- In older infants and children, the knee is more commonly affected. Patients old enough to ambulate may begin to walk with a limp or may refuse to walk altogether. Unlike the hip, where significant swelling may be absent, septic arthritis of the knee and most other joints is characterized by warmth, the presence of an effusion, and in most cases, significant limitation in range of motion.
- Gonococcal arthritis is likely in any postpubertal patient with joint pain and fever. It usually accompanies asymptomatic disease of the genitourinary tract. The knee, ankle, and especially the joints of the wrist, hand, and finger are affected.

DIAGNOSTIC EVALUATION

- The laboratory evaluation of suspected septic arthritis includes a complete blood count, erythrocyte sedimentation rate, blood culture, and joint fluid analysis. In most patients, the white blood count and the erythrocyte sedimentation rate will be elevated. Many patients, especially neonates and young infants, will have positive blood cultures.
- No single test or finding is sufficient to predict the presence of a septic joint, but, by using four clinical

TABLE 76-1   Analysis of Joint Fluid

CHARACTERISTIC	NORMAL	BACTERIAL	INFLAMMATORY
Appearance	Clear	Turbid, purulent	Clear or turbid
Leukocytes (cells/mL)	<100	>50,000	500–75,000
Neutrophils (%)	25	>75	50
Glucose (synovial/blood)	>50%	<50%	>50%

predictors, investigators have shown 99 percent accuracy in predicting the presence of a septic joint:

- ○ History of fever
- ○ Inability to bear weight
- ○ Elevated erythrocyte sedimentation rate (>40 mm/h)
- ○ Elevated white blood cell count (>12,000/mm³)
- The mainstay in the diagnosis of septic arthritis is analysis of joint fluid. Fluid is usually obtained by percutaneous aspiration. In the case of a suspected septic hip joint, aspiration is facilitated by sonographic guidance. Table 76-1 contrasts the characteristics of joint fluid under various conditions.
- Radiographic studies may be useful in demonstrating the presence of a joint effusion and to rule out other etiologies, such as trauma, but normal plain films do not rule out a septic joint. Ultrasound is most useful in evaluating the potentially septic hip.
- In infants, if clinical findings are indicative of or cannot exclude meningitis, a lumbar puncture is also indicated.

DIFFERENTIAL DIAGNOSIS

- The differential diagnosis of septic arthritis includes transient synovitis, cellulitis, traumatic hemarthrosis, osteomyelitis, collagen vascular diseases, Henoch-Schönlein purpura, and acute leukemia.
- In the hip, a number of problems specific to that joint must be considered. These include Legg-Calvé-Perthes disease, slipped capital femoral epiphysis, psoas abscess, obturator internus abscess, and diskitis. In the knee, the possibility of referred pain from the hip must be considered.

TREATMENT

- Treatment of septic arthritis consists of antibiotic therapy directed at the likely bacterial organisms (Table 76-2) and drainage of the involved joint.
- Serial aspiration is generally indicated for joints that are easily accessible, such as the knee. Incision and drainage procedures are preferred in joints that are

more difficult to access frequently for serial aspiration, such as the hip or shoulder, or when serial aspiration has not resulted in resolution of fluid accumulation.

OSTEOMYELITIS

PATHOPHYSIOLOGY

- Seeding of the bone with bacteria occurs by hematogenous spread, direct inoculation, or extension from an adjacent septic joint. Neonates subjected to invasive procedures in the setting of the intensive care unit are especially prone to develop osteomyelitis.

ETIOLOGY

- Overall, the most common etiology of osteomyelitis is *S. aureus.*
- In neonates, group B *Streptococcus* and enteric gram-negative organisms are also possible etiologies.
- *Pseudomonas aeruginosa* is often associated with osteomyelitis after puncture wounds of the foot.
- *Salmonella* is a consideration in sickle cell anemia patients.

CLINICAL MANIFESTATIONS

- Neonates may demonstrate few clinical findings other than irritability, fever, and some resistance to movement.
- Older infants and children may be able to localize discomfort over the affected site. Limp is a common finding in ambulatory patients.

DIAGNOSTIC TESTING

- Assessment includes:
  - ○ Complete blood count
    - White blood cell count may be normal or elevated
  - ○ Erythrocyte sedimentation rate
    - Usually increased
  - ○ Blood culture
    - Positive about 50 percent of the time
  - ○ Radiograph of the affected area
    - Usually unremarkable during the first week of the illness
    - Mottling and demineralization are usually observed a week after the initial symptoms.

TABLE 76-2   Treatment of Septic Arthritis and Osteomyelitis

AGE OR CONDITION GROUP	ORGANISMS	INITIAL ANTIBIOTICS
Neonates	Group B *Streptococcus* *Staphylococcus aureus* Gram-negative enteric bacilli *Candida* *Neisseria gonorrhoeae*	Oxacillin, 150–200 mg/kg/24 hr in 3–4 divided doses *and* Cefotaxime, 100–150 mg/kg/24 h in 3–4 divided doses
Infants and children <5 years of age	*Staphylococcus aureus* Group A *Streptococcus* *Haemophilus influenzae* type B (HiB)—if unimmunized	Ceftriaxone, 50 mg/kg/24 h given once daily
Children >5 years of age	*Staphylococcus aureus*	Nafcillin, 150 mg/kg/24 h in 4 divided doses *or* Cephalothin, 100–150 mg/kg/24 h in 4 divided doses *or* Vancomycin, 40 mg/kg/24 h in 4 divided doses—if suspicion of methicillin-resistant staphylococcal infection
Children >5 years of age without HiB immunization	*Staphylococcus aureus* *Haemophilus influenzae* type B	Cefuroxime, 100–150 mg/kg/24 h in 3 divided doses
Adolescents	*Neisseria gonorrhoeae* *Staphylococcus aureus*	Ceftriaxone, 50 mg/kg/24 h given once daily
Immunocompromised	Gram-negative enteric bacilli *Staphylococcus aureus* *Pseudomonas aeruginosa*	Ceftazidime, 100–150 mg/kg/24 h in 3 divided doses *and* Vancomycin, 40 mg/kg/24 h in 4 divided doses
Sickle cell disease	*Salmonella* spp. Gram-negative enteric bacilli *Staphylococcus aureus*	Ceftriaxone, 50 mg/kg/24 h given once daily *and* Nafcillin, 150 mg/kg/24 h in 4 divided doses *or* Cephalothin, 100–150 mg/kg/24 h in 4 divided doses
Puncture wounds of the foot	*Pseudomonas aeruginosa* *Staphylococcus aureus*	Ceftazidime, 100–150 mg/kg/24 h in 3 divided doses *and* Nafcillin, 150 mg/kg/24 h in 4 divided doses

- New periosteal bone formation is often evident after 10 days of symptoms
  - Radionuclear scanning with technetium-99m is often utilized because it is more sensitive than radiography early in the course of disease. Increased uptake is usually observed within 1 to 2 days after the onset of infection.
  - Ultrasound is able to detect subperiosteal abscesses accurately and simply early in the course of the disease and may be the only imaging test required in uncomplicated cases.
  - MRI has the highest sensitivity and specificity for detecting osteomyelitis.
  - The diagnosis is confirmed by needle aspiration of infected material. A steel needle is needed to penetrate the cortex.

TREATMENT

- Treatment for osteomyelitis is directed at eradicating the infection (Table 76-2).

INTERVERTEBRAL DISKITIS

- Intervertebral diskitis is an acute infection of the vertebral disk occasionally seen in children. Affected patients are usually younger than 5 years old. The lumbar area is most commonly involved.
- Most cases are preceded by an upper respiratory infection.
- Infants may become irritable and refuse to sit. Toddlers may refuse to walk. Older children may

complain of back or leg pain and may develop a limp.

- The physical examination may show a loss of lordosis. If the cervical vertebrae are involved, torticollis can occur.
- Tenderness along the vertebrae, mild fullness of the paraspinal muscles secondary to irritation, and occasionally hip pain and stiffness can occur.
- Fever may be present.
- The erythrocyte sedimentation rate is usually elevated.
- In about 40 percent of cases, blood cultures are positive.
- Radiographs of the involved area may demonstrate a narrowing of the disk space and, eventually, erosion of the vertebral end plates.
- Technetium-99m bone and MRI scans are able to diagnose the disease early in the course.
- Affected children can usually be managed as outpatients, with antibiotic therapy directed against *S. aureus*.

LYME DISEASE

- Lyme disease is caused by the spirochete *Borrelia burgdorferi* and is transmitted by *Ixodes scapularis*, commonly called the deer tick. In the United States, most cases are seen in southern New England, the Middle Atlantic states, and the upper Midwest.
- The overall risk of acquiring Lyme disease is low even in endemic areas. Prevention efforts center around the use of protective clothing and insect repellants, followed by close checking for ticks after exposure.
- Lyme disease is divided into two stages: early and late illness.
  - The early stage is further split into an early localized phase and an early disseminated phase. The early localized phase begins around 1 week after inoculation by the tick and is marked by a characteristic rash known as erythema migrans. The lesion starts as an erythematous papule or macule that spreads outward to form an enlarging circle with a red rim and central clearing.
  - Those with early disseminated disease will often develop secondary erythema migrans, presenting with several lesions that are smaller than the initial lesion. These lesions appear several days to weeks after the original lesion and are often accompanied by fever, myalgias, headache, malaise, conjunctivitis, and lymphadenopathy.
  - The late stage of Lyme disease consists of arthritis and, rarely, fever and encephalopathy. Large joints are most commonly affected, especially the knee, although virtually any joint can be involved.

- The differential diagnosis of Lyme arthritis includes:
  - Septic joint
  - Acute rheumatic fever
  - Juvenile rheumatoid arthritis
  - Postinfectious virally induced arthritis
- Diagnostic studies include:
  - Complete blood count
  - Antinuclear antibody
  - Rheumatoid factor
  - Urinalysis
  - Electrocardiogram
  - Throat culture
  - Lyme disease titers
  - Joint fluid in patients with active arthritis may contain up to 100,000 white blood cells/mL, with a preponderance of polymorphonuclear leukocytes.
- Antibiotic treatment of Lyme disease shortens the course of disease and can prevent the development of chronic illness. In some cases it effectively treats established chronic arthritis and neurologic symptoms. Erythema migrans and disseminated early disease without focal findings are treated with oral doxycycline or amoxicillin for 21 days.
  - Children younger than 8 years of age should not receive doxycycline.
  - Erythromycin can be substituted for allergic patients.
  - Cranial nerve palsies and arthritis are treated with the same medication, but for 30 days.
  - Intravenous or intramuscular treatment is used for patients with carditis or neurologic disease other than cranial nerve palsy. Treatment is with ceftriaxone or penicillin for 14 to 21 days.
- Treatment of early localized infection will stop progression of the disease, and the prognosis is excellent, even if treatment is not begun until the late phase. In contrast to studies in adults, long-term follow-up studies of children with Lyme disease do not show an increased risk of cognitive impairment.

ACUTE SUPPURATIVE TENOSYNOVITIS

- The palmar surface of the hand is vulnerable to suppurative tenosynovitis, because the flexor tendons of the finger are surrounded by a synovial sheath that localizes an infection and, if treatment is delayed, can provide a conduit for spread to deep spaces of the palm. It usually occurs as an extension of a localized infection.
- Physical examination of the hand reveals erythema and tenderness along the tendon sheath. Patients hold the affected finger in a flexed position, and active or passive extension provokes intense pain. The affected finger is diffusely swollen.

- The most common bacterial etiologies are *S. aureus* and group A *Streptococcus*. In adolescents and sexually abused children, *N. gonorrhoeae* is a likely possibility.
- Management consists of therapy with antibiotics and surgical drainage.

BIBLIOGRAPHY

Adams WV, Rose CD, Eppes SC, et al: Long-term cognitive effects of Lyme disease in children. *Appl Neurospsychol* 6:39–45, 1999.

Bachman DT, Srivastava G: Emergency department presentations of Lyme disease in children. *Pediatr Emerg Care* 14:356–361, 1998.

Fernandez M, Carrol CL, Baker CJ: Discitis and vertebral osteomyelitis in children: An 18-year review. *Pediatrics* 105:1299–1304, 2000.

Kaiser S, Jorulf H, Hirsch G: Clinical value of imaging techniques in childhood osteomyelitis. *Acta Radiol* 39:523–531, 1998.

Klein DM, Barbera C, Gray ST, et al: Sensitivity of objective parameters in the diagnosis of pediatric septic hips. *Clin Orthop* 338:153–159, 1997.

Kleinman PK: A regional approach to osteomyelitis of the lower extremities in children. *Radiol Clin North Am* 40:1033–1059, 2002.

Kocher MS, Zurakowski D, Kasser JR: Differentiating between septic arthritis and transient synovitis of the hip in children: An evidence-based clinical prediction algorithm. *J Bone Joint Surg [Am]* 81:1662–1670, 1999.

Lee SK, Suh KJ, Kim YW, et al: Septic arthritis versus transient synovitis at MR imaging: Preliminary assessment with signal intensity alterations in bone marrow. *Radiology* 211:459–465, 1999.

Nelson JD: Osteomyelitis and suppurative arthritis. In: Behrman RE, Kliegman RM, Jenson HB, eds. *Nelson Textbook of Pediatrics,* 16th ed. Philadelphia: Saunders, 776–780, 2000.

Perlman MH, Patzakis MJ, Kumar PJ, et al: The incidence of joint involvement with adjacent osteomyelitis in pediatric patients. *J Pediatr Orthop* 20:40–43, 2000.

Shapiro ED: Lyme disease (*Borrelia burgdorferi*). In: Behrman RE, Kliegman RM, Jenson HB, eds. *Nelson Textbook of Pediatrics*, 16th ed. Philadelphia: Saunders, 911–914, 2000.

Willis AA, Widmann RF, Flynn JM, et al: Lyme arthritis presenting as acute septic arthritis in children. *J Pediatr Orthop* 23:114–118, 2003.

QUESTIONS

1. A 3-year-old is brought to the ED for evaluation of an inability to bear weight on his left leg. The parents deny any history of trauma, and report the toddler was previously walking fine. There is a history of a low grade fever at home. On exam you note, a warm slightly swollen left knee. There is moderate pain with movement. Examination of the hip is unremarkable. You suspect septic arthritis. Which of the following findings would **NOT** be consistent with the diagnosis of septic arthritis?
   A. Elevated erythrocyte sedimentation rate
   B. Normal radiographs of the hip and knee
   C. Predominance of lymphocytes on manual differential
   D. History of fever
   E. Cloudy fluid aspirate

2. A 14-year-old girl is brought to the ED for evaluation of continued evaluation of foot pain. Upon further questioning, you learn that the patient stepped on a nail while cleaning out an attic 2 weeks earlier. Radiographs obtained demonstrate some mild periosteal bone formation. The **MOST** appropriate antibiotic coverage for this patient would be which of the following?
   A. Bicillin LA 1.2 million units IM
   B. Levaquin 500 mg IV
   C. Vancomycin 1 g IV
   D. Ceftriaxone 1 g IV
   E. Erythromycin 500 mg IV

3. A 4-year-old boy is brought to the ED for evaluation of new onset of a limp. According to the parents, the child was well except for an upper respiratory infection 1 week ago. Physical exam reveals an otherwise normal appearing child with a normal lower extremity examination. You do note that there is a mild amount of tenderness along palpation of the lower vertebrae and some fullness of the paraspinal muscles. An MRI of the lumbar spine is consistent with intervertebral diskitis. The **MOST** appropriate disposition in this patient would be which of the following?
   A. Inpatient admission for intravenous steroids
   B. Neurosurgical consultation
   C. Inpatient admission for intravenous antibiotics
   D. Outpatient therapy with oral antibiotics
   E. Outpatient therapy with oral prednisone

4. A 6-year-old girl is brought for evaluation of a rash and low-grade temperature after returning from a camping trip with her family. On examination you note several erythematous papules and macules in a circular configuration with central clearing. Which of the following treatment options would be **MOST** appropriate for this patient?
   A. Prophylactic amoxicillin for family members for 10 to 14 days
   B. Oral doxycycline for 21 days
   C. Oral amoxicillin for 21 days

D. Intramuscular penicillin for 21 days

E. Intramuscular ceftriaxone for 21 days

5. You receive a call from a local ED concerning the referral of a child with a swollen finger. Per the referring physician, the symptoms have gradually worsened over the last 3 days. The child now is holding the digit in slight flexion. There is marked erythema, swelling, and pain with both active and passive movement. You inform the physician that the patient will need antibiotics and surgical drainage. The most likely bacterial etiology would be which of the following?

A. *S. aureus*

B. Gram-negative organisms

C. *N. gonorrhoeae*

D. Group B Streptococcus

E *Pseudomonas aeruginosa*

ANSWERS

1. C. A predominance of lymphocytes on a manual differential would not be consistent with the diagnosis of septic arthritis. One would expect to see an elevated white blood cell count and a predominance of neutrophils on manual differential. Other findings that would heighten the suspicion of a septic joint include the following: history of fevers, elevated erythrocyte sedimentation rate, and turbid joint fluid.

2. B. In cases of osteomyelitis occurring after puncture wounds, *Pseudomonas aeruginosa* is the usual organism. These patients require intravenous antibiotics and a quinolone would be an acceptable choice in this situation. In the majority of cases of general osteomyelitis, *S. aureus* infection is the most common etiology.

3. D. Intervertebral diskitis is an acute infection of the vertebral disk in children less than 5 years of age. Most cases are preceded by an upper respiratory infection. If the diagnosis is made early by MRI, the nontoxic appearing patient may be managed as an outpatient with antibiotic therapy directed against *S. aureus*.

4. C. This patient is presenting with signs and symptoms consistent with the early stages of Lyme disease. Treatment at this stage involves oral antibiotic treatment amoxicillin or doxycycline for 21 days. Doxycycline is contraindicated in patients younger than 8 years of age. Intramuscular or intravenous treatment is reserved for patients with neurologic or cardiac involvement.

5. A. This patient is presenting with an acute suppurative tenosynovitis. The most common bacterial etiologies are *S. aureus* and group A *Streptococcus*. Management consists of intravenous antibiotics and surgical drainage.

77 INFLAMMATORY MUSCULOSKELETAL DISORDERS

Gary R. Strange
Diana Mayer
Valerie A. Dobiesz

REACTIVE AND POSTINFECTIOUS ARTHRITIS

• In many inflammatory and infectious disorders, arthritis is an associated finding in which joint manifestations appear to be secondary to an immunologic reaction to the disease process.

• Both ulcerative colitis and Crohn's disease can be associated with arthritis, as can gastroenteritis caused by *Shigella, Salmonella, Yersinia, Giardia*, and *Campylobacter*.

• Many viral infections, including hepatitis and infections due to Epstein-Barr virus, adenovirus, and rubella, are also associated with arthritis.

• The treatment of reactive arthritis is with antiinflammatory agents. Antibiotic therapy has not been shown to be helpful for full-blown reactive arthritis, but antibiotics probably are helpful in preventing the development of reactive arthritis when the primary problem is diagnosed prior to the development of arthritis.

TRANSIENT SYNOVITIS

• Transient synovitis of the hip is an inflammatory process that often follows an upper respiratory infection. The disorder is usually seen in children between the ages of 18 months and 7 years, with a presenting complaint of refusal to walk.

• Laboratory studies are mostly useful in distinguishing transient synovitis from a septic hip. In transient synovitis, the white blood cell count and erythrocyte sedimentation rate are usually normal or only slightly elevated, in contrast to septic arthritis, in which both are usually significantly elevated.

• The treatment of transient synovitis is bed rest and therapy with antiinflammatory agents.

• The prognosis is excellent.

JUVENILE RHEUMATOID ARTHRITIS

• The differential diagnosis of juvenile rheumatoid arthritis (JRA) includes:

- ○ Acute rheumatic fever
- ○ Systemic lupus erythematosus
- ○ Bacterial arthritis
- ○ Reactive arthritis
- ○ Neoplastic diseases, especially leukemia
- In the emergency department, the workup of suspected JRA includes a complete blood count, renal function studies, and a rapid streptococcal screen. Tests for antinuclear antibodies and rheumatoid factors are indicated but not immediately available in the emergency department.

SYSTEMIC LUPUS ERYTHEMATOSUS

- Complaints in patients with systemic lupus erythematosus (SLE) include fever, malaise, weight loss, and fatigue. Skin manifestations are common, including the characteristic erythematous rash extending from the malar regions across the bridge of the nose.
- In all patients with suspected SLE, a complete blood count, prothrombin time (PT), partial thromboplastin time (PTT), and erythrocyte sedimentation rate are indicated. The prevalence of renal involvement requires serum electrolytes, blood urea nitrogen, and creatinine. A urinalysis will often reveal microscopic hematuria and proteinuria. Antinuclear antibody, rheumatoid factor, complement studies, and quantitative immunoglobulins are indicated, but the results will not be available in the emergency department.

RHEUMATIC FEVER

- Acute rheumatic fever (ARF) is a systemic inflammatory condition that is a complication of group A β-hemolytic streptococcal pharyngitis. The exact path ology of the disease is unknown, but it is thought to be autoimmune in nature.
- The cardiac involvement of ARF results in carditis, which can affect all layers of the heart, including the pericardium, and is responsible for most of the morbidity associated with the disease. The carditis can be clinically silent or severe enough to result in congestive heart failure. Involvement of the valves, especially the mitral and aortic, results in significant long-term morbidity.
- Chorea occurs in up to 10 percent of patients, usually in preadolescent girls, and can be the only manifestation of disease. It consists of random, purposeless movements, most commonly involving the muscles of the extremities and face that in some cases are preceded by behavioral changes. The duration of chorea varies, but it is a self-limited process.

TABLE 77-1 Diagnosis of Rheumatic Fever (Revised Jones Criteria)[a]

LEVEL OF SIGNIFICANCE	MANIFESTATION
Major	Carditis
	Polyarthritis
	Chorea
	Erythema marginatum
	Subcutaneous nodules
Minor	Fever
	Arthralgias
	Elevated erythrocyte sedimentation rate or C-reactive protein
	Prolonged PR interval

[a] For formal diagnosis of acute rheumatic fever, either two major or one major and two minor manifestations must be accompanied by supporting evidence of streptococcal infection (positive throat culture or elevated antistreptolysin O titer).

- The dermatologic manifestations of ARF include erythema marginatum, which is an intermittent, red, slightly raised rash that occurs most commonly on the trunk and extremities. Subcutaneous nodules are painless, movable lesions that may develop later during the course of illness. They are rare.
- The diagnosis of rheumatic fever is usually made by utilizing a combination of clinical and laboratory findings. These are summarized in the modified Jones criteria (Table 77-1). The presence of two major and one minor or one major and two minor criteria is highly correlated with ARF. In addition to the criteria, virtually all children have serologic evidence of an antecedent streptococcal infection.
- Patients with arthritis but without carditis are managed with high-dose aspirin.
- Patients with evidence of significant carditis are treated with prednisone.
- Chorea may respond to haloperidol.
- Patients who suffer one attack of rheumatic fever are especially vulnerable to recurrent attacks, which can exacerbate damage to previously affected heart valves. Recurrent attacks can be prevented by prophylactic administration of antibiotics, most commonly by injections of benzathine penicillin administered every 3 weeks.

ENTHESOPATHIES

- Enthesopathy, also known as enthesitis, is an inflammation of tendons, ligaments, and fascia at their sites of attachment.
- Tenderness from enthesopathy may be noted in the chest wall, iliac crest, ischial tuberosity, posterior or plantar surface of the heel, metatarsophalangeal area, and anterior tibial tuberosity.

• Pain resulting from enthesopathies is treated with NSAIDs.

ANKYLOSING SPONDYLITIS

• Ankylosing spondylitis (AS) is a rheumatic disorder that can present in later childhood or adolescence. It is most common in males.
• AS is predominantly characterized by involvement of the sacroiliac joints and lumbar spine. Many patients have associated peripheral arthritis.
• The primary treatment of AS is with NSAIDs.

BIBLIOGRAPHY

Arkachaisri T, Lehman TJ: Systemic lupus erythematosus and related disorders of childhood. *Curr Opin Rheumatol* 11:384–392, 1999.

Cron RQ, Sharma S, Sherry DD: Current treatment by United States and Canadian pediatric rheumatologists. *J Rheumatol* 26:2036–2038, 1999.

Eich GF, Superti-Furga A, Umbricht FS, et al: The painful hip: Evaluation of criteria for clinical decision-making. *Eur J Pediatr* 158:923–928, 1998.

Fendler C, Laitko S, Sorensen H, et al: Frequency of triggering bacteria in patients with reactive arthritis and undifferentiated oligoarthritis and the relative importance of the tests used for diagnosis. *Ann Rheum Dis* 60:337–343, 2001.

Ferrieri P, Jones Criteria Working Group: Proceedings of the Jones Criteria workshop. *Circulation* 106:2521–2523, 2002.

Newberg AH, Newman JS: Imaging the painful hip. *Clin Orthop* 406:19–28, 2003.

Saxena A: Diagnosis of rheumatic fever: Current status of Jones criteria and role of echocardiography. *Indian J Pediatr* 67(suppl):S11–14, 2000.

Toivanen A: Bacteria-triggered reactive arthritis: Implications for antibacterial treatment. *Drugs* 61:343–351, 2001.

Toivanen P: From reactive arthritis to rheumatoid arthritis. *J Autoimmun* 16:369–371, 2001.

Toussirot E, Wendling D: Therapeutic advances in ankylosing spondylitis. *Expert Opin Investig Drugs* 10:21–29, 2001.

Van Der Linden S, Van Der Heijde D: Clinical aspects, outcome assessment and management of ankylosing spondylitis and postenteric reactive arthritis. *Curr Opin Rheumatol* 12:263–268, 2001.

Visvanathan K, Manjarez RC, Zabriskie JB: Rheumatic fever. *Curr Treat Options Cardiovasc Med* 1:253–258, 1999.

QUESTIONS

1. Which of the following is true regarding reactive and postinfectious arthritis?
   A. Is a direct inoculation of the joint by the organism
   B. The treatment of reactive arthritis is antibiotics
   C. May be associated with ulcerative colitis and Crohn's disease
   D. Causes crystal formation within joints
   E. Not associated with viral infections

2. A 5-year-old male presents with a complaint of left hip pain for 3 days and a limp. He recently had an upper respiratory tract infection that has resolved. He denies trauma/injury. He is afebrile and is non-toxic appearing. Which of the following is true regarding the management of this patient?
   A. The patient must be admitted for IV antibiotics
   B. The main concern is differentiation from septic arthritis
   C. Laboratory tests are not indicated
   D. Plain radiographs are diagnostic
   E. The prognosis is poor if no infection present

3. Which of the following is true regarding systemic lupus erythematosus in children?
   A. Skin manifestations are rare
   B. Patients typically present with pathologic fractures
   C. Renal involvement is common
   D. Stat antinuclear antibody and rheumatoid factors should be ordered in the ED
   E. Is caused by an enzyme deficiency

4. A 10-year-old girl presents with the complaint of sudden, aimless, irregular movements of her arms, a raised fleeting rash to her trunk, and migratory polyarticular arthritis. She had a sore throat 3 weeks ago. Which of the following is true regarding her condition?
   A. Is a complication of group A β-hemolytic streptococcal infections
   B. Is thought to be due to exotoxins
   C. Does not affect the heart
   D. The rash is called erythema chronicum migrans
   E. Commonly associated with painful subcutaneous nodules

5. Which of the following is true regarding carditis in acute rheumatic fever (ARF)?
   A. Affects only the cardiac valves
   B. Occurs in one third of patients
   C. No significant morbidity occurs
   D. Treatment of carditis is with high-dose aspirin
   E. Treatment of carditis prevents recurrence of the disease

ANSWERS

1. C. In many inflammatory and infectious disorders, arthritis is an associated finding and appears to be

secondary to an immunologic reaction to the disease process. Both ulcerative colitis and Crohn's disease may be associated with arthritis. Many viral infections are associated with arthritis. The treatment is with anti-inflammatory agents.

2. B. This patient has transient synovitis but the main concern is to differentiate this from septic arthritis. Laboratory studies may be helpful as the WBC and ESR are usually normal in transient synovitis and elevated in septic arthritis. Radiographs are usually normal or show a mild to moderate effusion. The patient may need arthrocentesis to determine the diagnosis. The prognosis for transient synovitis is excellent and is treated with bed rest and antiinflammatory agents.

3. C. Complaints in patients with SLE include fever, malaise, weight loss, and fatigue. Skin manifestations and renal involvement are common. A urinalysis will often reveal microscopic hematuria and proteinuria. Antinuclear antibody, rheumatoid factor, complement studies, and quantitative immunoglobulins will not be available in the ED.

4. A. This girl has acute rheumatic fever, an inflammatory condition that is a complication of group A β-hemolytic streptococcal pharyngitis. This infection stimulates antibody production to host tissues and is autoimmune in nature. There may be cardiac involvement resulting in carditis. The rash, erythema marginatum, is red, fleeting, faint, and serpiginous. Subcutaneous nodules are painless and rare.

5. B. Carditis occurs in one third of patients and can affect all layers of the heart and is responsible for most of the morbidity associated with ARF. Treatment of carditis is prednisone. Patients who suffer one attack of rheumatic fever are especially vulnerable to recurrent attacks.

78 NONMALIGNANT TUMORS OF BONE

Gary R. Strange
Diana Mayer
Valerie A. Dobiesz

INTRODUCTION

- A number of histologically benign tumors of bone present in childhood. Since these tumors may be painless, they are often found incidentally on routine radiographs.
- Another common presentation is that of pathologic fracture. Pathologic fractures are treated as are traumatic fractures, followed by specific treatment of the bone tumor as indicated.

- Some benign tumors are associated with pain that is usually relieved by aspirin or other nonsteroidal anti-inflammatory drugs (NSAIDs).

OSTEOID OSTEOMAS

- Osteoid osteoma is a relatively common benign tumor that frequently causes pain, especially at night, and which is responsive to NSAIDs. The most commonly affected areas are the femur and tibia, but osteoid osteoma may involve the vertebral bodies as well. Osteoid osteoma occurs primarily in boys between the ages of 5 and 20 years.
- Radiographs demonstrate a radiolucent center of osteoid tissue encircled by sclerotic bone.
- Surgical removal of the lesion is curative.

NONOSSIFYING FIBROMAS

- Non-ossifying fibromas are often incidental findings, but they can also cause chronic pain. Occasionally, pathologic fractures can occur.
- Radiographs reveal a characteristic scalloped lesion.
- Treatment is not required.

OSTEOCHONDROMAS

- Osteochondromas may result in a nonpainful mass or pathologic fracture, but many are completely asymptomatic.
- Radiographs demonstrate sessile or pedunculated lesions.
- These lesions should be biopsied and usually require removal.

ENCHONDROMAS

- Patients with enchondromas may present with a mass or pathologic fracture, but most are asymptomatic.
- Radiographs show thinning bone with cortical bulging and stippled calcification.
- Orthopedic consultation is indicated since curettage and bone grafting may be considered for larger or symptomatic lesions.

SOLITARY BONE CYSTS

- Solitary bone cysts are prone to associated fracture and require excision, especially in the lower extremity.

- Steroid injection into the lesion is another possible treatment.

ANEURYSMAL BONE CYSTS

- Radiographs show eccentric lytic lesions of the metaphysis.
- The usual treatment is curettage and bone grafting.

BIBLIOGRAPHY

Lefton DR, Torrisi JM, Haller JO: Vertebral osteoid osteoma masquerading as a malignant bone or soft-tissue tumor on MRI. *Pediatr Radiol* 31:72–75, 2001.

Levine SM, Lambiase RE, Petchprapa CN: Cortical lesions of the tibia: Characteristic appearances at conventional radiography. *Radiographics* 23:157–177, 2003.

Shaughnessy WJ, Arndt CAS: Benign tumors. In: Behrman RE, Kliegman RM, Jenson HB, eds. *Nelson Textbook of Pediatrics*, 16th ed. Philadelphia: Saunders, 1567–1569, 2000.

QUESTIONS

1. Which of the following is not a benign bone tumor?
   A. Osteoid osteoma
   B. Osteochondromas
   C. Enchondromas
   D. Nonossifying fibromas
   E. Osteosarcoma

2. A 12-year-old male presents with complaint of mild distal left leg pain for several months. He denies trauma or injury. On examination there is mild tenderness to the distal tibia. Radiographs reveal an eccentric, radiolucent, thin reactive shell of bone. A nonossifying fibroma is diagnosed. The most appropriate treatment would be:
   A. Emergent referral to an orthopedic surgeon for biopsy
   B. Symptomatic treatment with nonsteroidal anti-inflammatory medications
   C. A short leg splint and crutches
   D. Thorough evaluation for child abuse
   E. Admission for initiation of chemotherapy and possible amputation

3. A 10-year-old male presents with a complaint of pain to his right tibia worse at night for several weeks but now worse for one day after sliding in a baseball game yesterday. Physical exam is unremarkable except point tenderness to the distal tibia. A radiograph demonstrates a radiolucent center of osteoid tissue encircled by sclerotic bone with a non displaced linear fracture to the distal tibia. The most appropriate management of this patient would be:
   A. Symptomatic treatment with nonsteroidal anti-inflammatory medications
   B. Bucks traction and admission
   C. A short leg immobilization splint, analgesics, crutches, and orthopedic follow up
   D. Emergent orthopedic consultation for bone biopsy
   E. Oncology consult and referral for radiation therapy

ANSWERS

1. E. Osteoid osteomas, osteochondromas, endochondromas, and nonossifying fibromas are all nonmalignant tumors of the bone.

2. B. Non-ossifying fibromas are often incidental findings and have a classic radiographic appearance. These are usually asymptomatic but may cause chronic pain and present with pathologic fractures. Treatment is symptomatic such as aspirin or nonsteroidal anti-inflammatory medications.

3. C. This patient has an osteoid osteoma, which is a relatively common benign tumor and a pathologic fracture. These tumors frequently cause pain especially at night. The most commonly affected areas are the femur and tibia. It primarily occurs in boys between the ages of 5 and 20. The pathologic fracture is treated like a traumatic fracture with immobilization, analgesics, crutches and orthopedic follow up. The tumor may need to be surgically removed.

TOXICOLOGIC EMERGENCIES

79 GENERAL PRINCIPLES OF POISONING: DIAGNOSIS AND MANAGEMENT

Timothy Erickson
Gary R. Strange

EPIDEMIOLOGY

- There has been a 95 percent decline in the number of pediatric poisoning deaths in children under 6 years of age over the past few decades. Child-resistant product packaging, heightened parental awareness of potential household toxins, and more sophisticated medical intervention at the poison control and emergency and intensive care levels have all contributed to reduce morbidity and mortality.
- Of the over 1.4 million exposures involving individuals under 20 years of age reported to poison control centers in 1999, 2700 patients (0.2 percent) experienced a major outcome defined as a life-threatening effect or residual disability, with 85 fatalities (0.004 percent). Although responsible for the majority of pediatric poisonings, children under 6 years of age comprised only 2.7 percent of the fatalities.

HISTORY

- Although it may be difficult to obtain an accurate and complete history regarding an ingestion, this is an essential part of the proper evaluation of poisoned pediatric patients. All sources of information are explored in children who are comatose or too young to provide details.

PHYSICAL EXAMINATION

- A comprehensive physical examination may provide valuable clues regarding the ingestion or exposure.
- Since many drugs and toxic agents have specific effects on the heart rate, temperature, blood pressure, and respiratory rate, monitoring the vital signs may direct the clinician toward the proper diagnosis (Table 79-1).
- Additionally, the level of consciousness, pupillary size, and potential for seizures may be directly affected by the poison in a dose-dependent fashion.
- Other diagnostic clues are obtained from the skin examination and breath odor (Table 79-2).
- Several groups of toxins consistently present with recognizable patterns or signs. Recognizing these toxic syndromes, or toxidromes, may expedite not only the diagnosis of the toxic agent, but also its management (Table 79-3).

DIAGNOSTIC AIDS AND LABORATORY

- In children with significant or unknown ingestion, baseline laboratory studies include a complete blood cell count, renal functions, serum electrolytes, glucose, and arterial blood gases. In patients with known ingestion demonstrating no overt signs of toxicity, a more selective approach to diagnostic studies is acceptable.
- If the arterial blood gas value reveals a metabolic acidosis, calculating the anion gap can assist in formulating a differential diagnosis. A metabolic acidosis with an increased anion gap results from the presence of organically active acids and is characteristic of several toxins and various disease states (Table 79-4). The anion gap can be calculated as follows:

$$\text{Anion Gap} = Na - (Cl + HCO_3)$$

TABLE 79-1 Toxic Vital Signs

Bradycardia (PACED)
P	Propranolol (beta blockers)
A	Anticholinesterase drugs
C	Clonidine, calcium channel blockers
E	Ethanol and alcohols
D	Digoxin, Darvon (opiates)

Tachycardia (FAST)
F	Free base (cocaine)
A	Anticholinergics, antihistamines, amphetamines
S	Sympathomimetics
T	Theophylline

Hypothermia (COOLS)
C	Carbon monoxide
O	Opiates
O	Oral hypogylcemics, insulin
L	Liquor
S	Sedative hypnotics

Hyperthermia (NASA)
N	Neuroleptic malignant syndrome, nicotine
A	Antihistamines
S	Salicylates, sympathomimetics
A	Anticholinergics, antidepressants

Hypotension (CRASH)
C	Clonidine
R	Reserpine (antihypertensive agents)
A	Antidepressants
S	Sedative hypnotics
H	Heroin (opiates)

Hypertension (CTSCAN)
C	Cocaine
T	Theophylline
S	Sympathomimetics
C	Caffeine
A	Anticholinergics, amphetamines
N	Nicotine

TABLE 79-2 Toxic Physical Findings

Miosis (COPS)
C	Cholinergics, clonidine
O	Opiates, organophosphates
P	Phenothiazines, pilocarpine, pontine bleed
S	Sedative hypnotics

Mydriasis (AAAS)
A	Antihistamines
A	Antidepressants
A	Anticholinergics, atropine
S	Sympathomimetics (cocaine, amphetamines)

Seizures (OTIS CAMPBELL)
O	Organophosphates	C	Camphor, cocaine
T	Tricyclic antidepressants	A	Amphetamines
I	INH, insulin	M	Methylxanthines (theophylline, caffeine)
S	Sympathomimetics	P	PCP
		B	Beta-blockers, botanicals
		E	Ethanol withdrawal
		L	Lithium, lindane
		L	Lead, lidocaine

Diaphoretic skin (SOAP)
S	Sympathomimetics
O	Organophosphates
A	ASA (salicylates)
P	PCP

Red Skin:	Carbon monoxide, boric acid
Blue Skin:	Cyanosis, methemoglobinemia
Breath odors	

Bitter almonds	Cyanide
Fruity	DKA, Isopropanol
Oil of wintergreen	Methyl salicylates
Rotten eggs	Sulfur dioxide, hydrogen sulfide
Pears	Chloral hydrate
Garlic	Organophosphates, arsenic, DMSO
Mothballs	Camphor

INH, isonicotinic acid hydrazide (isoniazid); ASA, acetylsalicyclic acid; PCP, phencyclidine; DKA, diabetic ketoacidosis.

The normal anion gap ranges from 8 to 12 mEq/L.

- If ingestion of a toxic alcohol, such as methanol or ethylene glycol, is suspected, calculation of the osmolal gap is critical. The osmolal gap is the difference between the actual osmolality, best measured by freezing-point depression, and that calculated from major osmotically active molecules in the serum (sodium, glucose, and blood urea nitrogen). It is normally below 10.

$$\text{Calculated Osmolality} = 2(\text{Na}) + \text{Glucose}/18 - \text{BUN}/2.8 + \text{ETOH}/4.6$$

- When a particular drug or toxin is known or highly suspected, blood or serum can be tested for specific drug levels. These levels confirm the ingestion and often guide medical management. Commonly available tests are listed in Table 79-5.
- Toxicology screening can be helpful in the diagnosis of the unknown ingestion if the clinician is aware of its limitations. The urine toxicology screen may be of greater value, since the drug's metabolites continue to

be excreted in the urine for 48 to 72 h following the ingestion. Toxicology panels typically screen for drugs of abuse such as narcotics, amphetamines, cannabinoids, phencyclidine (PCP), and cocaine.

- Radiologic testing can prove valuable with certain ingestions, particularly those that are radiopaque or those that may induce a noncardiogenic pulmonary edema or chemical pneumonitis (Table 79-6).

MANAGEMENT

STABILIZATION

- The cornerstone of management of patients with a suspected overdose is supportive care, with particular attention to airway, breathing, and circulation.
- In children with an altered level of consciousness or in whom a bedside glucose oxidase test documents

TABLE 79-3   Toxic Syndromes

Anticholinergic (tricyclic antidepressants, antihistamines)

Hot as a hare	Hyperthermia
Dry as a bone	Dry mouth
Red as a beet	Flushed skin
Blind as a bat	Dilated pupils
Mad as a hatter	Confused delirium

Cholinergic (organophosphates)

D	Diarrhea, diaphoresis
U	Urination
M	Miosis, muscle fasciculations
B	Bradycardia, bronchosecretions
E	Emesis
L	Lacrimation
S	Salivation

Sympathomimetic (cocaine, amphetamines)
  Mydriasis
  Tachycardia
  Hypertension
  Hyperthermia
  Seizures

Narcotic
  Miosis
  Bradycardia
  Hypotension
  Hypoventilation
  Coma

Withdrawal
  Alcohol
  Benzodiazepines
  Barbiturates
  Antihypertensives
  Opioids

hypoglycemia, the physician should administer intravenous dextrose at 0.5 to 1.0 g/kg, given as 2 to 4 mL/kg of $D_{25}W$ in children or 50 mL (1 ampul) of $D_{50}W$ in the adolescent. If intravenous access is difficult or unobtainable, glucagon, 1 mg, is administered intramuscularly.

- Naloxone, a specific opiate antagonist with minimal side effects, is given to children or adolescents with lethargy or coma. The initial dose is 0.1 mg/kg intravenously or 2 mg for children weighing more than 20 kg.

TABLE 79-4   Metabolic Acidosis and Elevated Anion Gap

Methanol, **M**etformin
Ethylene glycol
Toluene, **T**heophylline
Alcoholic ketoacidosis
Lactic acidosis

Aminoglycosides (uremic agents)
Cyanide, **C**arbon monoxide
Isoniazid, **I**ron
DKA (diabetic ketoacidosis)

Grand mal seizures (toxic-related)
ASA (salicylates)
Paraldehyde, **P**henformin

SOURCE: Adapted from Bryson PD: *Comprehensive Review of Toxicology,* 2d ed. Rockville, MD: Aspen Publishing, 1989.

TABLE 79-5   Serum Drug Levels

Acetaminophen	Lithium
Carbon monoxide	Methanol
Cholinesterase	Methemoglobin
Digitalis	Phenobarbital
Ethanol	Phenytoin
Ethylene glycol	Salicylate
Iron	Theophylline
Lead	

GASTRIC DECONTAMINATION

- Whether patients are managed with syrup of ipecac, gastric lavage, cathartics, or activated charcoal depends on the toxicity of the particular drug, the quantity and time of ingestion, and the patient's condition. If the ingestion is recent and the child is symptomatic, or the toxin ingested may cause delayed toxicity, gastric evacuation is recommended.

GASTRIC EVACUATION

Induction of Emesis

- Syrup of ipecac is the most commonly used emetic agent. The recovery of ingested material in the vomitus is approximately 30 percent if ipecac is administered within 1 h of ingestion. Unfortunately, most children experience more than 3 episodes of vomiting, which delays the administration of activated charcoal. Ipecac is contraindicated in children less than 6 months of age, in patients with evidence of a diminished gag reflex and potential for coma or seizures, and in the ingestion of most hydrocarbons, acids, alkalis, and sharp objects. (See Table 79-7 for dosage.)

Gastric Lavage

- Gastric lavage mechanically removes toxins from the stomach using a large-bore orogastric tube irrigated with aliquots of normal saline. This mode of gastric decontamination is preferred in intoxicated children with a depressed level of consciousness who present within 1 h or have ingested a potentially life-threatening

TABLE 79-6   Toxicology and Radiology

Noncardiogenic pulmonary edema (MOPS)

M	Meprobamate, mountain sickness
O	Opiates
P	Phenobarbital
S	Salicylates

Toxins radiopaque on radiographs (CHIPES)

C	Chloral hydrate
H	Heavy metals
I	Iron
P	Phenothiazines
E	Enteric-coated preps (salicylates)
S	Sustained-release products (theophylline)

TABLE 79-7 Doses for Gastric Decontamination

Syrup of ipecac:	6–12 months of age: 5–10 mL with 15 mL/kg clear fluids 12 months–12 years: 15 mL ipecac plus 8 oz of clear fluids >12 years: 30 mL ipecac plus 16 oz water
Activated charcoal:	1–2 g/kg prepared as a slurry in water or sorbitol to achieve a 25% concentration For repetitive dosing: 1 g/kg every 2–4 h without sorbitol or cathartic
Cathartics:	Sorbitol (35% solution): 4 mL/kg of commercial solution diluted 1:1 Magnesium citrate (10% solution): 4 mL/kg Magnesium sulfate: (10% solution): 1–2 mL/kg

agent. In most cases, airway protection by endotracheal intubation prior to the lavage is indicated.

CHEMICAL DECONTAMINATION

Activated Charcoal

- The majority of poisoned children who are not critically ill can be managed safely and effectively in the emergency department with charcoal alone. The recommended initial dose of activated charcoal is summarized in Table 79-7.

Cathartics

- Cathartics are osmotically active agents that eliminate toxins from the gastrointestinal tract by inducing diarrhea. The most common agents are sorbitol, magnesium citrate, and magnesium sulfate. In the pediatric population, cathartic agents can result in hypermagnesemia, dehydration, and severe electrolyte imbalances if used excessively or repeatedly.

Whole Bowel Irrigation

- Whole bowel irrigation is now used in the overdose setting to "flush" the toxin down the gastrointestinal tract and prevent further absorption. The solution used is a polyethylene glycol electrolyte solution that does not appear to create fluid or electrolyte disturbances. The dose is 0.5 L/h for small children and 1 to 2 L/h for adolescents.

Antidotes

- Although the majority of poisonings in the pediatric population respond to supportive care and gastric decontamination alone, there are a few toxins that require antidotes (Table 79-8).

HEMODIALYSIS AND HEMOPERFUSION

- Although hemodialysis is recommended for a wide variety of toxins, it is necessary in only a few severely poisoned patients.

TABLE 79-8 Antidotes

TOXIN	ANTIDOTE
Acetaminophen	N-acetylcysteine
Benzodiazepines	Flumazenil
Beta blockers	Glucagon
Calcium channel blockers	Calcium, glucagon, and insulin and glucose
Carbon monoxide	Oxygen
Cyanide	Amyl nitrate, sodium nitrate, sodium thiosulfate
Digitalis	F(AB) fragments
Ethylene glycol/methanol	Ethanol, (4-MP)
Iron	Deferoxamine
Lead	(EDTA), (BAL), (DMSA)
Mercury/arsenic	BAL, D-Penicillamine
Methemoglobinemia	Methylene blue
Opiates	Naloxone
Organophosphates	Atropine, (2-PAM)
Tricyclic antidepressants	Sodium bicarbonate

4-MP, 4-methylpyrazone; EDTA, calcium ethylenediamine tetraacetate; BAL, British antilewisite; DMSA, dimercaptosuccinic acid; 2-PAM, 2-pralidoxime.

- Drugs that may be adequately dialyzed include those with a low molecular weight, low volume of distribution, low protein binding, and high water solubility.
- Examples include isopropanol, salicylates, theophylline, methanol, barbiturates, lithium, and ethylene glycol. Theophylline is responsive to charcoal hemoperfusion.

DISPOSITION

- Disposition of poisoned pediatric patients depends on the clinical condition of the child, as well as the potential toxicity of the agent. Clearly, all children demonstrating clinical instability are best monitored in an intensive care setting. Emergency department observation for 6 to 8 h is adequate if patients demonstrate no overt signs of toxicity and the ingestion does not involve a sustained release formulation. However, if the child has ingested a potentially dangerous dose of a toxin, is manifesting mild-to-moderate toxicity, requires antidotal therapy, or has a home environment not considered safe, a general pediatric admission is indicated.

BIBLIOGRAPHY

American Academy of Clinical Toxicology, European Association of Poison Centres and Clinical Toxicologists: Position statements on gastric lavage, activated charcoal, syrup of ipecac, cathartics and whole bowel irrigation. *J Toxicol Clin Toxicol* 35:711–762, 1997.

Bond GR: The role of activated charcoal and gastric emptying in gastrointestinal decontamination: a state-of-the-art review. *Ann Emerg Med* 39: 273–289, 2002.

Brent J, McMartin K, Phillips S, et al: Fomepizole for the treatment of ethylene glycol poisoning. *N Engl J Med* 340:832–838, 1999.

Ford M, Delaney KA: Initial approaches to the poison patient. In: Ford M, Delaney KA, Ling L, et al, eds. *Clinical Toxicology.* Philadelphia, Harcourt-WB Saunders, pp 1–4, 2001.

Henretig FM: Special considerations in the poisoned pediatric patient. *Emerg Clin North Am* 12:549–567, 1994.

Litovitz TL, Schwartz-Klein W, White S, et al: 1999 Annual Report of the AAPCC Toxic Exposure/Surveillance System. *Am J Emerg Med* 18:517–574, 2000.

Yuan TH, Kerns WP, Tomaszewski CA, et al: Insulin-glucose as adjunctive therapy for severe calcium channel antagonist poisoning. *J Toxicol Clin Toxicol* 37:463–474, 1999.

QUESTIONS

1. Which of the following toxic agents produces hyperthermia?
   A. Toxic alcohols
   B. Salicylates
   C. Theophylline
   D. Sedative hypnotics
   E. Opiates

2. A metabolic acidosis with an increased anion gap results from the presence of organically active acids and is characteristic of which of the following toxins?
   A. Isopropanol
   B. Acetaminophen
   C. Isoniazid
   D. Glyburide
   E. Lead

3. Which of the following statements regarding osmolality or osmolal gap is correct?
   A. The calculated osmolal gap is critical if you suspect ingestion of a heavy metal.
   B. Osmolality is best measured by gas chromatography.
   C. Osmolality is calculated by adding together the concentrations of major osmotically active serum components, which includes sodium, potassium, BUN, and creatinine.
   D. The normal osmolal gap is less than 20.
   E. Osmolality = 2(Na) + glucose/18 + BUN/2.8 + ETOH/4.6

4. Urine toxicology screens typically screen for which of the following?
   A. Alcohol
   B. Acetaminophen
   C. Salicylates
   D. Cocaine
   E. Barbiturates

5. The mnemonic "Hot as a hare, dry as a bone, red as a beet, blind as a bat, mad as a hatter" refers to which of the following toxic syndromes?

   A. Anticholinergic syndrome
   B. Cholinergic crisis
   C. Sympathomimetic syndrome
   D. Narcotic syndrome
   E. Withdrawal syndrome

6. Which of the following statements is true with regard to induction of emesis?
   A. Ipecac can be expected to induce vomiting within 5 to 10 min.
   B. The recovery of ingested material is approximately 75 percent if ipecac is administered within 1 h of ingestion.
   C. Ipecac usually produces multiple episodes of vomiting, which can delay administration of activated charcoal.
   D. Ipecac is specifically indicated after ingestion of hydrocarbons, acids, and alkalis.
   E. Ipecac may be used in children of all ages as long as the gag reflex is intact.

7. The majority of poisoned children who are not critically ill can be managed safely and effectively in the ED setting with which of the following treatments?
   A. Ipecac alone
   B. Gastric lavage alone
   C. Activated charcoal alone
   D. Gastric lavage and activated charcoal
   E. Whole bowel irrigation

8. In the pediatric population, repeated use of cathartic agents premixed in charcoal preparations can result in which of the following conditions?
   A. Severe electrolyte imbalance
   B. Overhydration
   C. Hypomagnesemia
   D. Impaired palatability
   E. Constipation

9. A 3-year-old child is brought to the ED after possible ingestion of unknown medication while playing in a medicine cabinet. Physical examination is within normal limits. What is the best management option?
   A. Administer ipecac and activated charcoal
   B. Admit for overnight observation
   C. Counsel and educate the parents regarding poison prevention at home and discharge the child
   D. ED observation for 6 to 8 h and, if no overt signs of toxicity, discharge the patient home
   E. Take protective custody of the child and inform the parents that they are not providing a safe home environment

ANSWERS

1. B. Uncoupling of oxidative phosphorylation may lead to hyperthermia with severe salicylate intoxication.

Sedatives and opiates may lead to hypothermia. The other agents have no specific effect on body temperature.

2. C. The classic triad of seizures, coma, and metabolic acidosis refractory to bicarbonate therapy should alert the physician to the possibility of INH ingestion. Isopropanol is the only toxic alcohol that does not typically produce acidosis. Metformin and phenformin are oral hypoglycemic agents that produce metabolic acidosis but other oral agents, such as glyburide, do not. Salicylates produce metabolic acidosis but acetaminophen does not. Iron produces metabolic acidosis but lead does not.

3. E. This is the correct formula for calculated osmolality. Osmolal gap is critical when you suspect a toxic alcohol ingestion. Osmolality is best measured by freezing point depression. Osmotically active agents include sodium, glucose, BUN, and ethanol. The normal osmolal gap is less than 10.

4. D. Toxicology panels typically screen for drugs of abuse such as narcotics, amphetamines, cannabinoids, phencyclidine, and cocaine. A grave error can occur if the physician assumes that a child ingested nothing simply because the toxicology screen is reported as negative.

5. A. This mnemonic refers to the anticholinergic toxidrome, which can be seen with toxicity from tricyclic antidepressants and antihistamines.

6. C. Ipecac has fallen out of favor in the ED setting for a number of reasons but the delay in administration of activated charcoal, which is the most effective gastric decontamination agent, is the primary reason. Ipecac is typically effective within 20 to 60 min and recovers only about 30 percent of the ingested material if administered early. It is specifically contraindicated after ingestion of acids, alkalis, and hydrocarbons and is also contraindicated in children under 6 months of age.

7. C. The majority of poisoned children who are not critically ill can be managed safely and effectively in the ED setting with charcoal alone.

8. A. Repeated doses of cathartics can lead to dehydration and electrolyte disturbances due to excessive diarrhea. Cathartics increase the palatability of charcoal. Hypermagnesemia may develop.

9. D. If ingestion of a potentially dangerous agent or a sustained release agent is NOT suspected, 6–8 hours of observation is usually sufficient to rule out significant toxicity.

80   ACETAMINOPHEN

Leon Gussow
Gary R. Strange
Patricia Lee

PHARMACOLOGY AND PATHOPHYSIOLOGY

- The therapeutic dose of acetaminophen in children is 15 mg/kg given every 4 to 6 h, with a maximum recommended daily dose of 80 mg/kg. Therapeutic serum levels are 5 to 20 µg/mL.
- Acetaminophen is eliminated primarily by hepatic pathways. After a therapeutic dose, 90 percent of the drug is metabolized to inactive sulfate and glucuronide conjugates. In young children, unlike in adults and adolescents, the sulfate conjugate predominates.
- In the overdose setting, the sulfate and glucuronide pathways become saturated, and increased amounts of acetaminophen are shunted through the P450-MFO system. Glutathione becomes depleted and free N-acetyl-P-benzoquinoneimine (NABQI) forms covalent bonds with structures on the hepatocytes. Necrosis ensues, distributed in a centrilobular fashion, corresponding to the area of greatest MFO activity.
- The toxic dose of acetaminophen is generally considered to be 140 mg/kg, but susceptibility to hepatotoxicity after acetaminophen overdose varies significantly. Children are more resistant than are adults.

CLINICAL PRESENTATION: THE FOUR STAGES OF ACETAMINOPHEN TOXICITY

STAGE 1 (0 TO 24 HOURS): GASTROINTESTINAL IRRITATION

- Patients may be asymptomatic, but young children frequently vomit after acetaminophen overdose, which may partially explain their relative resistance to severe toxicity.

STAGE 2 (24 TO 48 HOURS): LATENT PERIOD

- As nausea and vomiting resolve, patients appear to improve, but rising transaminase levels may reveal evidence of hepatic necrosis.

STAGE 3 (72 TO 96 HOURS): HEPATIC FAILURE

- Severe hepatotoxicity presents with jaundice, hypoglycemia, renewed nausea and vomiting, right upper quadrant pain, coagulopathy, lethargy, coma, hyperbilirubinemia, and markedly elevated transaminase levels. Renal failure may occur.

STAGE 4 (4 TO 14 DAYS): RECOVERY OR DEATH

- Patients who ultimately recover show improvement in laboratory parameters of hepatic function starting at about day 5 and recover completely.

LABORATORY

- An acetaminophen level is drawn 4 h after an acute ingestion or immediately if more than 4 h have elapsed since the ingestion.

MANAGEMENT

GASTRIC DECONTAMINATION

- Standard doses of activated charcoal can be given if patients come in within 2 h of ingestion of acetaminophen alone or if other toxic substances are also involved.

ANTIDOTE

- A glutathione precursor, *N*-acetylcysteine (NAC) restores the liver's ability to detoxify NABQI and prevents hepatonecrosis. It is most effective if started within 10 h of ingestion
- The Rumack–Matthew nomogram indicates which patients will require treatment with NAC. Any patient with a level that falls in the range of possible or probable hepatotoxicity is treated with a full course of NAC.
- The oral protocol approved by the United States Food and Drug Administration requires a loading dose of 140 mg/kg and then 17 additional doses of 70 mg/kg.
- The commercial 20-percent solution (Mucomyst, Mead Johnson & Company) is unpalatable and is diluted with 3 parts fruit juice or soda. If vomiting occurs within 1 h of treatment, the dose is repeated.

CHRONIC ACETAMINOPHEN POISONING

- The Rumack–Matthew nomogram applies specifically to a single, acute overdose taken at a known moment in time. It is now clear that children can develop hepatotoxicity after even moderately supratherapeutic doses of acetaminophen administered over several days. Doses above 150 mg/kg per day can cause toxicity.

BIBLIOGRAPHY

Anker A: Acetaminophen. In: Ford MD, Delaney KA, Ling LJ, Erickson T. *Clinical Toxicology.* Philadelphia, Saunders, 265–274, 2001.

Day A, Abbott GD: Chronic paracetamol poisoning in children: A warning to health professionals. *N Z Med J* 107:201, 1994.

Heubi JE, Barbacci MB, Zimmerman HJ: Therapeutic misadventures with acetaminophen: Hepatotoxicity after multiple doses in children. *J Pediatr* 132:22, 1998.

James LP, Wells E, Beard RH, Farrar HC: Predictors of outcome after acetaminophen poisoning in children and adolescents. J Pediatr 140:495–498, 2002.

Kearns GL, Leeder JS, Wasserman GS: Acetaminophen overdose with therapeutic intent (editorial). *J Pediatr* 132:5,1998.

Litovitz TL, Klein-Schwartz W, White S, et al: 1999 Annual report of the American Association of Poison Control Centers toxic exposure surveillance system. *Am J Emerg Med* 18:517, 2000.

Perry HE, Shannon MW: Efficacy of oral versus intravenous *N*-acetylcysteine in acetaminophen overdose: Results of an open-label clinical trial. *J Pediatr* 132:149, 1998.

QUESTIONS

1. Acetaminophen toxicity in children is associated with which of the following?
   A. A serum level greater than 140 mg/kg
   B. Done nomogram indicating area of possible or probable toxicity
   C. A loading dose of *N*-acetylcysteine at 70 mg/kg, followed by 17 subsequent doses of 17 mg/kg
   D. Daily doses of acetaminophen greater than 70 mg/kg/day
   E. Glucoronide conjugation predominates over sulfate conjugates

2. A 14-year-old girl presents following multiple episodes of emesis 2 days ago. At presentation, she is found to be lethargic. Laboratory tests reveal bilirubin of 10.5 mg/dL, glucose of 48 mg/dL, SGOT of

1200, and SGPT of 1680. Which of the following is true regarding this condition?

A. A normal serum acetaminophen level indicates lack of toxicity.

B. Gastric lavage with charcoal can be effective.

C. Patients who ultimately recover will show improvement in laboratory parameters of hepatic function at about day 5 and recover completely.

D. The initial presentation is characterized by hyperbilirubinemia and hypoglycemia.

E. Treatment with alkalinized saline is useful in preventing toxicity.

3. *N*-acetylcysteine is useful in acetaminophen toxicity as described below.

A. If vomiting occurs within 1 h of ingestion, the dose is not repeatable.

B. If it is given within 10 h of acute ingestion.

C. If it is given when the acetaminophen level is greater than 70 mg/kg.

D. If the acetaminophen level is greater than 70 mg/kg at 4 h after ingestion.

E. If it is given in a single dose.

ANSWERS

1. A. The toxic dose of acetaminophen is generally considered to be 140 mg/kg, but susceptibility to hepatotoxicity after acetaminophen overdose varies significantly. Children are more resistant than are adults. The Rumack–Matthew nomogram applies specifically to a single, acute overdose taken at a known moment in time. Children can develop hepatotoxicity after even moderately supratherapeutic doses of acetaminophen administered over several days. Doses greater than 150 mg/kg per day can cause toxicity. Prompt administration of *N*-acetylcysteine (NAC) within 10 h of acetaminophen ingestion can prevent hepatonecrosis. A loading dose of NAC at 140 mg/kg followed by 17 doses of 17 mg/kg is the recommended oral protocol. Unlike adults, in young children, sulfate conjugation predominates over glucuronide conjugation in acetaminophen metabolism.

2. C. The four stages of acetaminophen toxicity are: stage I is present during the first 24 h after ingestion. Patients in stage I may be asymptomatic or may present with frequent emesis. Stage II, occurring over the next 24 to 48 h, is a period of quiescence and the child will appear improved. Stage III, at 72 to 96 h, is a period of hepatic failure and presents with jaundice, hypoglycemia, nausea and vomiting, right upper quadrant pain, coagulopathy, lethargy, coma, hyperbilirubinemia, and markedly elevated transaminase levels. Renal failure may occur. Stage IV, at 4

to 14 days, is a period of recovery in which laboratory values begin to improve about day 5 and then recover completely. Alkalinized saline is not effective in treatment of acetaminophen toxicity.

3. B. *N*-acetylcysteine is a glutathione precursor that restores the liver's ability to detoxify *N*-acetyl-P-benzoquinoneimine (NABQI) and prevent hepatonecrosis. NAC is recommended if the acetaminophen level is greater than 140 mg/kg at 4 h after ingestion. The loading dose is 140 mg/kg and is given within 10 h of ingestion followed by 17 subsequent doses of 70 mg/kg. If vomiting occurs within 1 h of treatment, the dose is repeated.

81 TOXIC ALCOHOLS

Timothy Erickson
Gary R. Strange
Heather M. Prendergast

ETHANOL

SOURCES

- In addition to alcohol-containing beverages, such as beer, wine, and hard liquors, children have access to mouthwashes that can contain up to 75 percent ethanol, colognes, and perfumes (40 percent to 60 percent ethanol) and over 700 medicinal preparations that contain ethanol.

PHARMACOKINETICS AND PATHOPHYSIOLOGY

- The alcohol dehydrogenase pathway is the major metabolic pathway and the rate-limiting step in converting ethanol to acetaldehyde. In children under 5 years of age, the ability to metabolize ethanol is diminished due to immature hepatic dehydrogenase activity.

CLINICAL PRESENTATION

- Ethanol is a selective central nervous system (CNS) depressant at low concentrations and a generalized depressant at high concentrations.
- Death from respiratory depression may occur at ethanol levels above 500 mg/dL. Convulsions and death have been reported in children with acute

- Respiratory elimination of the acetone causes a fruity, acetone odor on the patient's breath similar to diabetic ketoacidosis.
- Because 70-percent isopropanol is a potent inebriant and twice as intoxicating as ethanol, a level of 50 mg/dL is comparable to an ethanol level of 100 mg/dL.

CLINICAL PRESENTATION

- Isopropanol-intoxicated patients are classically lethargic or comatose, hypotensive, and tachycardiac, with the characteristic breath odor of rubbing alcohol or acetone. Coma develops at levels above 100 mg/dL.
- With isopropanol, unlike the other toxic alcohols, acidosis, ophthalmologic changes, and renal failure are classically absent. However, like ethanol, methanol, and ethylene glycol, isopropanol can produce a significant osmolal gap (Table 81-1).

LABORATORY

- Patients are tested for the presence of acetonemia and acetonuria.
- Indicated laboratory studies include a complete blood cell count; levels of electrolytes, arterial blood gas, glucose, and serum ethanol and isopropanol; serum osmolarity, and renal functions.
- Isopropanol levels above 400 mg/dL correspond to severe toxicity.

MANAGEMENT

- No ethanol drip is indicated since the metabolite acetone is relatively nontoxic and excreted through the lungs.
- Hemodialysis is effective in removing isopropanol, but is reserved for:
  ○ Prolonged coma
  ○ Hypotension
  ○ Isopropanol levels above 400 to 500 mg/dL

TABLE 81-1 Comparison of Toxic Alcohols

PARAMETER	METHANOL	ETHYLENE GLYCOL	ISOPROPANOL
Anion gap acidosis	+	+	−
Osmolal gap	+	+	+
CNS depression	+	+	+
Eye findings	+	−	−
Renal failure	+/−	+	−
Ketones	−	−	+
Oxalate crystals	−	+	−

BIBLIOGRAPHY

Barceloux DG, Krenzelor E, Olson K, et al: American Academy of Clinical Toxicology Ad Hoc Committee: Guidelines on the treatment of ethylene glycol poisoning. *J Toxicol Clin Toxicol* 37:537–560, 1999.

Brent J, McMartin K, Phillips S, et al: Fomepizole for the treatment of ethylene glycol poisoning. *N Engl J Med* 340: 832–838, 1999.

Erickson T: Toxic alcohol poisoning: When to suspect and keys to diagnosis. *Consultant* 40:1845–1856, 2000.

Jacobsen D, McMartin KE: Antidotes for methanol and ethylene glycol poisoning. *J Toxicol Clin Toxicol* 35:127, 1997.

Litovitz TL, Schwartz-Klein W, White S, et al: 1999 Annual Report of the AAPCC Toxic Exposure Surveillance System. *Am J Emerg Med* 18:517–574, 2000.

Liu JJ, Daya MR, Carrasquill O, et al: Prognostic factors in patients with methanol poisoning. *J Toxicol Clin Toxicol* 36:175, 1998.

Sutton TL, Foster RL, Liner SR: Acute methanol ingestion. *Pediatr Emerg Care* 18:360–363, 2002.

QUESTIONS

1. A 4-year-old child is brought to the ED following ingestion of generic mouthwash approximately 2 h ago. A management priority in this child would be which of the following?
   A. Syrup of ipecac
   B. Bedside glucose
   C. Urine toxicology screen
   D. Consultation with a poison control center
   E. Rectal temperature

2. A 15-year-old patient is brought to the ED for evaluation of acute onset of abdominal pain associated with nausea and vomiting. Laboratory findings reveal an elevated lipase, amylase, and a metabolic acidosis. Which of the following would be helpful in establishing a diagnosis of methanol toxicity?
   A. Stat methanol levels
   B. Respiratory acidosis on arterial blood gas
   C. Pulmonary edema on chest radiograph
   D. Calcium oxalate crystals in the urine
   E. Elevated osmolal gap

3. The purpose of ethanol use in the setting of significant methanol ingestion is which of the following?
   A. Permanent inactivation of hepatic alcohol dehydrogenase
   B. Delayed formation of formaldehyde
   C. Delayed absorption of methanol
   D. Enhance renal elimination of methanol
   E. Enhanced systemic absorption of formic acid

4. You suspect methanol intoxication in a patient brought to the ED. The patient has normal vitals signs and demonstrates a mild acidosis on arterial blood gas. You are told by your pharmacy that there are no ethanol preparations available. Other alternative treatment options include which of the following?
   A. Hemodialysis
   B. Bicarbonate administration
   C. Folate
   D. Thiamine
   E. Pyridoxine

5. A 4-year-old girl is brought in unconscious following accidental ingestion of a medicine preparation containing significant ethanol. The patient is intubated in the field by paramedics and vital signs are stabilized. Which of the following would be the most appropriate intervention?
   A. Normal saline, 20 mL/kg bolus
   B. Lactated Ringer's, 20 mL/kg bolus
   C. $D_{25}W$, 2 to 4 mL/kg
   D. $D_{10}W$, 5 to 10 mL/kg
   E. $D_{50}W$, 1 to 2 mL/kg

6. A 5-year-old child is brought for possible ingestion of antifreeze. Based upon the pharmacokinetics of ethylene glycol, you would expect to see signs and symptoms of intoxication within which of the following time frames?
   A. Almost immediately
   B. 30 min postingestion
   C. 60 min postingestion
   D. 90 min postingestion
   E. Absorption is variable and can be delayed up to 3 h.

7. Which of the following is a **TRUE** statement regarding significant ethylene glycol ingestion and mortality?
   A. Death is frequently seen in the earliest stage.
   B. Death frequently occurs at stage II.
   C. Death is frequently seen in stage III.
   D. Death is an uncommon occurrence with significant ethylene glycol ingestions.
   E. It is variable because of the direct relationship between amount ingested and fatal toxicity.

8. A 7-year-old boy is brought in by paramedics for evaluation of altered mental status. On arrival to the ED, you note a fruity odor on the breath. Which of the following would heighten your suspicion of a toxic ingestion in this patient?
   A. An bedside glucose of 500
   B. Polydipsia by history
   C. Child found in family bathroom
   D. Acute onset of renal failure
   E. Visual complaints

ANSWERS

1. B. Over the counter mouthwashes can contain significant amounts of alcohol. In a child with suspected ethanol intoxication, the most critical laboratory tests are serum ethanol and glucose level. Convulsions and death have been reported in children secondary to alcohol-induced hypoglycemia.

2. E. Measurement of methanol levels is critical in **MANAGING** methanol toxicity. To make the diagnosis, the clinician has to rely on history, clinical presentation, and laboratory findings. An elevated osmolal gap in the right clinical setting is a valuable clue for establishing the diagnosis.

3. B. Ethanol is the mainstay of treatment for significant methanol toxicity. Ethanol has a greater affinity for hepatic alcohol dehydrogenase than methanol and delays the formation of the toxic metabolites, formaldehyde and formic acid.

4. C. Folate is a coenzyme in the metabolic step converting formate to CO_2 and H_2O and is indicated in the methanol-intoxicated patient. Bicarbonate administration is reserved for patients with marked acidosis (less than 7.20). Indications for hemodialysis include visual impairment, renal failure, methanol levels above 50 mg/dL, and refractory metabolic acidosis. Another alternative when IV ethanol is not available is oral ethanol.

5. C. All obtunded patients with alcohol intoxication should receive 2 to 4 mL/kg of $D_{25}W$ after a specimen has been obtained for blood glucose. Children are very susceptible to alcohol-induced hypoglycemia.

6. B. Ethylene glycol undergoes rapid absorption from the gastrointestinal tract and initial signs of intoxication may occur as early as 30 min postingestion

7. B. Stage II occurs within 12 to 36 h postingestion and is characterized by a rapid deterioration, tachypnea, cyanosis, pulmonary edema, and adult respiratory distress syndrome. Death is most common during this stage.

8. C. A normal glucose and a fruity odor on the child's breath should increase the suspicion for isopropanol ingestion. The fact that the patient was found in the bathroom should further increase the suspicion for toxic ingestion. A reasonable scenario would include the accidental ingestion of rubbing alcohol, commonly kept in bathrooms.

82 ANTICHOLINERGIC POISONING

Steven E. Aks
Gary R. Strange
Valerie A. Dobiesz

INTRODUCTION

- Anticholinergic poisoning results from both pharmaceutic agents and natural toxins (Table 82-1).

PHARMACOLOGY AND PATHOPHYSIOLOGY

- Anticholinergics act by inhibiting the action of the neurotransmitter acetylcholine, which is found at the sympathetic and parasympathetic ganglia, at parasympathetic nerve endings, at neuromuscular junctions, and in the central nervous system. These agents competitively block the action of acetylcholine at the effector site.

CLINICAL PRESENTATION

- The central and peripheral manifestations of anticholinergic substances (the anticholinergic toxidrome) are described by the following phrases:
  - Hot as a hare
  - Blind as a bat
  - Dry as a bone
  - Red as a beet
  - Mad as a hatter

TABLE 82-1 Common Examples of Anticholinergics

Pharmaceuticals
  Astemizole
  Atropine
  Cyprohepatidine
  Dimenhydrinate
  Diphenhydramine
  Hyoscyamine
  Pyrilines

Natural products
  Deadly nightshade (belladonna)
  Jimson weed
  Mushrooms (*Amanita muscaria*)

Other drug categories with anticholinergic properties
  Antiparkinson agents
  Antipsychotics
  Antispasmodics
  Cyclic antidepressants
  Phenothiazones

DIAGNOSIS

- Diagnosis is generally based on the constellation of signs and symptoms of the anticholinergic toxidrome.

MANAGEMENT

- Decontamination by lavage is preferred, followed by the administration of activated charcoal. Lavage can be of value several hours after ingestion because of decreased gut motility seen with anticholinergic poisoning.
- Ipecac is contraindicated because of the potential of altered mental status and seizures.
- Supportive care is generally all that is needed to successfully treat anticholinergic poisoning. For agitation and seizures, benzodiazepines can be of value.
- Hyperthermia is treated aggressively with cooling measures.
- Cardiac dysrhythmias are treated by standard measures. However, wide complex tachycardia after diphenhydramine has been treated successfully with sodium bicarbonate.
- Magnesium has been used successfully to treat torsades de pointes after astemizole overdose.
- Physostigmine functions as an anticholinesterase and counteracts the effects of anticholinergic drugs.
  - It should probably be used only for pure anticholinergic poisoning and is reserved for those cases not manageable with supportive care and those that manifest the following:
    - Profound agitation
    - Persistent seizures
    - Tachydysrhythmias
    - Refractory hypotension
    - Malignant hypertension

BIBLIOGRAPHY

Burns MJ, Linden CH, Graudins A, et al: A comparison of physostigmine and benzodiazepines for the treatment of anticholinergic poisoning. *Ann Emerg Med* 35:374–381, 2000.

Hasan RA, Zureikat GY, Nolan BM: Torsade de pointes associated with astemizole overdose treated with magnesium sulfate. *Pediatr Emerg Care* 9:23–25, 1993.

Holger JS, Harris CR, Engebretsen KM: Physostigmine, sodium bicarbonate, or hypertonic saline to treat diphenhydramine toxicity. *Vet Hum Toxicol* 44:1–4, 2002.

Hyers JH, Moro-Sutherland D, Shook JE: Anticholinergic poisoning in colicky infants treated with hyoscyamine sulfate. *Am J Emerg Med* 15:532–535, 1997.

Litovitz TL, Klein-Schwartz W, White S, et al: 1999 Annual Report of Poison Control Centers Toxic Exposure Surveillance System. *Am J Emerg Med* 18:517–574, 2000.

QUESTIONS

1. A 15-year-old male presents to the ED after drinking jimsonweed tea. His parents were concerned, noting him to be confused, flushed, febrile, and having dilated pupils. Which of the following is true regarding this patient?
   A. Gastric lavage is contraindicated in this patient.
   B. Ipecac should be given.
   C. Physostigmine should be administered immediately.
   D. Atropine and pralidoxime are the antidotes.
   E. The diagnosis is based on the signs and symptoms of this toxidrome.

2. Which of the following is true regarding anticholinergic poisoning?
   A. Hyperthermia is best managed with acetaminophen.
   B. Agitation and seizures may be treated with benzodiazepines.
   C. All patients should be admitted to a monitored setting.
   D. Physostigmine should be given with overdoses of cyclic antidepressants.
   E. There are no known cardiac effects in toxic ingestions.

3. Which of the following is helpful in distinguishing an anticholinergic toxicity from a sympathomimetic toxicity?
   A. Dry skin
   B. Mydriasis
   C. Tachycardia
   D. Hypertension
   E. Agitation

ANSWERS

1. E. Jimsonweed is an anticholinergic and is ingested to induce a hallucinogenic experience. This patient is exhibiting the classic anticholinergic toxidrome. Diagnosis is based on the constellation of signs and symptoms. Decontamination can be of value several hours after ingestion because of delayed gut motility. Ipecac is contraindicated because of the potential altered mental status and seizures. Treatment is generally supportive and physostigmine is reserved for cases not manageable with supportive care.

2. B. Hyperthermia should be treated with rapid cooling measures. Agitation and seizures are treated with

benzodiazepines. Asymptomatic patients who are observed for a minimum of 6 h and have no anticholinergic signs may be safely discharged. Physostigmine is contraindicated with ingestions of cyclic antidepressants. Cardiac dysrhythmias may occur.

3. A. Only anticholinergic toxicity causes dry skin. Sympathomimetics cause warm, moist skin. Mydriasis, tachycardia, hypertension, and agitation are shared by both toxidromes.

83 ORAL ANTICOAGULANTS

Jerrold B. Leikin
Gary R. Strange
Valerie A. Dobiesz

INTRODUCTION

- Oral anticoagulants are commonly available in the home in the form of prescription medications, such as warfarin (Coumadin), and are the predominant agent in many rodenticides, which are often placed in areas accessible to small children (Table 83-1).
- Some rodenticides contain newer, extremely potent and long-acting superwarfarin anticoagulants that can result in severe toxicity even when ingested in very small amounts.

PATHOPHYSIOLOGY

- Although there are many substances that can be considered anticoagulants, it is the vitamin K antagonists

TABLE 83-1   Vitamin K–Antagonist Agents

COUMARIN DERIVATIVES	
Difenacoum (Ratak)	Phenprocoumon
Bromadiolone (Bromone)	Acenacoumarin
Brodifacoum (Talan)	Sodium warfarin
Coumatetralyl (Endox)	Prolin (Eraze)
Discoumacetate	Coumafene
Zoocoumarin (Rodex)	Fumarin
Valone (PMP Tracking Powder)	Coumapuryl
Bishydroxy-Coumarin	Tomarin

INDANDIONE DERIVATIVES	
Diphacione (Dipazin)	Diphenadione
Pindone (Pival)	Diphacin (Kill-ko Rat Killer)
Chlorphacione (Caid, Drat)	
Valone	Pival
Anisindione	Piraldione (Tri-Ban)
Phenindione	Radione

that cause most of the problems in the pediatric age group.

DIAGNOSIS

- The clinical toxicity of anticoagulants is almost entirely restricted to bleeding diathesis.
- For patients who ingest a rodenticide, it is essential to determine whether the compound contained a "normal" anticoagulant or one of the superwarfarins. Ingestion of the lower toxicity agents is more common, and usually does not require aggressive intervention, while ingestion of the superwarfarin compounds is cause for concern.

LABORATORY STUDIES

- In the acute ingestion, all laboratory studies are likely to be normal.
- In chronic exposures or in cases where a toxic dose has been ingested significantly prior to arrival to the emergency department, measurement of the prothrombin time (PT) or international normalized ratio (INR) correlates with the depression of the vitamin K-dependent clotting factors.
- In cases where the PT is prolonged, baseline hemoglobin and platelet count are necessary.
- Additionally, the urine and stool should be checked for blood.

MANAGEMENT

GASTRIC DECONTAMINATION

- Activated charcoal is indicated in acute ingestions.
- Vitamin K_1 is the specific antidote for anticoagulant toxicity and is indicated in the presence of a prolonged INR/PT or for patients who have bleeding (Table 83-2).
- Patients with severe bleeding or with evidence of intracranial hemorrhage require rapid reversal of coagulopathy and are treated with fresh frozen plasma (15 mL/kg) or pooled clotting factors.

DISPOSITION

- Hospitalization is usually not necessary for children who ingest warfarin tablets or rodenticides that do not

TABLE 83-2   Doses of Vitamin K_1

Oral dose	Adult: 15–25 mg
Larger daily amounts for superwarfarin poisoning	
For small ingestion	Child: 5–10 mg
Intravenous dose	Adult: about 10 mg
For rapid correction only; diluted in a saline or glucose at a rate not to exceed 5 percent of total dose per minute	Child 1–5 mg
Intramuscular dose	
Mild ingestions—where risk of hematoma is low	Child: 1–5 mg
Subcutaneous injection	Adult: 5–10 mg
	Child: 1–5 mg

contain superwarfarin compounds. However, they require close outpatient follow-up with an INR or PT measurement at 48 h, with observation for gastrointestinal bleeding and prolongation of PT for up to 5 days after the ingestion.
- After ingestions of more than 0.5 mg/kg of warfarin or more than 0.05 mg/kg of a superwarfarin compound and for patients with prolonged PTs or active bleeding, hospitalization is indicated until the coagulation profile normalizes.

BIBLIOGRAPHY

Bruno GH, Howland MA, McMeeking A, et al: Long-acting anticoagulant overdose (bodifacoum) kinetics and optimal vitamin K dosing. *Ann Emerg Med* 35:262–267, 2000.

Hung A, Tait RC: A prospective randomized study to determine the optimal dose of intravenous vitamin K in reversal of over-warfarinization. *Br J Hematology* 109:537–539, 2000.

Ingels M, Lai C, Tai W, et al: A prospective study of acute, unintentional, pediatric superwarfarin ingestions managed without decontamination. *Ann Emerg Med* 40:73–78, 2002.

Litovitz TL, Klein-Schwartz W, White S, et al: 1999 Annual report of the American Association of Poison Control Centers toxic exposure surveillance system. *Am J Emerg Med* 18:517–574, 2000.

Mullins MF, Branda CL, Daya R: Unintentional pediatric superwarfarin exposures. Do we really need a prothrombin time? *Pediatrics* 105:402–404, 2000.

Sheperd G, Klein-Schwartz W, Anderson B: Acute pediatric brodificoum poisoning. *J Toxicol Clin Toxicol* 30:464, 1998.

QUESTIONS

1. A 5-year-old girl presents after she accidentally ingested a rodenticide containing a superwarfarin

compound. Which of the following is true regarding this ingestion?

A. The clinical toxicity is related to CNS effects.
B. Superwarfarin anticoagulants are less toxic than normal anticoagulants.
C. It is important to follow bleeding times in this patient.
D. Activated charcoal is indicated in acute ingestions.
E. Protamine sulfate is the antidote for this toxin.

2. Which of the following is an appropriate disposition for a child with an anticoagulant ingestion?

A. All ingestions of warfarin in children should be hospitalized.
B. Ingestions in patients with prolonged PTs can be followed as outpatients with serial PT levels.
C. Ingestions in patients with active bleeding should be hospitalized.
D. A child who ingests warfarin and has a normal PT level can be discharged safely and needs no follow up.
E. Ingestion of a superwarfarin can be safely discharged if there is no bleeding and a normal PT with follow up at 24 h only.

ANSWERS

1. D. Some rodenticides contain an extremely potent and long-acting superwarfarin anticoagulant that can result in severe toxicity. The clinical toxicity of anticoagulants is almost entirely restricted to bleeding diathesis. Measurement of prothrombin time (PT) or INR correlates with depression of the vitamin K-dependent clotting factors. Activated charcoal is indicated in acute ingestions. Vitamin K_1 is the specific antidote for anticoagulant toxicity. If severe bleeding is present, treatment with fresh frozen plasma or pooled clotting factors is indicated.

2. C. Hospitalization is usually not necessary for children who ingest warfarin or rodenticides that contain no superwarfin compounds. However, they require close follow-up with an INR or PT checked at 48 h with observation for GI bleeding and prolongation of PT for up to 5 days after ingestion. In patients with prolonged PTs or active bleeding, hospitalization is indicated until the coagulation profile normalizes.

84 ANTIHYPERTENSIVES, BETA BLOCKERS, AND CALCIUM ANTAGONISTS

Gary R. Strange
Kenneth R. Bizovi
Valerie A. Dobiesz

BETA-ADRENERGIC BLOCKING AGENTS

PATHOPHYSIOLOGY

- Suppression of the cardiovascular system is the hallmark of β-blocker overdose. β_1-blockade leads to negative inotropic and chronotropic effects. Membrane-stabilizing activity further exacerbates cardiotoxicity.

CLINICAL PRESENTATION

- Due to the rapid absorption of many β-blockers, the onset of symptoms may be as rapid as 30 min after ingestion, but it most commonly occurs within 1 to 2 h.
- Cardiovascular manifestations include:
  ◦ Hypotension
  ◦ Bradycardia
  ◦ Heart block
  ◦ Congestive heart failure

MANAGEMENT

- Absorption of β-blockers can be decreased by gastric emptying and administration of activated charcoal. If the ingestion occurred less than 4 h prior to presentation, gastric emptying is indicated.
- For patients with symptomatic bradycardia and hypotension, glucagon has been shown to reverse the toxic effects of β-blockers. It is a positive inotrope that appears to work by increasing cyclic AMP.
- Patients who do not respond to glucagon are treated with aggressive fluid resuscitation and sympathomimetics. Epinephrine is the catecholamine of choice, given as a continuous infusion, starting at a rate of 1 µg/min and titrating to perfusion parameters.
- Extracorporeal membrane oxygenation (ECMO) or cardiac bypass is considered for patients with toxicity refractory to all other therapy.

DISPOSITION

- A patient with a history of non–sustained-release β-blocker ingestion is observed on a cardiac monitor for 6 h after ingestion. Patients with signs of cardiovascular, respiratory, or CNS toxicity are admitted to a monitored bed. A patient who ingested a β-blocker that is not a sustained-release product can be discharged home after the observation period if there is no suicidal ideation and there are no signs of toxicity found by clinical examination, ECG, or cardiac monitoring.

CALCIUM CHANNEL BLOCKERS

PHARMACOLOGY

- Calcium channel blockers decrease contraction of vascular muscle and myocardium by inhibiting the influx of calcium into the cell, thereby, decreasing activity of calcium-dependent actin-myosin ATPase.

PATHOPHYSIOLOGY

- In overdose, the pharmacologic effects of calcium channel blockers may lead to life-threatening physiologic sequelae.
  - Slowing of the sinus node leads to bradycardia.
  - Slowing of conduction leads to heart blocks and asystole.
  - Decreased contractility can cause heart failure and shock.
  - Lowered peripheral vascular resistance leads to hypotension.

CLINICAL EFFECTS

- The different pharmacologic profiles of calcium channel blockers will cause various presentations, but in all cases, the cardiovascular effects predominate. Verapamil and diltiazem typically cause bradycardia and hypotension. Nifedipine primarily affects the arterioles, causing decreased peripheral vascular resistance, which leads to hypotension and reflex tachycardia.

LABORATORY

- Hypoperfusion, inhibition of insulin release, and electrolyte abnormalities are the metabolic consequences of calcium channel blocker overdose.
  - Decreased insulin release can lead to hyperglycemia.
  - Hypoperfusion may lead to profound lactic acidosis.
  - Hypocalcemia is the most frequent electrolyte abnormality.

MANAGEMENT

- If the ingestion was less than 1 h prior to presentation, gastric lavage is indicated.
- For patients who have ingested sustained-release preparations, whole bowel irrigation is accomplished by administering polyethylene glycol solution at a rate of 25 mL/kg/h by mouth or nasogastric tube until the effluent is clear. A dose of charcoal is administered prior to initiating whole bowel irrigation.
- For bradycardia, atropine is administered at 0.02 mg/kg/dose for two doses. The minimum dose of atropine is 0.1 mg.
- The primary antidote for an overdose of a calcium channel blocker is calcium. Calcium indications include:
  - Hypotension
  - Bradycardia
  - Heart block
- Calcium is administered as calcium gluconate, 10-percent solution, 0.2 to 0.5 mL/kg/dose by slow IV push. The dose is repeated in 10 to 15 min for persistent hypotension or bradycardia.
- Glucagon is another proposed antidote for calcium channel blocker toxicity. It stimulates adenylate cyclase, which increases the formation of cyclic AMP and promotes intracellular calcium influx. Currently, glucagons should be reserved for toxicity refractory to other measures.
- For calcium channel blocker overdose with hypotension that persists despite the administration of fluids, calcium salts and glucagon therapy with vasopressors are indicated. Dopamine is a reasonable first-line option. Amrinone, a phosphodiesterase inhibitor used in treating congestive heart failure, has been reported to be effective in reversing hypotension secondary to calcium channel blocker overdose.
- High-dose insulin has been shown to be effective in the management of calcium channel blocker overdose, presumably by improving myocardial contractility and by improving conduction by lowering potassium concentrations. Insulin should be used early in the ED course and administered as a bolus of regular insulin, 1 U/kg, followed by 1 U/kg/h for the first hour, then 0.5 U/kg/h thereafter until no longer needed.

CLONIDINE

PATHOPHYSIOLOGY

- Clonidine is an α_2-agonist that functions at the level of the brainstem by blocking sympathetic flow. It decreases heart rate, cardiac output, and peripheral vascular resistance.
- The effects of an overdose of clonidine are variable but largely reflect CNS toxicity.

MANAGEMENT

- After ventilation is stabilized, gastric lavage is indicated.
- Clonidine-induced bradycardia is treated with atropine if it is associated with hypotension.
- Hypotension is treated with aggressive fluid resuscitation. Moderate-dose dopamine may also be useful for hypotension and may also ameliorate bradycardia.
- There may be a role for naloxone in reversing the opiate-like side effects of clonidine on mental status and respiration and there is some indication that it can reverse clonidine-mediated hypotension.

BIBLIOGRAPHY

BETA BLOCKERS

Love JN, Enlow B, Howell JM, et al: Electrocardiographic changes associated with beta-blocker toxicity. *Ann Emerg Med* 40:603–610, 2002.
Love JN, Tandy TK: Beta-adrenoreceptor antagonist toxicity: A survey of glucagon availability. *Ann Emerg Med* 22:267, 1993.
Reith DM, Dawson AH, Epid D, et al: Relative toxicity of beta blockers in overdose. *J Toxicol Clin Toxicol* 34:273–278, 1996.

CALCIUM CHANNEL BLOCKERS

Kerns JA: Calcium channel antagonists. In: Ford MD, Delaney KA, Ling LJ, Erickson T, eds. *Clinical Toxicology.* Philadelphia: Saunders, 370–378, 2001.
Kline JA, Raymond RM, Schroeder JD, Watts JA: The diabetogenic effects of acute verapamil poisoning. *Toxicol Appl Pharmacol* 145:357–362, 1997.
Kozlowski JH, Kozlowski JA, Schuller D: Poisoning with sustained release verapamil. *Am J Med* 85:127, 1996.
Litovitz TL, Klein-Schwartz W, White S, et al: 1999 Annual Report of the American Association of Poison Control Centers Toxic Exposure Surveillance System. *Am J Emerg Med* 18: 517–574, 2000.
Yuan TH, Kerns WP, Tomaszewski CA, et al: Insulin-glucose as adjunctive therapy for severe calcium channel antagonist poisoning. *J Toxicol Clin Toxicol* 37:463–474, 1999.

CLONIDINE

Maloney MJ, Schwam JS: Clonidine and sudden death. *Pediatrics* 96:1176–1177, 1995.
Seger DL: Clonidine toxicity revisited. *J Toxicol Clin Toxicol* 40:145–155, 2002.

QUESTIONS

1. Which of the following is true regarding β-blocker overdose?
   A. The onset of symptoms is typically delayed 10 to 12 h.
   B. Respiratory depression is the hallmark of overdose.
   C. The treatment of choice is calcium gluconate.
   D. Cardiovascular effects include hypotension and heart block.
   E. All ingestions must be admitted to a monitored bed.
2. Which of the following is **NOT** indicated in the treatment of a calcium channel blocker overdose?
   A. Naloxone
   B. Glucagon
   C. Atropine
   D. Calcium gluconate
   E. High-dose insulin
3. Which of the following is an indication for giving calcium in a calcium channel blocker overdose?
   A. A history of a massive ingestion
   B. A polypharmacy overdose with digoxin
   C. Hypocalcemia
   D. Ingestion of a sustained-release preparation
   E. Bradycardia
4. A 3-year-old child presents with a history of taking 10 of her grandmother's clonidine pills accidentally. The child has a BP 60/P, P 50, and RR 14 and appears somnolent. Which of the following is true regarding this ingestion?
   A. Clonidine is a central α_2-agonist and stimulates sympathetic flow.
   B. Calcium and glucagon should be administered.
   C. Naloxone may be indicated in this patient.
   D. A temporary cardiac pacemaker should be placed.
   E. Vasopressors, such as dopamine, are contraindicated.
5. Which of the following is true regarding calcium channel blocker toxicity?

A. Decreased insulin release can lead to hyper-glycemia.
B. Hypercalcemia is the most frequent electrolyte abnormality.
C. The effects of an overdose are largely CNS toxicity.
D. All calcium channel blocker preparations have the same clinical presentation in overdose settings.
E. There is an increase in myocardial contractility.

ANSWERS

1. D. The onset of symptoms may be as rapid as 30 min but it most commonly occurs within 1 to 2 h. Suppression of the cardiovascular system is the hallmark of β-blocker overdose. Cardiovascular manifestations include hypotension, bradycardia, heart block, and congestive heart failure. The treatment of choice is glucagon in symptomatic patients. Asymptomatic patients that ingested a non–sustained-release product may be discharged home after a 6-h observation period if there is no suicidal ideation or signs of toxicity.

2. A. The primary antidote for an overdose is calcium, administered as calcium gluconate, 10-percent solution. Glucagon is used in refractory cases and increases the formation of cyclic AMP and promotes intracellular calcium influx. Atropine may be used for bradycardia. High-dose insulin has been shown to be effective in the management of calcium channel blocker overdose, presumably by improving myocardial contractility and by improving conduction by lowering potassium concentrations. Naloxone is not indicated.

3. E. The indications for giving calcium in a calcium channel blocker overdose are hypotension, bradycardia, or heart block. Calcium is dangerous to give with digoxin toxicity and may cause asystole and cardiac arrest.

4. C. Clonidine is a centrally acting α₂-agonist that blocks sympathetic flow. Calcium and glucagon are not indicated in this ingestion. Naloxone is useful in reversing the opiate-like side effects of clonidine on mental status and respiration and there is some evidence that it can reverse clonidine-mediated hypotension. Moderate-dose dopamine may also be useful for hypotension and may improve bradycardia. Bradycardia is treated with atropine if associated with hypotension and not a temporary pacemaker.

5. A. An inhibition of insulin release may lead to hyperglycemia. Hypocalcemia is the most frequent electrolyte abnormality. The different pharmacologic profiles of calcium channel blockers will cause various presentations, but in all cases, the cardiovascular effects predominate. Verapamil and diltiazem typically

cause bradycardia and hypotension. Nifedipine causes decreased peripheral vascular resistance leading to hypotension and reflex tachycardia. In general, there is a decrease in myocardial contractility leading to heart failure and shock.

85 ARSENIC

Jerrold B. Leikin
Gary R. Strange
Valerie A. Dobiesz

PATHOPHYSIOLOGY

- The toxicity of arsenic is twofold.
  - It combines reversibly with sulfhydryl groups of several enzymes of the Krebs cycle.
  - It can substitute as an anion for phosphate and disrupt oxidative phosphorylation.

CLINICAL MANIFESTATIONS

- The initial manifestations of arsenic poisoning are dominated by gastrointestinal symptoms:
  - Nausea
  - Abdominal pain
  - Vomiting
  - "Rice water" diarrhea.
  - Hypotension
  - Garlic odor to the breath or feces
- Other systemic manifestations are:
  - Diaphoresis
  - Renal failure
  - Hepatic dysfunction
  - Cardiac rhythm disturbances, including torsades de pointes
- In severe intoxications:
  - Seizures
  - Coma
- A peripheral neuropathy can develop 10 days to 3 weeks after ingestion, characterized by paresthesias of the extremities, followed by motor disability.
- Hypoglycemia can result from inhibition of gluconeogenesis in the citric acid cycle.
- Chronic arsenic toxicity can have a similar though less fulminant course, and is characterized by dermatologic manifestations.
  - Hyperpigmentation in a configuration similar to raindrops can occur on the eyelids, temples, and neck region.

○ Skin desquamation and brittle nails with transverse white striae (Aldrich Mees lines) can develop after 4 to 5 weeks of exposure.
○ Patchy and diffuse alopecia can develop.

DIAGNOSIS

• While serum arsenic levels greater than 7 µg/100 mL may be indicative of poisoning, urinary arsenic levels are more sensitive in demonstrating toxicity. Twenty-four-hour urinary arsenic levels above 100 µg are consistent with poisoning.

MANAGEMENT

• Initial therapy consists of stabilization of the airway and support of the circulatory system. Antiarrhythmic therapy may be required.
• If hemolysis is present, alkalinization of the urine is indicated.
• Gastric decontamination is performed by gastric lavage within 1 hour of ingestion or, if abdominal radiographs are positive, whole bowel irrigation.
• Chelation is indicated when the 24-hour urinary arsenic concentration exceeds 200 µg/L (Table 85-1).
• Hemodialysis is useful for enhancing arsenic elimination if renal failure develops.
• The management of arsine gas, which like arsenic has a characteristic garlic odor, is radically different from that of arsenic ingestion.
  ○ Chelation is not effective.
  ○ Treatment consists of dialysis or exchange transfusion.

BIBLIOGRAPHY

Angle CR, Centeno JA, Guha Maxumder DN: DMSA, DMPS treatment of chronic arsenicism. *J Toxicol Clin Toxicol* 36:495, 1998.

Flora SJS, Tripathi N: Treatment of arsenic poisoning; An update. *Indian J Pharmacol* 30:209–217, 1998.
Gebel TW: Arsenic and drinking water contamination. *Science* 283:1458–1459, 1999.
Gordon ME: Arsenics and old places. *Lancet* 356:170, 2000.
Henadez AF, Schiaffino S, Bullesteros JL, et al: Lack of clinical symptoms in an acute arsenic poisoning: An unusual case. *Veterinary Human Toxicol* 40:344–345, 1998.
Rusyniak DE, Furbee RB, Kirk MA: Thallium and arsenic poisoning in a small Midwestern town. *Ann Emerg Med* 39:307–311, 2002.
Subramanian KS, Kosnett ML: Human exposures to arsenic from consumption of well water in West Bengal, India. *Int J Occup Environ Health* 4:217–230, 1998.
Szincz L, Mueckter H, Gelgehauer N, et al: Toxicodynamic and toxicokinetic aspects of the treatment of arsenical poisoning. *J Toxicol Clin Toxicol* 38:214–216, 2000.
Wax PM: Features and management of arsenic intoxications. *J Toxicol Clin Toxico* 39:235–236, 2001.

QUESTIONS

1. A 10-year-old male is brought to the ED by his parents with a history of accidental arsenic ingestion. Which of the following is true regarding his condition?
   A. The toxicity of arsenic is caused by a toxic metabolite
   B. The initial manifestations are predominantly CNS
   C. Acute ingestions often have dermatologic manifestations
   D. Urinary arsenic levels are more sensitive than serum in demonstrating toxicity
   E. Alopecia may develop in the acute setting
2. Which of the following is **NOT** associated with arsenic poisoning?
   A. Rice water diarrhea
   B. Garlic odor to the breath or feces
   C. Paresthesias of the extremities
   D. Brittle nails with transverse white striae (Aldrich-Mees lines)
   E. Red discoloration of the skin and green color to emesis
3. Which of the following is true regarding the treatment of arsenic poisoning?

TABLE 85-1   Chelators of Arsenic

	ROUTE	DOSE	DOSING INTERVAL
Dimercaprol	IM	3–5 mg/kg	4–12 h
D-Penicillamine	PO	25 mg/kg	4 times/day
2,3 dimercaptosuccinic acid (DMSA or succimer)	PO	10 mg/kg	Every 8 h for 5 days, then every 12 h for 14 days or until urinary arsenic <50 µg/L
2,3 Dimercaptopropaine-1-sulfonic acid (sodium salt-DMPS-not FDA approved at present)	PO	5 mg/kg	Every 8 h
DMPS (not FDA approved at present)	IV	5 mg/kg	Every 2–6 h

IM, intramuscularly; IV, intravenously; PO, orally.

A. Initial therapy is stabilization of the airway and support of the circulatory system
B. Gastric decontamination is contraindicated in acute ingestions
C. Chelation is not effective in the management of acute ingestions
D. Charcoal is highly effective in binding arsenic
E. Nitrite-thiosulfate antidote therapy should be administered immediately

ANSWERS

1. D. The toxicity of arsenic occurs when it combines reversibly with sulfhydryl groups of several enzymes of the Krebs cycle and it substitutes as an anion for phosphate and disrupts oxidative phosphorylation. The initial manifestations of arsenic poisoning are dominated by GI symptoms. Chronic arsenic toxicity is characterized by dermatologic manifestations and alopecia can develop. Urinary arsenic levels are more sensitive in demonstrating toxicity.

2. E. Red discoloration of the skin and green color to emesis is associated with boric acid toxicity commonly found in roach powder. Rice water diarrhea and garlic odor to the breath or feces occur in acute arsenic poisoning. Paresthesias of the extremities and brittle nails with transverse white striae (Aldrich-Mees lines) can develop in chronic arsenic exposure.

3. A. Initial therapy consists of stabilization of the airway and support of the circulatory system as patients may present hypotensive. Gastric decontamination is performed by gastric lavage within 1 hour of ingestion or, if abdominal radiographs are positive, whole bowel irrigation. Chelation is indicated when the 24 hour urinary arsenic concentration exceeds 200 μg/L. Charcoal is not effective in binding arsenic. Nitrites and sodium thiosulfate are indicated in cyanide ingestions.

86 ASPIRIN

Michele Zell-Kanter
Gary R. Strange
Heather M. Prendergast

PHARMACOKINETICS

- At normal doses, aspirin is rapidly absorbed from the small intestine. If taken in large amounts, absorption can be delayed by the formation of concretions.
- Ingestions of less than 150 mg/kg are generally nontoxic. With ingestions of 150 to 300 mg/kg, mild to moderate toxicity occurs; and overdoses of over 300 mg/kg can be lethal.

PATHOPHYSIOLOGY AND CLINICAL PRESENTATION

- Children have a quicker onset of toxicity and exhibit more severe signs than adults.
  ○ Patients may complain of tinnitus and impaired hearing.
  ○ Direct stimulation of respiratory centers causes tachypnea, which in turn results in an early respiratory alkalosis.
  ○ Uncoupling of the Krebs cycle results in anaerobic metabolism and ketonemia, which causes the characteristic anion gap metabolic acidosis.
  ○ The acidosis can be exacerbated by hypovolemia, which results from vomiting, increased insensible losses from tachypnea and perspiration, and an osmotic diuresis. Fluid losses are especially severe in young children.
- An acidotic environment facilitates salicylate distribution into the brain, where it can cause agitation, delirium, seizures, and rarely coma.
- Patients can develop noncardiogenic pulmonary edema, most likely due to a toxic effect of salicylates on pulmonary endothelium.
- Uncoupling of oxidative phosphorylation can result in hyperthermia, which generally indicates significant toxicity.

LABORATORY STUDIES

- Required initial laboratory studies include complete blood count, electrolytes, and arterial blood gases. A toxicology screen is important, especially for patients with deliberate overdose.
- Plasma salicylate levels are easily obtainable and are best drawn 6 hours postingestion, when they reflect peak concentration. However, since the history of ingestion is often incorrect, a plasma salicylate level should be drawn upon presentation, and repeated every 2 hours to ensure that the level is decreasing.
- Patients with toxicity from chronic ingestion generally have a worse prognosis and clinical findings are more predictive of toxicity than the plasma level.

MANAGEMENT

- Treatment is based on symptomatology; the Done nomogram is no longer considered useful in predicating management.

- Intravascular volume is restored by boluses of crystalloid at doses of 10 to 20 mL/kg until adequate perfusion is assured. After urine output is established, potassium is added to the intravenous fluid for patients who are hypokalemic.
- Syrup of ipecac can be administered to induce emesis and evacuate gastric contents for patients who present within 1 hour of ingestion and who are alert and oriented.
- Patients who have any alteration in mental status are best managed by gastric lavage, after stability of the airway is established. Large amounts of aspirin have a tendency to form concretions in the stomach. Patients with significant ingestion can potentially benefit from gastric evacuation for several hours after ingestion.
- Activated charcoal is effective in adsorbing ingested aspirin and is administered as soon as gastric evacuation is accomplished.
- In conjunction with gastric decontamination, elimination of salicylate is enhanced by systemic alkalinization.
  - The goal of alkalinization is to increase the urine pH to 7.5 to 8.
  - This is accomplished by administering sodium bicarbonate in an initial bolus of 1 to 2 mEq/kg, followed by a bicarbonate drip titrated to the urine pH.
- Hypokalemia is common in salicylism and can impair attempts to alkalinize the urine, because potassium is exchanged for hydrogen in the tubular fluid when serum potassium is low. In hypokalemic patients, potassium is added to the intravenous solution once urine output is adequate.
- For patients with extreme toxicity, hemodialysis is an option
  - Indications for its use include:
    - Congestive heart failure
    - Noncardiogenic pulmonary edema
    - Central nervous system depression
    - Seizure
    - Metabolic acidosis refractory to alkalinization
    - Hepatic failure
    - Coagulopathy

BIBLIOGRAPHY

Donovan JW, Akhtar J: Salicylates. In: Ford MD, Delaney KA, Ling LJ, Erickson T, eds. Clinical Toxicology. Philadelphia, Saunders, 275–280, 2001.

Litovitz TL, Klein-Schwartz W, White S, et al: 1999 Annual report of the American Association of Poison Control Centers toxic exposure surveillance system. Am J Emerg Med 18:517, 2000.

QUESTIONS

1. A 16-year-old girl is brought to the ED for evaluation of an intentional aspirin ingestion following a breakup with her boyfriend. She is remorseful and embarrassed. Psychiatry has been consulted. A 6-hour post ingestion salicylate level demonstrates an ingestion of 140 mg/kg. Which of the following would be the MOST appropriate disposition for this patient?
   A. This is not a toxic ingestion. Discharge to home with parents and outpatient psychiatry follow-up
   B. This is not a toxic ingestion, but does require observation and should be admitted to pediatrics
   C. This is not a toxic ingestion, but does require inpatient psychiatric admission
   D. This is a potential toxic ingestion. The patient should have extended ED observation and a repeat level in 2 hours
   E. This is a potential toxic ingestion. The patient should be admitted and observed in the pediatric intensive care unit (PICU)

2. A child is brought to the ED for accidental ingestion of an unknown amount of chewable aspirin. The event was not witnessed. In the event of a significant ingestion expected physical and laboratory findings would include which of the following?
   A. Respiratory depression
   B. Lethargy with rapid progression to coma
   C. Respiratory alkalosis
   D. Gastrointestinal upset with profuse water diarrhea
   E. Significant hypothermia

3. You receive a call from EMS dispatch concerning a toddler being brought to your facility for a possible salicylate ingestion. The child was found near an open bottle of baby aspirin. Paramedics note there were several tablets found on the floor near the child. The MOST appropriate management would be which of the following?
   A. Syrup of Ipecac within 1 hour of ED presentation providing the child is alert and oriented
   B. Obtain a plasma salicylate level and repeat in 2 hours. If the levels are decreasing, the patient may be discharged without further treatment
   C. Treatment is based on symptomatology. If the child appears asymptomatic and has a negative salicylate level, no treatment is necessary
   D. Begin intravascular volume restoration with intravenous boluses of crystalloid.
   E. Administer activated charcoal

4. In patients found to have significant aspirin ingestion, which of the following is a management PRIORITY?
   A. Airway management with controlled hyperventilation

B. Systemic alkalinization
C. Urine Acidification
D. Intravenous potassium supplementation to offset hypokalemia
E. Hemodialysis

5. Which of the following conditions is NOT an indication for hemodialysis in the face of a toxic salicylate ingestion?
   A. Seizures
   B. Intractable vomiting
   C. Noncardiogenic pulmonary edema
   D. Refractory metabolic acidosis
   E. Altered mental status

ANSWERS

1. A. Ingestions of less than 150 mg/kg are generally nontoxic, and do not require admission. This patient appears to have a family support and would not meet criteria for inpatient psychiatry admission. This patient can be safely discharged home with her parents and outpatient psychiatry follow-up.

2. B. Children exhibit signs of toxicity much quicker than adults. Respiratory alkalosis is often an early sign. Often signs and symptoms include tinnitus, metabolic acidosis, vomiting, agitation, seizures, delirium, and hyperthermia. Coma is rarely seen.

3. C. Treatment in salicylate poisoning is based on symptomatology. Patients with evidence of salicylates should have initial lab studies performed and treatment started before discharge. A 6-hour postingestion level is recommended to determine the peak concentration. Syrup of Ipecac should only be given to patients who present within 1 hour of ingestion.

4. A. A management priority in salicylate poisoning is systemic alkalinization. This is accomplished with use of sodium bicarbonate titrated to urine pH of 7.5 to 8.0. Potassium supplementation can be added to intravenous fluids once urine output is adequate. Hemodialysis may be an option if the patient does not demonstrate improvement or experiences a deterioration in condition.

5. B. Vomiting can be common in salicylate ingestions, which increases fluid losses and worsens acidosis. It important to restore intravascular volume with boluses of crystalloid until adequate perfusion is demonstrated. Vomiting is not a recognized indication for hemodialysis. Current indications for hemodialysis in the face of salicylate poisonings include: congestive heart failure, noncardiogenic pulmonary edema, seizure, metabolic acidosis refractory to alkalinization, hepatic failure, and coagulopathy.

87 CARBON MONOXIDE

Timothy Turnbull
Gary R. Strange
Heather M. Prendergast

PATHOPHYSIOLOGY

- Carbon monoxide is a colorless, odorless, tasteless, and nonirritating gas formed as a by-product of incomplete combustion of fossil fuels or materials such as wood or charcoal. CO poisoning is most commonly caused by smoke inhalation. It also occurs from exposure to malfunctioning or improperly vented heating and cooking appliances, automobile exhaust fumes, and methylene chloride, a component of paint strippers that is metabolized to CO by the liver.

- The predominant toxic effect of CO poisoning is tissue hypoxia, since CO binds to hemoglobin with 250 times the affinity of oxygen and competitively displaces oxygen from the molecule. Carbon monoxide also alters the hemoglobin molecule in such a way that the remaining oxygen is bound with greater affinity, in effect displacing the oxyhemoglobin dissociation curve to the left.

- The most oxygen-sensitive organs of the body, the central nervous system and heart, are most susceptible to the effects of CO poisoning. Children, by virtue of their higher basal metabolic rates, are presumed to be more vulnerable to central nervous system damage at lower levels of CO than are adults.

CLINICAL PRESENTATION

- Clinical signs and symptoms of CO poisoning are notoriously nonspecific and correlate only roughly with the CoHb level at the scene (Table 87-1).

TABLE 87-1   Relationship of Carboxyhemoglobin (CoHb) Level and Clinical Manifestations of Carbon Monoxide Toxicity

CoHb LEVEL (%)	SIGNS AND SYMPTOMS
0–10	None
10–20	Mild headache, dyspnea on exertion
20–30	More severe headache, dyspnea
30–40	Severe headache, dizziness, nausea, vomiting, fatigue, poor judgment, dim vision
40–50	Confusion, tachypnea, tachycardia
50–60	Syncope, seizures, coma
60–70	Coma, hypotension, respiratory failure, death
>70	Rapidly fatal

- The best clues to the diagnosis are found in the history, and a correct assessment relies on a high index of suspicion, especially in the winter months when CO poisoning is more prevalent.
- It is axiomatic that any illness affecting more than one victim of a family or group from a common environment requires that CO poisoning be ruled out.
- As a rule, the physical examination is unrevealing and vital sign abnormalities are nonspecific. The cherry red skin commonly associated with CO poisoning is usually a postmortem finding.

LABORATORY STUDIES

- The diagnosis of CO poisoning is confirmed by measurement of the CoHb level, which can be obtained from an arterial or venous sample. A normal CoHb level is less than 1 percent, and is attributed to endogenous production during heme metabolism. Levels are as high as 5 percent in nonsmoking urban residents, and heavy smokers can have levels between 5 and 15 percent.
- In acute CO exposure, the CoHb level and the severity of toxicity correlate poorly.
- Arterial blood gas analysis provides information concerning acid–base status, and in severe cases of CO intoxication may reveal a metabolic acidosis. It may also reveal a "saturation gap." Since CO does not affect the PO_2 its level will be normal, but measured oxygen saturation will be decreased.
- It is important to note that oxygen saturation as measured by pulse oximetry is essentially unaffected by CO.

TREATMENT

- The cornerstone of treatment is high-flow supplemental oxygen.
- While the half-time of CoHb ranges from 4 to 6 hours on room air, it is decreased to 40 to 90 minutes at an FIO_2 of 100 percent.
- In more severely intoxicated patients or those at high risk for central nervous system toxicity, hyperbaric oxygen (HBO) therapy may be indicated. HBO can reduce the half-time of CoHb to 20 minutes while increasing the amount of dissolved oxygen in the plasma by 2 volumes-percent for every atmosphere.
- Specific indications for HBO vary among centers with hyperbaric chambers and are evolving. Generally accepted clinical indications include:
  - Coma or other signs of neurological impairment
  - Any period of unconsciousness including syncope
  - Evidence of myocardial ischemia
  - Pregnancy, especially when there is evidence of fetal distress.
- Aggressive use of HBO should also be considered in neonates and infants, given their greater vulnerability to the effects of CO intoxication and the difficulty in assessing symptoms.
- If HBO is not available locally, consideration should still be given to transfer of patients who meet the clinical criteria for HBO. The nearest HBO facility can be located by contacting Divers Alert Network at Duke University in North Carolina, telephone number (919) 684-8111.

DISPOSITION

- Children with mild poisoning (CoHb level below 5 percent) who are no longer symptomatic can be discharged. Prior to discharge, every effort should be made to locate the source of CO, since reexposure can be extremely harmful.
- Parents and caretakers should be advised of the potential for delayed neuropsychiatric sequelae, including persistent headaches, memory lapses, irritability, and personality changes. Occasionally, gait disturbances or incontinence can occur.
- Patients who require admission to the hospital include children with:
  - CoHb levels greater than 20 percent
  - Acidosis
  - Requirement for HBO

PROGNOSIS

- The mortality rate among patients with severe CO poisoning is about 30 percent. Most patients who die do so at the scene of exposure.
- Up to 11 percent of survivors have gross neurologic or psychiatric deficits. In addition, up to 25 percent of treated patients will experience delayed neurological deterioration following a period of apparent recovery.

BIBLIOGRAPHY

Ernst A, Zibrak JD: Carbon monoxide poisoning. *N Engl J Med* 339:1603–1608, 1998.
Rudge FW: Carbon monoxide poisoning in infants: Treatment with hyperbaric oxygen. *South Med J* 86:334, 1993.

Scheinkestel CD, Bailey M, Myles PS, et al: Hyperbaric or normobaric oxygen for acute carbon monoxide poisoning: A randomized controlled clinical trial. *Med J Aust* 170:203–210, 1999.

Tighe SQ: Hyperbaric oxygen in carbon monoxide poisoning. 100% oxygen is best option. *Br Med J* 321:110–111, 2000.

Weaver LK, Hopkins RO, Chan KJ, et al: Hyperbaric oxygen for acute carbon monoxide poisoning. *N Engl J Med* 347:1057–1067, 2002.

QUESTIONS

1. A 10-year-old girl is brought to the ED for evaluation of dizziness and headaches. Which of the following would heighten your suspicion for CO poisoning the most?
   A. Wood-burning fireplace at home
   B. Residence above an auto repair shop
   C. Family members with similar symptoms
   D. Occurrence in the winter months
   E. Attendance at an outdoor barbeque event 2 days prior

2. Paramedics bring a 7-year-old to the ED for possible smoke inhalation exposure at a suburban daycare facility. Which of the following tests results would be the MOST useful in excluding a significant CO exposure?
   A. Normal pulse oximetry result
   B. Normal pH on arterial blood gas
   C. Carboxyhemoglobin (CoHb) level of 5 percent
   D. Normal PO_2 on arterial blood gas
   E. Normal oxygen saturation on arterial blood gas

3. Several children are brought to the ED for evaluation following an adjacent apartment building fire. On arrival to the ED, the children are alert and oriented. Physical examination reveals normal vitals signs and no evidence of facial burns. The MOST appropriate treatment regimen would be which of the following?
   A. Observation on room air for 4 to 6 hours
   B. 100 percent oxygen by face mask for a minimum of 90 minutes
   C. 2 liters of oxygen by nasal cannula for 1 hour
   D. Transfer for hyperbaric oxygen therapy
   E. No additional treatment is necessary

4. Which of the following is NOT an absolute indication for hyperbaric oxygen treatment for CO poisoning?
   A. An asymptomatic first-trimester pregnancy
   B. Presence of chest pain
   C. Dizziness and a near syncopal episode
   D. Altered mental status
   E. Significant neonatal exposure

ANSWERS

1. C. Although CO poisoning is most often the result of smoke inhalation, significant exposure can occur from improper ventilation and malfunctioning appliances. A detailed history is extremely valuable in providing clues for the diagnosis. The majority of clinical signs and symptoms are nonspecific. While occurrence of such nonspecific complaints in winter months should increase your suspicion, occurrence of similar symptoms among family members mandates that CO poisoning is ruled out.

2. E. The diagnosis of CO poisoning is confirmed by COHb levels. In a nonsmoking urban residents, CoHb levels as high as 5 percent can be normal. A normal pulse oximetry reading does not rule out a CO exposure as this modality is unaffected by carbon monoxide. In cases of CO exposure the measured oxygen saturation on an arterial blood gas will be decreased.

3. B. The treatment of CO exposure is oxygen. The half-life of CoHb ranges from 4 to 6 hours on room air. However with 100 percent oxygen by face mask, this time can be reduced to 90 minutes. It would be most practical to place the children on 100 percent oxygen for approximately 90 minutes and observe in the emergency department during that time. If the children remain asymptomatic, they can be discharged to home with follow-up.

4. C. Dizziness is a common complaint with CO exposure. If there is no documented period of unconsciousness at any time during the exposure, there is no absolute indication for hyperbaric therapy. Generally accepted clinical indications include: evidence of myocardial ischemia, pregnancy, coma, and neurologic impairment.

88 CAUSTICS

Bonnie McManus
Gary R. Strange

INTRODUCTION

- Caustics are chemicals that cause injury on contact. Lye is the most frequent reported exposure.

PATHOPHYSIOLOGY

- Regardless of whether the caustic is an acid or an alkali, the severity of injury depends on:
  - The nature, volume, and concentration of the agent

- Contact time
- Presence or absence of stomach contents
- Tonicity of the pyloric sphincter
- Esophageal reflux after the ingestion
- Solids tend to produce intense localized upper esophageal injury.
- Liquids, especially strong bases, tend to produce circumferential lesions in the distal esophagus.

ALKALI BURNS

- Alkali burns cause liquefaction necrosis, a deep penetration injury associated with a pronounced exothermic reaction. Tissue destruction continues until the compound is significantly neutralized by tissue or the concentration is greatly decreased.
- Due to relatively prolonged contact time, solid alkalis tend to cause perioral, oropharyngeal, and upper esophageal injury. The injury may be severe with deep irregular linear burns.
- Liquid lye can cause severe esophageal injury with minimal oropharyngeal findings. The complications following liquid lye ingestion tend to be more severe than those from solid ingestions because the injury is circumferential and leads to stricturing.
- The stomach is involved about 20 percent of the time when there is esophageal injury. The incidence of stomach injury is relatively low because most of the lye is neutralized in the esophagus.
- There are three major phases of caustic esophageal injury:
  - Phase 1 is an acute inflammatory stage in which vascular thrombosis and cellular necrosis peak at 1 to 2 days, followed by sloughing of the necrotic tissue at approximately 3 to 4 days, resulting in an area of ulceration.
  - Phase 2 is the latent granulation phase, in which fibroplasia begins to fill in the ulcer with granulation tissue in the middle of the first week. By the end of the first week, collagen starts to replace the granulation tissue. Perforation is most likely during the second week when the esophageal wall is the weakest.
  - Phase 3 is the chronic cicatrization phase. It begins during weeks 2 to 4, producing variable degrees of scar formation and contractures.

ACID BURNS

- Acid burns cause coagulation necrosis with severe injury to superficial tissues, but penetration is avoided by the formation of an eschar that limits damage to deeper tissues. Unlike liquid alkali, which tends to produce injury very rapidly, acid injury may continue to evolve for up to 90 min after the ingestion.
- The nature of the injury is such that acid tends to reach the stomach without being buffered in the esophagus, which can cause severe gastric injury, including perforation.

PRESENTATION AND STABILIZATION

- Identification of the offending agent is crucial in determining the potential for harm. Caretakers who call the emergency department should be asked to bring the container, including labels, of the ingested substance.
- Many caustics, including highly alkaline laundry detergents, can cause life-threatening airway edema, which must be urgently addressed. Stridor, dyspnea, and dysphonia all indicate upper airway compromise that requires intervention. Patients with upper airway obstruction should be intubated under direct visualization or may need a surgical airway.
- Patients with a history of caustic ingestion, but without signs of airway compromise, are observed for excessive crying, drooling, or refusal to eat or drink, all of which indicate a significant injury.
  - The mouth is examined for signs of intraoral burns.
  - The chest is examined for retractions, wheezes, or rhonchi that indicate potential aspiration.
  - The abdomen is examined for tenderness, which in cases of acid ingestion suggests the possibility of gastric perforation. In cases of suspected perforation the patient is monitored carefully for the presence of intraabdominal hemorrhage and hypovolemic shock.
- In patients with signs of respiratory distress, oxygen saturation or arterial blood gases are critical in assessing lung function. Many caustics are powerful emetics and if aspirated, can cause severe pneumonitis or noncardiogenic pulmonary edema.
- Laboratory studies should include a complete blood count, serum electrolytes, renal functions, coagulation profile, and glucose.
- A chest radiograph is indicated in patients with signs of a significant ingestion or respiratory distress. Patients with abdominal pain or tenderness require an abdominal radiograph to exclude the presence of free air, indicating perforation.

MANAGEMENT

- After the airway is secured, an intravenous catheter is placed for use in the event that volume resuscitation is required.

- In the event of a large acid ingestion, a nasogastric tube is placed in an attempt to remove pooled acid and reduce injury.

DILUENTS AND BUFFERS

- Milk or water may be indicated after the ingestion of solid alkali in an attempt to move particulate material out of the oropharynx and esophagus. The amount given should be easily tolerated by the child so as not to induce emesis.
- There is no value in administering diluents in the case of liquid alkali ingestion because the injury is complete in a very short time and the risk of inducing emesis is great.

EMESIS

- Induction of emesis in caustic ingestions is contraindicated. Increased tissue damage occurs as the esophagus is reexposed to the offending agent.

GASTRIC ASPIRATION AND LAVAGE

- In general, gastric aspiration and lavage are not indicated in alkali injury because of the rapidity of the injury.
- Although there are no studies that show an advantage or disadvantage of gastric aspiration in strong acid ingestion, anecdotal reports suggest that potentially lethal acids should be removed through a soft catheter if the patient is seen within 90 min of ingestion.

CHARCOAL AND CATHARTICS

- The administration of charcoal and cathartics is contraindicated because caustics are poorly adsorbed by charcoal, the injury tends to occur prior to arrival in the emergency department, and charcoal creates a problem with visualization for the endoscopist.

ENDOSCOPY

- The challenge in managing the child with a caustic ingestion is in identifying the patient who is at risk for a serious injury. Since many patients have minimal clinical findings, clinical criteria are not reliable in identifying the presence or severity of burns.

- Endoscopy helps to define the extent of the injury and develop a prognosis. Because of the unreliability of clinical findings in predicting significant esophageal injury, the threshold for endoscopy is low. Any child with a history of significant ingestion, with oral lesions, or who is otherwise symptomatic, warrants endoscopy.
  - The optimal time for the procedure appears to be during the first several hours after the ingestion.
  - Endoscopy is not indicated for asymptomatic ingestion of household bleach, ammonia, or nonphosphate detergents. Evidence of perforation or shock is a contraindication to endoscopy.

STEROIDS

- Steroids are a controversial aspect of management of caustic ingestions. Theoretically, steroids decrease the incidence of esophageal strictures in patients with severe burns.

SPECIAL CONCERNS

BUTTON BATTERIES

- Button batteries frequently are swallowed by children. The batteries contain various combinations of zinc, cadmium, mercury, silver, nickel, or lithium in a concentrated alkaline medium, usually sodium or potassium hydroxide.
- Injury may occur due to pressure necrosis at the site where the battery becomes lodged. Lodging is most likely to occur at sites of anatomic narrowing, such as the cricopharyngeus, where the aorta or carina cross the esophagus, or in gut malformations such as a Meckel's diverticulum.
- A battery lodged in the esophagus requires urgent removal.
  - Burns have been reported as early as 4 h after ingestion and perforation as early as 6 h after.
  - The preferred method of extraction is endoscopy, which allows direct visualization of any esophageal injury.
- If the battery is intact and has passed through the esophagus, it does not need to be retrieved unless there are indications of intraabdominal injury, which include abdominal pain, tenderness, and hematochezia.
- A large battery ingested by a small child may also require removal.
  - If a battery greater than 15 mm in diameter is ingested by a child less than 6 years of age and has not passed the pylorus within 48 h, it is unlikely to do so.

- An asymptomatic patient with a gastrointestinal battery not lodged in the esophagus can be discharged and followed as an outpatient with serial radiographs to document passage of the battery. The parents can strain the child's stool until the battery has passed.
- Whole bowel irrigation is an alternative easily performed in the emergency department; it may promote passage of the battery in 4 to 8 h. This can be especially useful in cases in which follow-up is unreliable.

HYDROFLUORIC ACID

- Hydrofluoric acid is a weak acid found in some cleaning and rust-removing products. External contact can result in severe dermal or ocular injury. Death has been reported with exposures affecting as little as 2.5 percent of the body surface area.
- Severe pain and deep penetration despite minimal skin findings is the hallmark of a hydrofluoric acid burn. The mechanism of injury involves liquefaction necrosis and the formation of insoluble calcium and magnesium salts.
- Oral ingestions are frequently fatal.
- In cases of significant burns, systemic acidosis, hypocalcemia, hypomagnesemia, and hyperkalemia are common. Renal failure and hemolysis have been reported to occur.
- En route to the emergency department, copious irrigation to decrease diffusion is indicated.
- A gel of 3.5 g of calcium gluconate and 5 ounces of water-soluble lubricant or a 25-percent magnesium sulfate soak (epsom salt) will provide pain relief.
- Pain can also be alleviated by intradermal injection of calcium gluconate.
- In cases of oral ingestion, calcium and magnesium are given on a milliequivalent per milliequivalent basis.

BIBLIOGRAPHY

Ellenhorn MJ, Schowald S: *Medical Toxicology: Diagnosis and Treatment of Human Poisoning.* New York: Elsevier Science Publishing, 1083–1097, 1997.

Ford M, Delaney KA, Ling LJ, Erickson T, eds: *Clinical Toxicology.* Philadelphia: Saunders, 1002–1038, 2001.

Hojer J, Personne M, Hulten P, Ludwigs U: Topical treatments for hydrofluoric acid burns: A blind controlled experimental study. *J Toxicol Clin Toxicol* 40:861–866, 2002.

Homan CS, Singer A, Henry MC, et al: Thermal effects of neutralization and water dilution for acute alkali exposures in canines. *Acad Emerg Med* 4:27, 1997.

QUESTIONS

1. Strong liquid bases, such as lye, tend to produce which of the following patterns of injury?
   A. Intense localized upper esophageal injury
   B. Circumferential distal esophageal injury with minimal oropharyngeal findings
   C. Patchy lesions in the proximal esophagus
   D. Severe superficial injury with limited penetration
   E. Gastric injury in the absence of esophageal injury

2. Acid ingestions tend to be associated with which of the following complications?
   A. Esophageal perforation
   B. Severe metabolic acidosis
   C. Gastric perforation
   D. Esophageal strictures
   E. Aortic penetration

3. A 3-year-old child presents to the ED 30 min after ingesting a cup of dishwasher detergent. He is anxious, has a hoarse, stridorous cry, and is drooling. Which of the following is the best course of action for this presentation?
   A. Reassure the mother that this injury is likely to be oral only and proceed to rinse the mouth with water.
   B. Arrange for endoscopy to determine whether there is esophageal involvement.
   C. Administer vinegar or lemon juice to assist in neutralizing the alkaline detergent.
   D. Administer activated charcoal as soon as possible.
   E. Prepare for oral intubation, preferably in the operating room with anesthesia and ENT in attendance.

4. The optimal time for endoscopy to define the extent of injury and develop a prognosis after a caustic ingestion is:
   A. during the first several hours after the injury
   B. 4 to 6 h after injury, to assure that the full extent of injury is visible
   C. 24 to 48 h after the injury
   D. Timing is not crucial and endoscopy may take place anytime within a week of the injury.
   E. Endoscopy is used for treatment of complications but is not helpful in the acute phase to determine the extent of injury or to develop a prognosis.

5. Which of the following is true regarding removal of ingested button batteries?

A. Emetics are frequently successful in assisting the expelling of these batteries.

B. A battery lodged in the esophagus requires urgent removal.

C. A battery that is visualized radiographically in the stomach requires urgent removal if it has not passed into the intestine within 24 h.

D. Whole bowel irrigation is ineffective in facilitating passage of button batteries.

E. Once a battery is documented to have passed the pylorus, it is no longer necessary to follow the patient with serial radiographs and examinations.

ANSWERS

1. B. Strongly basic liquids tend to produce circumferential lesions of the distal esophagus associated with minimal oropharyngeal findings. Alkaline substances cause liquefaction necrosis and a deep penetrating injury. The incidence of stomach injury is relatively low because most of the base is neutralized in the esophagus.

2. C. With acid ingestions, the nature of the injury is such that acid tends to reach the stomach without being buffered in the esophagus and can cause severe gastric injury, including perforation. Significant esophageal injury is rare. Systemic acidosis is not generally seen. Solid alkalis, such as Clinitest tablets, have been reported to cause penetration of the esophageal wall with extension into the aorta but this is not seen with acids.

3. E. Many caustics, including highly alkaline laundry detergents, can cause life-threatening airway edema, which must be addressed urgently. Stridor, dyspnea, and dysphonia all indicate upper airway compromise that requires intervention. Patients with upper airway obstruction should be intubated under direct visualization and may need a surgical airway. Highly alkaline liquids do not tend to produce significant oral injury. Weak acids have not been shown to be helpful and charcoal is ineffective. Arranging for esophagoscopy is appropriate but attention to the airway takes precedence.

4. A. Endoscopy is used to define the extent of injury and to develop a prognosis. The optimal time for the procedure appears to be during the first several hours after the ingestion.

5. B. A battery lodged in the esophagus requires urgent removal. Once a battery passes into the stomach in an asymptomatic patient, the progress of the battery can be followed with serial radiographs and outpatient re-evaluations. Emetics have not been shown to be useful but whole bowel irrigation may be helpful in facilitating passage within 4 to 8 h.

89 COCAINE TOXICITY

Steven E. Aks
Gary R. Strange

PHARMACOLOGY AND PATHOPHYSIOLOGY

• Cocaine is a sympathomimetic agent that causes CNS stimulation. Use of it can result in agitation, hallucinations, abnormal movements, and convulsions. Paradoxically, children may present with lethargy. Both ischemic and hemorrhagic strokes have been reported.

• Cardiovascular manifestations of cocaine toxicity include sinus tachycardia and both supraventricular and ventricular dysrhythmias. Elevation in blood pressure can range from mild to fulminant hypertension associated with strokes. Myocardial ischemia, including myocardial infarction, has been described in otherwise healthy individuals as young as 17 years old having normal coronary arteries.

• Multiple pulmonary effects from inhalation of cocaine have been described, including exacerbation of asthma, pulmonary infarction, pneumomediastinum, pneumothorax, and respiratory failure.

• In association with agitation and hypertension, cocaine-induced hyperthermia can occur. A potential complication of hyperthermia is acute rhabdomyolysis. Cocaine-induced rhabdomyolysis can also occur in the absence of hyperthermia.

DIAGNOSIS

• Cocaine toxicity is likely in a patient who exhibits signs and symptoms consistent with sympathomimetic stimulation:
  ◦ CNS excitation
  ◦ Mydriasis
  ◦ Tachycardia
  ◦ Hypertension
  ◦ Hyperthermia

LABORATORY STUDIES

• For patients in whom cocaine toxicity is suspected, a toxicology screen can confirm the ingestion and rule out co-ingestants. Blood levels of cocaine and cocaine metabolites correlate poorly with signs and symptoms.

• Cardiac monitoring is essential to evaluate the patient for dysrhythmias.

- Patients who complain of chest pain require a 12-lead electrocardiogram. A chest radiograph is useful to exclude pneumothorax, pneumomediastinum, or infiltrate.
- If a urine dipstick is positive for blood but microscopy is negative for red blood cells, the patient is evaluated for rhabdomyolysis with a serum creatine kinase and urine myoglobin.
- For patients with severe headache or neurologic deficit, a computed tomographic (CT) scan of the brain is indicated to rule out the possibility of a cocaine-induced cerebrovascular accident.

MANAGEMENT

- Mildly toxic patients generally require no specific therapy.
- Moderate to severe agitation responds to benzodiazepines, which are also the drugs of choice for seizures.
- Benzodiazepines are also effective treatment for most patients with mild to moderate hypertension. In more severe cases, labetalol, which has both alpha- and beta-blocking characteristics, has been effective, as has sodium nitroprusside. Beta blockers are contraindicated, since unopposed alpha stimulation can exacerbate hypertension.
- Patients with severe hyperthermia are treated with aggressive cooling.
- The urine is alkalinized in patients with rhabdomyolysis.
- Activated charcoal adsorbs unpackaged orally ingested cocaine and is useful for the treatment of gastric contamination.

BODY STUFFERS

- Body stuffers may swallow cocaine in an attempt to hide the drug to avoid prosecution when accosted by law enforcement officers. Often the cocaine is poorly wrapped, and even carefully packaged packets can rupture with fatal results.
- Abdominal radiographs may be useful if the ingested packets are radiopaque.
- In body stuffers, gastric decontamination with syrup of ipecac or gastric lavage is contraindicated, since both may cause rupture of the packets.
- Whole bowel irrigation with polyethylene glycol electrolyte lavage solution can be used to enhance transit through the gastrointestinal tract. All ingested packets should be passed before the patient is discharged. A gastrograffin swallow or abdominal CT may be required before discharge to make sure all packets have been passed.
- In symptomatic body stuffers, a surgical consultation is indicated since laparotomy may be necessary.

DISPOSITION

- In asymptomatic or mild cases of cocaine toxicity, 4 to 6h of observation in the emergency department is adequate.
- Patients with moderate to severe symptoms are admitted to a monitored bed. Body stuffers are observed in a monitored setting until all packets have passed.

BIBLIOGRAPHY

Blaho K, Logan B, Winbery S, et al: Blood cocaine and metabolite concentrations: Clinical findings, and outcome of patient presenting to an ED. *Am J Emerg Med* 18:593–598, 2000.

June R, Aks SE, Keys N, et al: Medical outcome of cocaine bodystuffers. *J Emerg Med* 18:221–224, 2000.

Kneupfer MM: Cardiovascular disorders associated with cocaine use: Myths and truths. *Pharmacol Ther* 97:181–222, 2003.

Litovitz TL, Klein-Schwartz W, White S, et al: 1999 Annual Report of Poison Control Centers toxic exposure surveillance system. *Am J Emerg Med* 18:517–574, 2000.

Richman PB, Nashed AH: The etiology of cardiac arrest in children and young adults: Special considerations for ED management. *Am J Emerg Med* 17:264–270, 1999.

QUESTIONS

1. The clinical effects of cocaine most closely resemble which of the following toxidromes?
   A. Anticholinergic toxicity
   B. Parasympathetic hyperstimulation
   C. Sympathomimetic stimulation
   D. Cholinergic excess
   E. Narcotic syndrome
2. A 20-year-old male presents to the ED with a complaint of chest pain. He admits to cocaine use 4h prior to arrival. Which of the following statements is correct regarding his work-up?
   A. Urine toxicology screen is not helpful.
   B. Blood levels for cocaine correlate closely to hyper-metabolic signs and symptoms.
   C. ECG has been shown to be unnecessary due to the low prevalence of coronary artery disease in this age group.

D. Chest radiograph is useful to exclude pneumothorax, pneumomediastinum or infiltrate.

E. Computed tomographic (CT) scan of the brain is indicated to rule out the possibility of CVA.

3. A 30 year-old male is brought to the ED by paramedics after being observed to be acting in a threatening and aggressive manner in a public place. He is uncooperative and thrashing about on the ambulance cart. His blood pressure is 145/95 with pulse rate of 120 and respiratory rate of 30. The most appropriate initial pharmacologic intervention is:

A. Labetalol

B. Metoprolol

C. Haloperidol

D. Midazolam

E. Chlorpromazine

4. After the patient above is medicated, the temperature is noted to be 106°F. His toxicology screen is negative except for cocaine. The microscopic urinalysis is completely normal but the dip urine reveals moderate blood. What further diagnostic studies are indicated?

A. Noncontrast CT of the abdomen

B. Serum CPK and urine myoglobin

C. CT of the brain

D. CK-MB and Troponin-I

E. Arterial blood gases and blood lactate

ANSWERS

1. C. Cocaine toxicity presents with signs and symptoms of sympathomimetic stimulation. This toxidrome may be difficult to distinguish from that caused by anticholinergic toxicity. However, unlike sympathomimetic toxicity, anticholinergics cause urinary retention and decreased bowel sounds.

2. D. Chest radiographs are indicated to rule out pulmonary pathology. Urine toxicology screen is useful to confirm the ingestion and rule out co-ingestants. Blood levels of cocaine and cocaine metabolites correlate poorly with signs and symptoms. ECG is indicated, regardless of age, since myocardial ischemia and infarction have been described in otherwise healthy individuals as young as 17 years old having normal coronary arteries. CT of the brain is not indicated on a routine basis but is indicated when there is severe headache or neurologic deficit.

3. D. Moderate to severe agitation responds to benzodiazepines, which are also the drugs of choice for seizures. Benzodiazepines are also effective treatment for most patients with mild to moderate hypertension. In more severe cases, labetalol, which has

both alpha- and beta-blocking characteristics, has been effective, as has sodium nitroprusside. Beta-blockers are contraindicated, since unopposed alpha stimulation can exacerbate hypertension. Haloperidol and chlorpromazine lower the seizure threshold and are relatively contraindicated.

4. B. The hyperactivity of cocaine toxicity can result in rhabdomyolysis with or without associated hyperthermia. It is suspected when a urine dipstick is positive for blood (actually myoglobin) but microscopy is negative for red blood cells. The syndrome is confirmed by the presence of creatine phosphokinase (CPK) in the blood and myoglobin in the urine, both of which are produced by muscle breakdown. This patient would be treated with aggressive cooling and alkalinization of the urine. Myoglobin is prevented from precipitating out in the renal tubules by maintaining an alkaline urine, thus preventing the development of renal failure.

90 CYANIDE POISONING

Mark Mycyk
Anne Krantz
Gary R. Strange

INTRODUCTION

- There are a variety of sources of cyanide exposure in the pediatric population.
  - In fires, hydrogen cyanide gas is formed as a combustion product of wool, silk, synthetic fabrics, and building materials. Cyanide exposure by this route is now recognized as a major cause of toxicity among fire victims previously thought to be poisoned by carbon monoxide.
  - Acetonitrile, or methyl cyanide, is found in agents used to remove sculpted nails and is converted in vivo to hydrogen cyanide. Cyanide poisoning due to acetonitrile ingestion has occurred in children, resulting in at least one reported death.
  - Poisoning has also occurred from accidental ingestion of cyanide-containing metal cleaning solutions imported from Southeast Asia.
  - Amygdalin and other cyanogenic glycosides, found in the seeds and pits of certain plants such as apples, apricots, and peaches, are hydrolyzed in the gut to cyanide. Fruit pit ingestion has led to outbreaks of cyanide poisoning in children in Turkey and Gaza.
  - These and other sources of cyanide exposure are summarized in Table 90-1.

TABLE 90-1 **Sources of Cyanide Exposure**

Cyanogenic plants
   Prunus species (leaves, stem, bark, seed pits)
      American plum, wild plum
      Apricot
      Cherry laurel, Carolina cherry laurel
      Cultivated cherry
      Peach
      Wild black cherry
      Chokecherry
      Bitter almond
   Other
      Apple (seeds)
      Pear (seeds)
      Crabapple (seeds)
      Elderberry (leaves and shoots)
      Hydrangea (leaves and buds)
      Cassava (beans and roots)
Household agents
   HCN-containing fumigants
   Rodenticides
   Insecticides (aliphatic thiocyantes: Lethane 60, Lethane 302, Thanite)
   Sculpted nail removers containing acetonitrile (eg, Nailene Glue
      Remover)
   Silver and metal polish
Combustion products
   Silk, wool
   Polyurethane
   Polyacrylonitrile
Other
   Nitroprusside

TOXICOKINETICS

- Hydrogen cyanide gas is rapidly absorbed in the lungs and may cause profound toxicity within seconds.
- Ingested cyanide salts, such as sodium cyanide and potassium cyanide, are also rapidly absorbed across the gastric mucosa and may result in toxicity within min.
- Ingestion of amygdalin and other cyanogenic glycosides requires hydrolysis to release cyanide, so toxicity may be delayed up to several h after ingestion.
- Acetonitrile appears to release cyanide through oxidative metabolism by the hepatic cytochrome P450 system, thus delaying clinical manifestations of toxicity for 2 to 6 h from the time of ingestion.
- The widely distributed endogenous enzyme rhodanase (sulfurtransferase) in the presence of thiosulfate converts cyanide to nontoxic thiocyanate. This accounts for the majority (80 percent) of elimination with thiosulfate availability being the rate-limiting factor.

PATHOPHYSIOLOGY

- Cyanide inhibition of cytochrome oxidase prevents efficient cellular oxygen use and disrupts ATP production. This shift to anaerobic metabolism results in a severe lactic acidosis. Cyanide also shifts the oxygen-hemoglobin dissociation curve to the left, further impairing oxygen delivery to the tissues.

CLINICAL PRESENTATION

- Inhalation of cyanide gas causes loss of consciousness within seconds, whereas symptoms from an oral exposure develop anywhere from 30 min to several hours from the time of ingestion.
- Since cyanide poisoning causes profound tissue hypoxia, it makes clinical sense that the central nervous system and the cardiovascular system (the two organ systems most dependent on oxygen) are affected the earliest.
- Initial symptoms in victims not experiencing rapid loss of consciousness include headache, anxiety, confusion, blurred vision, palpitations, nausea, and vomiting. With progression of toxicity patients may experience a feeling of neck constriction, suffocation, and unsteadiness.
- Early clinical signs of cyanide poisoning are CNS stimulation or depression, tachycardia or bradycardia, hypertension, dilated pupils, bright red retinal veins on funduscopy, and declining mental status.
- Late signs of poisoning are seizures, coma, apnea, cardiac arrhythmias, and complete cardiovascular collapse.

LABORATORY EVALUATION

- Arterial blood gases will typically show a marked metabolic acidosis. Obtaining a venous blood gas analysis for comparison may demonstrate a diminished arterial-venous O_2 difference (A_{O_2} - V_{O_2} approaching zero) since the tissues' ability to extract oxygen from the blood is severely impaired.
- Serum chemistries may demonstrate an elevated anion gap due to the presence of a lactic acidosis from anaerobic metabolism.
- Numerous electrocardiographic changes may occur in cyanide toxicity.

TREATMENT

- The management of cyanide poisoning requires immediate supportive care as well as specific antidotal therapy.
- Airway management with 100-percent oxygen should be initiated and an intravenous line established in all patients.

- Fluid resuscitation should be administered to patients with hypotension, and sodium bicarbonate should be considered in profound acidosis.
- Mouth-to-mouth resuscitation by primary rescuers should be avoided because of the theoretical risk of secondary cyanide exposure. Contaminated clothing should be removed and skin and eyes should be copiously irrigated.

CYANIDE ANTIDOTES

- The only antidote currently approved for use in the United States is the Lilly Cyanide Antidote Kit, which contains:
  ∘ Amyl nitrite perles
  ∘ Sodium nitrite solution
  ∘ Sodium thiosulfate
- Nitrites produce methemoglobin, which has a higher affinity for cyanide than does cytochrome oxidase. This combination of methemoglobin and cyanide forms cyanomethemoglobin.
- Sodium thiosulfate provides a sulfur donor for the rhodanase-mediated conversion of cyanomethemoglobin to methemoglobin and thiocyanate. Thiocyanate is minimally toxic and is excreted by the kidneys.
- The recommended regimen and pediatric doses for the Lilly kit components is summarized in Table 90-2.
  ∘ Amyl nitrite perles are administered first while establishing an intravenous line and preparing the sodium nitrite solution. The perles should be crushed in gauze and held near the nose and mouth for 30 s. Amyl nitrite administration will produce a methemoglobin level of 3 to 7 percent.
  ∘ Once an intravenous line is established and the sodium nitrite solution prepared, administration of amyl nitrite perles may be stopped. Sodium nitrite (9 mg/kg, or 0.3 mL/kg of a 3-percent solution, not to exceed 10 mL) is administered at a rate of 2.5 mL/min. In an unstable or hypotensive patient, or when there is concomitant CO poisoning, the dose may be given more slowly, over 30 min.

- Following the nitrite administration, sodium thiosulfate is given to enhance clearance of cyanide as thiocyanate. Alternately, the thiosulfate may be administered concurrently at a separate site. The pediatric dose is 1.6 mL/kg of a 25-percent solution up to 50 mL (12.5 g).
- Typically, symptoms and signs of cyanide poisoning begin to respond within minutes of the administration of nitrites. When symptoms recur following antidote administration, both the sodium nitrite and sodium thiosulfate may be given again at half the original doses.
- Because there is no diagnostic test for cyanide poisoning that can be obtained in a timely manner, the diagnosis in the acute setting needs to be made clinically. In a situation in which cyanide poisoning is being considered but the diagnosis is uncertain, the use of sodium thiosulfate alone may be considered. If the patient remains critically ill, sodium nitrite should be administered slowly while blood pressure is monitored.

SMOKE INHALATION

- Several studies suggest a correlation between elevated carboxyhemoglobin levels and cyanide levels in smoke inhalation victims. Thus, when an elevated carboxyhemoglobin level is found in a severely ill, fire victim, cyanide poisoning is possible and it needs to be considered early and treated appropriately. This is particularly true in a fire victim who requires intubation or has a persistent metabolic acidosis, abnormal mental status, or cardiovascular instability not resolving with conventional therapy for carbon monoxide poisoning.

DISPOSITION

- Patients who are asymptomatic and whose exposure has apparently been minimal are observed for 4 to 6 h.
- Those who have ingested cyanogenic glycosides are observed for at least 6 h for evidence of the onset of toxicity.

TABLE 90-2 Recommended Usage of the Lilly Cyanide Antidote Kit

ANTIDOTE	QUANTITY AND FORM	PEDIATRIC DOSE
Amyl nitrite	12 perles (0.3 mL/perle)	Crush 1–2 perles in gauze and hold under patient's nose or over ET tube for 15–30 s each min[a]
Sodium nitrite	2 ampules of 3% solution (300 mg/10 mL)	0.3 mL/kg (9 mg/kg) not to exceed 10 mL (300 mg), intravenously at 2.5 mL/min, or over 30 min in smoke inhalation victims with carbon monoxide poisoning[b]
Sodium thiosulfate	2 ampules of 25% solution (12.5 g/50 mL)	1.6 mL/kg (400 mg/kg) up to 50 mL (12.5 g) at rate of 3–5 mL/min

[a] Check expiration date of all components. Shelf life for amyl nitrite is 1 year.
[b] Infuse more slowly when hypotension occurs. Monitor for blood pressure and be prepared to treat severe hypotension with fluids and vasopressors as needed. Monitor methemoglobin levels.

- Those ingesting acetonitrile-containing compounds are observed for 12 to 24 h.
- Patients requiring antidotal treatment are cared for in an intensive care unit where vital signs, mental status, arterial blood gases, methemoglobin, and carboxyhemoglobin levels can be checked frequently.

BIBLIOGRAPHY

Chin RG, Caldern Y: Acute cyanide poisoning: A case report. *J Emerg Med* 18:441–445, 2000.

Delaney KA: Cyanide. In: Ford MD, Delaney KA, Ling LJ, et al, eds. *Clinical Toxicology.* Philadelphia: Saunders, 705–711, 2001.

Kirk MA, Gerace R, Kulig KW: Cyanide and methemoglobin kinetics in smoke inhalation victims treated with the cyanide antidote kit. *Ann Emerg Med* 22:1413–1418, 1993.

Yen D, Tsai J, Wang LM, et al: The clinical experience of acute cyanide poisoning. *Am J Emerg Med* 13:524–528, 1995.

QUESTIONS

1. Two middle-aged victims are brought to the ED after being trapped in a burning building for approximately 15 min. Neither appears to have any significant thermal injury. Both victims are unconscious, have carbonaceous material in the nose but have normal oxygen saturation by pulse oximetry. Vital signs are stable with tachypnea at 28 but irregular cardiac rhythm at a rate of 110 is noted. Arterial blood gases show normal oxygenation but severe metabolic acidosis with bicarbonate of 5 mEq/L and P_{CO_2} of 25. Treatment with 100 percent oxygen is initiated but the patients do not appear to be responding. Which of the following approaches is most appropriate?
   A. Continue 100 percent oxygen therapy and order carboxyhemoglobin level
   B. Sodium bicarbonate, 2 amps IV push, followed by a bicarbonate drip
   C. Continue to observe, treat presumptively with glucose and naloxone, while awaiting comprehensive toxicology screens
   D. Continue 100 percent oxygen therapy, order carboxyhemoglobin level, and add thiosulfate therapy
   E. Reduce the oxygen concentration to 40 percent and initiate treatment with nitrites and thiosulfate

2. Which of the following statements regarding cyanide antidotes is correct?
   A. Amyl nitrite is unnecessary if sodium nitrite is used.
   B. Nitrites work in part by producing methemoglobin, which combines with cytochrome oxidase with greater affinity than cyanide.
   C. Cyanmethemoglobin is nontoxic and excreted by the kidneys.
   D. Sodium thiosulfate provides a sulfur donor for the rhodanase-mediated conversion of cyanmethemoglobin to methemoglobin and thiocyanate.
   E. Methemoglobin is produced in levels that do not result in significant toxicity.

ANSWERS

1. D. When an elevated carboxyhemoglobin level is found in a severely ill fire victim or a victim has been trapped in a closed burning building, cyanide poisoning is possible and it needs to be considered early and treated appropriately. This is particularly true in a fire victim who requires intubation or has a persistent metabolic acidosis, abnormal mental status, or cardiovascular instability not resolving with conventional therapy for carbon monoxide poisoning. In the situation in which cyanide poisoning is being considered but the diagnosis is uncertain, the use of sodium thiosulfate alone may be considered. Given the scenario in this question, other toxins, such as opiates and sedatives, are considered but the more pressing concern is the more immediately life-threatening possibility of cyanide gas inhalation. Treatment for presumed carbon monoxide toxicity while awaiting carboxyhemoglobin levels is also appropriate but insufficient treatment. Treatment of the metabolic acidosis with bicarbonate is unlikely to be effective. Treatment should continue presumptively for both carbon monoxide and cyanide, so 100-percent oxygen should be continued.

2. D. Due to the potentially very rapid toxicity of cyanide, amyl nitrite perles are crushed and held under the nose to begin the antidotal action immediately. This is followed by IV sodium nitrite as soon as possible. Nitrites work in part by producing methemoglobin, which binds cyanide more strongly than cytochrome oxidase. The cyanmethemoglobin produced is then converted to methemoglobin and thiocyanate by a rhodanase-mediated reaction. This step requires an available sulfur donor, which is provided by administration of sodium thiosulfate. The thiocyanate is nontoxic and is excreted by the kidney. Toxic levels of methemoglobin are often produced, however, and there is at least one report of a pediatric death due to methemoglobin produced by the antidotes for cyanide.

91 TRICYCLIC ANTIDEPRESSANT OVERDOSE

Steven E. Aks
Gary R. Strange

PHARMACOLOGY

- Toxic effects can be grouped as follows:
  - A *quinidine-like effect* accounts for cardiac dysrhythmias by inducing conduction blocks that manifest clinically with a widened QRS interval and QT abnormalities.
  - *Anticholinergic side effects* cause tachycardia and the anticholinergic overdose syndrome of mydriasis, dry mucous membranes, hyperthermia, decreased gastrointestinal motility, urinary retention, and mental status changes that can range from agitation to stupor and coma.
  - *Blockade of norepinephrine reuptake* augments tachycardia and can cause hypertension. Upon depletion of norepinephrine stores, hypotension can occur.
  - *Alpha blockade* causes hypotension by decreasing peripheral vasomotor tone.
- In toxic doses, absorption can be delayed because anticholinergic effects delay gastrointestinal motility.

CLINICAL PRESENTATION

- The clinical presentation of tricyclic antidepressant overdose is related primarily to the effects on the central nervous and cardiovascular systems.
- Patients can present to the emergency department with mental status changes that range from anxiety and agitation to confusion, delirium, and coma. Seizures can occur, and are of ominous clinical significance.
- Tachycardia is the most common cardiovascular manifestation of tricyclic antidepressant toxicity. Other abnormal rhythms include ventricular dysrhythmias, bradydysrhythmias, and cardiac arrest. The patient's blood pressure can be high or low.
- A patient who has taken an overdose of a tricyclic antidepressant is likely to arrive at the emergency department appearing clinically stable and may then suddenly deteriorate. The majority of patients who develop life-threatening problems do so within 2 h of arrival in the ED.

DIAGNOSIS

- When the diagnosis of tricyclic antidepressant overdose is entertained, cardiac monitoring is an essential first step. Persistent tachycardia is consistent with an overdose, and raises the suspicion that toxicity will progress. Several electrocardiographic parameters have been identified as markers of significant toxicity. The QRS duration has received much attention as a marker for overdose. In adults, a QRS duration less than 100 ms is correlated with a low risk of developing toxicity, while a QRS between 100 and 160 ms is sometimes associated with seizures and dysrhythmias, and a QRS greater than 160 ms with a high risk of seizures and dysrhythmias. However, in children, the QRS duration has not been well studied.
- It is useful to obtain a qualitative drug screen in suspected cases of tricyclic antidepressant overdose to confirm the ingestion. Because of the large volume of distribution of tricyclic antidepressants, the serum level does not accurately reflect clinical toxicity.
- In children, arterial blood gas monitoring is critical in the treatment of tricyclic antidepressant overdose. Acidemia may increase the proportion of drug released from binding sites, and contributes significantly to the propensity toward dysrhythmias.

MANAGEMENT

STABILIZATION

- Proper airway management is the first step in managing a patient with tricyclic antidepressant overdose. Intubation is necessary for patients with depressed mental status and for those with an absent gag reflex. It is also justified for patients who appear to be deteriorating clinically or for patients with doubtful mental status in whom gastric lavage is necessary.
- In intubated patients hyperventilation is indicated, since alkalemia can potentially reverse the cardiac toxicity of tricyclic antidepressant overdose.
- Hypotension is treated initially with boluses of crystalloid. If fluid resuscitation does not stabilize the blood pressure, pharmacologic support is indicated. Norepinephrine has theoretical advantages over dopamine because of its potential to directly reverse the alpha blockade caused by tricyclic antidepressants.

GASTRIC DECONTAMINATION

- Activated charcoal is administered along with a single dose of sorbitol. Multiple doses of charcoal are probably useful.

TREATMENT OF SEVERE TOXICITY

- If the QRS interval is greater than 100 ms, most investigators agree that alkalinization is indicated. This can be accomplished by administering sodium bicarbonate as a 1 to 2 mEq/kg bolus, followed by an infusion of sodium bicarbonate in D_5W. If the child is intubated, alkalinization can be obtained by a combination of bicarbonate administration and hyperventilation. The goal of alkalinization is to achieve a pH between 7.45 and 7.50.
- Alkalinization is believed to work by reversing the quinidine-like effects of tricyclic antidepressants.
- Ventricular dysrhythmias unresponsive to boluses of bicarbonate are treated with lidocaine. If the patient is hypotensive with a tachydysrhythmia, cardioversion is appropriate.
- Seizures are an ominous sign in the setting of a tricyclic antidepressant overdose. While generally short, seizures have been associated with incipient cardiac dysrhythmias. Seizures usually require no treatment, but benzodiazepines are effective if needed.
- Physostigmine should be viewed as a last line of therapy in cases of uncontrolled seizures, supraventricular dysrhythmia, and severe hypotension.

DISPOSITION

- Patients who do not develop tachycardia, QRS widening, anticholinergic symptoms, or drowsiness can be discharged after 6 h of monitoring in the emergency department.

BIBLIOGRAPHY

Litovitz TL, Klein-Schwartz W, White S, et al: 1999 Annual Report Of Poison Control Centers toxic exposure surveillance system. *Am J Emerg Med* 18:517–574, 2000.

McCabe JL, Cobaugh DJ, Menegazzi JJ, et al: Experimental tricyclic antidepressant toxicity: A randomized, controlled comparison of hypertonic saline solution, sodium bicarbonate, and hyperventilation. *Ann Emerg Med* 32:329–333, 1998.

McFee RB, Mofenson HC, Caraccio TR: A nationwide survey of the management of unintentional low dose tricyclic antidepressant ingestions involving asymptomatic children: Implications for the development of evidence-based clinical guideline. *Clin Toxicol* 38:15–19, 2000.

Teece S, Hogg K, Mackway-Jones K: Gastric lavage in tricyclic antidepressant overdose. *Emerg Med J* 20:64, 2003.

QUESTIONS

1. The cardiovascular toxicity of tricyclic antidepressants is due to which of the following pharmacologic effects?
   A. Quinidine-like effect
   B. Anticholinergic side effects
   C. Blockade of norepinephrine reuptake
   D. Alpha-adrenergic blockade
   E. All of the above

2. A 30-year-old depressed patient is brought to the ED 2 h after reportedly ingesting an unknown quantity of amitriptyline. On presentation, she is alert with stable vital signs and has no complaints. She now denies ingestion. Which of the following statements regarding her expected ED course and management is correct?
   A. Her mental status, symptomatology, and cardiac rhythm should be observed for 6 h and if no abnormality is detected, she can safely be discharged pending psychiatric evaluation.
   B. Since there is no change in mental status or cardiac rhythm on presentation, she is unlikely to develop a problem and she can be safely referred to Psychiatry without further medical attention.
   C. She must be admitted for continued observation since toxic effects are often delayed for up to 24 h.
   D. Activated charcoal is unlikely to be effective since the patient did not present within 1 h of reported ingestion.
   E. In spite of the delayed presentation, ipecac for induction of emesis is indicated to reduce the load of potentially highly toxic drug.

3. A 16-year-old boy is brought to the ED by his parents after taking 20 to 30 amitriptyline tablets that belonged to his mother. On presentation, his airway is clear but he is somnolent. Blood pressure is 90/50, pulse rate is 130, and respiratory rate is 20. His temperature is 101°F. An ECG is done and reveals tachycardia with wide QRS complexes. What is the most appropriate course of action?
   A. Initiate a dopamine drip at 2 to 5 µg/kg/min
   B. Administer activated charcoal, 50 g PO and continue to observe
   C. Intubate, hyperventilate, and administer sodium bicarbonate, 1 to 2 mg/kg as a bolus, followed by an infusion of sodium bicarbonate in D_5W
   D. Physostigmine, 0.02 mg/kg slow IV push
   E. Phenytoin, 18 mg/kg IV over 1 h as a prophylaxis for seizures

ANSWERS

1. E. The quinidine-like effect is responsible for cardiac dysrhythmias but the anticholinergic effects, blockage

of norepinephrine reuptake, and alpha blockage all contribute to the tachycardia and hypertension.

2. A. The majority of patients who develop life-threatening problems do so within 2 h of arrival in the ED. Toxic patients are likely to arrive appearing clinically stable and then may suddenly deteriorate. If no toxic effects are observed during a 6-h period of observation, medical monitoring can be discontinued. Psychiatric evaluation is indicated to assess for the suicide risk. Ipecac is contraindicated due to the risk for sudden deterioration, but charcoal is indicated even for delayed presentations, since the anticholinergic effects of the drug results in decreased gut motility.

3. C. If the QRS complex is greater than 100 ms, most investigators agree that alkalinization is indicated. This can be accomplished by a combination of intubation and hyperventilation, along with IV bicarbonate. The goal of alkalinization is to achieve a pH between 7.45 and 7.50. The initial approach to hypotension is fluid administration, followed by pressors if fluids are ineffective. There is a theoretical advantage to norepinephrine over dopamine due to its ability to reverse the alpha blockade caused by the drug. Seizures are usually self-limited and may not require treatment. Phenytoin is not effective prophylactically. Physostigmine should be reserved for patients who do not respond to first-line therapy for seizures, dysrhythmias, or severe hypertension.

92 DIGOXIN TOXICITY

Steven E. Aks
Jerrold B. Leikin
Gary R. Strange
Heather M. Prendergast

PHARMACOLOGY AND PATHOPHYSIOLOGY

- Digoxin is a positive inotrope that increases the force and velocity of myocardial contractions. In the failing heart, it can increase the cardiac output and decrease elevated end-diastolic pressures.
- On the cellular level, digoxin presumably functions by binding to and inactivating the Na^+-K^+ ATPase pump in the heart. This results in increased intracellular sodium concentration.
- There are numerous factors that predispose the patient to digoxin toxicity, the most common of which is electrolyte imbalance. Hyperkalemia in particular can result in significant conduction delays.

CLINICAL PRESENTATION

- The presentation of digoxin toxicity is highly varied, and depends largely on whether it results from an acute overdose or is a manifestation of chronic toxicity.
- Symptoms can be abrupt, with severe nausea, vomiting, and diarrhea. Associated complaints include weakness, headache, paresthesias, and altered color perception. Cardiovascular symptoms include palpitations and dizziness that may be secondary to hypotension.
- Patients with chronic toxicity tend to have more vague complaints, though many of the symptoms of acute overdose also occur. Malaise, anorexia, and low-grade nausea and vomiting are common.
- Cardiovascular toxicity is the most important factor in determining morbidity and mortality.
  - There are multiple dysrhythmias associated with digoxin toxicity, the most common being frequent premature ventricular beats. Other dysrhythmias can be supraventricular, nodal, or ventricular. Common disturbances are junctional escape beats and accelerated junctional rhythm, paroxysmal atrial tachycardia with AV block, and AV block of varying degrees. There is no single pathognomonic rhythm.

DIAGNOSIS

- A history of the exact amount of digoxin ingested is extremely helpful. A dose greater than 0.1 mg/kg has been suggested as an indication for the use of digoxin-specific Fab fragments.
- A digoxin level is indicated whenever there is clinical suspicion of toxicity.
  - In an overdose situation, the level is most accurate if obtained at 6 or more h after the ingestion.
  - The therapeutic digoxin range is between 0.8 and 1.8 ng/mL. Unfortunately, there is poor correlation between the digoxin level and clinical manifestations.
  - In a chronic overdose, toxicity can occur at lower levels.
- Other necessary laboratory studies include a complete blood count, serum electrolytes, calcium, magnesium, blood urea nitrogen, and creatinine.
- Cardiac monitoring is essential, as is a 12-lead electrocardiogram.

MANAGEMENT

- Digoxin-intoxicated patients can be highly unstable. All patients require a secure airway, intravenous access, and cardiac monitoring.

GASTRIC DECONTAMINATION

- Gastric lavage is indicated after an adequate airway is assured, which may require intubation.
- Activated charcoal along with a cathartic is indicated as a single dose.

ANTIDOTAL THERAPY

- Digoxin immune Fab fragments (Digibind) are specific antidigoxin antibodies derived from sheep. To decrease the risk of immunogenicity, only the Fab fragment is used. Specific indications include:
  ◦ Ingestion of greater than 0.1 mg/kg
  ◦ Digoxin level of greater than 5.0 ng/ml
  ◦ Presence of a life-threatening dysrhythmia
- Allergic reactions to Fab fragments are rare. Skin testing can be performed, but is usually not necessary.
- In addition to the administration of Fab fragments, standard treatment of dysrhythmias or AV blocks is indicated.
  ◦ Atropine or temporary pacing may be necessary to temporize while Fab fragments are taking effect.
  ◦ Cardioversion and lidocaine are appropriate in the event of ventricular tachycardia or fibrillation.
  ◦ Treatment with intravenous phenytoin or magnesium sulfate has been shown to be particularly useful in digoxin-induced tachydysrhythmias.
  ◦ Drugs to avoid in the treatment of digoxin-induced cardiac toxicity include calcium, sotalol, isoproterenol, and quinidine.
  ◦ Direct-current cardioversion should only be used as a last resort for life-threatening arrhythmia. If utilized, it should be dosed at the lowest energy possible.

DISPOSITION

- Children with trivial ingestions who are asymptomatic and have no detectable levels of digoxin 4h after the ingestion can be discharged from the emergency department after 6h of observation.

BIBLIOGRAPHY

Eddleston M, Rajapapakse S, Rajakanthan S, et al: Antidigoxin Fab fragments in cardiotoxicity induced by ingestion of yellow oleander: A randomized controlled trial. *Lancet* 355: 967–972, 2000.

Kinlay S, Buckley NA: Magnesium sulfate in the treatment of ventricular arrhythmias due to digoxin toxicity. *J Toxicol Clin Toxicol* 33:55, 1995.

Litovitz TL, Klein-Schwartz W, White S, et al: 1999 Annual Report of Poison Control Centers toxic exposure surveillance system. *Am J Emerg Med* 18:517–574, 2000.

Sekkul EA, Kaminer S, Sethi KD: Digoxin-induced chorea in a child. *Mov Disord* 14:877–879, 1999.

Valdes R Jr, Jortani SA: Monitoring of unbound digoxin in patients treated with anti-digoxin antigen-binding fragments: A model for the future? *Clin Chem* 44:183–185, 1998.

Williamson KM, Thrasher KA, Fulton KB, et al: Digoxin toxicity: An evaluation in current clinical practice. *Arch Intern Med* 158:2444–2449, 1998.

QUESTIONS

1. A 10-year-old child is brought to the emergency department for severe nausea, vomiting, and diarrhea. The parents are concerned because the child is on digoxin. Symptoms began 2 days after having the dosage increased. On examination, you find a mildly dehydrated but otherwise normal-appearing child. Which of the following is the **MOST** appropriate management?
   A. Obtain a stat digoxin level, if within therapeutic range, brief ED observation and discharge is all that is required.
   B. Obtain a stat digoxin level and administer charcoal; observe in ED for 6h and discharge to home if stable
   C. Obtain a stat digoxin level, begin supportive care, and admit for 23-h observation regardless of level
   D. Obtain a stat level, begin treatment with digoxin-specific Fab fragments, and admit for 23-h observation
   E. Obtain a stat level, perform a gastric lavage, and admit for 23-h observation

2. Which of the following is the **MOST** common dysrhythmia associated with digoxin toxicity?
   A. Multifocal atrial tachycardia
   B. Second degree AV block
   C. Premature ventricular beats
   D. Supraventricular tachycardia
   E. Paroxysmal atrial tachycardia with AV block

3. A 5-year-old is brought by paramedics after ingestion of an unknown quantity of his grandmother's digoxin. On arrival to the ED, the child is hypotensive, weak, and pale-appearing. You recognize the patient is unstable and immediately secure the airway, obtain intravenous access, and begin cardiac monitoring. Which of the following would **NOT** be recommended in management of digoxin toxicity?

A. Gastric lavage
B. Activated charcoal
C. Digoxin immune Fab fragments
D. Calcium gluconate
E. Atropine

ANSWERS

1. C. A digoxin level is indicated whenever there is clinical suspicion of toxicity. The therapeutic digoxin range is between 0.8 and 1.8 ng/mL. However, there is poor correlation between the digoxin level and clinical manifestations. Cardiac monitoring is essential for patients with signs and symptoms suggestive of digoxin toxicity.
2. C. There are multiple dysrhythmias associated with digoxin toxicity; however, the most common is frequent premature ventricular beats.
3. D. Patients with digoxin toxicity can be very unstable. Drugs to avoid in the treatment of digoxin-induced cardiac toxicity include calcium, sotalol, isoproterenol, and quinidine.

93 FISH POISONING

Timothy Erickson
Gary R. Strange
Heather M. Prendergast

INTRODUCTION

- Hazardous marine life can be classified into four major groups:
  - Venomous bites and stings, such as those inflicted by scorpion fish and the Portuguese man-of-war
  - Shock injuries, as from electric eels
  - Traumatogenic bites (sharks and barracudas)
  - Toxic ingestions or fish poisoning
    - Ciguatoxin
    - Scombrotoxin
    - Paralytic shellfish saxitoxin
    - Tetrodotoxin

CIGUATERA

PATHOPHYSIOLOGY

- Ciguatera fish poisoning is a serious public health problem in the Caribbean and Indo-Pacific regions.

- Ciguatoxin is produced by a dinoflagellate, *Gambierdiscus toxicus*, and concentrated in the food chain of predator reef fish such as barracuda, grouper, red snapper, parrotfish, jacks, and moray eels.
- When humans ingest contaminated fish, poisoning can cause distinct neurological and gastrointestinal symptomatology, due to the toxin's anticholinesterase activity.

CLINICAL PRESENTATION

- Within hours of ingestion, the patient may complain of neurologic symptoms such as circumoral tingling, headache, tremor, diffuse paresthesias, and classically, reversal of hot and cold sensations. Younger children may only present with discomfort and irritability.
- The patient also commonly suffers gastrointestinal symptoms, such as watery diarrhea, vomiting, and abdominal cramping, making it difficult to differentiate from typical pediatric gastroenteritis.
- Potentially fatal cardiovascular manifestations such as severe bradycardia, hypotension, and respiratory depression are possible but uncommon.

MANAGEMENT

- Treatment of ciguatera poisoning is primarily supportive.
- If the child presents within 1 hour of ingestion of the suspected fish and has not already vomited, decontamination with gastric lavage followed by activated charcoal is indicated.

SCOMBROTOXIN

PATHOPHYSIOLOGY

- Scombroid poisoning is a food-borne illness associated with the consumption of improperly handled dark-meat fish, such as tuna, bonito, skipjack, mackerel, and mahimahi (dolphin fish). Unlike ciguatoxin, scombrotoxin is not contracted from the marine environment but rather directly from the flesh of the fish, which has undergone bacterial decomposition due to improper refrigeration.

CLINICAL PRESENTATION

- Within minutes to hours following ingestion of a fish containing scombrotoxin, the patient experiences a histamine-like syndrome with diffuse erythema, pruritus, urticaria, dysphagia, and headache.

MANAGEMENT

- Although scombroid poisoning is typically self-limited, supportive measures and fluid resuscitation are indicated, as is gastric decontamination if the ingestion was recent.
- Antihistamines such as diphenhydramine have been reported to shorten the duration of symptoms. Intravenous infusion of a histamine H_2-receptor antagonist such as cimetidine has proven effective in patients with inadequate responses to diphenhydramine.

PARALYTIC SHELLFISH POISONING

PATHOPHYSIOLOGY

- Specific neurotoxic species of the dinoflagellate *Gonyaulax* form red tides and concentrate the toxin saxitoxin in bivalve shellfish such as mussels, clams, and scallops. Humans who consume contaminated shellfish can develop profound muscle weakness via a curare-like effect mediated through blockage of sodium conduction channels.

CLINICAL PRESENTATION

- Gastrointestinal symptoms may develop within minutes to hours after ingestion, with vomiting, diarrhea, and abdominal cramping.
- The patient may experience headache, ataxia, facial paresthesias, and on rare occasions muscle paralysis resulting in respiratory paralysis up to 12 hours after ingestion.

MANAGEMENT

- Supportive measures include fluid resuscitation, and in recent ingestions gastric decontamination.
- If paralytic shellfish poisoning is suspected, the patient is admitted for a 24-hour period for observation for respiratory depression.

TETRODOTOXIN

PATHOPHYSIOLOGY

- Tetrodotoxin, one of the most potent poisons known, results in poisoning after the ingestion of the puffer fish, California newt, Eastern salamander, or blue-ringed octopus.

- Intoxication produces profound neurologic symptoms and muscle weakness due to its inhibition of the sodium-potassium pump and subsequent blockade of neuromuscular transmission.
- In some reported studies mortality rates have approached 60 percent.

CLINICAL PRESENTATION

- Symptoms following ingestion of fish or amphibians containing tetrodotoxin begin within 30 minutes of ingestion.
- Early manifestations include circumoral and throat paresthesias.
- These findings are followed by GI complaints of vomiting and abdominal cramping.
- If the patient has consumed a large amount of the toxin, within minutes to hours they may experience a "feeling of doom" heralding ascending paralysis, respiratory depression, dilated pupils, hypotension, bradycardia, and a classic "locked-in" or zombie-like syndrome.
- Death results from either respiratory paralysis or cardiovascular collapse.
- Typically, if the patient survives beyond 24 hours, recovery occurs.

MANAGEMENT

- Treatment includes rapid stabilization and gastric decontamination with gastric lavage.
- Atropine has been recommended for bradycardia and hypotension.
- Edrophonium and neostigmine may be beneficial in restoring motor strength.
- Most importantly, the patient's airway and respiratory status should be supported aggressively.

BIBLIOGRAPHY

Attaran RR, Probst F: Histamine fish poisoning: A common but frequently misdiagnosed condition. *Emerg Med J* 19:474–475, 2002.

Isbister GK, Son J, Wang F, et al: Puffer fish poisoning: a potentially life-threatening condition. *Med J Aust* 177:650–653, 2002.

McInerney J, Shagal P, Bogel M: Scombroid poisoning. *Ann Emerg Med* 8:235, 1996.

Shoff WH, Shepherd SM: Scombroid, ciguatera, and other seafood intoxications. In: Ford M, Delaney K, Ling L, et al, eds. *Clinical Toxicology*, Philadelphia: Saunders, 959–969, 2001.

Swift AE, Swift TR: Ciguatera. *Clin Toxicol* 31:1–29, 1993.

QUESTIONS

1. A 5-year-old is brought to the emergency department for evaluation of watery diarrhea and gastrointestinal upset without vomiting. While obtaining the history, you learn that the family has just returned from a Caribbean vacation where the family enjoyed a variety of seafood. Which of the following would be an indication for aggressive treatment?
   A. Blood-tinged stools
   B. Circumoral tingling
   C. Paraesthesias
   D. Abdominal cramping
   E. Presentation within 1 hour of ingestion

2. A 9-year-old is brought to the ED for evaluation of an allergic reaction. Parents report the child was eating a tuna steak sandwich from an outdoor seafood vendor when he developed diffuse erythema, pruritus, and urticaria. The parents deny any previous episodes. On arrival, the child has no respiratory complaints. Based on the symptoms, the patient has MOST LIKELY ingested which of the following?
   A. Ciguatera toxin
   B. Scrombrotoxin
   C. Paralytic shellfish poisoning
   D. Tetrodotoxin
   E. Gambierdiscus toxicus

3. A 14-year-old boy is brought to the emergency department for evaluation of gastrointestinal symptoms and a mild headache. You learn that the symptoms began 2 hours after eating scallops from a local vendor. You recall several cases earlier that day involving seafood obtained from the same vendor. You suspect paralytic shellfish poisoning. What is the MOST appropriate management?
   A. Decontamination with gastric lavage and activated charcoal
   B. Fluid resuscitation
   C. Intravenous antihistamines
   D. Admit for 24 hour observation
   E. Extended ED observation for a minimum of 6 hours

4. Which of the following mechanisms is responsible for the toxicity seen with the tetrodotoxin?
   A. Inhibition of the sodium-potassium pump
   B. Anticholinesterase activity
   C. Inhibition of the calcium channels
   D. Stimulation of the dopamine receptors
   E. Selective uptake of serotonin

ANSWERS

1. E. The child has most likely ingested contaminated fish. Ciguatera fish poisoning is a serious health problem in the Caribbean and Indo-Pacific regions. Younger children tend to have presentations of gastrointestinal symptoms. Other symptoms include circumoral tingling, headache, tremor, paraesthesias, and reversal of hot and cold sensations. Treatment is primarily supportive unless the patient presents within 1 hour of ingestion and has not vomited.

2. B. Scromroid poisoning is commonly associated with a histamine-like syndrome with diffuse erythema, pruritus, urticaria, dysphagia, and headache. Scombroid poisoning is typically self-limited. Antihistamines have been shown to be beneficial.

3. D. In a patient with suspected paralytic shellfish poisoning, admission for a 24-hour period for observation for respiratory depression is recommended.

4. A. Tetrodotoxin intoxication causes profound neurologic symptoms and muscle weakness due to its inhibition of the sodium-potassium pump and subsequent blockade of neuromuscular transmission.

94 HYDROCARBONS

Bonnie McManus
Gary R. Strange
Patricia Lee

INTRODUCTION

- There are three major classes of hydrocarbons.
  - The aliphatic, or straight-chain compounds, include kerosene, mineral seal oil, gasoline, solvents, and paint thinners. Aliphatic compounds include halogenated hydrocarbons, such as carbon tetrachloride and trichloroethane, which are typically found in industrial settings as solvents. The halogenated hydrocarbons are well absorbed by the lung and gut, making them particularly dangerous. Centrilobular hepatic necrosis and renal failure are associated with ingestion of halogenated hydrocarbons, especially carbon tetrachloride. Fatal liver injury has been reported after ingestion of as little as 3 mL of carbon tetrachloride.
  - The cyclic or aromatic compounds contain a benzene ring and are used in industrial solvents. The aromatics are highly volatile, and unlike the straight-chain hydrocarbons, benzene and its major derivatives toluene and xylene are well absorbed from the gastrointestinal tract. Of the aromatics, benzene is the most toxic, with death reported after ingestion of as little as 15 mL.
  - The terpene compounds consist mainly of cyclic terpene rings and include compounds such as turpentine and pine oil.

- Viscosity, volatility, and surface tension are physical properties that affect the type and extent of toxicity.
  - *Viscosity* is defined as the resistance to flow, and is the most important property in determining the risk of aspiration.
  - *Volatility* describes the propensity of a substance to become a gas.
  - *Surface tension* describes the propensity of a compound to adhere to itself at the liquid's surface.
- Gaseous hydrocarbons such as methane and butane can act as asphyxiants by displacing air in the lungs and causing hypoxia.

PATHOPHYSIOLOGY

- The principal concern after most hydrocarbon ingestions is pulmonary toxicity. The lungs are spared unless there is direct contact with the hydrocarbon via aspiration.
- Fever is seen on presentation in 30 percent of cases. It does not correlate with clinical symptoms and is possibly of central origin.
- Many anticholinesterase pesticides are combined with kerosene vehicles.
  - A cholinergic crisis is likely in patients with excessive bronchorrhea, salivation, lacrimation, or urinary incontinence. The classic bradycardia and miosis may be obscured by the tachycardia and mydriasis from hydrocarbon-induced hypoxia.

CLINICAL PRESENTATION

- A history of coughing or gagging is consistent with aspiration. In addition to cough, early signs of pulmonary toxicity include gasping, choking, tachypnea, and wheezing. Bronchospasm may contribute to ventilation-perfusion mismatch and exacerbate hypoxia.
- In any patient with a history of hydrocarbon ingestion, it is essential to try to identify the compound, since this information can have profound implications for management and prognosis.

MANAGEMENT

- The mainstay of treatment for hydrocarbon exposure is supportive care.
- Airway patency is evaluated and established. Intravenous lines and cardiac monitors are indicated in symptomatic patients. Any patient with respiratory symptoms, including grunting, tachypnea, or cyanosis, is treated with humidified oxygen and requires an arterial blood gas evaluation.

GASTRIC EVACUATION

- Currently, gastric evacuation is not recommended in patients with minimal or no symptoms after ingestion of a pure petroleum distillate or turpentine.
- Gastric evacuation of most types of hydrocarbons is reserved for massive ingestions, which usually occur in adults or adolescents involved in a suicide attempt.
  - While still controversial, ingestions of 4 to 5 mL/kg of naphtha, gasoline, kerosene, or turpentine should probably be removed.
  - Other ingestions in which gastric evacuation is indicated are for those that contain dangerous additives such as benzene, toluene, halogenated hydrocarbons, heavy metals, camphor, pesticides, aniline, or other toxic compounds.
- Currently there is no overwhelming support for either emesis with ipecac or gastric lavage as a superior mode of gastric evacuation.
  - In the awake, alert patient with an intact gag reflex, ipecac is appropriate.
  - Emesis is contraindicated if there is previous unprovoked emesis or any degree of neurologic, respiratory, or cardiac compromise. In these cases gastric lavage is indicated after endotracheal intubation with a cuffed tube. If the child is younger than 8 years old, inflate the cuff only during lavage.
  - Activated charcoal is not indicated in the vast majority of hydrocarbon ingestions.

LABORATORY STUDIES

- In about 90 percent of patients with respiratory symptoms on presentation, the initial chest radiograph will be abnormal. Radiographic abnormalities can occur as early as 20 minutes or as late as 24 hours after ingestion.

DISPOSITION

- A patient who accidentally ingests a hydrocarbon and presents to the emergency department without symptoms should be observed for 6 hours. If during that time they remain asymptomatic and oxygen saturation and a chest radiograph are normal, discharge is appropriate.

VOLATILE SUBSTANCE ABUSE

- Among adolescents, inhalation abuse of volatile hydrocarbons is a significant health hazard. Typically, solvent-containing fluids such as typewriter correction fluid and adhesives, and other halogenated hydrocarbons, such as those found in gasoline and cigarette lighter fluid, are abused.

- The predominant acute risk of inhalation abuse is "sudden sniffing death." It is believed that the myocardium is hypersensitized and a sudden outpouring of sympathetic stimulation leads to fatal cardiac dysrhythmias.

- As with alcohol, acute poisoning with volatile substances involves an initial period of euphoria and disinhibition, with further intoxication leading to dysphoria, ataxia, confusion, and hallucinations. There is rapid onset and recovery, but repeated inhalations can prolong the altered state.

BIBLIOGRAPHY

Esmail A, Meyer L, Pottier A, et al: Deaths from volatile substance abuse in those under 18 years: Results from a national epidemiological study. *Arch Dis Child* 69:356, 1993.

Goldfrank LR, Kulgberg AG, Bresnitz EA: Hydrocarbons. In: Goldfrank LR, Flomenbaum NE, Lewin NA, et al, eds. *Goldfrank's Toxicologic Emergencies.* Norwalk, CT, Appleton & Lange, 1383–1398, 1998.

Litovitz TL, Klein-Schwartz W, White S, et al: 1999 Annual report of the American Association of Poison Control Centers toxic exposure surveillance system. *Am J Emerg Med* 18:517, 2000.

Widmer LR, Goodwin SR, Berman LS, et al: Artificial surfactant for therapy in hydrocarbon-induced lung injury in sheep. *Crit Care Med* 24:1524–1529, 1996.

QUESTIONS

1. The most important property in determining the risk of aspiration is:
   A. Volatility
   B. Surface tension
   C. Viscosity
   D. Molecular weight
   E. Type of hydrocarbon

2. The principle concern after most hydrocarbon ingestions is which target organ?
   A. Liver
   B. Bone marrow
   C. Intestines
   D. Lungs
   E. Skin

3. Management of a symptomatic patient with a moderate hydrocarbon ingestion may include all of the following except:
   A. Gastric lavage
   B. Activated charcoal
   C. Arterial blood gas
   D. Intubation
   E. Ipecac

4. A patient who accidentally ingests a hydrocarbon and presents to the emergency department without symptoms may be discharged home if all of the following are true EXCEPT:
   A. Abnormal chest radiography
   B. ED observation for 6 hours
   C. Normal pulse oximetry
   D. Normal mental status
   E. Normal respiratory examination

5. A 17-year-old male is brought to the ED in full cardiopulmonary arrest. On examination an odor of gasoline is noted to his clothes. The most likely cause of death is:
   A. Cardiac dysrhythmia
   B. Hydrocarbon ingestion
   C. Cardiac ischemia
   D. Opiate overdose
   E. Prolonged QT syndrome

ANSWERS

1. C. Viscosity is defined as the resistance to flow, and is the most important property in determining the risk of aspiration.

2. D. The principle concern after most hydrocarbon ingestions is pulmonary toxicity. The lungs are spared unless there is direct contact with the hydrocarbon via aspiration. In addition to cough, early signs of pulmonary toxicity include gasping, choking, tachypnea, and wheezing.

3. B. Activated charcoal is not indicated in most hydrocarbon ingestions. Gastric evacuation is reserved for massive ingestions. Ipecac should be reserved for alert patients with an intact gag reflex.

4. A. A person who accidentally ingests a hydrocarbon and presents to the emergency department without symptoms should be observed for 6 hours. If during that time they remain asymptomatic and oxygen saturation and a chest radiograph are normal, discharge is appropriate.

5. A. The predominant acute risk of inhalation abuse is "sudden sniffing death." It is believed that the myocardium is hypersensitized and a sudden outpouring of sympathetic stimulation leads to fatal cardiac dysrhythmias.

95 IRON POISONING

Steven E. Aks
Gary R. Strange
Patricia Lee

INTRODUCTION

- Iron is one of the most important pediatric toxins. It is an extremely common cause of poisoning and has a high potential for morbidity and mortality.
- The FDA has required unit dose packaging (blister-packs) for most products containing more than 30 mg of elemental iron per tablet. This new packaging of iron supplements is expected to decrease the frequency of pediatric iron overdose incidents.

PATHOPHYSIOLOGY

- Iron is absorbed through the gastrointestinal mucosa in the ferrous (Fe^{2+}) state. It is oxidized to the ferric (Fe^{3+}) state and attaches to ferritin.
- Toxicity occurs when ferritin and transferrin are saturated, and serum iron exceeds the total iron binding capacity (TIBC). Circulating free iron can damage blood vessels and can cause transudation of fluids from the intravascular space, resulting in hypotension.

CLINICAL PRESENTATION

- It is useful to attempt to identify the exact preparation, since content of elemental iron, which is the toxic ingredient, varies. If the preparation is identified, the number of pills ingested is important information, since the ratio of elemental iron ingested to the weight of the patient is critical in estimating the potential for toxicity (Table 95-1).
- It is useful to describe iron overdose in terms of the known stages of toxicity.
  - Stage 1 begins at the time of ingestion and lasts for about 6 h. More severe ingestions suffer vomiting, diarrhea, hematemesis, altered mental status, and possibly hypotension.
  - Stage 2 occurs from about 6 to 12 h postingestion, and is referred to as the quiescent or "danger" phase because the patient can appear to be improving, or may even be asymptomatic.
  - Stage 3, from about 12 to 24 h postingestion, is marked by the patient exhibiting major signs of toxicity.
    - Gastrointestinal hemorrhage
    - Cardiovascular collapse

TABLE 95-1   Iron Preparations

IRON PREPARATION	ELEMENTAL IRON (%)
Ferrous sulfate	20
Ferrous fumarate	33
Ferrous gluconate	12

INGESTED DOSE (mg/kg)	TREATMENT RECOMMENDATION
<20	Dilute and observe
20–40 mg/kg	Ipecac at home and observe
>40 mg/kg	Refer to health care facility

  - Altered mental status, ranging from lethargy to coma
  - Renal failure
  - Hepatic failure
  - Severe metabolic acidosis
  - Stage 4 is a latent phase in which the patient has recovered from the acute insult. It occurs 4 to 6 weeks after the ingestion when the patient develops symptoms due to strictures that develop in the gastrointestinal tract as a result of formation of scar tissue.

DIAGNOSIS

- Iron levels can be obtained between 2 and 6 h after ingestion, but are optimally drawn at 4 h postingestion.
  - A level greater than 300 to 350 µg/dL is considered toxic.
  - Levels greater than 500 µg/dL suggest potentially life-threatening toxicity.
- Abdominal radiographs can locate iron-containing tablets in the gut, and may reveal the presence of concretions.
  - If pills are identified, the patient is at risk for delayed absorption of iron.
  - Obtaining serial levels every 2 to 4 h until the iron level peaks is appropriate.
  - A positive radiograph after gastric lavage has recently been suggested as an indication for whole bowel irrigation.
- Deferoxamine is a compound that chelates free iron.
- The deferoxamine challenge test can be administered to patients who have ingested an unknown or borderline quantity of iron.
  - The challenge is conducted by administering 40 to 90 mg/kg intramuscularly of deferoxamine, up to a maximum of 1 g in children and 2 g in adults.
  - Classically, a positive test is indicated by the patient's urine developing a "vin rose" color 4 to 6 h after receiving deferoxamine.

However, the classical appearance is seen in a minority of patients. A subtle change in the color of the urine may be more easily detected by obtaining a baseline urine specimen prior to administering the challenge. Even a slight change in color to an orange or red indicates a positive test.

TREATMENT

GASTRIC EMPTYING

- Since neither activated charcoal nor any other substance is capable of absorbing iron in the gastrointestinal tract, gastric emptying is the sole method of gut decontamination.
- While syrup of ipecac can be used in children older than 6 months of age, there is a trend toward gastric lavage for patients in whom it is technically feasible.
- Lavage is performed with saline. Previous recommendations included adding bicarbonate to the lavage solution, since it was felt it would bind iron and make it insoluble and easier to remove. This has not been shown to be effective in the clinical setting.
- Whole bowel irrigation with polyethylene glycol electrolyte solution should be initiated if pills are noted on abdominal radiographs after gastric lavage.

CHELATION

- Chelation with deferoxamine is used for significant iron ingestions. Standard indications for therapy include a peak iron level of 300 to 350 µg/dL or a patient who exhibits signs of toxicity in the absence of an available iron level.
  - Deferoxamine is administered at 6 h intervals.
  - The intramuscular dose is 90 mg/kg/dose, with a maximum single dose in children not to exceed 1 g.
  - Intravenous administration is indicated for patients with moderate to severe toxicity.
  - Hypotension is the most common side effect of intravenous therapy, and can usually be treated by slowing down the drip or making the solution more dilute.
  - The end point of chelation is reached when the color of the patient's urine returns to normal.

DISPOSITION

- Children with peak serum iron levels less than 300 µg/dL approximately 4 h post-ingestion and without symptoms of toxicity may be discharged in the care of reliable caretakers.

BIBLIOGRAPHY

Ben Mokhtar H, Thabet H, Brahmi N, et al: Acute iron poisoning. *Vet Hum Toxicol* 44:219–220, 2002.
Black J, Zenal JA: Child abuse by intentional iron poisoning presenting as shock and persistent acidosis. *Pediatrics* 111: 197–199, 2003.
Morris CC: Pediatric iron poisonings in the United States. *South Med J* 93:352–358, 2000.

QUESTIONS

1. A 2-year-old girl is brought to the Emergency Department 6 h after ingestion of 30 chewable vitamins with iron. The parents state that several hours after ingestion, the child vomited once but now appears to be improved. Your advice to the parents should be:
   A. The danger period is over. The child will do well.
   B. The child is in the danger phase.
   C. If no pills are identified by abdominal radiograph, the child is in no danger.
   D. The child should be lavaged.
   E. Activated charcoal should be given the child.
2. Iron levels which suggest life-threatening toxicity are:
   A. Greater than 100 to 200 µg/dL
   B. Greater than 200 to 300 µg/dL
   C. Greater than 300 to 400 µg/dL
   D. Greater than 400 to 500 µg/dL
   E. Greater than 500 µg/dL
3. All of the following are true regarding deferoxamine **EXCEPT:**
   A. Indicated if a peak iron level of 300 to 350 µg/dL
   B. Administered at 6 h intervals
   C. Intravenous administration is used for severe toxicity.
   D. The end point of chelation is when the color of the patient's urine turns from yellow to red.
   E. Hypotension is a common side effect of intravenous therapy.

ANSWERS

1. B. Stage 1 of iron toxicity begins at time of ingestion and lasts for 6 hours. Severe ingestions may present with vomiting, diarrhea, hematemesis, altered mental status, and possibly hypotension. Stage 2 occurs at 6 to 12 h postingestion and is referred to as the quiescent or "danger" phase because the child can appear to be improving or asymptomatic. Stage 3 from 12 to 24 h,

is marked by major symptoms of toxicity including bleeding, cardiovascular collapse, altered mental status, renal and hepatic failure and metabolic acidosis. Stage 4 is a latent or recovery phase. Although iron pills may be identified by radiograph, the physician should not rely on the absence of pill identification to continue treatment. Time of presentation of this child is too late for lavage. Lavage must be done within 1 to 2 h postingestion to be effective. Activated charcoal is not effective in absorbing iron in the gastrointestinal tract.

2. E. A level greater than 300 to 350 μg/dL is considered toxic but levels greater than 500 μg/dL suggest potentially life-threatening toxicity.

3. D. The end point of chelation is reached when the color of the patient's urine turns from wine red to yellow (normal).

96 ISONIAZID TOXICITY

Timothy J. Rittenberry
Michael Green
Gary R. Strange
Heather M. Prendergast

PHARMACOLOGY

• The metabolic degradation of isoniazid (INH) is complex and occurs primarily via hepatic acetylation. The ability to inactivate INH via acetylation is genetically determined in an autosomal dominant fashion, resulting in two groups of patients: fast acetylators and slow acetylators, the latter being autosomal recessive for the acetylation gene. Fifty to sixty percent of the American population undergoes slow acetylation.

PATHOPHYSIOLOGY

• INH is an inhibitor of several cytochrome P450-mediated functions, such as demethylation, oxidation, and hydroxylation.
• Its inhibition of pyridoxine phosphokinase impairs conversion of pyridoxine to the physiologically active pyridoxal phosphate, a necessary cofactor in the formation of the inhibitory brain peptide gamma aminobutyric acid (GABA).
• INH also combines with most active forms of pyridoxine, forming inactive INH-pyridoxal hydrazones, which undergo renal excretion.

• Pyridoxine depletion and reduced GABA levels in the brain lead to the lower seizure threshold seen in acute INH toxicity.
• The toxic dose of INH is highly variable.

CLINICAL PRESENTATION OF ACUTE TOXICITY

• Due to its rapid gastrointestinal absorption, symptoms can occur within 30 min of ingestion.
• Nausea, vomiting, dizziness, ataxia, slurred speech, and tachycardia may be quickly followed by metabolic acidosis, generalized seizures, and coma.
• The clinical triad of seizures, coma, and metabolic acidosis refractory to bicarbonate therapy should alert the emergency physician to the possibility of INH ingestion.
• INH toxicity should be strongly considered in any child or adolescent that presents with seizures who is undergoing treatment with or has access to INH.

TREATMENT

STABILIZATION

• In the symptomatic patient with an INH overdose, aggressive supportive care and monitoring is necessary.
• In the patient presenting with protracted seizures or coma, endotracheal intubation is indicated.

DECONTAMINATION

• Even in asymptomatic patients, the induction of emesis is not recommended, since seizures may occur abruptly and without warning.
• Gastric lavage performed within 1 h of ingestion is useful in achieving gut decontamination, with the contents sent for toxicologic analysis.
• Activated charcoal and a cathartic, such as sorbitol, are then administered to further decrease absorption.

ANTIDOTAL THERAPY

• The mainstay of treatment in INH toxicity is pyridoxine.
  ○ If the INH dose is known, an equal dose of pyridoxine on a gram-for-gram basis is administered over 5 to 10 min.
  ○ If the dose of INH is unknown, pyridoxine is given initially at 70 mg/kg up to a total of 5 g and repeated in 15 min for the persistently comatose or convulsing patient.

- Commonly used anticonvulsants alone may be ineffective in controlling INH-induced seizures. However, there is evidence that benzodiazepines may act synergistically with pyridoxine and have a protective effect.
- Hemodialysis, hemoperfusion, and exchange transfusion have all been described as useful, but are reserved for the most severe, refractory cases or for patients with renal failure.

DISPOSITION

- Patients with suspected INH poisoning who remain asymptomatic after 6 hours following ingestion or patients without a seizure disorder who have ingested less 20 mg/kg may be discharged from the ED.

BIBLIOGRAPHY

Ellenhorn MJ, Barceloux DG: Anti-infective drugs. In: Ellenhorn MJ, Barceloux DG, eds. *Ellenhorn's Medical Toxicology: Diagnosis and Treatment of Human Poisoning*, 2d ed. Baltimore, Williams & Wilkins, 240–243, 1997.

Litovitz TL, Klein-Schwartz W, White S, et al: 1999 Annual report of the American Association of Poison Control Centers toxic exposure surveillance system. *Am J Emerg Med* 8:517–574, 2000.

Osborn HH: Antituberculous agents. In: Goldfrank LR, Flomenbaum NE, Lewin NA, et al, eds. *Goldfrank's Toxicologic Emergencies*, 6th ed. Stamford, CT: Appleton & Lange, 727–733, 1998.

Romero JA, Kuczler FJ: Isoniazid overdose. Recognition and management. *Am Fam Physician* 57:749–752, 1998.

Shah BR, Santucci K, Sinert R, et al: Acute isoniazid neurotoxicity in an urban hospital. *Pediatrics* 95:700–704, 1995.

Shannon MW: Isoniazid. In: Haddad LM, Shannon MW, Winchester JF, eds. *Clinical Management of Drug Overdose*, 3d ed. Philadelphia: Saunders, 721–726, 1998.

Sullivan EA, Geoffrey P, Weisman R, et al: Isoniazid poisonings in New York City. *J Emerg Med* 16:57–59, 1998.

QUESTIONS

1. A 5-year-old child is brought to the emergency department following an unknown ingestion of his grandfather's medication. Open bottles of isoniazid and ibuprofen are found on the floor. Shortly after arrival, the child begins vomiting and complaining of dizziness. His speech is slurred. Which of the following would **NOT** be consistent with an acute toxicity secondary to isoniazid?

   A. Delirium
   B. Refractory seizures
   C. Refractory acidosis
   D. Ataxia
   E. Coma

2. You suspect isoniazid toxicity in a patient based on signs and symptoms on presentation. You immediately begin aggressive supportive care and monitoring. Which of the following reflects the correct usage of pyridoxine?

   A. 4 g of pyridoxine : 1 g of isoniazid
   B. 3 g of pyridoxine : 1 g of isoniazid
   C. 2 g of pyridoxine : 1 g of isoniazid
   D. 1 g of pyridoxine : 1 g of isoniazid
   E. In unknown ingestions, a minimum of 5 g of pyridoxine

ANSWERS

1. A. The toxic dose of isoniazid (INH) is highly variable. Due to its rapid gastrointestinal absorption, symptoms can occur within 30 min of ingestion. Clinical presentations include: nausea, vomiting, dizziness, ataxia, slurred speech, metabolic acidosis refractory to bicarbonate therapy, seizures, and coma.

2. D. In the symptomatic patient with INH overdose, aggressive supportive care and monitoring is mandatory. Endotracheal intubation is indicated for protracted seizures and coma. The mainstay of treatment in INH toxicity is pyridoxine. Pyridoxine should be given on a gram-for-gram basis over 5 to 10 min. In cases of unknown ingestion, pyridoxine should be given at 70 mg/kg up to a total of 5 g.

97   LEAD POISONING

Mark Mycyk
Yona Amatai
Daniel Hryhorczuk
Gary R. Strange
Valerie A. Dobiesz

INTRODUCTION

- The average blood lead level of American children has decreased by more than 80 percent since the 1970s because of early screening initiatives and hazard reduction. In spite of this progress, several long-term studies have shown an association of lead levels once thought to be nontoxic with impaired growth and behavioral and neurocognitive development.

SOURCES

- Ingestion of leaded paint is the most common and clinically relevant source of lead poisoning in children. Most homes built before 1978 were painted with lead-based paint. Renovation of old buildings and poorly controlled lead abatement pose a risk for lead poisoning through inhalation and ingestion of contaminated dust and soil.
- Lead exposure can occur through ingestion of drinking water contaminated by lead in plumbing.

PHARMACOKINETICS AND PATHOPHYSIOLOGY

- The absorption rate of lead through the gastrointestinal tract in infants and children is about 50 percent. Iron deficiency and dietary calcium deficiency increase the absorption of lead in the gut. Lead dust and fumes can also be absorbed through the respiratory tract.
- Lead toxicity results from interaction of lead with sulfhydryl and other ligands on enzymes and other macromolecules.
- The major target organs of lead are:
  - Bone marrow
  - Central nervous system
  - Peripheral nervous system
  - Kidneys.

CLINICAL MANIFESTATIONS

- Symptoms and signs of lead toxicity are often not noticeable or may be subtle and nonspecific.
- With the improvement in preventing childhood lead poisoning in the United States, the most likely cause for ED referral in such children is a high blood lead level (BLL) found during a screening program.
- Lead toxicity is grossly correlated with BLL (Table 97-1), but is more pronounced in young children and in those with prolonged exposure to lead.
- Overt lead encephalopathy may ensue after days or weeks of symptoms and present with ataxia, forceful vomiting, lethargy, or stupor, and can progress to coma and seizures.
- Since lead poisoning is so frequent and may present with a variety of signs and symptoms, a high index of suspicion is required. This is particularly true among populations at risk, such as inner city dwellers, African Americans, all children from low socioeconomic classes, and those who live in old houses that have been recently renovated.
- The differential diagnosis of lead poisoning includes iron deficiency, behavior and emotional disorders, abdominal colic and constipation, mental retardation, afebrile seizures, subdural hematoma, central nervous system neoplasms, sickle cell anemia, and Fanconi's syndrome.

TABLE 97-1   Class of Child, Toxic Effect, and Recommended Action According to Blood Lead Measurement

CLASS	BLOOD LEAD LEVEL (μg/dL)[a]	TOXIC EFFECT	RECOMMENDED ACTION
I	0–5	No noticeable effect	
	5–9	Inhibition of ALAD	
IIA	10–14		Rescreen every 3 months; educate parents
IIB	15–19	Inhibition of ferrochelatase	Retest in 2 months, nutritional and educational intervention, environmental investigation
III	20–44	Reduced growth, hearing, nerve conduction, neuropsychological deficits, reduced heme synthetase, increased EP, urine d-ALA	All of the above plus pharmacologic treatment: DMSA, penicillamine, or CaNa$_2$EDTA (following a positive lead mobilization test)
IV	45–69	Anemia, abdominal colic, reduced IQ, lead lines in x-ray	Immediate chelation: CaNa$_2$EDTA or DMSA
V	>70	Encephalopathy risk, nephropathy (>100 μg/dL)	Medical emergency: chelate with BAL plus EDTA, increased ICP precautions

[a] Conversion factor: 1.0 μg/dL = 0.04826 Mmol/L.
ALAD, aminolevulinic acid dehydratase; EP, erythrocyte protoporphyrin; ALA, aminolevulinic acid.
SOURCE: Adapted from Centers for Disease Control and Prevention: Screening young children for lead poisoning: Guidance for state and local public health officials. US Dept. of Health and Human Services, Public Health Service, *Federal Register*, February 21, 1997.

- Radiographic evidence of lead poisoning consists of bands of increased density at the metaphyses of long bones that are best seen in radiographs of the distal femur and proximal tibia and fibula. The popular term "lead lines" is a misnomer, since the increased radiopacity is caused by abnormal calcification from the disrupted metabolism of bone matrix rather than actual deposition of lead in the metaphysis.
- Other essential tests include measurement of hemoglobin and hematocrit, evaluation of the patient's iron status, examination of the blood smear for basophilic stippling of the erythrocytes, and a urinalysis to exclude glycosuria or proteinuria.
- A spinal tap is avoided in children with lead encephalopathy due to the concern for herniation.

MANAGEMENT

- The principles of management in lead poisoning include:
  - Identification and removal of the lead source
  - Correction of dietary deficiencies that enhance lead absorption
  - Pharmacologic chelation
  - Supportive therapy
  - Long-term follow-up.
- For patients with lead levels between 10 and 20 µg/dL, treatment consists of environmental management, nutritional evaluation, and repeated screening. In many cases, this involves removing the child from the home until the source of lead exposure is identified and removed.
- For patients with BLLs between 20 and 44 µg/dL, environmental evaluation and remediation are required. Pharmacologic intervention may be indicated and is accomplished on an outpatient basis if the child is asymptomatic.
- The decision to treat may be aided by a CaNa$_2$EDTA immobilization test. CaNa$_2$EDTA is administered in a dose of 500 mg/m^2 in 5-percent dextrose infused over 1 h, or the same dose may be given intramuscularly. The amount of lead is measured in urine collected over the next 8 h. A ratio of lead excreted (in micrograms) to the CaNa2EDTA dose (in milligrams) greater than 0.6 is considered positive.
- Oral dimercaptosuccinic acid (DMSA) is currently the only treatment approved for oral chelation of childhood lead poisoning. It is given 30 mg/kg/d in three divided doses for the first 5 days, then 20 mg/kg/d in two divided doses for 14 more days.
- Outpatient treatment is also possible with oral D-penicillamine (Cuprimine). Currently, it is not approved by the FDA for the treatment of lead poisoning, but is approved for other uses and has been successful in children not able to tolerate DMSA therapy.
- Children with asymptomatic lead poisoning and BLLs of 45 to 69 µg/dL are admitted to the hospital for chelation therapy with either CaNa$_2$EDTA or DMSA.
- Children with *symptomatic* lead poisoning with or without encephalopathy who have BLLs higher than 45 µg/dL, and all patients with BLLs higher than 70 µg/dL are treated with BAL at a dose of 25 mg/kg/d in six divided doses given by deep intramuscular injection. Once the first dose is given and adequate urine flow is established, CaNa$_2$EDTA is added as a continuous intravenous infusion at 50 mg/kg/d in dextrose or saline.
- When treating a child with encephalopathy, the intramuscular route for CaNa$_2$EDTA with procaine 0.5 percent is preferred to reduce the amount of fluid administered. This combined treatment is given for 5 days, with daily monitoring of blood urea nitrogen (BUN), creatinine, liver enzymes, and electrolytes.
- **Lead encephalopathy** should always be considered in young children with mental status changes and no other clinical evidence of infection. Lead encephalopathy is treated with fluid restriction, controlled ventilation, and furosemide. Mannitol is avoided because it may leak from the compromised vessels into the cerebellar interstitial spaces and cause a rebound of the intracranial pressure.
- Lead poisoning is most commonly a consequence of chronic exposure, and a rebound elevation of BLL is expected after each course of chelation therapy as lead is mobilized from body stores. Repeat BLLs 2 weeks after the completion of chelation gives a reasonable peak rebound level.

BIBLIOGRAPHY

American Academy of Pediatrics, Committee on Drugs: Treatment guidelines for lead exposure in children. *Pediatrics* 96:155–160, 1995.

Angle CR: Childhood lead poisoning and its treatment. *Ann Rev Pharmacol Toxicol* 33:409–434, 1993.

Liebelt EL, Shannon MW: Oral chelators for childhood poisoning. *Pediatr Ann* 23:616–626, 1994.

Manton WI, Angle CR, Stanek SL, et al: Acquisition and retention of lead by young children. *Environ Res* 82:60–80, 2000.

Piomelli S: Childhood lead poisoning. *Pediatr Clin North Am* 49:1285–1304, 2002.

Pirkel JL, Brody DJ, Gunter EW, et al: The decline in blood lead levels in the United States—The National Health and Nutrition Examination Surveys (NHANES). *JAMA* 272: 284–291, 1994.

Rogan J, Dietrich KN, Ware JH, et al: The effect of chelation therapy with succimer on neuropsychological development in children exposed to lead. *N Engl J Med* 344:1421–1426, 2001.

QUESTIONS

1. The most common source of lead poisoning in children in the United States is from what source?
   A. Ingestion of drinking water contaminated by lead in plumbing
   B. Ingestion of lead-based paint
   C. Ingestion of lead-based toys
   D. Contaminated well water
   E. Ingestion of fish contaminated with lead
2. The major target organs in lead toxicity are which of the following?
   A. Heart, central nervous system, kidneys, and GI tract
   B. Bone marrow, central nervous system, peripheral nervous system, and kidneys
   C. Reproductive organs, heart, central nervous system, and kidneys
   D. GI tract, heart, central nervous system, and skin
   E. Skin, GI tract, kidneys, and heart
3. Which of the following is true regarding the signs and symptoms of lead toxicity in children?
   A. Ataxia, lethargy, or stupor may occur
   B. May present with abdominal pain and constipation
   C. Basophilic stippling of the erythrocytes may occur
   D. Radiographic changes with bands of increased density at the metaphyses of long bones may occur
   E. All of the above
4. Which of the following is **NOT** an important principle in the management of lead poisoning?
   A. Identification and removal of the lead source
   B. Correction of dietary deficiencies that enhance lead absorption
   C. Chelation therapy
   D. Supportive therapy
   E. Admission for all patients with abnormal lead levels
5. A 1-year-old male is brought in by his mother with an elevated lead level on routine screening. The blood lead level is 60 µg/dL and the child has been slightly fussier over the last several weeks with constipation. The family lives in an inner-city housing development in need of repairs. Which of the following is the optimal treatment of this child?

   A. Outpatient chelation with oral dimercaptosuccinic acid (DMSA) and close follow up
   B. Admission for supportive care
   C. Admission and treatment with dimercaprol (BAL) IM every 4 h
   D. Admission and treatment with dimercaprol (BAL) IM every 4 h followed by CaNa$_2$EDTA in a continuous infusion
   E. Admission with serial lead levels if increasing treatment with dimercaprol (BAL) IM every 4 h

ANSWERS

1. B. Ingestion of leaded paint is the most common and clinically relevant source of lead poisoning in children. Most homes built before 1978 were painted with lead-based paint. Renovation of old buildings and poorly controlled lead abatement pose a risk for lead poisoning through inhalation and ingestion of contaminated dust and soil.
2. B. The major target organs of lead are: bone marrow, central nervous system, peripheral nervous system, and kidneys.
3. E. Symptoms and signs of lead toxicity may be subtle or nonspecific. CNS symptoms may occur such as ataxia, vomiting, lethargy, stupor, coma, and seizures. Abdominal symptoms, such as colicky pain, constipation, or diarrhea, may occur. The blood smear may show basophilic stippling of the erythrocytes. Radiographic evidence of lead poisoning consists of horizontal bands of increased density at the metaphyses of long bones especially around the knee.
4. E. The principles of management of lead poisoning include: identification and removal of the lead source, correction of dietary deficiencies that enhance lead absorption (iron deficiency and dietary calcium deficiency), chelation therapy, supportive therapy, and long-term follow-up. Environmental management and remediation is important for removal of lead-based paint but is not considered child abuse. Populations at risk include inner city dwellers, African Americans, all children from low socioeconomic classes, and those who live in old houses that have recently been renovated.
5. D. Admission is indicated for all symptomatic patients and asymptomatic patients with lead levels >45 µg/dL. Children with symptomatic lead poisoning who have blood lead levels 45 µg/dL and all patients with levels >70 µg/dL are treated with BAL IM every 4 hours (3 to 5 mg/kg) followed by CaNa$_2$—EDTA in a continuous intravenous infusion. The child should be removed from the home until the source of lead exposure is identified and removed.

98 METHEMOGLOBINEMIA

Timothy Erickson
Michele Zell-Kanter
Gary R. Strange

INTRODUCTION

- Methemoglobin is formed when iron in hemoglobin is oxidized from the ferrous (Fe^{++}) state to the ferric (Fe^{+++}) state. Under normal physiologic conditions, methemoglobin is present in red blood cells at concentrations of 1 to 2 percent.
- Hereditary methemoglobinemia is found in 2 forms:
  - Deficiency in NADH-dependent methemoglobin reductase
  - Hemoglobin M, which is a structural abnormality in hemoglobin.
- Acquired methemoglobinemia results from exposure to drugs or chemicals that accelerate the oxidation of hemoglobin beyond the cell's capacity to reduce it (Table 98-1).
- Infants are more sensitive than adults to methemoglobin-producing agents, such as nitrites, nitrates, or contaminated foods. The infant's high gastric pH allows bacterial proliferation and increased production of nitrites.

CLINICAL PRESENTATION

- The classic, chocolate brown coloration of blood is usually seen at concentrations of 15 to 20 percent. Although pediatric patients may have clinical signs of cyanosis at this level, they are typically asymptomatic.
- Concentrations ranging from 30 to 40 percent may produce generalized symptoms such as poor feeding, lethargy, and irritability. The older child may complain of fatigue, dizziness, headaches, and weakness.

TABLE 98-1 Causes of Acquired Methemoglobinemia

Acetanilid	Lidocaine	Phenacetin
Aminophenols	Menthol	Phenols
Aniline compounds	Nitrates	Phenylazopyridine
Antimalarials	Nitrites	Phenylhydroxyamine
Benzocaine	Nitrofurans	Prilocaine
Bismuth subnitrite	Nitroglycerin	Pyridine
Chlorates	Nitrous oxide (contaminated)	Quinones
Cobalt preparations	Paraaminosalicylic acid	Resorcinol
Copper sulfate	Paratoluidine	Shoe polish
Dapsone	Pesticides (propham, fenuron)	Sulfonamides
Dinitrobenzene		Sulfones
Fuel additives		Trinitroluene

- At levels above 55 percent, patients may experience respiratory depression, cardiac arrhythmias, seizures, and coma.
- Concentrations over 70 percent are potentially lethal.

MANAGEMENT

- Initial treatment of any drug- or chemical-induced methemoglobinemia involves supportive care consisting of airway control, supplemental oxygen, and removal of the patient from the source of exposure.
- Oral exposure is managed with gastric emptying and charcoal administration.
- The skin is decontaminated if dermal absorption is suspected.
- If methemoglobin levels exceed 30 percent or the patient exhibits clinical signs of hypoxia, administration of methylene blue is recommended.
  - The initial dose is 1 to 2 mg/kg of a 1-percent solution given intravenously over 5 min.
  - If clinical signs persist, the dose is repeated in 1 h and every 4 h thereafter, to a maximum dose of 7 mg/kg.

DISPOSITION

- Most investigators concur that patients who have methemoglobin concentrations below 20 percent and are asymptomatic require only admission and close observation, as their hemoglobin levels should normalize within 24 to 72 h.
- Any symptomatic pediatric patient with levels over 20 percent or those requiring methylene blue administration should be monitored in an intensive care setting.

BIBLIOGRAPHY

Aepfelbacher FC, Breen P, Manning WJ: Methemoglobinemia and topical pharyngeal anesthesia. *N Engl J Med* 348:85–86, 2003.

Coleman MD, Coleman NA: Drug-induced methemoglobinemia. *Drug Safety* 14:394–405, 1996.

Gilman CS, Veser FH, Randall DR: Methemoglobinemia from topical oral anesthetic. *Acad Emerg Med* 4:1011–1013, 1997.

Hanukoglu A, Danon PN: Endogenous methemoglobinemia associated with diarrheal disease in infancy. *J Pediatr Gastroenterol Nutr* 23:1–7, 1996.

Nakajima W, Ishida A, Arai H: Methemoglobinemia after inhalation of nitric oxide in an infant with pulmonary hypertension. *Lancet* 350:1002–1003, 1997.

Osterhoudt KC: Methemoglobinemia. In: Ford M, Delaney K, Ling L, et al, eds. *Clinical Toxicology.* Philadelphia: Saunders, 211–217, 2000.

Wright RO, Lewander WT, Woolf AD: Methemoglobin: Etiology, pharmacology, and clinical management. *Ann Emerg Med* 34:646–656, 1999.

QUESTIONS

1. Which of the following is true regarding methemo-globinemia?
   A. Blood appears chocolate brown rather than red when iron in hemoglobin is in the ferrous state.
   B. Normal methemoglobin concentrations in red blood cells is on the order of 15 to 20 percent.
   C. The classic, chocolate brown coloration of blood is usually seen at concentrations of 15 to 20 percent methemoglobin.
   D. The classic, chocolate brown coloration of blood is rarely seen.
   E. The chocolate brown coloration may be seen but only with concentrations over 70 percent.
2. Which of the following statements regarding the treatment of methemoglobinemia is correct?
   A. Treatment with oxygen is ineffective and not indicated.
   B. Decontamination is rarely feasible regardless of whether the skin or gastrointestinal tract was the route of exposure.
   C. Specific treatment for symptomatic patients is with methylene blue.
   D. Methemoglobin levels above 30 percent require treatment with exchange transfusion or hyperbaric oxygen.
   E. Methemoglobinemia is self-limited and rarely requires treatment.

ANSWERS

1. C. The classic, chocolate brown coloration of blood in methemoglobinemia is usually seen at concentrations of 15 to 20 percent. Methemoglobin is formed when the iron in hemoglobin is oxidized from the ferrous state to the ferric state. Methemoglobin is present in normal blood cells up to a level of 1 to 2 percent. Levels over 70 percent are potentially lethal.
2. C. Specific treatment for methemoglobinemia is with methylene blue and it is indicated for patients with levels above 30 percent or who are symptomatic. Exchange transfusion and hyperbaric oxygen therapy are indicated for patients with levels above 70 percent who are not responding to methylene blue. Oxygen and decontamination are both indicated.

99 MUSHROOM POISONING

Timothy J. Rittenberry
Jaime Rivas
Gary R. Strange

IDENTIFICATION

- Exact mushroom identification is difficult or unlikely in most cases and is not critical to initiating emergency care. However, identification is possible if specimens are available.
- Even when identification is accomplished, toxin concentrations can be highly variable, depending on species, season, locale, and the specific part of the mushroom ingested.

CLASSIFICATION

- Categorization based on the predominant toxin, conveniently groups North American mushroom ingestions into eight groups:
  - Gastroenteric irritants
  - Cyclopeptides
  - Gyromitrin group
  - Muscarine group
  - Coprine-containing group
  - Those containing ibotenic acid and muscimol
  - Hallucinogenic indole–containing mushrooms
  - Orellanine group

GASTROENTERIC IRRITANTS

- Gastroenteric irritant mushrooms are the most commonly encountered mushroom ingestions in children.
  - The grouping includes a myriad of mushroom species, which have in common the ability to cause marked gastrointestinal irritation without specific end organ injury or CNS manifestations.
  - These include the "little brown mushrooms," found commonly in yards, and *Chlorophyllium molybdides*, probably the most frequently reported toxic mushroom exposure in North America.
- The physician should ensure gut decontamination with gastric lavage and early administration of activated charcoal.

CYCLOPEPTIDES

- This group of mushrooms is responsible for most North American deaths.

○ It includes various members of the *Amanita, Lepiota*, and *Galerina* genera containing amatoxins, which cause severe hepatorenal dysfunction and gastritis.

○ *Amanita phalloides*, known as "the death cap," is responsible for more than 50 percent of all serious mushroom poisonings, with several other *Amanita spp*, such as *A. virosa* ("destroying angel"), *A. vernal*, and *A. ocreata* also involved.

PRESENTATION, DIAGNOSIS, AND TREATMENT

• The clinical presentation of ingestion of the cyclopeptide group of mushrooms occurs in four stages.

○ The initial latent phase is characterized by a 6- to 12-h asymptomatic period, during which time, protein synthesis is being disrupted.

○ A gastroenteritis-like phase follows, as phalloidin-induced nausea, vomiting, bloody diarrhea, and abdominal pain predominate. This phase may last up to 24 h.

○ The following latent phase is marked by an apparent remission of 6 to 24 h, as overt symptomatology is absent but hepatocellular damage continues.

○ The final hepatorenal phase follows, within 36 to 72 h of ingestion, during which, jaundice, hypoglycemia, confusion, coagulopathy, and hepatorenal failure develop.

• The key to treatment is early gut decontamination, but the typical latent phase preceding symptoms will often delay presentation and preclude effective removal of the toxin.

○ The immediate home use of ipecac in the pediatric patient is important in all suspected mushroom ingestions, and concerned parents who make immediate telephone contact are advised to give the appropriate dose of ipecac, followed by immediate medical evaluation.

○ Gastric lavage is employed with the aspirate saved for possible use in identification.

○ Activated charcoal is administered, with or without a cathartic, depending on the level of gastroenteric disturbance. Repeated doses of activated charcoal and duodenal drainage may be useful during the first 24 to 72 h to enhance elimination and interrupt enterohepatic circulation of the amatoxins, thus, ameliorating liver damage.

• Supportive care to maintain fluid and electrolyte balance is appropriate, as is the supportive treatment of any developing hepatic and renal insufficiency.

• Severe toxicity may require liver transplantation.

INDOLE-CONTAINING MUSHROOMS

• *Psilocybe semilanceata, Psilocybe coprophila*, and *Paneolus* are the most commonly ingested mushrooms in this group, which contain psychoactive indoles that are similar to lysergic acid (LSD).

• Presenting symptoms may include labile mood, muscle weakness, panic, and hallucinosis.

• Treatment consists of gut decontamination and supportive care.

• Hospitalization for observation in a low-stimulus environment, with repeated doses of activated charcoal, is appropriate.

MONOMETHYLHYDRAZINE GROUP

• *Gyromitrin* is a toxic hydrazone, which is responsible for most of the effects of this group. It is a hemolysin, neurotoxin, and hepatotoxin that inhibits pyridoxal phosphate, causing reactions in a manner similar to isoniazid. It is toxic due to action at the level of gamma aminobutyric acid synthesis in the central nervous system.

• In severe cases, methemoglobinemia, hemolysis with hemoglobinuria, confusion, lethargy, seizures, acidosis, and hypoglycemia may develop.

• As in all mushroom ingestions, treatment is elimination and supportive care.

○ Gastric lavage may be useful with an immediate presentation, but this scenario is unlikely in light of the typical 6- to 12-h delay in onset of symptoms.

○ Ipecac-induced emesis is potentially dangerous in light of an increased likelihood of seizures.

○ Activated charcoal is indicated, and the clinical similarity to cyclopeptide ingestion suggests that repeated administration of activated charcoal and duodenal aspiration for the first 24 to 72 h may be useful.

○ Seizures are treated with pyridoxine in a manner similar to isoniazid toxicity. Pyridoxine is administered parenterally at an initial dose of 25 mg/kg, increasing to a maximum dose of 300 mg/kg, or until seizure activity resolves.

MUSCARINE

• Ingestion of mushrooms, such as *Clitocybe dealbata* or *Inocybe fastigiata*, results in a muscarine-induced cholineric crisis.

• Symptoms occur rapidly, usually within 15 to 60 min, and are those expected of cholinergic stimulation. Salivation, lacrimation, urinary frequency, increased gastroenteric motility, diarrhea, diaphoresis, miosis, blurred vision, bronchospasm, bronchorrhea, bradycardia, and even hypotension may occur. Symptoms are typically mild and short-lived, lasting up to 6 h.

- Treatment consists of gut decontamination using gastric lavage followed by activated charcoal.
  - A cathartic is not necessary in the presence of increased gastroenteric motility.
- Cardiac monitoring is necessary due to the potential for bradyarrhythmias.
- The use of atropine in the face of severe cholinergic crisis is indicated with an initial dose of 0.01 mg/kg IV. The total dose of atropine is based on the drying of secretions, rather than pupillary dilation.

COPRINE GROUP

- The common alcohol inky (*Coprinus atramentarius*) is an edible mushroom without toxic effects when eaten in the absence of ethanol. However, when ethanol is coingested, a disulfiram-like reaction may occur. The biochemical events involved are not identical to that seen with Antabuse, but the clinical picture is similar.
- Patients presenting acutely after coprine exposure and ethanol use exhibit facial flushing, paresthesias, diaphoresis, headache, nausea, and vomiting. Severe reactions can result in hypotension or acidosis.

IBOTENIC ACID AND MUSCIMOL

- *Amanita muscaria* and *Amanita pantherina* contain the psychoactive isoxazoles, ibotenic acid and muscimol, which are responsible for the toxicologic profile of this ingestant. In spite of its name, *Amanita muscaria* carries insignificant amounts of muscarine and does not result in a syndrome of cholinergic excess.
- Within 30 min to 2 h of ingestion of mushrooms of this group, symptoms resembling ethanol intoxication occur, with ataxia, confusion, irritability, bizarre behavior, euphoria, and hyperkinetic activity.
- Supportive care is the mainstay of treatment. Gastric lavage, followed by activated charcoal, is followed by observation.

ORELLENINE

- Ingestion of *Cortinarius orellanus* causes tubulointerstitial nephritis, which can lead to acute or chronic renal failure.
- Due to the prolonged latency period, the use of gut decontaminations and activated charcoal is of no benefit. Supportive care should center on fluid management and monitoring renal function.

BIBLIOGRAPHY

Enjalbert F, Rapior S, Nouguier-Soule J, et al: Treatment of amatoxin poisoning: 20-year retrospective analysis. *J Toxicol Clin Toxicol* 40:715–757, 2002.

Litovitz TL, Klein-Schwartz W, White S, et al. 1999 annual report of the American Association of Poison Control Centers toxic exposure surveillance system. *Am J Emerg Med* 2000;18:517–574.

Schneider SM: Mushrooms. In: Ford MD, Delaney KA, Ling LJ, Erickson T, eds. *Clinical Toxicology.* Philadelphia: Saunders, 899–908, 2001.

QUESTIONS

1. The most commonly encountered toxic mushroom ingestions in children are due to which group of mushrooms?
   A. Gastrointestinal irritants, such as the little brown mushroom
   B. Amatoxin-producing mushrooms such as *Amanita, Lepiota*, and *Galerina*
   C. Psychoactive indole-containing mushrooms
   D. Gyromitrin-producing mushrooms
   E. Coprine mushrooms, such as the common alcohol inky

2. Which group of mushrooms is responsible for most deaths due to mushroom ingestion?
   A. Gastrointestinal irritants, such as the little brown mushroom
   B. Amatoxin-producing mushrooms, such as *Amanita, Lepiota*, and *Galerina*
   C. Psychoactive indole-containing mushrooms.
   D. Gyromitrin-producing mushrooms
   E. Coprine mushrooms, such as the common alcohol inky

3. A 6-year-old boy presents to the ED with a report of ingesting several mushrooms of an unknown variety about 2 h ago. He complains of nausea, one episode of vomiting, crampy abdominal pain, weakness, and anxiety. No further information is available. Which of the following statements is true regarding his treatment?
   A. Gastric decontamination is unlikely to be of help.
   B. Enhancement of elimination and supportive care are indicated in all mushroom intoxications.
   C. Activated charcoal is ineffective in adsorbing mushroom toxins.
   D. Prophylactic treatment with a benzodiazepine or haloperidol is indicated, since this is a likely prodrome to the hallucinogenic phase due to indole-containing mushroom ingestion.

E. The likely cause of the symptoms is a gastrointestinal irritant mushroom and no treatment is required.

4. A 16-year-old girl is on a group camping trip when she suddenly becomes ill and is transported to the nearest ED for evaluation. She is diaphoretic, anxious, tremulous, crying profusely, drooling, has been incontinent of urine and feces. A friend tells you that she and some other campers may have eaten some mushrooms. Of the following conclusions, which is most likely to explain her symptoms?
  A. This symptom complex is unlikely to be due to mushroom ingestion.
  B. These symptoms are due to anticholinergic exposure and are most likely due to exposure to insecticides.
  C. These symptoms are likely due to muscarine, which is present in high concentrations in *Amanita muscarina*.
  D. These are symptoms of cholinergic stimulation that may result from ingestion of *Clitocybe, Inocybe* and *Amanita*.
  E. These symptoms are most likely due to co-ingestion of coprine group mushrooms along with alcohol.

ANSWERS

1. A. The most commonly encountered mushroom ingestions in children are due to gastrointestinal irritants that cause marked gastrointestinal irritation without specific end-organ injury or CNS manifestations.
2. B. The cyclopeptide- or amatoxin-producing mushrooms, including the genera *Amanita, Lepiota*, and *Galerina*, cause severe hepatorenal dysfunction and gastritis. They are responsible for most North American deaths due to mushroom ingestion.
3. B. Mushroom identification is difficult and unlikely. Specific identification is usually not critical since treatment is supportive with enhancement of elimination of the toxic substances from the GI tract.
4. D. These symptoms are of cholinergic excess and may be due to muscarine, which is present in mushrooms of these three genera. Muscarine is present in only trace amounts in *Amanita muscarina*, however. It contains the psychoactive isoxazoles, ibotenic acid and muscimol, which produce an intoxication similar to ethanol. Coprine group mushrooms in combination with ethanol produce a disulfarim-like reaction.

100 NEUROLEPTICS

Timothy Erickson
Gary R. Strange

INTRODUCTION

- Neuroleptics or phenothiazines are a group of major tranquilizers or antipsychotic drugs that are therapeutically designed to treat schizophrenia and other psychiatric disorders.

PATHOPHYSIOLOGY

- Neuroleptics act by blocking dopaminergic, alpha-adrenergic, muscarinic, histaminic, and serotonergic neuroreceptors. Blockade of the dopamine receptors results in the desired behavior modification, but also produces extrapyramidal side effects, such as dystonic reactions.

DYSTONIC REACTIONS

CLINICAL PRESENTATION

- Dystonic reactions are characterized by slurred speech, dysarthria, confusion, dysphagia, hypertonicity, tremors, and muscle restlessness. Other reactions or dyskinesias include oculogyric crisis (upward gaze), torticollis (neck twisting), facial grimacing, opisthotonos (scoliosis), and tortipelvic gait disturbances.

MANAGEMENT

- If a child exhibits signs of acute muscular dystonia, intravenous diphenhydramine (2 mg/kg up to 50 mg over several minutes) is rapidly administered.
- Alternatively, the patient can be given benztropine intramuscularly in a dose of 0.05 to 0.1 mg/kg (up to 2 mg).

ACUTE OVERDOSE

CLINICAL PRESENTATION

- Following an acute overdose of neuroleptics, mild CNS depression is common, usually occurring within 1 to 2 hours of the ingestion. Children are more susceptible to these sedative effects than adults.

- Like the tricyclic antidepressants, poisoning from neuroleptics can result in orthostatic hypotension and cardiac dysrhythmias.

MANAGEMENT

- Initial management of an acute neuroleptic overdose includes stabilizing the airway and circulation.
  - If the patient remains hypotensive despite adequate amounts of IV fluid, a vasopressor with alpha-agonist activity, such as norepinephrine, may be considered.
  - Vasopressors with both alpha and beta-agonist activity, such as dopamine, may actually exacerbate hypotension because of unopposed beta-adrenergic stimulation, during which alpha-receptors are being blocked by the neuroleptic.
  - Because of the potential cardiotoxicity of phenothiazines, patients require close cardiac monitoring.
- Since phenothiazine toxicity classically demonstrates central nervous system depression and pupillary miosis, adequate doses of naloxone are indicated to treat potential coexistent opioid toxicity.
- Most children presenting after acute neuroleptic toxicity do well with supportive care alone.

NEUROLEPTIC MALIGNANT SYNDROME

CLINICAL PRESENTATION

- Less than 1 percent of patients exhibit the life-threatening extrapyramidal dysfunction known as neuroleptic malignant syndrome, characterized by skeletal muscle rigidity, coma, and severe hyperthermia following the use of phenothiazines or haloperidol.

MANAGEMENT

- The neuroleptic syndrome results in a high mortality rate and is treated aggressively with rapid cooling and administration of dantrolene at 0.8 to 3.0 mg/kg intravenously every 6 hours, up to 10 mg/kg per day.

DISPOSITION

- Any symptomatic child presenting with acute neuroleptic poisoning is admitted and observed for CNS and respiratory depression as well as for cardiotoxicity or thermoregulatory problems.

- Patients with minor, asymptomatic ingestions can be observed for up to 6 hours.

BIBLIOGRAPHY

Buckley P, Hutchinson M: Neuroleptic malignant syndrome. *J Neurol Neurosurg Psychiatry* 58:271–273, 1995.

Deroos FJ: Neuroleptics. In: Ford M, Delaney K, Ling L, et al, (eds):. *Clinical Toxicology.* Philadelphia: Saunders, 539–545, 2001.

Gupta S, Mosnik D, Black DW, et al: Tardive dyskinesia: Review of treatments past, present, and future. *Ann Clin Psychiatry* 11:257–265, 1999.

Kane JM: Newer antipsychotic drugs. *Drugs* 46:585–593, 1993.

Litovitz TL, Klein-Schwartz W, White S: Annual report of the American Association of Poison Control Centers toxic exposure surveillance system. *Am J Emerg Med* 18:517–574, 2000.

Owens DGC: Adverse effects of antipsychotic agents: Do newer agents offer advantages? *Drugs* 51:895–930, 1996.

Raja M: Managing antipsychotic induced acute and tardive dystonia. *Drug Safety* 19:57–72, 1998.

Van Harten PN, Hoek H, Kahn RS: Acute dystonia induced by drug treatment. *BMJ* 319:623–626, 1999.

Viejo LF, Morales V, Punal P, et al: Risk factors in neuroleptic malignant syndrome: A case control study. *Acta Psychiatr Scand* 107:45–49, 2003.

QUESTIONS

1. The desired behavioral modification and extrapyramidal side effects of neuroleptics result from the blockade of which of the following?
   A. Alpha-adrenergic receptors
   B. Muscarinic receptors
   C. Serotonergic neuroreceptors
   D. Histaminic receptors
   E. Dopamine receptors
2. The neuroleptic malignant syndrome (NMS) is characterized by which of the following findings?
   A. Muscular flaccidity
   B. Central nervous system hyperexcitability
   C. Severe hyperthermia
   D. History of neuroleptic use in presence of high ambient temperature
   E. Dysarthria
3. Which of the following is the most appropriate treatment for a patient who presents with NMS?
   A. Diphenhydramine, 2 mg/kg IV push, maximum 50 mg
   B. Benztropine, 0.05 to 0.1 mg/kg IM, maximum 2 mg

C. Bromocryptine, 1 mg/kg IV push
D. Dantrolene, 0.8 to 3.0 mg/kg IV every 6 h, maximum 10 mg/kg per day
E. Haloperidol, 0.1 mg/kg IM, maximum 5 mg

ANSWERS

1. E. Neuroleptics have all of these effects, but it is the blockade of dopamine receptors that produce the desired therapeutic effect as well as the major extrapyramidal side effects.
2. C. NMS is characterized by skeletal muscle rigidity, coma, and severe hyperthermia. It is unrelated to ambient temperature. Dysarthria is characteristic of an acute dystonic reaction that may develop in response to use of a neuroleptic but is not related to the development of NMS.
3. D. NMS results in a high mortality rate and is treated aggressively with rapid cooling and administration of dantrolene at 0.8 mg to 3.0 mg/kg IV every 6 h , up to 10 mg/kg per day. Dantrolene acts peripherally by treating skeletal muscle rigidity. Bromocryptine can be used but it is an oral preparation. Diphenhydramine and benztropine are effective for acute dystonic reactions but not for NMS. Haloperidol is a cause of NMS.

101 NONSTEROIDAL ANTI-INFLAMMATORY DRUGS

Michele Zell-Kanter
Gary R. Strange

INTRODUCTION

• In the overdose setting, NSAIDs are relatively devoid of toxicity.

CLINICAL PRESENTATION

• Typically, patients who ingest NSAIDs exhibit only central nervous system (CNS) or gastrointestinal (GI) toxicity.
• An exception to this is phenylbutazone, which has been associated with significant toxicity and death, especially in children.
• Long-term use of NSAIDs is associated with nephrotoxicity, including acute tubular necrosis, acute interstitial nephritis, and acute renal failure. Renal toxicity is not associated with acute overdose.

LABORATORY STUDIES

• Infrequently, overdose of NSAIDs has been associated with an anion-gap acidosis. For patients with severe clinical symptoms, an arterial blood gas is indicated.

MANAGEMENT

• After the patient is stabilized, gastric decontamination is indicated. In a patient presenting within 1 hour of ingestion, syrup of ipecac or gastric lavage can be used in a patient with a stable airway and who has not ingested an NSAID known to cause seizures.
• Activated charcoal is administered after ipecac-induced emesis ceases, gastric lavage is terminated, or for the patient who presents more than 1 hour after ingestion.

BIBLIOGRAPHY

Litovitz TL, Klein-Schwartz W, White S, et al: 1999 Annual report of the American Association of Poison Control Centers toxic exposure surveillance system. *Am J Emerg Med* 18:517, 2000.

Sung J, Russell RI, Chan FK, et al: Non-steroidal anti-inflammatory drug toxicity in the upper gastrointestinal tract. *J Gastroenterol Hepatol* 15:G58–68, 2000.

Skeith KJ, Wright M, Davis P: Differences in NSAID tolerability profiles: Fact or fiction? *Drug Safety* 10:183, 1994.

Vane JR, Botting RM: Anti-inflammatory drugs and their mechanism of action. *Inflamm Res* 47(Suppl 2): S78, 1998.

QUESTION

1. Which of the following statements regarding toxicity of NSAIDs is correct?
   A. A major concern with acute overdose is renal toxicity
   B. In the overdose setting, NSAIDs are relatively devoid of toxicity
   C. The most common symptoms of toxicity are cardiovascular in origin
   D. While the availability of plasma ibuprofen measurement is limited, levels correlate closely with signs and symptoms of toxicity
   E. NSAID overdose may be associated with non-anion gap acidosis

ANSWER

1. **B.** In the overdose setting NSAIDs are relatively devoid of toxicity. The most common manifestations are gastrointestinal and central nervous system related. While chronic use can result in nephrotoxicity, renal problems are not seen in acute overdose. Assay procedures for measuring plasma ibuprofen levels are readily available but there is poor correlation between the absolute level and toxicity. Infrequently, NSAID overdose can be associated with anion-gap acidosis.

102 OPIOIDS

Timothy Erickson
Gary R. Strange

INTRODUCTION

• Opioids are naturally occurring or synthetic drugs that have activity similar to that of opium or morphine. They are used clinically for analgesia and anesthesia and are widely available for illicit oral, inhalational, or parenteral abuse.

CLINICAL PRESENTATION

• The classic triad of acute toxicity consists of:
  ◦ CNS depression
  ◦ Respiratory depression
  ◦ Pupillary constriction (miosis)

MANAGEMENT

• The primary management of opioid poisoning includes urgent stabilization of the airway and administration of the pure opioid antagonist naloxone.
• If adequate doses of the antidote are given in a timely fashion, intubation can be avoided, since the onset of action for naloxone is usually within 1 minute after administration.
  ◦ In addition to intravenous administration, naloxone can be given via the endotracheal tube subcutaneously, or intralingually with a comparably rapid onset of action.

◦ In the overdose setting, the dose of naloxone is 0.1 mg/kg in children from birth to 5 years or 20 kg body weight, at which time a 2-mg dose is given. If there is no response, repeat doses of 2 mg are given to older children and adolescents, up to a maximum of 10 mg.
◦ An exception to this rule is in the chronic opioid-abusing adolescent or dependent neonate, in whom a withdrawal syndrome can be precipitated. In this setting, the patient receives supportive care, since opioid withdrawal is not a life-threatening situation.
◦ Due to the short half-life of naloxone (20 to 30 min) repeated doses may be indicated, particularly when dealing with opioids with longer duration of action, such as codeine, methadone, and diphenoxylate-atropine. If repeat doses of naloxone are required, a continuous intravenous infusion of naloxone is instituted.
• Gastric lavage can be performed if the child presents within 1 hour after an oral ingestion. The airway must be protected since there is potential for CNS and respiratory depression. Additionally, an initial dose of activated charcoal with cathartic is advised following any oral ingestion.

DISPOSITION

• Any pediatric patient presenting with CNS and respiratory depression from opioid poisoning that is responsive to naloxone is admitted for observation, since most of the opioids demonstrate longer duration of action than naloxone and require repetitive administration or continuous naloxone infusion.

BIBLIOGRAPHY

Chamberlain JM, Klein BL: A comprehensive review of naloxone for the emergency physician. *Am J Emerg Med* 12:650–660, 1994.

Kaplan JL, Mark JA, Calabro JJ, et al: Double-blind, randomized study of nalmefene and naloxone in emergency department suspected narcotic overdose. *Ann Emerg Med* 34:42–50, 1999.

Kleinschmidt KC, Wainscott M, Ford M: Opioids. In: Ford M, Delaney KA, Ling L, et al, eds. *Clinical Toxicology.* Philadelphia: Saunders, 2001, pp 627–639.

Litovitz TL, Schwartz-Klein W, White S, et al: 1999 Annual report of the AAPCC toxic exposure surveillance system. *Am J Emerg Med* 18:517–574, 2000.

Sporer KA: Acute heroin overdose. *Ann Intern Med* 130:584–590, 1999.

QUESTIONS

1. Opioid poisoning may be associated with all of the following findings EXCEPT:
   A. CNS depression
   B. Respiratory depression
   C. Miosis
   D. Non-cardiac pulmonary edema
   E. Mydriasis
2. All of the following statements regarding naloxone are correct EXCEPT:
   A. Naloxone is a pure opioid antagonist
   B. If adequate doses of naloxone are given in a timely fashion, intubation can be avoided even in the presence of a significant opioid overdose
   C. Onset of action is within 1 minute
   D. The dose is 0.1 mg/kg in infants and young children, with a maximum of 5 mg
   E. In the chronic opioid-abusing adolescent, naloxone may precipitate the narcotic withdrawal syndrome

ANSWERS

1. E. The classic presentation is CNS depression, respiratory depression, and pupillary constriction (miosis). In massive overdoses, the respiratory toxicity can also cause noncardiac pulmonary edema.
2. D. The maximum dose is often given as 10 mg, but even larger doses are associated with minimal or no side effects.

103 ORGANOPHOSPHATES AND CARBAMATES

Jerrold B. Leikin
Gary R. Strange

INTRODUCTION

- The organophosphates, and to a lesser extent the carbamate compounds, are particularly toxic chemicals. They are widely distributed throughout industry, agriculture, and the home, where they are used predominantly as pesticides.

PATHOPHYSIOLOGY

- Organophosphate toxicity results from the linking with and inactivating of acetylcholinesterase, and this inactivation is essentially permanent.

- The inactivation of acetylcholinesterase leads to the accumulation of acetylcholine at cholinergic receptor sites.
- Excess acetylcholine initially stimulates, then paralyzes cholinergic transmission at parasympathetic nerve endings, certain sympathetic nerve endings, and the neuromuscular junction.
- Organophosphates penetrate the central nervous system (CNS), where they paralyze cholinergic transmission.

CLINICAL PRESENTATION

- The initial signs and symptoms of cholinergic excess are usually muscarinic in nature. This constellation of findings is characterized by the mnemonic *SLUDGE:*
  ○ *S*alivation
  ○ *L*acrimation
  ○ *U*rination
  ○ *D*efecation
  ○ *G*astrointestinal cramps
  ○ *E*mesis
- The mnemonic does not include the pulmonary findings, which can cause life-threatening hypoxia and require urgent intervention (Table 103-1).
- Nicotinic manifestations include hypertension, pallor, and tachycardia.
- Striated muscle can be severely affected. Initially cholinergic excess stimulates fasciculations, which

TABLE 103-1   Clinical Effects of Organophosphate and Carbamate Intoxication

MUSCARINIC EFFECTS (ORGANOPHOSPHATES AND CARBAMATES)	
Salivation	Bradycardia
Diaphoresis	Miosis (late finding)
Lacrimation	Bronchorrhea
Defecation	Bronchospasm
Abdominal cramps	
Rhinorrhea	

NICOTINIC EFFECT (ORGANOPHOSPHATES ONLY)	
Fasciculations/twitching	Tachycardia
Weakness	Hypertension
Tremors	Pallor
Areflexia	Cramps

CENTRAL NERVOUS SYSTEM EFFECTS (ORGANOPHOSPHATES PREDOMINANTLY; CARBAMATES RARELY)	
Headache	Seizures
Restlessness	Coma
Confusion	Respiratory depression
Bizarre behavior	Ataxia

INTERMEDIATE SYNDROME (ORGANOPHOSPHATES ONLY)
Paralysis of head, neck, extremity muscles 3.5–7 days after resolution of cholinergic symptoms

are followed by weakness that can range from very mild to full paralysis.

DIAGNOSIS

LABORATORY STUDIES

- In the acute phase, there is no test that can identify organophosphate toxicity, and the initial management of the patient is based on clinical findings.
- Organophosphates cause depression of red blood cell cholinesterase and plasma pseudocholinesterase. Red blood cell cholinesterase represents cholinesterase found in nerve tissue, brain, and erythrocytes. It is a better indicator of toxicity than plasma pseudocholinesterase, which is a liver protein.

TREATMENT

STABLIZATION

- The most important aspect of stabilization is to assure adequate oxygenation and ventilation. In cases where there is severe bronchospasm, copious secretions, or marked weakness of respiratory muscles, urgent intubation and ventilation is indicated until antidotal therapy takes effect.
- Fluid resuscitation may be required for patients who have suffered significant volume loss from the gastrointestinal tract.

DECONTAMINATION

- Decontamination is vital in a patient with organophosphate or carbamate toxicity.
  - The patient is completely undressed, including removal of any jewelry, and the skin cleansed with soap and water.
  - Contaminated clothing is discarded.
  - The hospital staff must take care that they are not contaminated by contact with patients with dermal exposure.
- Since emesis and diarrhea is common in organophosphate and carbamate intoxication, ipecac or lavage is rarely useful. Activated charcoal is indicated to adsorb toxin remaining in the gastrointestinal tract.

ANTIDOTAL THERAPY

- Atropine is the antidote for the muscarinic effects of organophosphate toxicity, and it also relieves the CNS manifestations.

  - An initial dose of 0.05 mg/kg is indicated, and this may be doubled every 5 to 10 min until symptoms are relieved.
  - The goal of therapy is the drying of airway secretions so that oxygenation and ventilation are maintained.
  - Treatment with atropine must usually continue for at least 24 h.
- Endotracheal or nebulized administration of ipratropium bromide (0.5 mg every 6 h) may also assist in drying secretions.
- The specific antidote for the nicotinic manifestations of organophosphate toxicity is pralidoxime. It also relieves the central nervous system effects.
  - Pralidoxime works by restoring the activity of acetylcholinesterase.
  - Pralidoxime is administered at a dose of 25 to 50 mg/kg diluted to a 5-percent concentration in normal saline and infused over a 5- to 30-min period. It is repeated at 6- to 12-h intervals until there is relief of muscle weakness.
- Charcoal hemoperfusion is effective in removing parathion, demeton-*S*-methyl sulfoxide, dimethioate, and malathion. Exchange transfusion also has been utilized in parathion toxicity.

CARBAMATES

- Carbamates are commonly found in flea and tick powders and in ant killers.
- Toxicity with carbamates is primarily restricted to muscarinic effects, which are often the only manifestations of the poisoning (see Table 103-1).
- The initial management of the muscarinic effects of carbamate toxicity is the same as for organophosphates, with stabilization of the airway and breathing and complete decontamination of the patient. The skin is washed, although dermal exposure is less likely with carbamates than with organophosphates. Atropine is administered as antidotal therapy.

BIBLIOGRAPHY

Aaron CK: Organophosphates and carbamates. In: Ford MD, Delaney KA, Ling LJ, et al, . *Clinical Toxicology.* Philadelphia: Saunders, 819–828, 2001.

Ekins BR, Geller RJ, Khasigian PA, et al: Severe carbamate poisoning caused by methomyl with clinical improvement produced by pralidoxime. *Veterinary Hum Toxicol* 35:358, 1993.

Guven H, Tuncok Y, Gidener S, et al: The absorption of parathion by activated charcoal in vitro. *Veterinary Hum Toxicol* 35:359, 1993.

Kuffner E, Morasco R, Hoffman RS, et al: Human plasma cholinesterase protects against parathion toxicity in mice. *Veterinary Hum Toxicol* 35:332, 1993.

Litovitz TL, Schwartz-Klein W, White S, et al: 1999 Annual report of the American Association of Poison Control Centers toxic exposure surveillance system. *Am J Emerg Med* 18: 517–574, 2000.

Mattingly JE, Sullivan JE, Spiller HA, et al: Intermediate syndrome after exposure of chlorpyrofos in a 16 month old female. *J Toxicol Clin Toxicol* 39:305, 2001.

Medicis JJ, Stork CM, Howland MA, et al: Pharmacokinetics following a loading dose plus a continuous infusion of pralidoxime compared with the traditional short infusion regimen in human volunteers. *J Toxicol Clin Toxicol* 34:289–295, 1996.

Rotenberg M, Shefi M, Dany S, et al: Differentiation between organophosphate and carbamate poisoning. *Clin Chim Acta* 234:11–21, 1995.

Walker B Jr, Nidiry J: Current concepts: Organophosphate toxicity. *Inhal Toxicol* 14:975–990, 2002.

QUESTIONS

1. Which of the following are the initial signs and symptoms of organophosphate pesticide toxicity?
   A. Primarily nicotinic manifestations
   B. Limited to the manifestations represented by the mnemonic *SLUDGE*
   C. Include the *SLUDGE* manifestations but may also include life-threatening pulmonary findings
   D. Predominately related to skeletal muscle rigidity
   E. Predominately related to peripheral neuropathy

2. Which of the following statements regarding decontamination in the setting of organophosphate poisoning is most accurate?
   A. Most cases of severe toxicity are due to oral ingestion and decontamination is limited to the use of activated charcoal.
   B. Most cases of severe toxicity are due to inhalation of pesticide dust and decontamination is not possible.
   C. Severe toxicity can occur after dermal exposure, and careful removal of clothing and cleansing of the skin, while using protective equipment for the caregivers, is indicated.
   D. Either ipecac or lavage should be initiated early in the course of treatment.
   E. Activated charcoal is ineffective.

3. Which of the following statements regarding antidotal therapy in organophosphate toxicity is correct?
   A. Atropine is the antidote for the muscarinic effects of organophosphate toxicity but cannot be used if the patient is significantly tachycardic.

   B. Atropine is an effective antidote in a dose of 0.02 mg/kg with a maximum dose of 2 mg.
   C. Ipratropium bromide is not effective in the setting of organophosphate toxicity.
   D. Pralidoxime is the antidote for the nicotinic effects of organophosphate toxicity and is administered as a loading dose, usually followed by repeated doses or by continuous infusion for at least 48 h.
   E. Pralidoxime is given as a 1-time standard dose of 50 mg/kg.

ANSWERS

1. C. The initial signs and symptoms of organophosphate toxicity are those of cholinergic excess and are usually muscarinic in nature. The constellation of symptoms is described by the mnemonic *SLUDGE*, but the mnemonic does not include the pulmonary findings, which can cause life-threatening hypoxia and require urgent intervention.

2. C. Decontamination is vital in a patient with organophosphate toxicity. Neither ipecac nor lavage is usually practical due to the emesis and diarrhea that are common. Activated charcoal is indicated to adsorb toxin remaining in the GI tract. Dermal exposure is a major route leading to toxicity and great care to remove contaminated clothing and jewelry as well as to protect healthcare providers must be taken.

3. D. Atropine is the primary antidote for the muscarinic effects and is given even in the presence of tachycardia. Very large doses of atropine may be required and there is no specific maximum dose. The end point is drying of airway secretions. Ipratropium bromide may be used as an alternative to atropine and is given endotracheally or by inhalation. Pralidoxime is the antidote for the nicotinic effects of organophosphates and usually must be continued by repeat dosing or continuous infusion for at least 48 h.

104 PHENCYCLIDINE TOXICITY

Steven E. Aks
Gary R. Strange

INTRODUCTION

- Phencyclidine (PCP) is a common drug that is used for recreational purposes by adolescents and adults. PCP is commonly used with marijuana, and is sometimes used along with alcohol, cocaine, or other substances.

PHARMACOLOGY

- Phencyclidine is a cyclohexylamine structurally related to ketamine that was developed as a dissociative anesthetic.

CLINICAL PRESENTATION

- The neurologic effects of PCP overdose include excitation, hyperreflexia, blank stares, nystagmus, hallucinations, seizures, and psychosis.
- Phencyclidine can cause acute behavioral toxicity.
- A hallmark is its ability to cause a fluctuating level of consciousness, characterized by periods of lethargy and coma alternating with aggressive or assaultive activity.

MANAGEMENT

- The mainstay of management of the patient with phencyclidine intoxication is good supportive care.
- It is essential that health care providers take necessary measures to assure the safety of the patient and the emergency department staff. It is erroneous to view the psychosis and abnormal behavior as similar to that caused by the hallucinogens. Attempts to "talk the patient down" will be fruitless. Physical and appropriate chemical restraints should be used as necessary.
- Pharmacologic agents, such as benzodiazepines and haloperidol, have been used successfully in cases of PCP intoxication. They are titrated to effect, with meticulous attention paid to the integrity of the airway.
- Phenothiazines are contraindicated in the setting of PCP intoxication because of their ability to lower the seizure threshold and the possibility of causing hypotension.
- Although acidification of the urine has been suggested to enhance elimination of PCP, it is contraindicated because of the potential to worsen renal insufficiency should rhabdomyolysis develop.

DISPOSITION

- Patients with severe toxicity and evidence of prolonged coma, seizures, hyperthermia, rhabdomyolysis, or unstable vital signs should be admitted to an intensive care unit for monitoring and supportive care.
- Patients with minor manifestations of toxicity can be observed in the emergency department for 6 to 8 h and discharged in the care of responsible caretakers when the patient's mental state returns to baseline.

BIBLIOGRAPHY

Litovitz TL, Klein-Schwartz W, White S, et al: 1999 Annual report of the American Association of Poison Control Centers toxic exposure surveillance system. *Am J Emerg Med* 18: 517–574, 2000.

Moriarty AL: What's "new" in street drugs: "Illy." *J Pediatr Health Care* 10:41–42, 1996.

Shannon M: Letter. *Pediatr Emerg Care* 14:180, 1998.

Weiner AL, Vieira L, McKay CA: Ketamine abusers presenting to the emergency department: A case series. *J Emerg Med* 18:447–451, 2000.

QUESTION

1. Which of the following statements regarding appropriate management of phencyclidine toxicity is correct?
   A. A calm reassuring approach will usually allow the caregiver to "talk the patient down."
   B. Phenothiazines are the preferred drugs for use as tranquilizers in these patients.
   C. Physical restraints are frequently required.
   D. Acidification of the urine is indicated to enhance elimination.
   E. Gastric lavage is the first-line approach for reducing toxicity.

ANSWER

1. C. Attempts to talk PCP-intoxicated patients down are fruitless and potentially dangerous. Phenothiazines are contraindicated since they decrease the seizure threshold. Acidification of the urine is effective in enhancing elimination but it is dangerous due to the frequent association of PCP toxicity with rhabdomyolysis. Myoglobin precipitation in renal tubules is enhanced in an acid urine. Gastric lavage, while it may be effective, is impractical with these patients, who are frequently wildly agitated. Physical restraints are frequently required.

105 POISONOUS PLANTS

Andrea Carlson
Kimberly Sing
Gary R. Strange

INTRODUCTION

- There is considerable overlap in the clinical manifestations of toxicity of many plants, and for most patients the treatment is supportive.

GASTROINTESTINAL IRRITANTS

- Most toxic plants primarily cause nausea, vomiting, and diarrhea.
- The phytolaccine alkaloid found in *pokeweed* primarily causes irritation of the skin, mucous membranes, and gastrointestinal tract. The green berries contain more toxin than the purple berries, which are attractive to children.
- The toxalbumins of the *rosary pea* and *castor beans* inhibit protein synthesis and are the most toxic substances known. The bright scarlet seed of the rosary pea is very appealing to children. The seed must be masticated to liberate the toxalbumin. Decontamination should be attempted even 4 hours after ingestion.
- During the Christmas holidays, children are often exposed to *mistletoe* and *holly*. The leaves are more toxic than the berries and mainly cause gastroenteritis, which is usually not very severe.
- The *Arum* spp., *Dieffenbachia* and *Philodendron*, are houseplants that toddlers tend to ingest and are the most common cause of symptomatic plant ingestions. They can cause severe oral and pharyngeal burns secondary to insoluble calcium oxalate crystals.

CARDIOVASCULAR TOXINS

- Plants that contain cardiac glycosides inhibit the Na^+-K^+-ATPase pump, causing an increase in serum potassium and a decrease in intracellular potassium, thereby changing the membrane potential. Each of the following plants contains glycosides, in increasing potency: *lily of the valley < foxglove < oleander < yellow oleander*.
- Toxicity can consist predominantly of gastrointestinal symptoms, with vomiting and diarrhea. In severe cases, cardiac toxicity results, mainly in the form of arrhythmias that include first, second, and third-degree heart block.
- For patients who have not vomited, gastric decontamination is indicated.
- For patients with bradydysrhythmias, atropine and cardiac pacing are indicated, but may be ineffective.
- For severe cardiac instability, a trial of Digibind can be given.

NEUROLOGIC TOXINS

- *Water hemlock* is easily confused with the wild carrot or Jerusalem artichoke. Patients may progress to status epilepticus, respiratory distress, rhabdomyolysis, and death.

NICOTINE-LIKE TOXINS

- Plants that contain nicotine-like toxins cause a toxidrome consisting of nausea, vomiting, salivation, abdominal cramps, confusion, tachycardia, mydriasis, and fever. Seizures may occur in this initial stimulatory stage.
- *Poison hemlock* contains coniine, which causes a curare-like paralysis at the neuromuscular junction and a strychnine-like convulsant activity. Death occurs from respiratory paralysis.
  - Whole bowel irrigation may prove helpful if large amounts have been ingested.

ANTICHOLINERGIC AGENTS

- *Jimsonweed, black henbane*, and *mandrake* all contain varying amounts of both hyoscyamine and scopolamine.
  - Decontamination is attempted even 12 to 24 hours after ingestion because there is delayed gastric emptying.
  - Physostigmine is reserved for patients with seizures, severe hallucinations, hypertension, or arrhythmias.

RENAL FAILURE

- The stalk of the *rhubarb* is edible, but the leaves are toxic because of the high content of soluble calcium oxalate, which is concentrated in the kidneys and can cause renal failure.
  - Symptoms usually begin 6 to 12 hours after ingestion but may be delayed for 24 hours.
  - Because of the precipitation of calcium, patients may develop hypocalcemia, resulting in electrocardiographic changes, paresthesias, tetany, hyperreflexia, muscle twitches, muscle cramps, and seizures.

BIBLIOGRAPHY

Krenzelok EP: American mistletoe exposures. *Am J Emerg Med* 15:516–520, 1997.

Krenzelok EP, Mrvos R, Jacobsen TD: Contrary to the literature, vomiting is not a common manifestation associated with plant exposures. *Vet Hum Toxicol* 44:298–300, 2002.

Hung OL, Lewin NA, Howland MA: Herbal preparations. In: Goldfrank LR, Flomenbaum NE, Lewin NA, et al, eds. *Goldfrank's Toxicologic Emergencies*, 6th ed. Stamford, CT: Appleton & Lange, 1221–1242, 1998.

Litovitz TL, Klein-Schwartz W, White S, et al: 1999 Annual Report of the American Association of Poison Control Centers Toxic Exposure Surveillance System. *Am J Emerg Med* 18:517–574, 2000.

Meda HA, Diallo B, Buchet J, et al: Epidemic of fatal encephalopathy in preschool children in Burkina Faso and consumption of unripe akee (*Blighia sapida*) fruit. *Lancet* 353:536–540, 1999.

Shih RD, Goldfrank LR: Plants. In: Goldfrank LR, Flomenbaum NE, Lewin NA, et al, eds. *Goldfrank's Toxicologic Emergencies,* 6th ed. Stamford, CT: Appleton & Lange, 1243–1260, 1998.

QUESTIONS

1. *Dieffenbachia* and *Philodendron* are common houseplants that are commonly ingested by toddlers. The most common manifestations of toxicity are:
   A. Nausea, vomiting, and diarrhea
   B. Severe oral and pharyngeal burns
   C. Bradydysrhythmias
   D. Status epilepticus
   E. Respiratory distress

2. Plants such as foxglove and oleander, which contain cardiac glycosides, when ingested can cause dysrhythmias, including heart blocks. In a patient unresponsive to atropine and cardiac pacing, which of the following interventions is indicated?
   A. Magnesium
   B. Phenytoin
   C. Digibind
   D. Sodium bicarbonate
   E. Physostigmine

3. Water hemlock is often confused with wild carrot or Jerusalem artichoke and ingested by children. Severe intoxication typically presents in which of the following patterns?
   A. Renal failure
   B. Anticholinergic toxidrome: hot as a hare, blind as a bat, dry as a bone, red as a beet, mad as a hatter
   C. Nausea, vomiting, salivation, abdominal cramps, and confusion
   D. Status epilepticus, respiratory distress, and rhabdomyolysis
   E. Sympathomimetic toxidrome: tachycardia, hypertension, hyperthermia

4. A 10-year-old boy presents with an anticholinergic toxidrome after ingesting jimsonweed about 18 hours prior to arrival. He had a temperature of 104°F and exhibits confusion and agitation, but his blood pressure and pulse rate are only modestly elevated. Which of the following interventions is indicated?
   A. Physostigmine, 0.02 mg/kg IV
   B. Haloperidol, 2 mg IM
   C. Decontamination by gastric lavage, followed by administration of activated charcoal.
   D. Observation and supportive care only
   E. Magnesium, 2 g IV

5. The stalk of the rhubarb plant is edible but the leaves are toxic due to which of the following effects?
   A. The leaves contain a high content of calcium oxalate, which is concentrated in the kidneys and produces renal failure
   B. The leaves contain the toxin hypoglycin A which causes profound and persistent hypoglycemia
   C. The leaves contain a small amount of cyanide
   D. The leaves contain hyoscyamine, an atropine isomer
   E. The leaves contain cardiac glycosides

ANSWERS

1. B. *Dieffenbachia* (dumb cane) and *Philodendron* produce burns in the mouth and throat but do not cause gastroenteritis, cardiopulmonary or neurologic problems.

2. C. Patients who have ingested plant material containing cardiac glycosides may develop cardiac dysrhythmias, including heart blocks. They may respond to atropine or cardiac pacing but they may also be unresponsive. In the presence of cardiac instability, Digibind can be used and has been reported to be effective.

3. D. Water hemlock toxicity may progress to status epilepticus, respiratory distress, rhabdomyolysis, and death.

4. C. Jimsonweed has anticholinergic effects, including slowed gastrointestinal motility. Gastric decontamination is indicated even 12 to 24 hours after ingestion. Physostigmine is reserved for patients with seizures, severe hallucinations, hypertension or dysrhythmias.

5. A. The leaves of the rhubarb plant contain calcium oxalate, which can precipitate out in the renal tubules and produce renal failure.

106 SEDATIVE HYPNOTICS

Timothy Erickson
William B. Ignatoff
Gary R. Strange

BARBITURATES

PHARMACOLOGY AND PATHOPHYSIOLOGY

- The barbiturates are classified as:
  - Ultra-short-acting (thiopental)
  - Short-acting (pentobarbital)
  - Long-acting (phenobarbital)

- These agents are primarily used as anticonvulsants and for induction of anesthesia.
- Barbiturates are primarily central nervous system depressants that mediate their effect through inhibition of aminobutyric synapses of the brain.

CLINICAL PRESENTATION

- In the overdose setting, the pediatric patient will present with sedation and coma, often accompanied by respiratory depression.
- Vital signs may reveal hypotension, bradycardia, and hypothermia.

LABORATORY

- In addition to baseline laboratory studies, a quantitative serum phenobarbital level is obtained to document the toxicity, but is not mandatory for definitive management.
- Therapeutic concentrations of phenobarbital range between 15 and 40 µg/mL. Patients with levels above 50 µg/mL will exhibit mild toxicity, while those with levels above 100 µg/mL are typically unresponsive to pain and suffer from respiratory and cardiac depression.

TREATMENT

- The primary management of barbiturate toxicity is support and stabilization of the airway and circulation.
- Comatose patients may require intubation.
- Hypotensive patients are managed with fluid resuscitation, and if necessary, pressors.
- Gastric lavage may be useful up to 1-h post-ingestion. Since most barbiturate ingestions cause CNS and respiratory depression, syrup of ipecac is contraindicated.
- Several investigations have demonstrated the efficacy of multidosing of activated charcoal in children, since the barbiturates, particularly phenobarbital, undergo enterohepatic circulation.
- Urinary alkalinization with sodium bicarbonate to a pH of 7.5 to 8.0 can hasten the renal excretion of phenobarbital, which is a weak acid. This procedure is recommended in severe toxicity.
- Alkalinization is not effective for toxicity from shorter-acting agents.

BENZODIAZEPINES

- Benzodiazepines are among the most commonly prescribed drugs in the world and they cause the majority of sedative hypnotic overdoses. They are used for their anxiolytic, muscle relaxant, and anticonvulsant properties.

PATHOPHYSIOLOGY

- The benzodiazepines act by facilitating the neurotransmission of gamma-aminobutyric acid (GABA). Pure benzodiazepine overdoses result in a mild to moderate CNS depression.

CLINICAL PRESENTATION

- Following an acute overdose, the patient classically presents with sedation, somnolence, ataxia, slurred speech, and lethargy. Profound coma is rare, and its presence should prompt a search for other coingestions or reasons for coma.

TREATMENT

- The most critical management intervention is stabilization of respiration.
- Ipecac is contraindicated due to the CNS effects of these agents.
- Gastric lavage is indicated for patients presenting within 1 h of ingestion, and activated charcoal is recommended in all significant overdoses.
- Flumazenil is an antidotal agent that reduces or terminates benzodiazepine effects by competitive inhibition at the central nervous system GABA sites. In comatose children, initial doses of 0.01 mg/kg intravenously have been recommended. If no response is elicited, this dose can be repeated.

CHLORAL HYDRATE

PATHOPHYSIOLOGY

- Chloral hydrate is an effective sedative hypnotic that produces minimal respiratory and circulatory depression when given in therapeutic doses.
- Although most authorities recommend regimens of 25 to 50 mg/kg per dose, doses up to 80 to 100 mg/kg have been reported as safe and effective for pediatric sedation.

CLINICAL PRESENTATION

- Signs and symptoms of chloral hydrate toxicity are very similar to those seen in barbiturate overdoses, with respiratory, CNS, and cardiovascular manifestations.

TREATMENT

- As with the other sedative hypnotics, the child's airway is stabilized.
- Close attention is paid to the cardiovascular status due to the potential for cardiotoxicity.
- Gastric decontamination considerations are similar to those of the other sedative hypnotic agents.
- If the patient is unstable, hemodialysis should be considered since this method effectively removes the active metabolite trichloroethanol.

BIBLIOGRAPHY

Frenia ML: Multiple dose activated charcoal compared to urinary alkalinization for the enhancement of phenobarbital elimination. *J Toxicol Clin Toxicol* 34:169–175, 1996.

Litovitz TL, Klein-Schwartz W, White S: 1999 Annual report of the American Association of Poison Control Centers toxic exposure surveillance system 2000. *Am J Emerg Med* 18:517–574, 2000.

Olshaker JS, Flanigan J: Flumazenil reversal of lorazepam-induced acute delirium. *J Emerg Med* 24:181–183, 2003.

Sugarman JM, Paul RI: Flumazenil: A review. *Pediatr Emerg Care* 10:37–49, 1994.

Waltzman ML: Flunitrazepam: A review of "roofies." *Pediatr Emerg Care* 15:59–60, 1999.

QUESTIONS

1. In addition to supportive care and gastric decontamination, which of the following interventions is specifically indicated for severe toxicity due to phenobarbital?
   A. Urinary acidification
   B. Urinary alkalinization
   C. Intubation and controlled ventilation to a P_{CO_2} end point of 30 to 35
   D. Gastric lavage with sodium bicarbonate
   E. Administration of methylene blue
2. In addition to supportive care and gastric decontamination, which of the following interventions is specifically indicated for severe toxicity due to benzodiazepines?
   A. Forced diuresis
   B. Hemodialysis
   C. Hemoperfusion
   D. Flumazenil
   E. Nalmefine
3. Potential adverse effects of chloral hydrate include which of the following?
   A. Hypertension
   B. Respiratory alkalosis
   C. Depression of cardiac contractility
   D. Paradoxical hyperexcitability
   E. Hyperthermia

ANSWERS

1. B. Urinary alkalinization, with sodium bicarbonate, to a pH of 7.5 to 8.0 can hasten the renal excretion of phenobarbital, which is a weak acid. This procedure is recommended in severe toxicity.
2. D. Flumazenil is an antidotal agent that reduces or terminates benzodiazepine effects by competitive inhibition at the central nervous system GABA sites. Forced diuresis, hemodialysis, and hemoperfusion are not effective since benzodiazepines are highly bound to plasma proteins. Nalmefine is a long-acting opioid antagonist.
3. C. In large overdoses, chloral hydrate can depress myocardial contractility, resulting in dysrhythmias. It may also produce hypotension, respiratory depression, coma, and hypothermia.

107 THEOPHYLLINE

Frank P. Paloucek
Gary R. Strange

INTRODUCTION

- Important factors contributing to the toxicity of theophylline are its widespread use, narrow therapeutic index, the proliferation of dosage forms, its availability as a nonprescription product, and multiple drug–drug, drug–disease, and drug–food interactions.

PHARMACOLOGY AND PHARMACOKINETICS

- The exact mechanism of action of theophylline is unknown but the majority of its effects appear to reflect its actions as a direct adenosine antagonist.
  - Central nervous system stimulation
  - Medullary vomiting center stimulation
  - Positive inotrope and chronotrope
  - Reduction of peripheral arteriolar resistance
  - Increase in renal blood flow and glomerular filtration rate
  - Stimulation of secretion of gastric acid and pepsin
- Theophylline is predominantly marketed and used in sustained-release dosage forms, which leads to

significant delays in presentation or development of symptoms and prolonged absorption times.

ACUTE THEOPHYLLINE TOXICITY

- The clinical manifestations of acute theophylline toxicity are primarily gastrointestinal, cardiovascular, and neurologic. Disturbances in serum electrolytes are also produced.
  - Gastrointestinal manifestations include nausea, vomiting, and gastrointestinal bleeding.
  - Cardiovascular manifestations include tachyarrhythmias, hypotension, and cardiac arrest. Sinus and supraventricular tachycardias, along with nausea and vomiting, are the most common presenting features of theophylline toxicity, regardless of etiology. These are not life-threatening in the absence of other underlying cardiac disease.
  - Neurologic manifestations include mental status changes, tremor, seizures, and coma. Seizures are a very ominous event. Status epilepticus can occur and is associated with more significant morbidity and mortality than other causes of status epilepticus in children. A predisposing factor for seizures in acute toxicity is a serum theophylline concentration above 100 mg/L.
  - Electrolyte disturbances are fairly typical in the acutely toxic patient and can include hypokalemia, hypophosphatemia, and hypercalcemia.
  - Miscellaneous manifestations of theophylline toxicity include diuresis secondary to transient increase in renal blood flow in acute pediatric exposures, rhabdomyolysis, and tachypnea. Hyperglycemia can also occur.
- Increased mortality is associated with those aged less than 2 years or serum theophylline concentrations above 100 mg/L in acute pediatric overdoses.
- The single most important laboratory evaluation for suspected theophylline toxicity is serum theophylline concentration. The normal range is 10 to 20 mg/L and the toxic range is above 20 mg/L, although toxic symptoms can occur at concentrations of 10 to 20 mg/L.

MANAGEMENT

- Patients presenting with acute theophylline toxicity are managed with conventional supportive care and treatment of specific complications as they arise. There is no specific antidote for theophylline toxicity.
- Activated charcoal is the gastric decontamination treatment of choice. The initial dose is calculated to deliver 10 g of charcoal for every 1 g of ingested theophylline, up to a maximum of 100 g of charcoal. It is important to note that achieving a 10 : 1 ratio may require multiple doses. The initial dose is administered with sorbitol in a 1.5 g/kg dose.
- An alternative to gastric decontamination with charcoal is whole bowel irrigation with a high-molecular weight polyethylene glycol dosed at 15 to 40 mL/kg/h. This is equally efficacious for acute ingestions when administered within 1 h of ingestion, but it is not effective in late presentations of acute ingestions, in which charcoal is the treatment of choice.
- Elimination enhancement is an important consideration for theophylline toxicity. Effective modalities include:
  - Multiple-dose oral activated charcoal
    - Oral activated charcoal at 25 g every 2 h is initiated and continued until concentrations are below 20 mg/L or gastrointestinal complications occur.
  - Hemodialysis
    - Indicated prophylactically for patients with theophylline concentrations above 100 mg/L in an overdose
  - Charcoal hemoperfusion
    - Indicated prophylactically for patients with theophylline concentrations above 100 mg/L in an overdose
  - Exchange transfusions
  - Plasmapheresis

ACUTE-ON-CHRONIC THEOPHYLLINE TOXICITY

- Patients with acute-on-chronic theophylline toxicity present with the same clinical manifestations as those with acute toxicity, but toxicity develops at lower levels. If not diagnosed by the history, acute-on-chronic toxicity is suspected in patients taking theophylline who develop multifocal atrial tachycardias, hypotension, or hypokalemia.
- Management is similar to that of acute toxic overdose.
  - The only variation occurs with the use of elimination-enhancing treatment. The end point of multiple-dose activated charcoal is 30 mg/L, not 20 mg/L, if theophylline therapy remains indicated.
  - Hemodialysis and charcoal hemoperfusion are indicated prophylactically in patients with theophylline concentrations above 100 mg/L in an acute or acute-on-chronic overdose.

CHRONIC THEOPHYLLINE TOXICITY

- For chronic overdose patients with theophylline concentrations above 30 mg/L, oral activated charcoal at 25 g every 2 h is initiated and continued until concentrations are below 30 mg/L or gastrointestinal complications occur.

• Gastric decontamination is not indicated for the chronic patient.

• Either hemodialysis or charcoal hemoperfusion is indicated in the chronic patient when serum theophylline concentration is above 60 mg/L, especially for patients older than 60 years of age, although there are fewer data supporting this recommendation than for acute ingestions and concentrations above 100 mg/L.

BIBLIOGRAPHY

Cooling DS: Theophylline toxicity. *J Emerg Med* 11:415–425, 1993.

Kempf J, Rusterholtz T, Ber C, et al: Hemodynamic study as guideline for the use of beta blockers in acute theophylline poisoning. *Intensive Care Med* 22:585–587, 1996.

Osborn HH, Henry G, Wax P, et al: Theophylline toxicity in a premature neonate—Elimination kinetics of exchange transfusion. *J Toxicol Clin Toxicol* 4:639–644, 1993.

Polak M, Rolon MA, Chouchana A, et al: Theophylline intoxication mimicking diabetic ketoacidosis. *Diabetes Metab* 25:513–516, 1999.

Paloucek FP: Theophylline toxicokinetics. *J Pharm Pract* 6:57–62, 1993.

Shannon M: Predictors of major toxicity after theophylline overdose. *Ann Intern Med* 119:1161–1167, 1993.

Shannon MW: Comparative efficacy of hemodialysis and hemoperfusion in severe theophylline intoxication. *Acad Emerg Med* 4:674–678, 1997.

Shannon MW: Life-threatening events after theophylline overdose. *Arch Intern Med* 159:989–994, 1999.

QUESTIONS

1. The most common presenting features of acute theophylline toxicity are which of the following?
   A. Nausea, vomiting, and gastrointestinal bleeding
   B. Ventricular dysrhythmias and hypotension
   C. Hyperkalemia and hypocalcemia
   D. Nausea, vomiting, and sinus or supraventricular tachycardia
   E. Generalized tonic-clonic seizures

2. Which of the following interventions has **NOT** been shown to be effective in the management of acute theophylline toxicity?
   A. Adenosine can serve as a specific antidote to theophylline toxicity.
   B. Activated charcoal is the gastric decontamination treatment of choice.
   C. Whole bowel irrigation with polyethylene glycol may be used to enhance elimination.
   D. Hemodialysis or charcoal hemoperfusion is indicated prophylactically in patients with theophylline concentrations above 100 mg/L.
   E. The preferred pharmacologic treatment for seizures is a benzodiazepine.

3. Management of chronic theophylline toxicity varies from that of acute theophylline toxicity in which of the following ways?
   A. Hemodialysis and charcoal hemoperfusion are not indicated for chronic toxicity.
   B. The end point of multiple-dose activated charcoal is 30 mg/L, not 20 mg/L, if theophylline therapy remains indicated after a chronic overdose.
   C. Gastric decontamination requires prolonged, high-volume lavage after chronic overdose.
   D. Seizures are less likely to occur in chronic toxicity and usually require no specific treatment if they do occur.
   E. Electrolyte disturbances are more frequent in chronic overdose situations and often do not respond to conventional therapy.

ANSWERS

1. D. The common presenting features are nausea, vomiting, and supraventricular tachycardias. These are not life-threatening in the absence of cardiac disease. Electrolyte disturbances are common, with hypokalemia, hypophosphatemia, and hypercalcemia most common. Significant ventricular dysrhythmias are rare. Seizures are frequent but not the most common presentation.

2. A. There is no specific antidote for theophylline toxicity. The other interventions listed are all appropriate in an acute theophylline intoxication.

3. B. The end point of multiple-dose activated charcoal is 30 mg/L, not 20 mg/L, if theophylline therapy remains indicated after a chronic overdose. Either hemodialysis or charcoal hemoperfusion **IS** indicated in the chronic patient when serum theophylline concentration is above 60 mg/L, especially in patients older than 60 years of age. Gastric decontamination with lavage is not indicated in chronic overdoses. Seizures, including status epilepticus, may occur in chronic overdoses and should be treated with benzodiazepines or barbiturates. Electrolyte disturbances are less frequent in chronic overdoses but they do respond to conventional therapy.

108 LETHAL TOXINS IN SMALL DOSES

Leon Gussow
Gary R. Strange

CAMPHOR

- Camphor is present in many over-the-counter liniments and cold preparations. As little as 1 g has been reported to cause death in an 18-month-old child.
- Clinical symptoms of camphor toxicity, which occur rapidly with onset 5 to 120 min after ingestion, typically begin with a feeling of generalized warmth progressing to pharyngeal and epigastric burning, followed by mental status changes. Muscle twitching and fasciculations may herald the onset of seizures, which have also been reported to occur suddenly, without preceding symptoms.
- Management of ingestion of camphor consists of supportive care and gastric decontamination. Seizures are managed with benzodiazepines or phenobarbital.
- Asymptomatic patients should be observed for 8 h after ingestion of camphor prior to discharge from the emergency department.

BENZOCAINE

- Benzocaine is present in many local anesthetics, including first aid ointments and infant teething formulas. Benzocaine is metabolized to aniline and nitrosobenzene, both of which can cause methemoglobinemia, especially in infants under 4 months of age, who are deficient in methemoglobin reductase.
- Clinical signs and symptoms of benzocaine toxicity begin 30 min to 6 h after ingestion, with tachycardia, tachypnea, and a characteristic cyanosis that does not respond to oxygen.
- Treatment of toxicity consists of gastric emptying, general support, and in selected cases, the administration of the antidote, methylene blue, which is indicated for methemoglobin levels above 30 percent and symptoms of respiratory distress or altered mental status.

LOMOTIL

- Lomotil is an antidiarrheal preparation that combines an opiate (diphenoxylate) with an anticholinergic (atropine). After ingestion, respiratory depression can occur as late as 24 h and there appears to be no correlation between dose ingested and severity of symptoms.

Therefore, any child with known or suspected ingestion of any amount of Lomotil is admitted and monitored for at least 24 h, no matter what the initial clinical condition.
- Syrup of ipecac is contraindicated, since CNS depression may supervene and induced emesis will delay the administration of activated charcoal. In any patient with CNS or respiratory depression, gastric lavage is indicated, even if many hours have passed since ingestion.
- Multiple-dose activated charcoal (1 g/kg every 4 h) is recommended because difenoxine undergoes enterohepatic recycling. A cathartic can be given with the first dose of charcoal, but is not repeated with every dose.

CHLOROQUINE

- Chloroquine, an antimalarial agent, is a powerful, rapidly acting cardiotoxin capable of causing sudden cardiorespiratory collapse. The interval between ingestion and cardiac arrest is often less than 2 h.
- Chloroquine causes myocardial depression and vasodilation, producing sudden profound hypotension. Automaticity and conductivity of heart muscle is also decreased, resulting in bradycardia and ventricular escape rhythms.
- Induction of emesis should be avoided; gastric lavage is the preferred method of gastric emptying. Activated charcoal (1 g/kg) and a cathartic should be given by mouth or via orogastric tube.
- Treatment is largely supportive.
- Intubation, ventilation, defibrillation, and cardiac pacing may be required.
- Class IA antiarrhythmics (quinidine, procainamide, and disopyramide) are contraindicated.

METHYL SALICYLATE

- Methyl salicylate is a concentrated liquid that is absorbed quickly and can produce early-onset severe salicylate toxicity. Ingestion of less than 1 teaspoon has been fatal in a child.
- Clinical presentation and treatment of this overdose is similar to that of other types of salicylate poisoning.

BIBLIOGRAPHY

Couper RT: Methemoglobinemia secondary to topical lignocaine/prilocaine in a circumcised neonate. *J Paediatr Child Health* 36:406, 2000.

Gouin S, Patel H: Unusual cause of seizure. *Pediatr Emerg Care* 12:298, 1996.

Koren G: Medications which can kill a toddler with one tablet or teaspoonful. *Clin Toxicol* 31:407–413, 1993.

Liebelt EL, Shannon MW: Small doses, big problems: A selected review of highly toxic common medications. *Pediatr Emerg Care* 9:292–297, 1993.

Spiller HA, Revolinski DH, Winter M, et al: Multi-center retrospective evaluation of oral benzocaine exposure in children. *Vet Hum Toxicol* 42:228–231, 2000.

QUESTIONS

1. A 2-year-old asymptomatic child is brought to the emergency department by concerned parents who found the child with an open container of Campho-Phenique. During the observation period in the ED, what specific toxic signs would you concerned about?
   A. Oropharyngeal burns with upper airway obstruction
   B. Sudden onset of seizures
   C. Nausea, vomiting and gastrointestinal bleeding
   D. Tachypnea and cyanosis poorly responsive to oxygen therapy
   E. Respiratory depression and pin-point pupils

2. Benzocaine is present in many local anesthetic creams and first aid ointments. Ingestion of small quantities of this substance can result in which of the following?
   A. Respiratory acidosis
   B. Severe hypoxia at the cellular level
   C. Methemoglobinemia
   D. Metabolic alkalosis
   E. Salicylism

3. Lomotil is an antidiarrheal preparation that contains a combination of two ingredients that are toxic in very small quantities. These are:
   A. Methyl salicylate and scopolamine
   B. Metaclopromide and hydrocodone
   C. Paregoric and lidocaine
   D. Diphenoxylate and atropine
   E. Bismuth subsalicylate and aluminum hydroxide

4. Chloroquine is used in the treatment and prophylaxis of malarial disease. Its primary toxicity is which of the following?
   A. Gastrointestinal upsets
   B. Respiratory depression
   C. Cardiac toxicity
   D. Neurological depression
   E. Metabolic disturbances

5. An 18-month-old child has ingested about a teaspoon of oil of wintergreen. You advise the parents to do which of the following?
   A. Observe the child at home for tachypnea or hyperthermia and bring the child to the ED if these signs develop.
   B. Administer syrup of ipecac at home and bring the patient to the ED for evaluation after vomiting has ceased.
   C. Reassure the parents that this is a nontoxic dose, requiring no special action.
   D. Bring the child immediately to the ED for gastric evacuation, activated charcoal administration, and evaluation for severe salicylate intoxication.
   E. Bring the child to the ED for measurement of a 6-h salicylate level, anticipating a nontoxic level and that no further treatment will be necessary.

ANSWERS

1. B. Clinical symptoms of camphor toxicity begin rapidly, with onset 5 to 120 min after ingestion. Initially, a feeling of generalized warmth progresses to pharyngeal and epigastric burning sensation. No actual oral or upper airway burns are seen. Mental status changes can follow, with confusion, restlessness, delirium, and hallucinations. Muscle twitching and fasciculations may herald the onset of seizures, which have been reported to occur suddenly, without preceding symptoms.

2. C. Benzocaine is metabolized to aniline and nitrosobenzene, both of which can cause methemoglobinemia, especially in infants under 4 months of age, who are deficient in methemoglobin reductase.

3. D. Lomotil contains an opiate (diphenoxylate) and an anticholinergic (atropine). Ingestions of 1/2 to 1 tablet have been reported to cause toxic signs and symptoms. Respiratory depression can occur as late as 24 h after ingestion, making prolonged observation necessary for all possible ingestions.

4. C. Chloroquine is a powerful, rapidly acting cardiotoxin capable of causing sudden cardiorespiratory collapse.

5. D. One teaspoon of oil of wintergreen contains 7 g of salicylate (equivalent to 21 aspirin tablets) and ingestion of this amount has been reported to kill a small child.

109 HUMAN AND ANIMAL BITES

Gary R. Strange
David A. Townes
Patricia Lee

HISTORY AND PHYSICAL EXAMINATION

- It is important to obtain a complete history of the injury, including what type of animal caused the wound and the age of the wound. One must also elicit host factors that may affect wound healing; especially important is a history of diabetes, peripheral vascular disease, chronic use of glucocorticoids, or other immunocompromised states.
- The physical examination should include a full examination and exploration of the wound. The type of wound (laceration, crush, or puncture) and the extent of involvement of deep structures must be determined. If the wound occurs over a joint, the joint should be examined through the full range of motion.
- When appropriate, radiographs should be obtained to look for fractures, foreign bodies, and air in the joint or soft tissues. One should keep in mind that the canine jaw can generate forces up to 450 pounds per square inch. In children this force may be sufficient to penetrate the cranium. Computed tomography of the head should be considered in bite wounds to the scalp.

WOUND CARE

- One of the best methods of reducing the risk of infection is adequate irrigation of the wound. An acceptable method is to irrigate the wound with 1 to 2 L of normal saline through a 19 or 20-gauge vascular catheter.
- The decision to close the wound depends on its age, type, and location. Under no circumstances should a wound that appears infected be closed.
- In most cases, bite wounds on the hand should be left open because of the high potential for morbidity if these wounds become infected.
- Dog bites may be safely closed if they are not located on the hands.
- Cat bites, which are usually puncture wounds, should not be closed because they cannot be adequately cleaned.
- In general, wounds that are more than 8 to 12 hours old should be left open. Potentially disfiguring bite wounds on the face may be closed even when more than 12 hours old; however, these patients must be followed very carefully for evidence of infection.
- All bite wounds treated on an outpatient basis should be reevaluated within 48 hours.

ANTIBIOTICS

- Wounds that have evidence of infection should be treated with antibiotics. The use of antibiotics in prophylaxis remains controversial. The type of animal, location of the wound, and host factors must be considered.
- Wounds on the hands and feet should be treated with antibiotics, while those on the face and scalp are less likely to become infected and do not need prophylactic antibiotic coverage.
- In general, bite wounds caused by cats and humans should be treated prophylactically, while those caused

by dogs and rodents may not need treatment with antibiotics.

- If the decision to treat with prophylactic antibiotics is made, the initial treatment should be for 3 days. If at the end of this time there is no evidence of infection, the wound is very unlikely to become infected and the antibiotics may be discontinued.
- Dog bites tend to become infected with *Staphylococcus aureus, Streptococcus* species, and *Pasteurella canis*, but *Pseudomonas* species, *Enterobacter cloacae*, and many others have been identified.
- Cat bites are likely to become infected with *Pasteurella multocida*.
- Human bite wounds tend to become infected with *Staphylococcus aureus, Streptococcus* species, and *Eikenella corrodens. Pasteurella* species are unlikely infectious agents in human bite wounds.
- In the case of dog and cat bites *Staphylococcus* and *Streptococcus* species may be covered by dicloxacillin or a first-generation cephalosporin. *Pasteurella* species are covered by penicillin, ampicillin, amoxicillin, amoxicillin/clavulanic acid, second and third-generation cephalosporins, doxycycline, trimethoprim-sulfamethoxazole, clarithromycin, and azithromycin.
- Empiric therapy for dog and cat bites should include a beta-lactam antibiotic and a beta-lactamase inhibitor, a second-generation cephalosporin with anaerobic activity, or a combination of penicillin and a first-generation cephalosporin.
- For human bite wounds, *Eikenella corrodens* is covered by penicillin or amoxicillin/clavulanic acid, and dicloxacillin can be used to cover *Staphylococcus* and *Streptococcus*. It may be necessary to use a two-antibiotic regimen for human bite wounds.

RABIES PROPHYLAXIS

- Rabies is a viral infection transmitted in the saliva of infected animals. It is caused by the rhabdovirus group and may lead to encephalomyelitis. The disease is almost universally fatal.
- In determining the need for rabies prophylaxis, the physician must consider the type of animal causing the injury and the prevalence of rabies in the region. If rabies is not suspected, no treatment is indicated.
- In the case of dogs, cats, and ferrets, the animal should be captured and quarantined for 10 days. If the animal remains healthy, no treatment is necessary. If the animal becomes ill or if rabies is suspected, the animal should be sacrificed and the brain examined for evidence of rabies. If the animal is infected the child should be immediately vaccinated.
- Most other carnivores including skunks, raccoons, and foxes should be considered infected unless proven

negative by laboratory testing. Livestock, large rodents, lagomorphs, and other mammals should be considered on an individual case basis. If the animal cannot be located, decisions regarding prophylaxis must be based on the prevalence of rabies in the area and the species of biting animal.

- Post-exposure prophylaxis is indicated for bite, scratch, or mucous membrane exposure to a bat if the animal cannot be collected and tested. Post-exposure prophylaxis may be indicated in cases in which contact is likely to have occurred but is not documented. This includes a child sleeping in a room where a bat is found.
- Post-exposure prophylaxis includes the administration of one of the available vaccines and human rabies immune globulin. The vaccine, such as human diploid cell vaccine (HDCV), is given in five 1-mL intramuscular injections on days 0, 3, 7, 14, and 28. It should be administered in the deltoid or anterolateral thigh. It should not be administered in the gluteal area. Human rabies immune globulin (HRIG) is dosed at 20 IU/kg.

TETANUS PROPHYLAXIS

- Tetanus immunoprophylaxis should also be considered. Refer to Chapter 23 for guidelines.

BIBLIOGRAPHY

Edwards MS: Infections due to human and animal bites. In: Geigin RD, Cherry JD, eds. *Textbook of Pediatric Infectious Diseases*, 4th ed. Philadelphia: Saunders, 2841–2855, 1998.

Human Rabies Prevention—United States, 1999. Recommendations of the Advisory Committee on Immunization Practices (ACIP). *MMWR* 48:1–21, 1999.

Jackson SC: Mammalian bites. In: Surpure JS, ed. *Synopsis of Pediatric Emergency Care.* Boston: Andover Medical, 393–401, 1993.

Talan DA, Citron DM, Abrahamian FM, et al: Bacteriologic analysis of infected dog and cat bites. *N Engl J Med* 340: 85–92, 1999.

Trott A: Bite wounds, in Trott A (ed): *Wounds and Laceration: Emergency Care and Closure*, 2nd ed. St. Louis: Mosby-Year Book, 1997, pp 265–284.

Wilkerson JA: Clinical updates in wilderness medicine—rabies update. *Wilderness Environ Med* 11:31–39, 2000.

QUESTIONS

1. An 18-month-old child is brought to the ED by concerned parents who state that their child was bitten by the neighbor's pit bull dog after the child slapped

at the dog. The neighbor states that the dog is up to date on his immunizations. A check with the local health department reveals no case of rabies from dog bite within your community for the past 25 years. Physical examination reveals a full-thickness 3-cm scalp wound over the right temporal area. The child is alert and appropriately interactive. No other injuries are noted. The most appropriate next step in management should be:
A. Suture wound. Discharge home with prescription for cephalexin and follow up in 1 week
B. CT of head
C. Administration of 1 mL of human diploid cell vaccine IM and 20 IU/kg of human rabies immune globulin IM
D. Do not suture. Explain to the parents that a dog bite has a high likelihood of becoming infected and the wound should be allowed to heal by intention
E. Contact local health authorities to sacrifice the dog and examine the dog's brain for evidence of rabies

2. A 14-year-old male presents with a 1-cm laceration located on the dorsum of his right hand. He states he sustained the injury during a fight at a party last night. He does not remember the date of his last tetanus immunization. He denies numbness, weakness, or other injury. The most appropriate management course would be:
A. Irrigate wound, tetanus 0.5 mL IM, and discharge home. Explain to patient that wound is too old to suture
B. Irrigate wound, tetanus 0.5 mL IM, suture wound, and discharge home with prescription for cefixime
C. X-ray hand to evaluate for fracture, irrigate wound, tetanus 0.5 mL IM, discharge home with prescription for amoxicillin/clavulanate
D. Admit for IV antibiotics
E. Explain to patient that the wound may be infected with *Pasturella multocida* and treatment with antibiotics is appropriate

3. A 13-year-old woman presents 4 hours after she was bitten on the hand by her own cat. The best management of this injury would be:
A. Reassure the patient that cat bites are frequently benign and follow-up is generally not necessary
B. Suture the wound and discharge home on amoxicillin/clavulanic acid
C. Explain that cat bite wounds are generally puncture wounds and should not be sutured
D. Explain that antibiotics are not necessary
E. Begin a 3-day antibiotic course of treatment targeted against *Eikenella corrodens*

4. A 9-year-old boy is brought by his mother following a camping trip in which the patient and a group of other boys unsuccessfully attempted to capture a

wild raccoon. While reaching for the animal, the boy sustained a bite to his right hand. The mother is concerned that that her son might need a tetanus booster injection. The most appropriate course of action should be:
A. Capture the raccoon and bring to the state laboratory for testing
B. Administer tetanus immunization, clean the wound, and discharge home on a beta-lactam antibiotic
C. Administer human rabies immune globulin and discharge home
D. Administer tetanus toxoid, human rabies immune globulin and begin human diploid cell vaccine (HDCV) injection
E. Administer tetanus immune globulin and tetanus toxoid

ANSWERS

1. B. The canine jaw can generate forces up to 450 pounds per square inch. In children, this force can be sufficient to penetrate the cranium. Computed tomography of the head should be considered in bite wounds to the scalp. Dog bites may be safely closed if they are not located on the hands and have no evidence of infection. Empiric therapy for dog bites should include a beta-lactam antibiotic and a beta-lactamase inhibitor. In this case, the dog has not been shown to reside in a rabies endemic area and the dog was provoked into aggression by the child's action, so treatment for rabies or sacrificing the animal is not required. All bite wounds treated on an outpatient basis should be reevaluated within 48 hours for infection.

2. C. In most cases, bite wounds over the hand should be left open because of the high potential for infection and morbidity should the wound become infected. In addition, wounds that are more than 8 to 12 hours old should be left open. Human bite wounds tend to become infected with *Staphylococcus aureus* and *Streptococcus* species and *Eikenella corrodens*. *Pasturella* species are unlikely infectious agents in human bite wounds. For human bite wounds, *Eikenella corrodens* is covered by penicillin, amoxicillin/clavulanic acid or dicloxicillin. A two-antibiotic regimen for human bite wound may be necessary.

3. C. Cat bites are usually puncture wounds and should not be closed because they cannot be adequately cleaned. All bite wounds treated on an outpatient basis should be reevaluated within 48 hours. Wounds on the hands and feet should be treated with antibiotics. Cat bites are likely to become infected with *Pasturella multocida*.

4. D. Most carnivores, including skunks, raccoons, and foxes, should be considered infected unless proven negative by laboratory testing. If the animal cannot be located, decisions regarding prophylaxis must be based on the prevalence of rabies in the area and the species of the biting animal. Post-exposure prophylaxis includes the administration of one of the available vaccines and human rabies immune globulin. The vaccine such as human diploid cell vaccine (HDCV) is given in five 1 mL intramuscular injections on days 0, 3, 7, 14 and 28. It should be administered in the deltoid or anterolateral thigh. It should not be administered in the gluteal area. Human rabies immune globulin HRIG is dosed at 20 IU/kg.

110 SNAKE ENVENOMATIONS

Timothy Erickson
Bruce E. Herman
Mary Jo A. Bowman
Gary R. Strange
Valerie A. Dobiesz

INTRODUCTION

- Snake bites usually occur when people venture into the snake's natural habitat, but bites have been reported among religious sects that handle snakes, as well as in pet owners and zoo workers.
- Families of venomous snakes indigenous to the United States include:
  ○ Crotalidae (pit vipers)
  ○ Elapidae (coral snakes)

PIT VIPERS

ANATOMY

- Pit vipers classically possess:
  ○ Triangular or arrow-shaped head
  ○ Facial pits between the nostril and eye that serve as heat and vibration sensors
  ○ Vertical or elliptical pupils

PATHOPHYSIOLOGY

- Because of their small body weight, infants and young children are relatively more vulnerable to severe envenomation.

- Bites on the head or trunk are more severe than extremity bites. Bites on the upper extremities are most common and potentially more dangerous than those on the lower extremities, whereas lower extremity bites may result in delayed clinical signs of toxicity. Direct envenomation into an artery or vein is associated with a much higher mortality rate.
- The venom itself is a complex mixture of enzymes that primarily function to immobilize, kill, and digest the snake's prey. The major toxic effects occur within the surrounding tissue, blood vessels, and blood components.

CLINICAL PRESENTATION

- Local cutaneous changes classically include 1 or 2 puncture marks with pain and swelling at the site, while nonvenomous snakes usually leave a horseshoe-shaped imprint of multiple teeth marks.
- If the envenomation is severe, swelling and edema may involve the entire extremity within an hour. Ecchymosis, hemorrhagic vesicles, and petechiae may appear within several hours.
- Systemic signs and symptoms include paresthesias of the scalp, periorbital fasciculations, weakness, diaphoresis, nausea, dizziness, and a minty or metallic taste in the mouth.
- Severe bites can result in coagulopathies and disseminated intravascular coagulation (DIC). Rapid hypotension and shock, with pulmonary edema and renal and cardiac dysfunction, can also result, particularly if the victim suffers a direct intravenous envenomation.

MANAGEMENT

- The victim's extremity should be immobilized and physical activity minimized.
- To maintain renal flow and intravascular volume, oral fluids are vigorously administered.
- To guide therapy, wounds are graded as:
  ○ Minimal (local cutaneous swelling and tenderness at the bite site)
  ○ Moderate (significant extremity swelling and evidence of systemic toxicity)
  ○ Severe (obvious systemic findings, unstable vital signs, and laboratory evidence of coagulopathy)
- The patient's tetanus prophylaxis should be updated if needed.
- Broad-spectrum antibiotics are administered in moderate or severe envenomations.
- Crotalidae antivenin is the fundamental treatment for pit viper envenomation. The conventional equine

antivenin has been supplanted by Crotalinae polyvalent immune Fab (ovine) antivenom (crotaline Fab). Crotaline Fab appears to be safe and effective for use in children. Control of coagulopathy may require repeat dosing. The incidence of hypersensitivity reactions is much lower than with the equine antivenin.

- In comparison with adults, pediatric patients are given proportionately more antivenin, since children receive a greater amount of venom per kilogram of body weight.
- Antivenin is most efficacious if given within 4 to 6 hours of the bite. It is of less value if delayed for 8 hours, and is of questionable value after 24 hours.

DISPOSITION

- The prognosis following pit viper envenomation is generally good, with an overall mortality rate below 1 percent if the antivenin is given in adequate amounts without delay.
- If a pediatric patient only has a suspected bite, develops no signs or symptoms of envenomation during 6 to 12 hours of observation, and has normal laboratory studies, the child can be discharged. Exceptions to this rule are bites from the Mojave rattlesnake, which can cause delayed neurologic and respiratory depression several hours after envenomation.
- If the child exhibits moderate to severe envenomation, has evidence of coagulopathy, or requires antivenin administration, admission to an intensive care unit is indicated.

CORAL SNAKES

- Two members of the coral snake family (Elapidae) are indigenous to the United States.
  - The western coral snake (*Micrurus euryoxanthus*) is found in Arizona and New Mexico.
  - The eastern coral snake (*Micrurus fulvius fulvius*) is found in the Carolinas and the Gulf states.
- A mnemonic quote to help distinguish the coral snakes from nonpoisonous snakes in the United States is "red on yellow, kill a fellow; red on black, venom lack," which refers to order of the colored bands that run vertically down the body of the coral snake.

CLINICAL PRESENTATION

- The venom of the coral snake is primarily neurotoxic.
- Within several hours the patient may experience paresthesias, vomiting, weakness, diplopia, fasciculations, confusion, and occasionally respiratory depression.

- The fatality rate from eastern coral snake bites is as high as 10 percent.

MANAGEMENT

- The coral snake antivenin is effective against bites of the eastern coral snake, but not against western coral snake bites. Fortunately the venom of the western coral snake is less toxic than that of its eastern counterpart.
  - Three to five vials of the antivenin are generally recommended following skin testing. Adverse side effects include anaphylaxis and serum sickness.

EXOTIC SNAKES

- Several bites occur each year from nonindigenous snakes. Physicians encountering victims of exotic snake envenomation may receive assistance in treatment by calling the local zoo's herpetologist or regional poison control center.

BIBLIOGRAPHY

Chippaux JP: Snake bites: Appraisal of the global situation. *Bull World Heath Org* 76:515–524, 1998.

Clark RF, Williams SR, Nordt SP, Boyer-Hassen LV: Successful treatment of crotalid-induced neurotoxicity with new polyvalent FAB antivenom. *Ann Emerg Med* 30:54–57, 1997.

Dart RC, McNally J: Efficacy, safety and use of snake antivenoms in the United States. *Ann Emerg Med* 37:181–188, 2001.

Gold BS, Dart RC, Barish RA: Bites of venomous snakes. *N Engl J Med* 347:347–356, 2002.

Holstege CP, Miller A, Wermuth M, et al: Crotalid envenomation. *Crit Care Clin* 13:889–921, 1997.

Lawrence WT, Giannopoulos A, Hansen A: Pit viper bites: Rational management in locales in which copperheads and cottonmouths predominate. *Ann Plastic Surg* 36:276–285, 1996.

Litovitz TL, Schwartz-Klein W, White S, et al: 1999 Annual report of the American Association of Poison Control Centers toxic exposures surveillance system *Am J Emerg Med* 18:517–574, 2000.

Norris RL, Bush SP: North American venomous reptile bites. In: Auerbach PS, ed. *Wilderness Medicine: Management of Wilderness Emergencies*, 4th ed. St. Louis: Mosby, 896–926, 2001.

Offerman SR, Bush SP, Moynihan JA, Clark RF: Crotaline Fab antivenom for the treatment of children with rattlesnake envenomation. *Pediatrics* 110: 968–971, 2002.

Ruha AM, Curry SC, Beuhler M, et al: Initial postmarketing experience with crotalidae polyvalent immune Fab for treatment of rattlesnake envenomation. *Ann Emerg Med* 39: 648–650, 2002.

Whitley RE: Conservative treatment of copperhead snakebites without antivenin. *J Trauma* 41:219–221, 1996.

QUESTIONS

1. Which of the following statements is correct regarding snake envenomations?
   A. There is only one family of venomous snakes indigenous to the United States
   B. The venom of coral snakes is primarily neurotoxic
   C. Incision of the bite and suctioning out the venom is indicated in pit viper bites
   D. Tourniquets have been shown to be effective when applied immediately after a venomous snake bite
   E. Antivenin should be given to all snake bites

2. A 10-year-old male presents to the ED with a history of being bitten on the arm by a rattlesnake while on a camping trip with his family. He appears ill with significant progressive swelling to his left arm, nausea, and dizziness. He is hypotensive and tachycardic. Which of the following would be appropriate in the management of this patient?
   A. Fluid restriction
   B. Observation in the ED for 6 to 12 hours
   C. Administration of Crotalidae antivenin
   D. Admission to the general pediatric ward
   E. Routine blood work is not necessary

3. Which of the following is correct regarding snake envenomations?
   A. Pediatric patients are given proportionately less antivenin than adults
   B. Antivenin is highly efficacious if given after 24 hours of the bite
   C. A coral snake in the United States with red bands next to black is most likely to be venomous
   D. The venom of western coral snakes is more toxic than the eastern and has an effective antivenin
   E. If the patient suffers a snake bite from a nonindigenous snake the local zoo herpetologist may be consulted

4. Pit viper bites in children have which of the following characteristics?
   A. Children are less vulnerable to severe envenomations than adults
   B. Bites on the lower extremity are more severe than on the head or trunk
   C. Severe bites can result in coagulopathies and disseminated intravascular coagulation
   D. The fatality rate is as high as 20 percent even with optimal treatment

   E. The hallmark of a pit viper bite is multiple teeth marks with no pain or swelling

5. Which of the following is correct regarding coral snake envenomations?
   A. Coral snakes are distinguished by a triangular head, facial pits and vertical pupils
   B. They are dull in color typically brown or green
   C. Symptoms may include cardiac dysrhythmias
   D. Skin testing should be done prior to administration of the antivenin
   E. There are no serious side effects to the administration of antivenin

ANSWERS

1. B. The two families of venomous snakes indigenous to the United States are Crotalidae (pit vipers) and Elapidae (coral snakes). Incision and suctioning of the snake bite and tourniquet placement is contraindicated. Antivenin therapy is guided by the type of snake and the severity of symptoms.

2. C. To maintain renal flow and intravascular volume, fluids should be given. This bite would be considered moderate to severe. Crotalidae antivenin is the fundamental treatment for pit viper envenomation. There is now a Crotalidae polyvalent immune Fab Antivenom available. If the child exhibits moderate to severe envenomation, has evidence of coagulopathy, or requires antivenin administration, admission to an intensive care unit is indicated. Laboratory studies such as a CBC, INR, coagulation profile, and UA should be obtained for evaluation of systemic effects.

3. E. In comparison with adults, pediatric patients are given proportionately more antivenin since children receive a greater amount of venom per kg of body weight. Antivenin is most efficacious if given within 4 to 6 hours of the bite and of less value with delays in treatment. The mnemonic for coral snakes to help distinguish poisonous snakes is "red on yellow, kill a fellow; red on black venom lack." The venom of the western coral snake is less toxic than the eastern and the antivenin is not effective in western coral snake bites. Calling the local zoo herpetologist or regional poison control center may be helpful for exotic snake bites.

4. C. Because of their small body weight, infants and young children are relatively more vulnerable to severe envenomation. Bites on the head or trunk are more severe than extremity bites. A severe bite can result in coagulopathies and DIC. The overall mortality rate is generally good at less than 1% if the antivenin is given in adequate amounts without delay. The hallmark of pit viper bites is fang marks with local pain and swelling.

5. D. Pit vipers classically possess a triangular head, facial pits, and vertical pupils. Coral snakes are brightly colored with black, red, and yellow rings. The venom is primarily neurotoxic and not cardiotoxic. A skin test should be done prior to administration of the antivenin as adverse effects include anaphylaxis and serum sickness.

111 SPIDER AND ARTHROPOD BITES

Timothy Erickson
Bruce E. Herman
Mary Jo A. Bowman
Gary R. Strange
Valerie A. Dobiesz

BLACK WIDOW SPIDERS

- The black widow spider, found throughout the temperate and tropical zones of the earth, is a shiny black spider with eight eyes, eight legs, fangs, and poison glands, with a characteristic red hourglass mark on the ventral surface of the abdomen.
- The bite typically produces a pinprick or burning sensation but may go unnoticed. Within the first few hours, the site may develop redness, cyanosis, urticaria, or a characteristic halo-shaped target lesion.
- More generalized symptoms, consisting of pain in the regional lymph nodes, chest, abdomen, and lower back, follow. The pain classically descends down the lower extremities, with burning of the soles of the feet. Abdominal rigidity along with vomiting is often severe enough to be mistaken for a surgical emergency.
- Flexor spasm of the limbs will cause the patient to assume a fetal position while writhing in pain. Patients may demonstrate hypertension, sweating, salivation, dyspnea with increased bronchosecretions, and convulsions. If untreated, symptoms may last for up to 7 days, with persistent muscle weakness and pain for several weeks. Although uncommon, death can result from respiratory or cardiac failure.

MANAGEMENT

- For local pain relief, early application of ice may be effective. A parenteral opiate such as morphine is recommended. Muscle relaxants such as diazepam may provide some relief.

- Because of the relative hypocalcemia induced by black widow spider bites, many recommend 10 percent calcium gluconate at 1 to 2 mL/kg up to 10 mL/dose, given slowly with careful cardiac monitoring as the first-line treatment in symptomatic patients. However, recent studies refute its effectiveness.
- The use of *Latrodectus*-specific antivenin is restricted to patients with severe envenomation and no allergic contraindications and in whom opioids and benzodiazepines are ineffective. Patients who should receive the antivenin early include the very young as well as those with cardiovascular disease. The antivenin provides relief within 1 to 2 hours and readministration is rarely indicated.

BROWN RECLUSE SPIDERS

- The brown recluse spider, *Loxosceles reclusa*, is a brown to fawn-colored spider, 1 to 5 cm in length, with a characteristic violin or fiddle-shaped marking on the dorsal cephalothorax (it is nicknamed the fiddleback spider). They have long, slender legs and have six eyes instead of the eight typical of most spiders.
- Envenomations typically occur during the months of April through October, at night, while the victim rummages through an old closet or attic, puts on a shoe, or uses a blanket containing a trapped spider. Humans are most commonly bitten on the extremities.
- The clinical response of loxoscelism ranges from a cutaneous irritation (necrotic arachnidism) to a life-threatening systemic reaction. Within a few hours the patient experiences itching, swelling, erythema, and tenderness over the bite site. Classically, erythema surrounds a dull blue-gray macule circumscribed by a ring or halo of pallor. Gradually, within 3 to 4 days, the wound forms a necrotic base with a central black eschar. Within 7 to 14 days the wound develops a full necrotic ulceration.
- The systemic reaction, which is much less common than the cutaneous reaction, is associated with higher morbidity. The reaction rarely correlates with the severity of the cutaneous lesion. Within 24 to 72 hours following the envenomation, the patient experiences fever, chills, myalgias, and arthralgias. If the systemic reaction is severe, the patient may suffer coagulopathies, disseminated intravascular coagulation (DIC), convulsions, renal failure, and hemolytic anemia, heralded by the passage of dark urine.

MANAGEMENT

- The wound should be cleaned, tetanus immunization updated, and the involved extremity immobilized to reduce pain and swelling. Early application of ice to the bite area lessens the local wound reaction, whereas heat will exacerbate the symptoms. Antihistamines may prove beneficial.

- Many experts advocate the use of a polymorphonuclear leukocyte inhibitor such as dapsone to diminish the amount of scarring and subsequent surgical complications. Its use is controversial and it has not been proven effective in any large study with human or animal control cases. Because of the potential for dapsone to induce methemoglobinemia, careful monitoring should be maintained if it is given.
- Although supported in the early literature, early excisional treatment can cause complications such as recurrent wound breakdown and hand dysfunction. A better approach is to wait until the necrotic process has subsided (usually several weeks) and perform secondary closure with skin grafting as indicated.
- Although not proven in clinical trials, glucocorticoids may provide a protective effect on the red blood cell (RBC) membrane, thus slowing hemolysis.
- The patient must be monitored closely for the development of DIC. Transfusion with RBCs and platelets may be necessary. Urine alkalinization with bicarbonate may lessen renal damage if the patient is experiencing acute hemolysis.

TARANTULAS

- Tarantulas are widely feared because they are the largest of all spiders. Found in the deserts of the western United States, these large, hairy spiders are relatively harmless.

SCORPIONS

- Worldwide, scorpions are responsible for thousands of deaths annually. In the United States there have been no reported deaths from scorpion stings in more than 25 years.
- Unless the scorpion is identified, the diagnosis is based on clinical symptoms. Most victims will have only local pain, tenderness, and tingling; however, young children and those who suffer more serious envenomations may experience the venom effects as overstimulation of the sympathetic, parasympathetic, and central nervous systems.
- Dysconjugate, "roving" eye movements are very common in children, along with other neurological findings, including muscle fasciculations, weakness, agitation, and opisthotonos.
- The treatment of *Centruroides* envenomations is supportive. Cool compresses and analgesics are used for

the local symptoms and pain. Wound care and tetanus prophylaxis are indicated. Tachydysrhythmias and hypertension may be treated with intravenous beta blockers. Benzodiazepines may be helpful for agitation and muscle spasms.

- A hyperimmune goat serum antivenin has been used with success for more severe envenomations with potentially life-threatening symptoms; however, it is available only in Arizona. Consultation for treatment is available through the Arizona Poison Control System.

HYMENOPTERA

- If present, the embedded stinger should be removed manually. Previous sources recommended cautiously scraping the stinger off with lateral pressure, rather than grasping it, in order to avoid compression of the venom sac resulting in further release of venom. However, recent studies have demonstrated that this is erroneous, because the venom has likely been completely released within seconds of envenomation.
- Treatment is symptomatic, with ice or cold compresses and an antihistamine.
- The swelling may spread to the entire extremity and persist for several days. A short course of prednisone (1 mg/kg per day for 5 days) may decrease the duration of symptoms.
- Multiple stings (usually over 25 to 50) may produce a toxic reaction with gastrointestinal symptoms being the principal feature; urticaria and bronchospasm are not usually present. Treatment is supportive.
- More severe reactions are manifested as bronchospasm, laryngeal edema, and hypotensive shock secondary to massive vasodilation. In all but the mildest of systemic reactions, the mainstay of treatment is epinephrine, given as a subcutaneous injection (0.01 mL/kg of 1:1000 solution).
- Glucocorticoids should be given for their antiinflammatory effects as well as their effect of preventing the late-phase response.
- Essential to the treatment of any systemic reaction is the prevention of future reactions. Patients who have had a systemic reaction should be instructed to wear protective clothing and avoid Hymenoptera-infested habitats. Portable epinephrine kits should be prescribed for the patient to carry at all times.

IMPORTED FIRE ANTS

- Fire ants sting in a two-phase process. The ant first bites the victim with powerful mandibles, then, if undisturbed, will arch the body and swivel around the attached mandibles to sting the victim repeatedly. This produces a characteristic circular pattern of papules/stings around two central punctures.

- These lesions are intensely pruritic, may resemble cellulitis, and persist for 24 to 72 hours.
- Topical glucocorticoid ointments, local anesthetic creams, and oral antihistamines may be useful for the itching associated with these reactions.
- Anaphylactic reactions have been estimated to occur after as many as 1 percent of fire ant stings. Anaphylaxis may occur several hours after a sting and is known to occur more frequently in children than in adults.

BIBLIOGRAPHY

Kim KT, Oguro J: Update on the status of Africanized honeybees in the western United States. *West J Med* 170:220–222, 1999.

Litovitz TL, Schwartz-Klein W, White S, et al: 1999 Annual report of the American Association of Poison Control Centers toxic exposures surveillance system. *Am J Emerg Med* 18:517–574, 2000.

Lovecchio F, Welch S, Klemmens J, et al: Incidence of immediate and delayed hypersensitivity to *Centruroides* antivenin. *Ann Emerg Med* 34: 615–619, 1999.

Minton S, Bechtel B, Erickson T: North American arthropod envenomation and parasitism. In: Auerbach PS, ed. *Wilderness Medicine*, 4th ed. St. Louis: Mosby, 863–887, 2001.

Philips S, Kohn M, Baker D, et al: Therapy of brown spider envenomation: A controlled trial of HBO, dapsone and cryoheptadine. *Ann Emerg Med* 25:363–368, 1995.

Sofer S, Shahak E, Gieron M: Scorpion envenomation and antivenin therapy. *J Pediatr* 124:973–978, 1994.

Vetter RS, Bush SP: Reports of presumptive brown recluse spider bites reinforce improbable diagnosis in regions of North America where the spider is not endemic. *Clin Infect Dis* 35:442–445, 2002.

Vetter RS, Visscher PK, Camizine S: Mass envenomation by honey bees and wasps. *West J Med* 170:223–227, 1999.

QUESTIONS

1. A 20-year-old male presents with a sudden onset of severe diffuse abdominal pain with nausea and vomiting. He is afebrile and his vital signs are stable. His abdominal examination reveals marked rigidity. He denies urinary symptoms, change in bowel habits, trauma, or previous episodes of abdominal pain. On exam the right leg is noted to have a halo-shaped target lesion. The most appropriate treatment for this patient would be:
   A. Immediate surgical consult for exploratory laparotomy
   B. Antivenin
   C. CT scan of the abdomen and pelvis
   D. Parenteral opiates, muscle relaxants, and possibly calcium gluconate
   E. Analgesics, fluid hydration, and an IVP

2. A 40-year-old woman presents with the complaint of being bitten by a spider while in the attic moving some old blankets. She now has swelling, erythema, and has a central blue-grey macule with a surrounding ring of palor. She denies any other symptoms. The most appropriate treatment of this wound would be:
   A. Apply local heat, and give topical antibiotics
   B. Apply local heat, analgesics, and consider antivenom
   C. Apply ice, consider dapsone, early excisional treatment
   D. Apply ice, consider dapsone, delayed excision
   E. Apply ice, dapsone, and steroids

3. A 30-year-old presents to the ED very anxious because he was just bitten by his pet tarantula he recently found on a camping trip in Arizona. He had mild tenderness at the bite site when bitten but denies any symptoms currently. Appropriate treatment would be:
   A. Make cruciate incisions and suction to withdraw the venom
   B. Apply ice, analgesics, and consider dapsone
   C. Apply ice, analgesics, and muscle relaxants
   D. Reassure the patient this is a harmless bite
   E. Apply ice, analgesics, consider antivenin

4. A patient was recently treated for a brown recluse spider bite and develops shortness of breath. She is noted to be cyanotic and hypoxic refractory to oxygen therapy. The nurse notes that her blood is brown colored when drawing her labs. What complication do you suspect in this patient?
   A. Hemolytic anemia
   B. Methemoglobinemia from treatment
   C. Disseminated intravascular coagulation
   D. Severe systemic reaction to the spider bite
   E. Acute adult respiratory distress syndrome

5. Which of the following is true regarding scorpion bites?
   A. There have been no reported deaths in the U.S. from scorpion stings in more than 25 years
   B. There is no known antivenin for life-threatening cases
   C. Hyperbaric oxygen has been shown to be effective in severe cases
   D. Dapsone may be considered for severe local reactions
   E. Scorpion bites are harmless and typically asymptomic

ANSWERS

1. **D.** This patient has a characteristic black widow spider bite, which can present with abdominal rigidity with vomiting mimicking a surgical emergency. The bite may produce a pinprick or burning sensation but may go unnoticed as in this patient. Within the first few hours the site may develop redness, cyanosis, urticaria, or a characteristic halo-shaped target lesion. Treatment includes early application of ice, parenteral opiates such as morphine, muscle relaxants such as diazepam, and possibly calcium gluconate for relative hypocalcemia. The use of Latrodectus-specific antivenom is restricted to severe envenomations refractory to other treatments.

2. **D.** This patient has a brown recluse spider bite. This is a classic scenario for a bite. She has a cutaneous reaction. Classically erythema surrounds a dull blue-grey macule circumscribed by a ring or halo of pallor. This may progress to form a necrotic base with a central black eschar. The wound should be cleansed, tetanus status addressed, and immobilized to reduce pain. Early ice application lessens the local wound reaction whereas heat will exacerbate symptoms. Early excision can cause complications such as recurrent wound breakdown and is not recommended; rather, delayed treatment after several weeks is recommended; perform secondary closure with skin grafting as needed.

3. **D.** Tarantulas, the largest of all spiders are relatively harmless. They are found in the western US. Local wound care, tetanus, and reassurance would be the appropriate management.

4. **B.** This patient has methemoglobinemia, a known complication of dapsone. Dapsone, a polymorphonuclear leukocyte inhibitor, has been recommended for brown recluse spider bites to decrease the amount of scarring and subsequent surgical complications. Its use is controversial and it has not been proven effective in any large study with human or animal control cases.

5. **A.** Worldwide scorpions are responsible for thousands of deaths annually but in the United States there have been no reported deaths from scorpion stings in more than 25 years. A hyperimmune goat antivenin is available for severe envenomations with potentially life-threatening symptoms in Arizona. Most victims have local pain, tenderness, and tingling. More severe cases may have dysconjugate, "roving" eye movements, muscle fasciculations, weakness, agitation, and opisthotonos. Treatment is supportive with cool compresses, analgesics, tetanus prophylaxis, and wound care. Hyperbaric oxygen and dapsone are not indicated.

112 MARINE ENVENOMATIONS

Timothy Erickson
Bruce E. Herman
Mary Jo A. Bowman
Gary R. Strange
Valerie A. Dobiesz

COELENTERATES

- Coelenterates include jellyfish, sea anemones, and corals.
- Coelenterates envenomate through organelles called nematocysts, which contain venom-coated threads. Even dead coelenterates can envenomate, as can fragmented tentacles and "unfired" nematocysts on the skin.
- Jellyfish stings are the most common marine envenomations.
- The Portuguese man-of-war is one of the most feared jellyfish. It produces a characteristic linear, spiral, painful urticarial lesion almost instantly. Symptoms peak within a few hours and persist for many more. Systemic symptoms may include nausea, vomiting, muscle cramps, diaphoresis, weakness, hemolysis, and rarely, vascular collapse and death.
- The box jellyfish (or sea wasp) of Australia is the most deadly coelenterate. Death can occur within minutes of envenomation. If the victim can be rescued from the water, an antivenin is available.
- The sea nettle is the most commonly encountered jellyfish. It is widely distributed in temperate as well as tropical waters. Sea nettles cause predominantly local effects consisting of painful urticarial lesions.
- Treatment of sea nettle envenomation includes reassurance, immobilization of the injured part, and ice. The area is rinsed with sterile saline or seawater to maintain isosmolar conditions and wash off unfired nematocysts. Remaining nematocysts are inactivated by rinsing with vinegar and are then removed by gentle scraping or shaving. Analgesics and antihistamines are helpful. Tetanus immunization is indicated, but prophylactic antibiotics are not.
- Sea anemones and corals are sessile creatures that cause local urticarial reactions upon contact. Contact with hard corals may cause lacerations that are treated with vigorous local wound care, tetanus prophylaxis, and broad-spectrum antibiotics.

VENOMOUS FISH

- Stingrays are the most commonly encountered venomous fish. They are flat, round-bodied fishes that burrow underneath the sand in shallow waters. When startled or stepped on, the stingray thrusts its spiny tail upward and forward, driving its venom-laden stinging apparatus into the foot or lower extremity of the victim. As the sting is withdrawn, the sheath surrounding it ruptures and the venom is released. Parts of the sheath may be torn away and remain in the wound.
- Stingray venom is short acting, heat-labile, and causes intense pain, peaking within 1 hour but lasting up to 48 hours. Signs and symptoms are usually limited to the injured area.
- Treatment of the stingray wound includes irrigation with sterile saline or seawater to dilute the venom and remove sheath fragments. The injured part is immersed in hot water, no warmer than 113°F, for 30 to 90 minutes to inactivate the heat-labile venom.
- Analgesics are usually required. Wounds are debrided and left open. Tetanus immunization is updated and broad-spectrum prophylactic antibiotics such as trimethoprim-sulfamethoxazole (TMP-SMX), ciprofloxacin, or a third-generation cephalosporin are administered.
- Scorpion fish envenomations occur from spines on their dorsal or pelvic fins and are often associated with lacerations. The venoms are heat-labile and cause immediate intense pain that peaks within 60 to 90 minutes and persists for up to 12 hours. Treatment is immersion of the affected limb in hot water for 30 to 90 minutes, or until pain is relieved. Wounds are irrigated with sterile saline, explored, and cleaned of debris. The wound is left open and treated with prophylactic antibiotics in addition to tetanus prophylaxis.
- Stonefish envenomations are similar to those of the other scorpion fish, but their clinical manifestations are more severe. Stonefish venom, a potent neurotoxin, can cause dyspnea, hypotension, and cardiovascular collapse within 1 hour and death within 6 hours. A specific stonefish antivenin is available in Australia.

CATFISH

- Catfish stings occur from spines contained within a sheath on their dorsal or pectoral fins. The hands and forearms of fishermen are the most common sites. The heat-labile venoms produce a stinging, burning, throbbing sensation that occurs immediately and usually resolves within 60 to 90 minutes. Treatment is immediate immersion in hot water for pain relief.
- Catfish spines may penetrate the skin and break off. The wound should be explored and debrided and any retained spines should be removed. The puncture wound should be left open and treated with prophylactic broad-spectrum antibiotics, in addition to tetanus prophylaxis.

ECHINODERMS

- Echinoderms include sea urchins, starfish, sand dollars, and sea cucumbers. Of these, sea urchins are the only ones that regularly cause medically significant envenomations. They are slow-moving, colorful, bottom dwellers that can puncture the skin when picked up or stepped on, break off, and be retained. Their venom can cause local pain that may persist for days. Treatment is immediate immersion in hot water, careful removal of spines, and vigorous local wound care. Tetanus immunization and broad-spectrum antibiotic prophylaxis are indicated.

SEA SNAKES

- Sea snakes are encountered throughout the Indo-Pacific region. They are among the deadliest snakes in the world, and will bite with little provocation. Envenomations result in severe neurotoxicity with rapid muscular and respiratory paralysis. An antivenin is commercially available.

BIBLIOGRAPHY

Aldred B, Erickson T, Lipscomb J, et al: Lionfish stings in an urban wilderness. *J Wilderness Environ Med* 4:291–296, 1994.

Auerbach P: Envenomation by aquatic animals. In: Auerbach PS, ed. *Wilderness Medicine*, 4th ed. St. Louis: Mosby, 1450–1487, 2001.

Cook L: Prehospital incident profiles: Gone fishin. *J Emerg Med Serv* 27:75–78, 2002.

Exton D, Moran PJ, Williamson J: Phylum *Echinodermata*. In: Williamson JA, Fenner PJ, Burnett JW, et al, eds. *Venomous and Poisonous Marine Animals.* Sydney: University of South Wales, 312–326, 1999.

Fenner PJ, Williamson JA: Worldwide deaths and severe envenomation from jellyfish stings. *Med J Aust* 165:658, 1996.

Tomaszewski C: Aquatic envenomations. In: Ford M, DeLaney K, Ling L, et al, eds. *Clinical Toxicology.* Philadelphia: Saunders, 970–984, 2000.

QUESTIONS

1. Which of the following is true regarding coelenterate envenomations?
   A. Dead jellyfish cannot envenomate
   B. Jellyfish envenomate via a stinger that injects venom
   C. Jellyfish are responsible for the most common marine envenomations
   D. The Portuguese man-of-war is a non-venomous coelenterate
   E. Treatment for coelenterate envenomations consists of immersion in hot water, analgesics, and antibiotics

2. A 6-year-old boy stepped on the tail of a stingray while walking in the swallow waters of a beach in Florida. Which of the following would be the most appropriate treatment of this injury?
   A. Irrigation with sterile saline, immersion in hot water, analgesics, tetanus, antibiotics
   B. Rinsing with vinegar, local wound care, analgesics, tetanus
   C. Surgical debridement to remove the sheath fragments, antibiotics, analgesics, tetanus
   D. Irrigation with sterile saline, analgesics, tetanus, antibiotics
   E. Irrigation with sterile saline, antivenin, tetanus

3. Which of the following is true regarding the treatment of a patient who presents after stepping on a sea urchin spine?
   A. A specific antivenin exists in Australia
   B. Treatment is by immersion in hot water, removal of spines, administration of tetanus toxoid and antibiotics
   C. Treatment is by irrigation with sterile saline, rinsing with vinegar, removal of spines, administration of tetanus toxoid and antibiotics
   D. Treatment is by removal of spines, administration of tetanus toxoid and antibiotics
   E. No treatment is indicated except for local wound care, tetanus toxoid and antibiotics

4. Which of the following paired items is correct?
   A. Catfish stings – rinse with vinegar
   B. Sea snake envenomation – local wound care
   C. Sea anemones envenomation – immersion in hot water
   D. Stonefish envenomation- antivenin
   E. Scorpion fish envenomation – rinse with vinegar

5. Which of the following is correct regarding marine envenomations?
   A. Scorpion fish are the most commonly encountered venomous fish
   B. The stingray uses nematocysts to inject venom
   C. The box jellyfish typically causes a minor localized urticarial lesion
   D. Sea snake injuries are common in the Southeastern United States
   E. Catfish stings occur from spines within a sheath on their fins

ANSWERS

1. C. The coelenterates envenomate through nematocysts, which contain venom coated threads. Dead colenterates can envenomate. Jellyfish are the most common marine envenomations. The Portuguese man-of-war is one of the most feared jellyfishes and characteristically causes linear, spiral, painful urticarial lesions but also may progress to systemic symptoms and death. Treatment includes immobilization of the injured part, ice, rinsing the area with sterile saline or seawater, rinsing with vinegar, analgesics, antihistamines, and tetanus as indicated.

2. A. The treatment of a stingray wound includes irrigation with sterile saline or seawater to dilute the venom and remove sheath fragments, immersion in hot water for 30 to 90 min to inactivate the heat-labile venom, analgesics, tetanus and prophylactic antibiotics such as trimethoprim-sulfamethoxazole, ciprofloxacin, or a third generation cephalosporin.

3. B. Treatment of these injuries includes immersion in hot water, careful removal of spines, and vigorous local wound care. Tetanus immunization and broad-spectrum antibiotics prophylaxis is indicated.

4. D. Stonefish envenomations can be severe as the venom is a potent neurotoxin which can cause dyspnea, hypotension, and cardiovascular collapse within 1 hour and death within 6 hours. A specific stonefish antivenin is available in Australia. Catfish venom is heat-labile and treatment is immersion in hot water. Sea snakes are among the deadliest snakes in the world and cause a severe neurotoxicity with rapid muscular and respiratory paralysis. An antivenin is available. Sea anemones are coelenterates and envenomate through nematocysts that are inactivated with vinegar. Scorpion fish venom is heat-labile and stings need to be immersed in hot water.

5. E. Stingrays are the most commonly encountered venomous fish. The stingray uses its tail to drive its venom-laden stinging apparatus into the extremity of the victim. The box jellyfish is the most deadly and venomous coelenterate causing death within minutes of envenomation. Sea snakes are typically found in the Indo-Pacific region. Catfish stings do occur from spines contained within a sheath on their dorsal or

pectoral fins. The hands and forearms of fisherman are the most common sites of injury.

113 NEAR DROWNING

Gary R. Strange
Simon Ros
Heather M. Prendergast

INTRODUCTION

- Drowning is the second most common cause of unintentional death in children and adolescents, second only to motor vehicle crashes. Two age groups in the pediatric population are especially at risk for submersion injuries:
  - Children under 5 years of age
  - Adolescents
- The primary injury following submersion occurs in the lung. Hypoxemia, the result of the pulmonary dysfunction, is then the cause of secondary injuries, especially to the brain and heart, where cerebral edema and myocardial failure may develop.
- Fluid aspiration occurs in 90 percent of drowning victims, but it is unusual for large quantities of water to be aspirated. Laryngospasm prevents aspiration in 10 percent of cases, resulting in "dry" drowning.
- When significant aspiration occurs, the pathophysiology of lung injury is dependent on the characteristics of the aspirated fluid. Aspiration of fresh water inactivates surfactant and damages the alveolar basement membrane. Aspiration of hypertonic seawater results in the movement of intravascular fluid into the alveoli, with subsequent edema and shunting.
- Hypothermia appears to exert a protective effect on drowning victims, especially when rapidly induced. The diving reflex, which results in preferential shunting of blood to the brain and the heart, has been suggested as an additional contributing factor to intact survival following extended submersion in very cold water (lower than 40°F).

MANAGEMENT

PREHOSPITAL CARE

- Early initiation of cardiopulmonary resuscitation in a submersion victim is of paramount importance. As cardiopulmonary resuscitation in the water is not effective, the patient must be extricated as soon as possible.

HOSPITAL MANAGEMENT

- All patients are placed on a cardiac monitor and pulse oximeter and 100 percent oxygen is administered by mask or endotracheal tube. Persistent hypoxemia suggests the need for continuous positive airway pressure (CPAP) or positive end-expiratory pressure (PEEP).
- Occult injury is common in drowning victims, especially injuries to the head and neck as a result of falls or diving accidents. Emergent cervical spine radiography and computed tomography of the head is indicated in all patients with suspected head and neck injury.
- Toxicologic studies should be considered in all victims of submersion. There is a very high correlation between submersion injury and alcohol intoxication in adolescents.
- In small children, the potential for intentional abuse or neglect must be considered.
- Hypothermia may not be detected unless a rectal temperature is obtained along with the rest of the vital signs.

PROGNOSIS

- The prognosis of near-drowning patients is determined by the severity of the anoxic brain injury and is generally good. Early institution of resuscitative efforts and the presence of spontaneous respirations and heartbeat upon presentation to the emergency department are the best predictors of intact neurological survival in drowning victims.

DISPOSITION

- Asymptomatic patients with normal arterial blood gases and chest radiography may be discharged after a 6-hour period of observation. All other patients are admitted to the hospital.

BIBLIOGRAPHY

Allen WC: The long-QT syndrome. *N Engl J Med* 342:514–515, 2000.
Causey AL, Tilelli JA, Swanson ME: Predicting discharge in uncomplicated near drowning. *Am J Emerg Med* 18:9–11, 2000.
Gheen KM: Near drowning and cold water submersion. *Semin Pediatr Surg* 10:26–27, 2001.
Hwang V, Shofer FS, Durbin DR, Baren JM: Prevalence of traumatic injuries in drowning and near-drowning in children and adolescents. *Arch Pediatr Adolesc Med* 157: 50–53, 2003.

Modell JH, Graves SA, Ketover A: Clinical course of 91 consecutive near drowning victims. *Chest* 70:231, 1976.

Pearn J: Successful cardiopulmonary resuscitation outcome reviews. *Resuscitation* 47:311–316, 2000.

Quan L: Near drowning. *Pediatr Rev* 20:255–259, 1999.

Sachdeva RC: Near drowning. *Crit Care Clin* 15:281–296, 1999.

Smith GS, Brenner RA: The changing risks of drowning for adolescents in the U.S. and effective control strategies. *Adolesc Med* 6:153–170, 1995.

Zuckerman GB, Conway EE Jr: Drowning and near drowning: A pediatric epidemic. *Pediatr Ann* 29:360–366, 2000.

Zuckerman GB, Gregory PM, Santos-Damiani SM: Predictors of death and neurologic impairment in pediatric submersion injuries: The pediatric risk of mortality score. *Arch Pediatr Adolesc Med* 152:134–140, 1998.

QUESTIONS

1. Which of the following pediatric groups is at the HIGHEST risk for submersion injuries?
   A. Infants
   B. Toddlers and preschoolers
   C. Elementary school children
   D. Young adults
   E. Risk is equal throughout the various stages

2. A 13-year-old is brought to the ED after a near-drowning episode in a local lake. The victim was playing unsupervised with friends and was pulled from the lake by bystanders. One of the friends states that "he swallowed a lot of water." Potential respiratory complications in this patient would MOST LIKELY be the result of which of the following?
   A. Laryngospasm
   B. Occult chest trauma
   C. Damage to the alveolar basement membrane from the inactivation of surfactant
   D. Excessive shunting and edema in the lungs from movement of intravascular fluid into the alveoli
   E. Anoxic injury

3. You are informed by EMS dispatch that a 5-year-old girl is being transported to your ED following a drowning incident at a nearby pool. The patient is unconscious and total submersion time is unknown.
   Part 1. The MOST important priority in the prehospital setting would be which of the following?
   A. Attempts to evacuate aspirated fluid by performing a modified Heimlich maneuver.
   B. Cervical spine immobilization
   C. Wrap the patient in warm blankets
   D. Initiate cardiopulmonary resuscitation (CPR) if the patient is pulseless
   E. Do nothing and continue rapid transport

Part 2. A management priority for this patient on arrival to your emergency department would be which of the following?
   A. Obtaining a rectal temperature
   B. Determining the presence of hypoxemia
   C. Cervical spine radiographs
   D. Toxicology studies
   E. Through evaluation for signs of abuse or neglect

4. A 14-year-old was brought to the ED following a near-drowning incident. On arrival to the ED, the patient was alert and asymptomatic. Arterial blood gases and chest radiographs obtained at presentation and several hours later were all normal. The MOST appropriate disposition for this patient would be which of the following?
   A. Discharge home after a 6-hour ED observation period
   B. Admit for 23-hour observation to a general pediatric floor
   C. Transfer to a comprehensive pediatric center
   D. Call for a pulmonary consult before discharging patient
   E. Admit to a monitored pediatric bed.

ANSWERS

1. B. The risk of submersion injuries has a bimodal distribution. It is highest in children under the age of 5, and then rises again during adolescence when risk-taking behavior tends to increase. Submersion injuries in adolescents are often associated with alcohol use.

2. C. Fluid aspiration occurs in 90 percent of drowning victims. The patient most likely aspirated fresh water from the lake and would be vulnerable because of the inactivation of lung surfactant. Aspiration of hypertonic seawater causes significant shunting and lung edema. Laryngospasm is somewhat of a protective measure and prevents aspiration in 10 percent of near drowning cases.

3. Part 1: D. In the prehospital setting, early initiation of CPR is a paramount importance and should take priority. Once CPR is initiated, there should be no further delays in transport. Occult injuries are common in drowning victims. It is recommended that all potential trauma victims be placed on a backboard with cervical spine immobilization.
   Part 2: B. Determining the presence of hypoxemia is a priority and will dictate further airway management. All patients should be placed on 100 percent oxygen either by mask or endotracheal tube. Persistent hypoxemia suggests the need for continuous positive airway pressure (CPAP) or positive end-expiratory pressure (PEEP). Obtaining a rectal temperature will be helpful

in identifying hypothermia and guiding rewarming efforts.

4. A. Asymptomatic patients with normal arterial blood gases and chest radiographs may be discharged after a 6-hour ED observation period. Patients with abnormalities in either test or those in which close follow-up is not possible should be admitted to the hospital.

114 BURNS AND ELECTRICAL INJURIES

Gary R. Strange
Barbara Pawel
Heather M. Prendergast

BURNS

• Thermal injuries are the second most common cause of death in children in the United States. Young children have a higher mortality rate from burns than older children and adults, but with modern advances in treatment, mortality rates have improved significantly.

CAUSES

• Scalding is the most common mechanism of thermal injury in the pediatric population. It most commonly results when children under 3 years of age reach and tip over hot liquids that are in containers on a stove or counter. Partial-thickness burns usually result (Fig. 114-1).

• Bathtub scalds are another common mechanism. These can be prevented by setting hot water temperature below 120°F.

• Contact of clothing with a flame may result in the ignition of fabrics. Flame-retardant fabrics, especially for pajamas and nightgowns, are now in common use and have reduced the incidence and severity of injury from "catching on fire."

• By far the most lethal cause of burns in children is the house fire, accounting for 45 percent of burn-related deaths. The type of burn varies from minor partial thickness injuries to full-thickness, total-body burns. Smoke inhalation and inhalation of other toxic gases (see Chaps. 87 and 90) also contribute to the morbidity and mortality of the house fire.

• The intentional inflicting of burns to a child is, unfortunately, a common form of abuse. Every burn

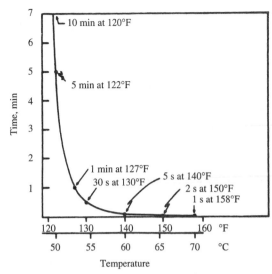

FIG. 114-1 Duration of exposure to hot water to cause full-thickness epidermal burns of skin at various water temperatures. (Reproduced with permission from Katcher ML: Scald burns from hot tap water. *JAMA* 246:1219, 1981. Modified from Moritz AR, Henriques FC Jr: Studies of thermal injury. *Am J Pathol* 23:695, 1947. Copyright 1981, American Medical Association.)

injury in a child should be evaluated for the potential for abuse or neglect (see Chap. 118).

PATHOPHYSIOLOGY

• The center of a burn is an area of coagulation necrosis and vascular thrombosis. There is intense vasoconstriction, caused by the release of vasoactive substance from injured cells, which may lead to ischemia and secondary injury. Surrounding this area are concentric areas of stasis and hyperemia. Later, there is vasodilation and development of gaps between endothelial cells.

• Burns of the hands, feet, and perineum should always be considered serious, and all significant burns in these locations should initially be managed in the hospital, preferably in a burn center.

• Depth of the burn is estimated by clinical criteria, which are used to classify the burn by degrees.
  ◦ First-degree burns involve only the epidermis. The skin is erythematous but there are no blisters.
  ◦ Second-degree burns are partial-thickness burns that involve the dermis to a variable degree. The dermal appendages are always preserved and provide a source for regeneration. Second-degree burns are characterized by the presence of marked edema, erythema, blistering, and weeping from the wound.
  ◦ Third-degree burns are full-thickness injuries. The dermis and dermal appendages are destroyed. The skin appears whitish or leathery.

○ Fourth-degree burns extend into deep tissues, such as muscle, fascia, nerves, tendons, vessels, and bone.
- The body surface area (BSA) involved is also important in determining treatment and disposition. The percentage surface area involved in the burn is estimated by the "rule of nines" in adults, but in children, the proportion of body surface area, made up by anatomic parts, especially the head, varies considerably with age (Fig. 114-2).

DIAGNOSTIC EVALUATION

HISTORY AND PHYSICAL EXAMINATION
- The history of the events leading to the burn may be helpful in assessing the degree of injury and the likelihood of other injuries, such as smoke inhalation and

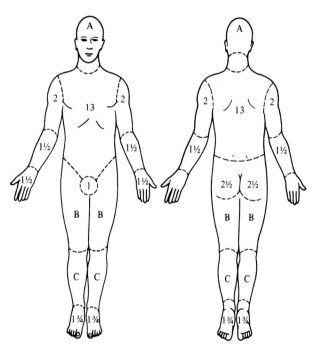

Relative Percentages of Areas Affected by Growth (Age in Years)

	0	1	5	10	15	Adult
A: half of head	$9\frac{1}{2}$	$8\frac{1}{2}$	$6\frac{1}{2}$	$5\frac{1}{2}$	$4\frac{1}{2}$	$3\frac{1}{2}$
B: half of thigh	$2\frac{3}{4}$	$3\frac{1}{4}$	4	$4\frac{1}{4}$	$4\frac{1}{2}$	$4\frac{3}{4}$
C: half of leg	$2\frac{1}{2}$	$2\frac{1}{2}$	$2\frac{3}{4}$	3	$3\frac{1}{4}$	$3\frac{1}{2}$

Second degree _____ and

Third degree _____ =

Total percent burned ____

FIG. 114-2 Classic Lund and Browder chart. (Reproduced with permission from Dimick AR: Burns, in Tintinalli JE, Kelen GD, Stapczynski JS (eds): *Emergency Medicine*, 5th ed. New York: McGraw-Hill, 2000.)

blunt trauma. Concomitant medical problems, medications, allergies, and tetanus immunization status should be ascertained.

PRIMARY SURVEY
- The airway is assessed immediately on presentation. The most common cause of death during the first hour after a burn injury is respiratory impairment. Intubation is indicated early in the emergency department course of patients who have signs of upper airway involvement (Table 114-1).
- Humidified oxygen is used to maintain oxygenation. Positive end-expiratory pressure or continuous positive airway pressure may be useful to improve oxygenation when there is pulmonary involvement.
- Bronchospasm is treated with β-adrenergic agonists. Close monitoring of oxygen saturation by pulse oximetry, supplemented by arterial blood gases, is indicated.
- Patients with over 15 percent BSA burns require a large-bore intravenous line for isotonic fluid administration. A second line is advisable for extensive burns and is essential if there are signs of cardiovascular instability.

SECONDARY SURVEY
- After stabilization, a thorough physical examination is needed to assess the burn injury completely and to evaluate for concomitant injury.
- Particular attention to the vascular status of extremities is imperative. Circumferential burns may result in vascular compromise and require escharotomy to prevent limb loss.
- Circumferential burns to the thorax may result in respiratory embarrassment, as indicated by poor chest expansion and declining oxygen saturation. Lateral thoracic escharotomy may be life-saving in this situation.

LABORATORY EVALUATION
- A complete blood count is indicated to establish baseline characteristics. The hematocrit will often be elevated secondary to fluid loss, and the white blood cell count is often elevated as a result of an acute-phase reaction.

TABLE 114-1   Indications for Early Intubation in Burn Patients

Stridor
Hoarseness
Rales
Wheezing
Singed nasal hairs
Carbonized sputum
Cyanosis
Altered mental status

- Serum electrolytes will often reveal an elevated potassium level due to the breakdown of cells, and depressed bicarbonate level due to metabolic acidosis resulting from fluid loss and hypovolemic shock.
- On urinalysis, the urine-specific gravity is helpful in assessing the hydration status.
- The presence of myoglobin in the urine is important to detect, since acute tubular necrosis can result. Myoglobin is indicated by a positive dip test for blood in the absence of red blood cells on the microscopic examination. When myoglobinuria is suspected, aggressive hydration is initiated and potent diuretics, such as furosemide and mannitol, are considered in efforts to maintain high urine flow and prevent tubular necrosis.

MANAGEMENT

- After assurance of airway integrity, the primary guiding principle in burn management is the restoration or maintenance of tissue perfusion. Using the Parkland formula, isotonic crystalloid, 4 mL/kg per percent BSA, is administered over the first 24 hours. Half is administered over the first 8 hours and the remainder over 16 hours. Maintenance fluid requirements must be added to the fluid amounts calculated by the Parkland formula (see Chap. 51).
- It must be remembered that burn fluid calculations provide only an estimation of fluid requirements. Sufficient fluid should be administered to maintain a urine flow of 1 to 1.5 mL/kg/h.
- Initial wound care consists of sterile saline-soaked dressings. Room-temperature solutions are sufficient. The application of ice or cold solutions is contraindicated due to the possibility of developing hypothermia in extensively burned patients and to the addition of cold injury to the burned surface.
- The burned surface can be cleaned with povidone-iodine solution and debris and devitalized tissue removed.
- If the patient is to be transferred to a burn unit, care should be taken to be in compliance with the burn unit protocol. Often, this will include simply covering the burn wound surface with dry sterile sheets after initial cleaning.
- Burns that are managed on an outpatient basis will require a bulky sterile dressing.
- Burns are often extremely painful. Once the patient is hemodynamically stabilized, consideration for analgesia with a potent narcotic analgesic, such as morphine, 0.1 to 0.2 mg/kg IV, is indicated. This dose can be repeated at 15 minutes intervals as needed, while monitoring the adequacy of respirations (rate and oxygen saturation), blood pressure, and mental status.

- Tetanus prophylaxis should be considered for all burns. Guidelines are given in Chap. 23.
- All jewelry on or distal to the burned area and any other constricting items should be removed immediately on presentation.
- Minor burns (Table 114-2) can be soaked in sterile saline, cleaned gently with povidone-iodine solution, and dressed with a topical antibiotic preparation. Silver sulfadiazine is commonly used.
- In outpatient management, it is reasonable to leave stable blisters intact. Flaccid blisters and those already broken should be debrided carefully and the surface covered with antibiotic cream and a sterile dressing.

DISPOSITION

- Criteria for outpatient management, admission, and transfer to a burn center are outlined in Table 114-2.

ELECTRICAL INJURIES

EPIDEMIOLOGY

- Two groups of children are at increased risk: exploring toddlers (12 to 24 months) who chew on extension cords and adventuresome adolescents.

TABLE 114-2 Guidelines for Burn Triage and Disposition

OUTPATIENT MANAGEMENT

Partial thickness burn—less than 10% body surface
Full thickness burn—less than 2% body surface

INPATIENT MANAGEMENT

Hospital (other than burn center)
   Partial thickness burn—less than 25% body surface
   Full thickness burn—less than 15% body surface
   Partial thickness burn—face, hands, feet, perineum
   Questionable burn wound depth or extent
   Chemical burn, minor
   Significant coexisting illness or trauma
   Inadequate family support
   Suspected abuse
   Fire in an enclosed space

BURN CENTER

   Partial thickness burn—more than 25% body surface
   Full thickness burn—more than 15% body surface
   Full thickness burn—face, hands, feet, perineum
   Respiratory tract injury
   Associated major trauma
   Major chemical and electrical burns

ELECTROPHYSIOLOGY

- The factors that determine the extent of electrical injuries are voltage, current (amperage), resistance, current type, duration, and pathway.
  - *Voltage* is a measurement of the electrical "pressure" in a system. Injuries are divided into low (less than 1000 V) and high (over 1000 V) voltage. The latter usually produces greater tissue destruction.
  - *Amperage* is a measure of the rate of flow of electrons. The margin between the household amperage (0.001 to 0.01 A) and that capable of causing respiratory arrest (0.02 to 0.05 A) and ventricular fibrillation (0.05 to 0.10 A) is narrow.
  - *Resistance* is a measure of the difficulty of electron flow. Specific tissues have defined resistances. Resistance increases in the following order: nerve < blood < muscle < skin < tendon < fat < bone.
    - The most severe injuries occur in extremities due to high internal resistance and small cross-sectional diameter.
    - Damage to internal organs is less frequent due to low tissue resistance and the large cross-sectional diameter of the torso.
  - *Current type* is either alternating or direct. Alternating current is much more dangerous than direct current at the same voltage.
  - The *current pathway* will determine the nature of injuries and complications. Once surface resistance is overcome, low-voltage current follows the path of least resistance. High-voltage current follows a direct course to ground, regardless of tissue type and resistance.
    - Hand-to-hand flow: carries a 60 percent mortality rate due to spinal cord transection at C4-8, myocardial injury, and tetanic muscle contractions of the thorax, resulting in suffocation.
    - Hand-to-foot flow: carries a 20 percent mortality rate from cardiac arrhythmias.
    - Foot-to-foot flow: generally not associated with fatalities.
    - Current passing through the head: likely to produce brain and brain stem damage.
    - Current passing through the thorax: likely to produce cardiorespiratory arrest.

TYPES OF INJURIES

- Victims of electrical injury may have very little external damage while sustaining serious underlying tissue damage.

SKIN AND UNDERLYING TISSUES

- Entry and exit burns are found commonly in all non-water-related electrical injuries. The most common entry points are the hands and skull. The most common exit points are the heels.
- Very young children often bite on electrical cords, sustaining severe oro-facial injuries. Burns are often full-thickness, involving the lips and oral commissure. These burns are initially bloodless and painless. As the eschar separates in 2 to 3 weeks, severe bleeding can occur from damage to the labial, facial, or even carotid arteries.

CARDIOVASCULAR SYSTEM

- Current passing directly through the heart can induce ventricular fibrillation. Lightning injury will frequently induce asystole. The most common electrocardiographic (ECG) abnormalities are sinus tachycardia and nonspecific STT changes.

KIDNEY

- Acute renal failure may occur from myoglobin released by extensively damaged muscle and hemoglobin from hemolysis.

NEUROLOGIC EFFECTS

- Immediate central nervous system effects include loss of consciousness, agitation, amnesia, deafness, seizures, visual disturbance, and sensory complaints.

EYES

- Cataracts can be seen in any electrical injury involving the head or neck.

SKELETAL SYSTEM

- Blunt trauma or tetanic muscle contractions can cause fractures or dislocations. Amputation of an extremity is necessary in 35 to 60 percent of survivors due to extensive underlying injuries.

PSYCHOLOGICAL SEQUELAE

- Victims often display depression, flashbacks, and general psychosocial dysfunction.

MANAGEMENT

PREHOSPITAL CARE

- Extrication is extremely dangerous until the power source is disconnected.
- Victims should be treated as multiple blunt trauma patients, with special attention given to spinal immobilization.

EMERGENCY DEPARTMENT CARE

- The greatest threats to life include cardiac arrhythmias, renal failure from myoglobin and hemoglobin precipitants, and hyperkalemia from massive muscle breakdown.
- Baseline ECG and cardiac monitoring is not indicated for children exposed to household current (120 to 240 V) unless there was loss of consciousness, tetany, wet skin, trans-thoracic current flow, or the event was unwitnessed. If the ECG is consistent with cardiac injury, further evaluation with echocardiography or nuclear scanning may be necessary.
- The usual fluid replacement formulas utilized for burn patients underestimate fluid requirements in electrical burn patients. Fluids should maintain a urine output of 1 to 2 mL/kg per hour.
- Alkalinization of the urine with bicarbonate and administration of mannitol or furosemide may be needed to treat myoglobinuria.
- Extensive muscle damage frequently requires fasciotomy.
- Debridement is best left to a burn surgeon.
- Recommendations for admission are varied. It is generally agreed that admission is not required for non-transthoracic low-voltage injuries in the asymptomatic child without ECG abnormalities. All other patients require admission and close observation. A multidisciplinary approach, including medical, psychiatric, and social services, is required.

LIGHTNING INJURIES

MORBIDITY AND MORTALITY

- The mortality rate of lightning-related injury approaches 30 percent, with 75 percent of survivors left with permanent sequelae.

MECHANISM OF INJURY

- There are several mechanisms by which lightning can cause injury.
  - Direct strike: the likelihood of direct strike is increased when the person is carrying or wearing metal objects.
  - Side flash or "splash": the victim is near an object that is struck, with object resistance greater than air resistance between the object and the person.
  - Ground current: lightning strikes the ground close to a victim, with the result that the ground current passes through the victim. When the victim stands with feet apart, a potential difference between the feet allows current to flow through the body to the ground (stride potential or step current).

- Thermal flash: temperatures between 8000 and 30,000°C of short duration cause burns that are generally not as severe as household or industrial electrical burns.
- Blunt injury: the shock wave can cause perforation of the tympanic membrane or damage to internal organs.
- Lightning acts as a direct-current countershock, with higher voltage and amperage than seen in high-voltage electrical accidents. The extremely short duration of lightning shock accounts for the small amount of skin damage usually seen. Most of the lightning energy flows around the outside of the body, with less energy actually flowing through the victim.

TYPES OF INJURIES

SKIN

- Skin damage is decreased by the short duration of contact and by lower skin resistance from rain or sweat. Entry wounds, exit wounds, and deep muscle damage are rare.
- Major types of burns include the following:
  - Feathering burns: arborescent, spidery, erythematous streaks that are pathognomonic of lightning injury. They appear up to several hours after injury and disappear within 24 hours.
  - Linear burns: partial-thickness burns in areas of high sweat concentration.
  - Punctate burns: multiple, discrete, circular burns in groups which can be full or partial thickness.
  - Thermal burns: heating of metal objects or ignition of clothing can cause thermal burns.

CARDIOPULMONARY EFFECTS

- Asystole can result from the massive direct-current countershock produced by a lightning strike. Respiratory arrest may occur from effects on the medullary respiratory center.

VASCULAR EFFECTS

- Arterial spasm and vasomotor instability result in cool, mottled, pulseless extremities.

NEUROLOGIC EFFECTS

- Transient loss of consciousness, retrograde amnesia, transient paralysis, and paresthesias are common.

EYES

- Cataracts are the most common injury and may develop immediately or over a prolonged period.

EARS

- Tympanic membrane rupture is common.

GASTROINTESTINAL TRACT
- Gastric dilatation is common.

PSYCHOLOGICAL SEQUELAE
- Anxiety, sleep disturbances, nocturnal enuresis, depression, and hysteria-related phenomena have all been reported.

MANAGEMENT

PREHOSPITAL CARE
- Lightning injury victims should be approached as blunt multiple trauma patients with attention to advanced life support protocols and cervical spine protection.

EMERGENCY DEPARTMENT CARE
- A thorough search for blunt trauma injuries is necessary. Radiographs are done as indicated but include cranial CT in all unconscious patients.
- Baseline ECG and continued cardiac monitoring is indicated. Arrhythmias should be treated by standard protocols.
- Fluid resuscitation must be approached cautiously; central monitoring lines may be helpful.
- Fasciotomy is rarely indicated, as the mottled, pulseless extremity associated with lightning injury often improves over several hours.

DISPOSITION

- Some authorities suggest admission for all victims of lightning injuries. Others suggest admission for all except those children with a completely normal examination, normal laboratory tests, and ECG, plus adequate home supervision and close follow-up care.

SEQUELAE

- Long-term sequelae may include paralysis, dysesthesia, and disturbances in mood, affect, and memory. Supportive psychotherapy may be necessary.

BIBLIOGRAPHY

Cooper MA, Andrews CJ, Holle RL, et al: Lightning injuries. In: Auerbach PS. *Wilderness Medicine*, 4th ed. St. Louis: Mosby, 73–110, 2001.

Koumbourlis AC: Electrical injuries. *Crit Care Med* 30(11 Suppl):S424–430, 2002.

Niazi ZV, Salzberg CA: Thermal, electrical and chemical injury to the face and neck in children. *Facial Plast Surg* 7:185–193, 1999.

Palmieri TL, Greenhalgh DG: Topical treatment of pediatric patients with burns: a practical guide. *Am J Clin Dermatol* 3:529–534, 2002.

Rabban JT, Blair JA, Rosen CL, et al: Mechanisms of pediatric electrical injury: New implications for product safety and injury prevention. *Arch Pediatr Adolesc Med* 151:696–700, 1997.

Sheridan RL, Remensnyder JP, Snitzer JJ, et al: Current expectations for survival in pediatric burns. *Arch Pediatr Adolesc Med* 154:245–249, 2000.

Smith ML: Pediatric burns: Management of thermal, electrical and chemical burns and burn-like dermatologic conditions. *Pediatr Ann* 29:367–378, 2000.

Stewart C: Emergency care of pediatric burns. *Pediatr Emerg Med Rep* 5:101–112, 2001.

Yowler CJ, Fratianne RB: Current status of burn resuscitation. *Clin Plast Surg* 27:1–10, 2000.

Zubair M, Besner GE: Pediatric electrical burns: Management strategies. *Burns* 23:413–420, 1997.

QUESTIONS

1. A 3-year-old is brought to your ED for evaluation of scalding burns to face, arms, and torso from hot coffee. On examination you note that the burns to the hands and face seem quite extensive. There is marked edema, erythema, and some blistering present. Which of the following is a management priority in this child?
   A. Estimate the percentage surface area involved in the burn. If the burn involves more than 15 percent BSA, begin aggressive fluid administration
   B. Assess the child's airway and oxygenation status
   C. Begin humidified oxygen and prepare for intubation
   D. Determine the vascular status of the child's extremities
   E. Empirically begin nebulized respiratory treatments to prevent bronchospasm
2. A 6-year-old is brought by her babysitter for evaluation of lower extremity burns sustained while in the bathtub. After a through assessment, you determine that the child's burns are primarily first and second degree partial-thickness burns with a total BSA of 15%. The child's parents have been notified and are en route to your facility. The next step in management of this patient would be which of the following?
   A. Determine whether child abuse is present by looking for signs of bruising and other burns
   B. Initiate wound care with sterile saline soaked dressings and topical silver sulfadiazine cream
   C. Begin intravenous fluids
   D. Debridement of devitalized tissue prior to transfer to the burn unit
   E. Do nothing at this time and contact the nearest burn center for transfer

3. Which of the following would **NOT** require immediate transfer to a burn center?
   A. Partial thickness burns to hands and feet
   B. Third and fourth degree burns to extremities
   C. Facial burns and hypoxia on presentation
   D. Partial-thickness burns with dermal involvement to the forearm with significant blistering
   E. Partial-thickness burn to perineum
4. A 12-year-old is transported to your facility by paramedics for evaluation following an electrical injury. The details surrounding the injury are unclear. Which of the following current pathways would be associated with the fewest complications?
   A. Hand-to-hand flow
   B. Hand-to foot flow
   C. Foot-to-foot flow
   D. Current passing through the head
   E. Current passing through the thorax
5. A toddler is brought to your ED for evaluation for a possible electrical injury. The parents state that the child was found with an electrical cord in her mouth. On exam, the child appears playful. A thorough examination would include all EXCEPT which of the following?
   A. Examination of hands and heels for entry and exit burns
   B. Examination of the lips and oral commissure for orofacial burns
   C. Estimation of fluid requirements if evidence of electrical injuries are found
   D. Baseline ECG and cardiac monitoring
   E. Baseline chemistries and urinalysis
6. You are informed by the EMS dispatcher that there was a lightning strike in your area, and you will be receiving two pediatric victims. Reports indicate that the children were not in the direct vicinity of the lightning strike, and were huddled near a tree when the injury occurred. A physician at the scene states one of the victims appears to have a perforated tympanic membrane. Based on your understanding of lightning injuries, what is the MOST likely mechanism of injury in these children?
   A. Direct strike from lightning
   B. Ground current
   C. Side flash
   D. Thermal flash
   E. Blunt injury

ANSWERS

1. B. The airway should be assessed immediately on presentation. The most common cause of death during the first hour following a burn is respiratory impairment. Humidified oxygen is used to maintain oxygenation. Intubation may be necessary if the airway appears compromised after assessment. Evaluation of vascular status is part of the secondary survey.
2. C. In a patient with extensive burns, the next management priority should be restoration and maintenance of tissue perfusion. Burns involving over15 percent BSA should have a large-bore intravenous catheter placed for administering fluids. Fluid requirements should be estimated using the Parkland formula at 4 mL/kg per percent BSA. It is best to avoid manipulation of burns prior to transport to a burn center. Covering the burns with dry sterile coverings is recommended.
3. D. Isolated burns to the extremities that are not circumferential and have no evidence of vascular compromise may be treated as an outpatient with close follow-up and do not necessarily require transfer to a burn center.
4. C. Foot-to-foot flow is generally not associated with fatalities. The mortality rates for the other current pathways mentioned range from 20 to 60 percent and are associated with complications that include brain and brainstem damage, paralysis, myocardial injury, and cardiopulmonary arrest.
5. D. Baseline ECG and cardiac monitoring is not indicated for children exposed to household current. Most victims of electrical injury have very little external damage while sustaining underlying tissue damage. A careful examination of this child is necessary. In cases of high suspicion, baseline chemistries can be useful.
6. E. In cases of blunt injury, the shock wave can cause perforation of the tympanic membrane. There may also be associated damage to internal organs as well. All lightning victims must undergo a thorough search for blunt trauma injuries. In the prehospital setting, victims should be immobilized and transported under advanced life support protocols.

115 HEAT AND COLD ILLNESS

Gary R. Strange
Heather M. Prendergast

HEAT ILLNESS

- Infants are predisposed to the development of heat illness due to their poorly developed thermoregulatory systems. An especially tragic situation, which is entirely preventable through parental education, is the development of heat illness in small children left in closed cars on hot days.

- Older children and adolescents are susceptible to heat illness when they exercise vigorously under hot, humid conditions. Adolescent zeal for competitive athletics, coupled with an often-held belief among the young in their invulnerability, can lead to serious heat illness.
- Acclimatization to a hot, humid environment allows the individual to perform harder and longer without developing heat illness. Full acclimatization takes 3 to 4 weeks, during which, the individual must limit exertion. Children take longer to acclimatize than adults.

PATHOPHYSIOLOGY

- The body can dissipate heat by four mechanisms:
  ◦ Radiation
  ◦ Conduction
  ◦ Convection
  ◦ Evaporation
    ▪ Evaporation of sweat from the skin is a major heat-dissipation mechanism, especially in conditioned athletes. This source of heat loss is relatively ineffective, however, when the relative humidity exceeds 85 percent.

TYPES OF HEAT ILLNESS

HEAT CRAMPS
- With heavy exertion, the muscles that are working the hardest may begin to go into spasm. The cause has long been described as dilutional hyponatremia, which usually occurs in conditioned athletes who replace fluid losses with water. However, there is no clear evidence that dilutional hyponatremia is the actual cause.

HEAT EXHAUSTION
- Heat exhaustion is a syndrome of dizziness, postural hypotension, nausea, vomiting, headache, weakness, and, occasionally, syncope, which may be associated with normal temperature or moderate temperature elevation (39 to 41.1°C). It tends to occur in unacclimatized individuals. The cause of heat exhaustion may be either salt or water depletion.

HEAT STROKE
- Heat stroke is the most severe form of heat illness. Patients present with disorientation, seizures, or coma.
- Classic heat stroke is typically seen in the elderly and develops over a period of days.
- With exertional heat stroke, which is much more likely in the pediatric population, the skin may be dry or sweating may continue. The temperature ranges from 41.1 to 42.2°C.

- There is no clear scientific evidence to indicate that heat stroke results from fluid and electrolyte abnormalities. Although dehydration is no doubt a predisposing condition, other predisposing factors that are poorly understood seem to be necessary for heat stroke to occur.
- Complications are common, leading to the high mortality rate. These include:
  ◦ Neurologic dysfunction (100 percent)
  ◦ Moderate to severe renal insufficiency (53 percent)
  ◦ Disseminated intravascular coagulation (45 percent)
  ◦ Adult respiratory distress syndrome (10 percent)
  ◦ Rhabdomyolysis (up to 25 percent)

MANAGEMENT

- Heat cramps are treated by removing the patient to a cool environment and providing rest and oral electrolyte solutions.
- Heat exhaustion is also treated by removal to a cool environment and providing rest. Intravenous rehydration is recommended, starting with 20 mL/kg of normal saline over 30 min.
- If heat exhaustion symptoms have resolved during emergency department treatment and observation, the patient may be released to continue rest and rehydration in a cool environment.
- Heat stroke is an immediately life-threatening entity. After assessment and stabilization of the airway, breathing, and circulation, cooling should be instituted immediately.
  ◦ Spraying the skin with room-temperature water and directing an electric fan onto the patient's skin will usually result in rapid reduction of the core temperature.
  ◦ Ice packs may be used in the groin and axilla, but ice water applied widely to the skin may cause vasoconstriction and impair the dissipation of heat.
  ◦ Submersion in cold water is very effective in lowering the temperature but makes other resuscitative efforts practically impossible.
  ◦ Invasive lavage to lower the body temperature has not been adequately studied and is not currently recommended.
  ◦ Core temperature should be monitored continuously during treatment and active cooling should continue until the core temperature falls to 39°C.
  ◦ Diazepam, 0.2 to 0.3 mg/kg/dose IV, may be required to prevent shivering.
  ◦ Intravenous fluids are required and should initially be given as isotonic crystalloid at a rate of 20 mL/kg over the first hour.
  ◦ Since the effects of heat stroke are widespread throughout essentially every system of the body and

the differential diagnosis is broad (Table 115-1), extensive diagnostic evaluation is indicated.

- Arterial blood gases are helpful in evaluating oxygenation, ventilation, and acid–base status. Changes in body temperature alter blood gas values, but whether corrections in the values are helpful before treatment decisions are made is controversial.
- The complete blood count will usually show an elevated white blood cell count. Counts above 20,000/mm^3 and elevated band counts are more consistent with an underlying infection and should prompt a complete septic work-up. Hemoglobin and hematocrit values are usually elevated due to dehydration.
- Electrolyte studies may reveal abnormal sodium levels. Elevated potassium levels may indicate the development of rhabdomyolysis.
- Renal function tests may initially be elevated due to dehydration and may rise later, as renal failure develops.
- Urinalysis will often show a high specific gravity as a reflection of the hydration status. If the urine

TABLE 115-1   Differential Diagnosis of Heat Stroke: Symptom Complex—Altered Mental Status, Hyperthermia

POTENTIAL DIAGNOSIS	PERTINENT HISTORY	PERTINENT FINDINGS ON PHYSICAL EXAMINATION	PERTINENT LABORATORY DATA
Encephalitis and meningitis	Fever Prodromal illness Severe headache Chills	Temperature Neck stiffness Kernig and Brudzinski signs positive	Lumbar puncture: elevated WBCs, positive Gram's stain, cultures
Malaria	Exposure Travel history Previous history	Fever pattern Confusion	Peripheral blood smear
Typhoid fever, typhus	Exposure Travel history	Fever pattern	Titers: Weil–Felix reaction, complement fixation
Sepsis	Fever Age extreme Immunocompromised	Fever Confusion Coma Focal infection	Chest x-ray WBC: elevated Cultures: blood, urine, spinal fluid
Hypothalamic hemorrhage	Hypertension Anticoagulant therapy	Coma Fever Focal neurologic findings	Brain CT: hemorrhage
Thyroid storm	Preexisting hyperthyroidism Risk factors Stress Surgery Trauma Infection Failure to take antithyroid medication	Goiter Tachycardia Seizures Hypotension	Thyroid function studies: T$_3$ and T$_4$
Malignant hyperthermia	Inhalation anesthetic Succinylcholine	Muscle fasciculation	Arterial blood gases: acidosis Electrolytes: hyperkalemia hypermagnesemia
Heat stroke	Risk factors Exposure to heat load Exercise	Hot, flushed skin Confusion Agitation Seizures Tachycardia Hypotension Vomiting Diarrhea Muscle tenderness	AST: elevated WBC: elevated Electrolytes: hyper- or hypo-kalemia, hyponatremia, hypocalcemia, hypophosphatemia Arterial blood gases: metabolic acidosis Urine: myoglobin Clotting factors: decreased Blood glucose: variable

Reproduced with permission from Barreca RS: Heat illness, in Hamilton GC, Sanders AB, Strange GR, Trott AT (eds): *Emergency Medicine: An Approach to Clinical Problem-Solving.* Philadelphia, Saunders, 1991, p 402.

is positive for hemoglobin in the absence of red blood cells on the microscopic evaluation, rhabdomyolysis should be suspected.

- Liver enzymes may be elevated, since the liver is very sensitive to heat stress. Transaminase levels peak in 24 to 48 hours and correlate well with the severity of injury. Very high levels (aspartate transaminase >1000 IU) are predictive of severe illness and complications.
- Computed tomographic scanning of the brain is indicated to rule out intracranial pathology, especially if the mental status does not promptly improve with lowering of the temperature.
- An electrocardiogram is indicated to evaluate for myocardial ischemia, which can result from severe cardiovascular stress.

- After evaluation and stabilization, patients with heat stroke are admitted to an intensive care setting for continued monitoring and aggressive treatment.

COLD ILLNESS

- Hypothermia is defined as a core temperature of <35°C. A low body temperature may develop as a result of exposure to low ambient temperature or may be secondary to a disease process (Table 115-2).
- Neonates are at high risk for developing hypothermia due to their large surface area compared with body mass and the relative paucity of subcutaneous tissue. The evaporation of warm amniotic fluid from the skin

TABLE 115-2 Causes of Hypothermia in Infants and Children

Environmental factors	CNS disorders
Exposure	Degenerative diseases
Near drowning	Head trauma
Infections	Spinal cord trauma
Meningitis	Subarachnoid hemorrhage
Encephalitis	Cerebrovascular accidents
Sepsis	Intracranial neoplasm
Pneumonia	Vascular factors
Metabolic and endocrine factors	Shock
Hypoglycemia	Pulmonary embolism
Diabetic ketoacidosis	Gastrointestinal hemorrhage
Hypopituitarism	Dermatologic factors
Myxedema	Burns
Addison's disease	Erythrodermas
Uremia	Iatrogenic factors
Malnutrition	Cold fluid factors
Toxicologic factors	Exposure during treatment
Alcohol	or postdelivery
Anesthetic agents	Prolonged extrications
Barbiturates	
Carbon monoxide	
Cyclic antidepressants	
Narcotics	
Phenothiazines	

of the newborn is a major source of heat loss that must be guarded against in all cases.

- In recent years, there has been an increase in exposure-related hypothermia in older children and adolescents; this is believed to be associated with the increased popularity of winter sports. Inexperience and lack of caution, which are common among adolescents, increase the likelihood of their becoming victims of hypothermia.

PATHOPHYSIOLOGY

- Exposure to cold stimulates skin receptors, resulting in peripheral vasoconstriction and conservation of heat. As the temperature of the blood declines, the preoptic anterior hypothalamus is stimulated. Heat production is then increased by shivering and by metabolic and endocrine means of thermogenesis, primarily mediated by thyroid and adrenal secretions (Fig. 115-1).
- Heat is lost from the body by four mechanisms:
  ○ Radiation accounts for 55 to 65 percent of heat loss. Radiation losses are reduced by insulation (clothing, subcutaneous fat) and by reduction in skin blood flow (vasoconstriction).
  ○ Conduction is not a major route of heat loss under normal conditions, but conductive heat loss increases 5 times in the presence of wet clothing and 25 to 30 times with submersion in cold water.
  ○ Convection heat losses are greatly increased by wind currents and bodily movement. The wind-chill effect significantly increases the likelihood of hypothermia developing at a given temperature.
  ○ Evaporation accounts for 20 to 25 percent of heat loss, primarily via respiration and insensible water loss from the skin. When the skin is wet, evaporative losses are increased.
- Essentially every part of the body is affected by hypothermia (Table 115-3).

CARDIOVASCULAR EFFECTS
- After an initial tachycardia, the heart rate falls as temperature falls.
- Atrial dysrhythmias commonly appear at temperatures below 32°C.
- Ventricular ectopy is seen with temperatures below 30°C and the risk of ventricular fibrillation is greatly increased.
- A J wave (Osborn wave) may be present at the junction of the QRS complex and ST segment (Fig. 115-2).

CENTRAL NERVOUS SYSTEM EFFECTS
- Brain enzymes are less functional with declining temperature, resulting in a linear decrease in cerebral

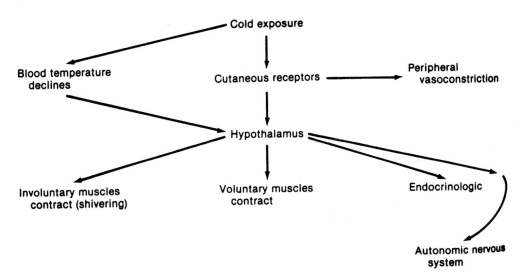

FIG. 115-1 Physiologic responses in hypothermia. (Reproduced with permission from Cooper MA, Danzl DF: Hypothermia, in Hamilton GC, Sanders AB, Strange GR, Trott AT (eds): *Emergency Medicine: An Approach to Clinical Problem-Solving.* Philadelphia, Saunders, 1991, p 410.)

metabolism. At 20°C, the electroencephalogram shows a flat line.

RESPIRATORY EFFECTS

- Cold initially stimulates the respiratory drive, but, as temperature falls, a progressive decline in minute ventilation supervenes.
- Bronchorrhea, due to the local effect of cold air, can be severe, simulating pulmonary edema.

RENAL EFFECTS

- The kidney produces a large "cold diuresis" of dilute glomerular filtrate.

GASTROINTESTINAL EFFECTS

- Gastrointestinal motility is decreased and gastric dilatation, ileus, constipation, and poor rectal tone, commonly result.

DIAGNOSIS

- The diagnosis of hypothermia may be obvious when a history of exposure is known. However, hypothermia may develop insidiously due to causes other than exposure or to exposure in relatively warm environments.
- Once hypothermia is known or suspected, a history of exposure is sought, including:
  - ◦ Circumstances
  - ◦ Location
  - ◦ Ambient temperature
  - ◦ Length of exposure

- ◦ Presence or absence of submersion or wet skin and clothing
- If significant exposure is unlikely, an extensive history is required to search for clues for other causes of hypothermia (see Table 115-1).
- The key physical findings in patients with hypothermia, and the temperature level at which they occur, are depicted in Table 115-3.
- Most thermometers for routine clinical use will record a temperature down to only 34.4°C. Special glass or electronic thermometers are required for accurate measurement of temperatures in hypothermic patients. Continuous monitoring of rectal, esophageal, or tympanic temperature is very useful during treatment.
- The skin is typically cold, firm, pale, or mottled. Localized damage due to frostbite may be present.
- Early neurologic signs of hypothermia include confusion, apathy, poor judgment, slurred speech, and ataxia. Coma usually supervenes by the time the temperature reaches 27°C. Focal neurologic defects may be present. The Glasgow Coma Scale can serve as a useful quantitative means of following the patient's response to treatment, but it is not as useful with the nonverbal infant.
- For patients with hypothermia not related to exposure and in those exposure-related individuals who present with temperatures below 32°C, extensive diagnostic testing is indicated.
  - ◦ Arterial blood gases are useful for evaluation of oxygenation, ventilation, and acid–base status. Although some authorities have recommended correcting blood gas results for body temperature,

TABLE 115-3 Pathophysiologic Changes During Hypothermia

CENTIGRADE TEMPERATURE	FARENHEIT TEMPERATURE	FINDINGS
37.6	99.6	Normal rectal temperature
37	98.6	Normal oral temperature
35	95.0	Maximal shivering
		Increased metabolic rate
33	91.4	Apathy
		Ataxia
		Anmesia
		Dysarthria
31	87.8	Decreased level of consciousness
		Bradycardia
		Hypotension
		Bradypnea
		Shivering stops
29	85.2	Dysrhythmias
		Insulin not effective
		Dilated pupils
		Poikilothermia
27	80.6	Areflexia
		No response to pain
		Comatose
25	77.0	Cerebral blood flow one-third normal
		Cardiac output one-half normal
		Significant hypotension
23	73.4	No corneal reflex
		Maximal ventricular fibrillation risk
19	66.2	Asystole
		Flat electroencephalogram
15	59.2	Lowest temperature survived from accidental hypothermia in an infant
9	48.2	Lowest temperature survived from therapeutic hypothermia

Reproduced with permission from Cooper MA, Danzl DF: Hypothermia, in Hamilton GC, Sanders AB, Strange GR, Trott AT (eds): *Emergency Medicine: An Approach to Clinical Problem-Solving.* Philadelphia, Saunders, 1991, p 415.

correction can lead to false elevation of P_{O_2} and subsequent under-treatment.

○ Toxicologic studies are frequently indicated to detect causative or predisposing agents.

○ Cultures of body fluids are indicated in all cases of moderate to severe hypothermia. Sepsis is a common cause of hypothermia in the infant and may also develop as a complication of hypothermia due to other causes.

○ Radiologic imaging will include:
   ▪ Chest radiograph in all cases of significant hypothermia. Pulmonary edema may develop during rewarming and aspiration is relatively common.
   ▪ Cervical spine films if there is suspicion of trauma.
   ▪ Cranial computed tomographic scanning may be indicated in the setting of trauma or to search for other etiologic factors, especially when mental status does not clear along with rewarming.

○ Electrocardiography is indicated for all patients with a core temperature below 32°C to detect dysrhythmias or evidence of myocardial ischemia. The J wave (see Fig. 115-2) is usually seen when the temperature falls below 32°C.

PREHOSPITAL CARE

• Great caution is needed to prevent hypothermia or to initiate its early treatment in neonates. The neonate should immediately be dried and wrapped in warm blankets. Alternatively, the neonate can be placed against the body of the mother and then covered.

• For other potentially hypothermic patients, wet clothing should be removed, and dry blankets applied.

• When prolonged extrications are required, hypothermia is particularly likely to develop.

• Resuscitation fluids should be warmed whenever possible.

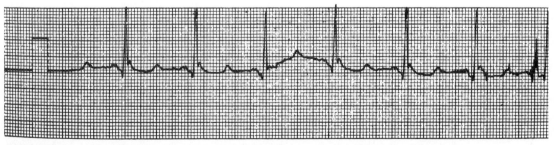

FIG. 115-2 Example of a J wave in a hypothermic patient. (Reproduced with permission from Cooper MA, Danzl DF: Hypothermia, in Hamilton GC, Sanders AB, Strange GR, Trott AT (eds): *Emergency Medicine: An Approach to Clinical Problem-Solving.* Philadelphia, Saunders, 1991, p 411.)

- Heated, humidified oxygen, if available, may minimize further core temperature loss and significantly add to other rewarming techniques.
- Cardiac monitoring is indicated to detect dysrhythmias. Because pulse and respiratory rates may be very slow in hypothermia, assessment for breathing and pulselessness is carried out over a 30- to 45-s period.
- If the patient is not breathing, ventilation is started immediately using warmed humidified oxygen whenever possible.
- If there is no pulse, chest compressions are started immediately. Do not withhold basic life support while the patient is being rewarmed.

EMERGENCY DEPARTMENT MANAGEMENT

- Obtunded patients without protective airway reflexes require endotracheal intubation after preoxygenation. Endotracheal intubation should be done as atraumatically as possible, but should not be withheld for fear of precipitating ventricular fibrillation.
- Intravenous lines are started and fluid resuscitation is guided by vital signs, urinary output, and pulmonary status.
- Cardiac monitoring is initiated.
- Continuous monitoring of rectal, esophageal, or tympanic temperature is very helpful during treatment.
- A urinary catheter and a nasogastric tube are inserted.
- A bedside glucose determination is done to assess the need for glucose supplementation.
- If narcotic intoxication is a possibility, naloxone, 2 mg IV, is administered.
- Cardiopulmonary resuscitation is started in the pulseless patient, and interventions are guided by cardiac monitor findings.
- The cold myocardium may be resistant to defibrillation and to pharmacologic agents. If the initial three defibrillation attempts fail to establish a rhythm, CPR is resumed and the patient is rewarmed to 30°C before defibrillation is repeated. Many patients spontaneously convert to an organized rhythm at a core temperature of 32 to 35°C.
- During hypothermia, protein binding of drugs is increased, and most drugs will be ineffective in normal doses. Pharmacologic attempts to alter the pulse or blood pressure are to be avoided because drugs can accumulate in the peripheral circulation and subsequently lead to toxicity as rewarming occurs.
- It is important to remember that infants and children who have sustained prolonged hypothermic cardiac arrest have recovered with little or no neurologic impairment. In general, resuscitative efforts should

continue until the hypothermic child is warmed to at least 30°C.
- In moderate to severe cases of hypothermia, active rewarming is started as soon as possible.
  ○ Heated, humidified oxygen and intravenous fluids heated to 40°C have been shown to be safe and efficacious and are used from the beginning.
  ○ Further heat loss is prevented by using radiant warmers for neonates and infants. The older child and adolescent should be covered with dry blankets.
  ○ Active external rewarming, as with hot packs and electric blankets, can be dangerous. The rewarming of cold extremities can result in the mobilization of cold peripheral blood to the central circulation, resulting in core temperature after-drop.
  ○ Active core rewarming is used in most cases of moderate to severe hypothermia.
    ▪ Heated humidified oxygen
    ▪ Heated intravenous fluids
    ▪ Irrigation of the stomach, bladder, or colon (heat transfer by these techniques is somewhat limited)
    ▪ Irrigation of the mediastinum or pleural cavity via a thoracostomy tube (effective but very invasive)
    ▪ Peritoneal lavage with heated fluid (40 to 45°C) is probably a more effective method.
    ▪ Extracorporeal rewarming is the most rapid and effective method and is indicated in hypothermic cardiac arrest and with patients who present with completely frozen extremities.
  ○ Forced air rewarming has recently been described as effective, noninvasive, and not associated with an afterdrop phenomenon.
  ○ Applying subatmospheric pressure to the hand and forearm, along with heat (described as immediately resulting in subcutaneous vasodilatation and rapid heat acquisition).
  ○ Previously healthy patients who are only mildly hypothermic (35 to 33°C) will usually reheat themselves safely if they are placed in a warm environment and given dry insulating coverings (passive external rewarming).
  ○ Beyond the neonatal period, sepsis is the most common cause of hypothermia in infants. All hypothermic patients should have a thorough evaluation to search for a source of infection and should have broad spectrum antibiotics initiated early.

DISPOSITION

- Most patients with hypothermia will require hospitalization for further treatment and evaluation.
- Those patients with a core temperature below 32°C will require cardiac monitoring.

- Profoundly hypothermic patients with cardiac arrest and those with completely frozen extremities are candidates for extracorporeal rewarming and may require transfer to a tertiary care facility with this capability.
- Patients with mild accidental hypothermia (35 to 32°C) may be rewarmed and discharged to a safe environment if there is no evidence of underlying disease.

FROSTBITE

- Predisposing factors
  - Environmental factors
    - Wind
    - Contact with metal objects
    - Poor insulation by clothing
    - Wet clothing
    - Tight clothing
    - Clothing permeable to wind
    - Lack of covering for cold-sensitive parts, such as the face and hands
  - Individual factors
    - Poor fitness
    - Fatigue
    - Dehydration
    - Prior cold injury
    - Acute or chronic illness
    - Poor peripheral circulation
  - Behavioral factors
    - Alcohol intoxication
    - Very young age with lack of awareness of behavior
    - Adolescent recklessness with feelings of invulnerability
    - Psychiatric disturbances
  - Occasion-linked factors
    - Mountain-climbing
    - Cross-country skiing
    - Accidents

PATHOPHYSIOLOGY

- Localized hypothermia is described in terms similar to those used for burns.
  - First degree frostbite is limited to the superficial epidermis. Erythema and edema occur and resolve without sequelae.
  - Second degree frostbite results in deeper epidermal involvement and presents with large, clear bullae.
  - Third degree injury consists of full thickness skin injury.

TREATMENT

- The treatment of frostbite is rapid rewarming. The preferred technique is immersion of the affected part in circulating warm water (40 to 42°C).

- Narcotic analgesics are often required to control pain during rewarming.
- It is very difficult to determine tissue viability after significant hypothermic injury. Debridement of nonviable tissue is best delayed for several days to weeks to preserve as much tissue as possible.
- Topical aloe vera cream and ibuprofen may be used for outpatient treatment after rewarming.
- Rewarmed body parts are highly susceptible to refreezing, leading to even greater tissue loss. If exposure is anticipated, it is better not to rewarm the tissue.

BIBLIOGRAPHY

HEAT ILLNESS

American Academy of Pediatrics Committee on Sports Medicine and Fitness: Climatic heat stress and the exercising child and adolescent. *Pediatrics* 106:158–159, 2000.

Backer HD, Shopes E, Collins SL, Barkan H: Exertional heat illness and hyponatremia in hikers. *Am J Emerg Med* 17:532–539, 1999.

Bouchama A, Knochel JP: Heat stroke. *N Engl J Med* 346:1978–1988, 2002.

Centers for Disease Control and Prevention: Heat-related illnesses and deaths—Missouri, 1998, and United States, 1979–1996. *MMWR Morb Mortal Wkly Rep* 48:469–473, 1999.

Dematte JE, O'Mara K, Buescher J, et al: Near-fatal heat stroke during the 1995 heat wave in Chicago. *Ann Intern Med* 129:173–181, 1998.

Noakes TD: Fluid and electrolyte disturbances in heat illness. *Int J Sports Med* 19(suppl 2):S146–S149, 1998.

COLD ILLNESS

Kornberger E, Schwarz B, Lindner KH, et al: Forced air surface rewarming in patients with severe accidental hypothermia. *Resuscitation* 41:105–111, 1999.

Murphy JV, Banwell PE, Roberts AH, et al: Frostbite: Pathogenesis and treatment. *J Trauma* 48:171–178, 2000.

Soreide E, Grahn DA, Brock-Utne JG, et al: A non-invasive means to effectively restore normothermia in cold stressed individuals: A preliminary report. *J Emerg Med* 17:725–730, 1999.

Walpoth BH, Walpoth-Aslan BN, Mattle HP, et al: Outcome of survivors of accidental deep hypothermia and circulatory arrest treated with extracorporeal blood warming. *N Engl J Med* 337:1500–1505, 1997.

Weinberg AD: The role of inhalation rewarming in the early management of hypothermia. *Resuscitation* 36:101–104, 1998.

QUESTIONS

1. A junior member of the outdoor track and field team is brought to your emergency department for acute onset of dizziness, nausea, and vomiting following a series of long-distance race events. He is alert and oriented. A rectal temperature is 39°C. The patient is found to be markedly orthostatic. Based on your assessment, this patient is presenting with signs and symptoms consistent with **WHICH** of the following?
   A. Heat cramps
   B. Gastroenteritis
   C. Heat exhaustion
   D. Heat stroke
   E. Heat syncope

2. A frantic mother brings her 7-year-old child to the emergency department for evaluation. The child was involved in an outdoor jump rope competition approximately 2 h ago. Since that time, the mother states her daughter has had several episodes of vomiting and now seems confused. While obtaining the history, the child begins seizing. A rectal temperature is 42°C. The child is most likely suffering from **WHICH** of the following?
   A. Heat cramps
   B. Child abuse
   C. Heat exhaustion
   D. Heat stroke
   E. Severe dehydration.

3. The patient in question 2 is stabilized and intubated for airway protection. Which of the following cooling methods would be the **MOST** effective in this patient?
   A. Submersion in a cold water bath
   B. Ice water generously applied to the patient's skin
   C. Cold water gastric and bladder lavage
   D. Ice packs to the groin and axilla
   E. Use of an electric fan while spraying the patient with room-temperature water

4. Which of the following laboratory findings would **NOT** be expected in the above patient?
   A. Elevated specific gravity
   B. Prerenal azotemia
   C. Mild leukocytosis
   D. Microcytic anemia
   E. Hyperkalemia

5. A 10-year-old child is pulled from a river following a submersion incident. Which mechanism of heat loss would account for the **GREATEST** heat dissipation in this patient?
   A. Radiation
   B. Conduction
   C. Convection
   D. Evaporation
   E. Wind-chill effects

6. A 12-year-old girl is brought to your emergency department for evaluation of cold weather exposure. The patient became separated from family members during a ski trip. On arrival to the ED, the patient is found to have a temperature of 34.4°C. A management priority in this patient would be which of the following?
   A. Active rewarming with warmed blankets and warm beverages by mouth
   B. Active rewarming with heated humidified oxygen and warmed intravenous fluids
   C. Active core rewarming with gastric lavage
   D. Hot water submersion baths for hands and feet
   E. Rectal temperature

7. A teenager is brought to the emergency department for cold weather exposure to his hands during mountain climbing. On evaluation of his hands, you find significant erythema and edema that extends to the deeper epidermal layer. The capillary refill is normal and there are scattered large clear bullae on the dorsum. Based on your assessment, the patient has which of the following?
   A. First degree frostbite
   B. Trench hands
   C. Second degree frostbite
   D. Third degree frostbite
   E. Partial thickness burns

ANSWERS

1. C. The patient is exhibiting signs of heat exhaustion. Heat exhaustion often presents as a syndrome of dizziness, postural hypotension, nausea, and vomiting with a normal mental status. It can be associated with normal or mildly elevated body temperatures. It is common in unacclimatized individuals.

2. D. The patient is a victim of heat stroke, which is the most **SEVERE** form of heat illness, and is a life-threatening emergency. Patients can present with disorientation, seizures, or coma. Rapid cooling is a priority after assessment and stabilization of the airway, breathing, and circulation.

3. E. Spraying the skin with room-temperature water and directing an electric fan onto the patient's skin is an effective method for rapid reduction of the core temperature. Ice water applied to the body can be counterproductive by causing vasoconstriction and impairment of heat dissipation. Submersion in cold water, while effective, may be impractical in this patient.

4. D. In heat stroke patients, laboratory abnormalities are reflective of a dehydrated state. Common

abnormalities include elevated white blood cell counts, hemoglobin and hematocrit, high specific gravity on urinalysis, and elevated renal function tests. The liver is very sensitive to heat and is common to see elevated transaminase levels.

5. B. Under normal conditions, radiation accounts for 55 to 65 percent of heat loss, and conduction is not a major route of heat loss. However, in the case of submersion in cold water, the conductive heat loss is increased 25 to 30 times.

6. E. It is imperative that a rectal temperature be obtained on all patients with suspected hypothermia. Most thermometers for routine clinical use will record a temperature down to only 34.4°C. Once an accurate rectal temperature is obtained, the most appropriate warming methods can be started.

7. C. The patient is suffering from second degree frostbite and will require rapid rewarming of his extremities. The preferred technique is immersion of his hands in a circulating warm water bath at 40 to 42°C. If there is a possibility of re-exposure, then rewarming should be delayed. Rewarmed body parts are highly susceptible to refreezing, and can lead to greater tissue loss.

116 HIGH-ALTITUDE ILLNESS AND DYSBARIC INJURIES

Ira J. Blumen
Gary R. Strange
Heather M. Prendergast

HIGH-ALTITUDE ILLNESS

- High-altitude illness most often affects young and otherwise healthy individuals. Symptoms may develop within hours or days after ascent.
- There are three major factors that influence the incidence, onset, and severity of high-altitude illness:
  ○ Rate of ascent
  ○ Altitude achieved
  ○ Length of stay
- Children, because of their physiologic differences, are at greater risk for developing both acute mountain sickness (AMS) and high-altitude pulmonary edema (HAPE).

PHYSIOLOGIC RESPONSE

- At high altitude, hypoxia results in increased cerebrospinal fluid (CSF) pressure, fluid retention, fluid shifts, and impaired gas exchange.

- Through acclimatization, a series of physiologic adjustments work to restore the tissue oxygen pressure to near its sea level value. Successful acclimatization will vary between individuals and cannot be predicted by physical conditioning, examination, or testing.
- A slow, graded ascent is the key to acclimatization. In the ideal setting, the first night's sleep occurs at less than 8000 ft, with the first day spent at rest. If the altitude of the desired climb is between 10,000 and 14,000 ft, then, the daily ascent is limited to 1000 ft. Above 14,000 ft, 2 days should be taken for each 1000 ft ascent.
- Pharmacologic agents may also be beneficial adjuncts to acclimatization. Acetazolamide (Diamox) has been shown to be very effective when staging is not possible or with individuals who are at an increased risk of high-altitude illness.

RESPIRATORY SYSTEM

- As an individual ascends, the hypoxic ventilatory response (HVR) will attempt to compensate for the decrease in arterial P_{O_2} through an increase in the ventilatory rate. An inadequate HVR, resulting in relative hypoventilation, has been suggested as the etiology for AMS and HAPE.

CARDIOVASCULAR SYSTEM

- The heart rate will begin to increase at an altitude of 4000 ft. There will also be a slight increase in blood pressure secondary to increased catecholamines and selective vasoconstriction.

HEMATOPOIETIC SYSTEM

- The hematopoietic response to high altitude is a critical element in an individual's ability to acclimatize. Within hours of ascent, erythropoietin output is increased in response to the hypoxia. In approximately 4 to 5 days, there will be an increase in circulating red blood cells.

CENTRAL NERVOUS SYSTEM

- Cerebral hypoxia begins when the P_{O_2} falls to 50 to 60 mm Hg. The potent vasodilatory effects of hypoxia will overcome hypocapnic vasoconstriction and result in an increased cerebral blood flow. This response, which increases oxygen delivered to the brain, also increases intracranial pressure and can lead to high-altitude cerebral edema (HACE).

RENAL SYSTEM

- Respiratory alkalosis stimulates renal excretion of bicarbonate, producing a metabolic acidosis to compensate for the respiratory alkalosis.

ACUTE MOUNTAIN SICKNESS

- AMS is the most common and mildest form of high-altitude illness. Up to 25 percent of individuals traveling to 8000 ft will become symptomatic, although nearly everyone who rapidly ascends to 11,000 ft will develop AMS.

PATHOPHYSIOLOGY
- Although normal acclimatization inhibits ADH and aldosterone, resulting in a high-altitude-induced diuresis, the opposite is seen with AMS. Aldosterone, ADH, and renin-angiotensin increase, resulting in fluid retention and a leakage from the vascular space to the extravascular space.

CLINICAL PRESENTATION
- The onset of AMS symptoms is usually within 4 to 8 h of a rapid ascent, but it can be delayed for up to 4 days. Symptoms develop following strenuous activity or sleeping at high altitude. In most cases, symptoms peak in 24 to 48 h and resolve by the third or fourth day.
- The clinical presentation of AMS includes the following symptoms, in order of prevalence:
  ◦ Headache
  ◦ Sleep disturbance
  ◦ Fatigue
  ◦ Shortness of breath
  ◦ Dizziness
  ◦ Anorexia
  ◦ Nausea
  ◦ Vomiting
- On physical examination, vital signs may be normal or slightly elevated. Fluid retention is exhibited as fine rales or peripheral edema. Retinal hemorrhages may also be seen.
- Sleep disturbance and periods of sleep apnea are common.

TREATMENT
- Once symptoms occur, activity should be minimized, with no higher ascent until signs and symptoms have resolved. Proceeding to a lower altitude is indicated for any individual who shows no signs of improvement within 1 to 2 days or worsens. Immediate descent is indicated if ataxia, decreased level of consciousness, confusion, dyspnea at rest, rales, or cyanosis are present.
- If descent is not an option, the use of supplementary oxygen will relieve most of the signs and symptoms of AMS. During sleep, 1 to 2 L/min can be of significant benefit.
- A Gamow bag is a portable, fabric hyperbaric bag that has been shown to relieve the central effects of AMS. Using a foot pump, it can be pressurized in excess of 100 torr for the physiologic equivalent of a 4000- to 5000-ft descent.
- Symptomatic treatment for the headache is with acetaminophen, which will have no impact on the hypoxic ventilatory response. Victims of AMS are to refrain from using narcotics, which depress this response.
- Prochlorperazine, given for nausea and vomiting, is also effective in *increasing* the respiratory drive. The dosage of prochlorperazine for children larger than 10 kg in weight, or older than 2 years, is 0.1 to 0.15 mg/kg/dose IM, PO, or PR.
- The carbonic anhydrase inhibitor acetazolamide may be used in the treatment or prophylaxis of AMS. It decreases the reabsorption of bicarbonate, forcing a renal bicarbonate diuresis and resulting in a mild metabolic acidosis. This increases the ventilation rate and arterial P_{O_2}. The pediatric dosage for acetazolamide is 5 to 10 mg/kg/day, given every 12 h.
- Dexamethasone is also used to treat AMS, although its mechanism of action is unknown. Dexamethasone minimizes the symptoms of AMS but does not impact acclimatization. Its use is reserved for those with sulfur allergies or intolerance to acetazolamide. A loading dose of 4 mg PO or IM is given, and improvement is generally noted within 2 to 6 h.

PREVENTION
- Prevention of AMS through acclimatization is not always possible for vacationing climbers, skiers, and other sport enthusiasts. Prevention includes:
  ◦ Slow graded ascent
  ◦ Diet high in carbohydrates
  ◦ Low salt intake
  ◦ Adequate fluid intake
  ◦ Alcohol avoidance
  ◦ Tobacco avoidance

HIGH-ALTITUDE CEREBRAL EDEMA

- HACE is the most severe, life-threatening form of high-altitude illness. HACE is uncommon, affecting less than 1 to 2 percent of individuals who ascend without acclimatization.

CLINICAL PRESENTATION

- HACE commonly begins with the symptoms of AMS and progresses to diffuse neurologic dysfunction.
  - Onset of severe symptoms is 1 to 3 days after ascent to altitude, but early signs of AMS may rapidly deteriorate to severe HACE in as few as 12 h.
  - Severe headaches, nausea, vomiting, and altered mental status are common symptoms associated with HACE.
  - Truncal ataxia is the cardinal sign. This alone warrants immediate descent. If not recognized, HACE will proceed to include confusion, slurred speech, diplopia, hallucinations, seizures, impaired judgment, cranial nerve palsies (third and sixth), abnormal reflexes, paresthesias, decreased level of consciousness, coma, and finally death.
  - A 60-percent mortality rate is associated with HACE once coma is present.

TREATMENT

- Definitive treatment of HACE is descent, and as quickly as possible.
- High-flow oxygen is indicated as soon as symptoms are recognized.
- Dexamethasone can produce dramatic improvement. An initial dose of 1 to 2 mg/kg PO or IM (maximum dose 8 mg) is given followed by a maintenance dose of 1 to 1.5 mg/kg/day (not to exceed 16 mg/day) divided q 4 to 6 h for 5 days. The dose is then tapered for 5 days before it is discontinued.
- Hyperbaric therapy with the Gamow bag has been reported to be useful in mild HACE and may be life-saving if descent is impossible.
- For severe cases, intubation and controlled ventilation are indicated to decrease intracranial pressure. Furosemide and mannitol are second-line treatments.

HIGH-ALTITUDE PULMONARY EDEMA

- HAPE is a life-threatening manifestation of high altitude illness and represents a unique form of noncardiogenic pulmonary edema. It is estimated that HAPE affects 0.5 to 15 percent of those who ascend rapidly to high altitudes. Other than trauma, it is the most common cause of death at altitude.
- Children and young adults are more susceptible to HAPE. Individuals younger than 20 years may be 10 to 13 times more prone to develop HAPE.

CLINICAL PRESENTATION

- The onset of HAPE usually occurs within 1 to 4 days after ascent to altitude, most commonly during the second night at altitude. However, initial symptoms may develop within hours following ascent.
- Early in the course, the victim will develop a dry cough, fatigue, and dyspnea on exertion.
- As HAPE progresses, the patient will have a productive clear cough, orthopnea, weakness, and altered mental status. This intensifies to severe dyspnea at rest, a cardinal sign of HAPE. The patient may be tachycardic, tachypneic, and febrile to 102°F. Rales become bilateral.
- A chest radiograph reveals bilateral fluffy asymmetric infiltrates and dilated pulmonary arteries. Without treatment, florid pulmonary edema and respiratory failure will develop.

TREATMENT

- Immediate descent may be life-saving and is not to be delayed. There is a delicate balance, however, between rapid descent and the amount of energy the victim expends to descend quickly. Individuals may deteriorate from overexertion as they proceed to a lower altitude.
- Supplemental oxygen effectively lowers pulmonary arterial pressure, which raises arterial oxygen saturation.
- High-flow oxygen at 6 to 8 L/min by mask is administered to anyone with significant symptoms.
- An end-expiratory airway pressure (EPAP) mask that can deliver 5- to 10-cm H_2O of end-expiratory pressure can be used to improve oxygen delivery. When oxygen is not available and descent is not possible, the portable Gamow bag may be used for hyperbaric treatment and has been shown to be effective in patients with HAPE.
- Pharmacologic agents play a limited role in the treatment of HAPE. Acetazolamide may be useful in the prevention of HAPE. Although furosemide has been shown to be helpful, caution must be used due to the prevalence of hypovolemia and dehydration. Nifedipine has been shown to decrease pulmonary arterial pressure. Again, caution must be exercised in the use in a potentially hypovolemic dehydrated patient.

ALTITUDE-RELATED SYNDROMES

HIGH-ALTITUDE RETINAL HEMORRHAGE

- It is estimated that 50 percent of individuals who ascend to 16,000 ft and 100 percent of those who ascend to 21,000 ft will develop high-altitude retinal hemorrhage (HARH) within 2 to 3 days after arrival to altitude.
- HARH presents with tortuous dilation of the retinal arteries and veins, retinal hemorrhages, and papilledema. The hemorrhages are most often throughout the fundus but spare the macula. It is painless and

usually asymptomatic, with no visual disturbances noted.

CHRONIC MOUNTAIN SICKNESS
- Chronic mountain sickness (CMS), also referred to as Monge's disease, is a rare complication of high-altitude illness. Some individuals will fail to acclimatize despite prolonged exposure or living at high altitude. Symptoms are similar to those of AMS and include headache, dyspnea, sleep disturbance, and fatigue.
- Treatment for CMS includes descent to a lower altitude, oxygen, phlebotomy, and the use of respiratory stimulants such as acetazolamide.

ULTRAVIOLET KERATITIS
- Snow blindness is caused by increased ultraviolet (UV) light exposure at higher altitudes secondary to the loss of the protective atmosphere and fewer pollutants.
- Patients develop a foreign body sensation or severe pain approximately 12 h after exposure.
- Treatment is with oral analgesics to alleviate the severe discomfort. Symptoms resolve within 24 h.
- Sunglasses with Polaroid lenses and side blinders are preventative.

HIGH-ALTITUDE PHARYNGITIS AND BRONCHITIS
- High-altitude bronchitis and pharyngitis are common at altitudes above 8000 ft, secondary to the excessive inhalation of dry, cold air that causes drying and cracking of the upper airway mucous membranes. Symptoms include a dry, hacking, and painful cough.
- Symptoms are prevented or minimized by ensuring adequate hydration and salivation. Throat lozenges and hard candy help to maintain oral secretions. Inhaled steam, gargling, and oral fluids will also keep the mucous membranes moist. A cloth worn over the mouth and nose helps to warm the inspired air and trap moisture.

DYSBARIC INJURIES

- Dysbaric injuries may be the result of several distinct events that expose an individual to a change in barometric pressure.
- The first possible etiology is an altitude-related event, which can be illustrated by the rapid ascent or descent during airplane transport or sudden cabin decompression at an altitude higher than 25,000 ft.
- The second type of dysbaric injury results from an underwater diving accident.
- A third dysbarism is caused by a blast injury that produces an overpressure effect.

BAROTRAUMA: DYSBARISMS FROM TRAPPED GASES

- While an individual is descending while scuba diving, a negative pressure develops within enclosed air spaces relative to the ambient surrounding pressure. If air is unable to enter these structures, equalization does not take place, and the air-filled cavities collapse. If the cavity is a rigid structure and unable to collapse, the negative pressure may result in fluid being displaced from the blood vessels of the surrounding mucosa into the cavity.

BAROTITIS
- **Barotitis media (middle ear squeeze)** is the most common diving-related barotrauma.
  ○ Equalization via the eustachian tube will occur when there is a pressure differential of approximately 15 to 20 mm Hg. The diver becomes symptomatic if equalization is unsuccessful and the pressure differential reaches or approaches 100 mm Hg.
  ○ The symptoms include a fullness in the ears, severe pain, tinnitus, vertigo, nausea, disorientation, and transient, conductive hearing loss.
  ○ The physical examination may reveal erythema or retraction of the tympanic membrane (TM), blood behind the TM, a ruptured TM, or a bloody nasal discharge.
  ○ Treatment should be directed toward its prevention, before pain develops.
  ○ Scuba divers should attempt to clear their ears every 2 to 3 ft during descent.
  ○ To decrease the incidence of ear discomfort and injury to the TM, a predive treatment of a topical vasoconstrictor nasal spray (oxymetazoline hydrochloride, 0.05 percent) may be beneficial when used about 15 min before beginning a dive. The recommended pediatric dosage for ages 6 years and up is 2 to 3 sprays in each nostril.
  ○ Pseudoephedrine may also be considered as a predive treatment. For ages 6 to 12 years, the recommended dose is 30 mg PO.
- **Alternobaric vertigo** may develop during descent, but it is more common during ascent. A sudden change in middle ear pressure or asymmetrical middle ear pressure may result in decreased perfusion, affecting vestibular function. Symptoms include transient vertigo, tinnitus, nausea, vomiting, and fullness in the affected ear. Decongestants, antiemetics, and medication for vertigo are recommended.
- **Barotitis externa** occurs when the external auditory canal, which is normally a patent air-filled cavity that communicates with the surrounding environment, is occluded during descent.

- **Barotitis interna**, or **inner ear squeeze**, is uncommon but may result in permanent injury to the structures of the inner ear. It often follows a vigorous Valsalva maneuver.
  - In addition to sudden sensorineural hearing loss, symptoms include severe pain or pressure, vertigo, tinnitus, ataxia, nausea, vomiting, diaphoresis, and nystagmus.

ALTITUDE-RELATED BAROTITIS

- **Barotitis media** is the most common barotrauma of air travel. During ascent to altitude, gas will normally escape through the eustachian tube every 500 to 1000 ft to equalize pressures. As altitude decreases, the gas within the middle ear will contract. As with diving, equalization may be accomplished by yawning, swallowing, or performing the Valsalva maneuver.

BAROSINUSITIS

- Normally, air can pass in and out of the sinus cavities without difficulty. However, if a person has a cold or sinus infection, air may be trapped and will be subject to the barometric pressure changes. Failure of the air-filled frontal or maxillary sinuses to equilibrate results in pain or pressure above, behind, or below the eyes, which is commonly referred to as **sinus squeeze**.
- The most effective treatment involves the use of a vasoconstrictor nasal spray before initiating a dive or before starting a descent from altitude in an airplane.
- **Reverse sinus squeeze** is felt during a diving ascent when an obstruction of the sinuses results in excessive pressure. A sharp pain will be felt in the affected sinus.

BARODONTALGIA

- **Barodontalgia**, or **tooth squeeze**, is often associated with recent dental extraction, dental fillings, periodontal infection, periodontal abscess, or tooth decay.
- Treatment is directed toward preventative dental care and pain control.

FACE MASK SQUEEZE

- During descent, the increased ambient pressure will tend to exert increasing pressure against the air-filled face mask of a scuba diver. The diver may develop facial or eye pain, subconjunctival hemorrhages, subconjunctival edema, epistaxis, and periorbital edema.

AEROGASTRALGIA

- Ingesting carbonated beverage, chewing gum (and swallowing air), eating large meals, and preexisting gastrointestinal problems increase the amount of gas in the intestines. Gas expansion will cause discomfort, abdominal pain, belching, flatulence, nausea, vomiting, shortness of breath, or hyperventilation.

PULMONARY OVER-PRESSURIZATION SYNDROME

- Pulmonary over-pressurization syndrome (POPS) is an example of the positive-pressure barotrauma that can be seen during ascent. The alveoli become over inflated and can rupture, causing a pneumothorax.

AIR EMBOLISM

- An air embolism is the most serious dysbaric injury. Due to the buoyancy of air and the fact that scuba divers are usually upright during ascent, the brain is most commonly affected. The onset of symptoms is immediately on ascent, or within 10 to 20 min of surfacing.
- Arterial air embolization to the brain is more common than to the heart or spinal cord. Neurologic symptoms are similar to those of a stroke and include numbness, dizziness, headaches, weakness, visual field deficits, confusion, behavioral changes, amnesia, paralysis, vertigo, blindness, aphasia, deafness, sensory deficit, seizures, focal deficits, and loss of consciousness.

PNEUMOTHORAX AND EMPHYSEMA

- A pneumothorax developing during a dive is a major problem since, on ascent; a simple pneumothorax may progress to a tension pneumothorax, shock, and loss of consciousness.
- These complications may also occur during air transport in an unpressurized aircraft.
- Treatment of a scuba diving pneumothorax is no different than the treatment of other traumatic or nontraumatic pneumothoraxes.

DECOMPRESSION SICKNESS: DYSBARISMS FROM EVOLVED GASES

- As ambient pressure increases, the positive-pressure gradient between the alveoli and the blood will result in more nitrogen being dissolved. As a dive progresses, the gas in the blood will equilibrate quickly with the gas in the alveoli. Nitrogen gas, however, is almost five times more soluble in fat. It will take longer to saturate these tissues. Therefore, the body will absorb more nitrogen gas at a rate that is dependent on the depth and duration of the dive. The longer and deeper the dive, the more nitrogen gas will be accumulated within the body. Since nitrogen is not metabolized, it remains dissolved until the nitrogen gas pressure in the lung decreases and the nitrogen can be removed. During a slow ascent, as the surrounding pressure decreases, the nitrogen that is absorbed into the tissues is released into the blood and the alveoli. If the ascent is too quick, nitrogen levels do not have the opportunity to equalize among the tissues, blood, and alveoli. The pressure outside the body will drop significantly below the sum of the partial pressures of the gases inside the body. This results in the gas coming out of solution and the formation of gas bubbles in the blood or tissue.

- Decompression sickness can be classified as follows:
  ○ Type I, which typically involves extravascular gas bubbles and causes joint pain, skin rashes, and lymphedema.
  ○ Type II, which is caused by intravascular nitrogen gas emboli. The presentation may be very similar to that of air emboli. Children are more prone to type II injuries.
- Symptoms usually develop within 6 to 12 h after the conclusion of a dive. A sharp, throbbing, or dull achy pain is a common presentation. There may also be associated numbness or tingling (paresthesia). The pain commonly is diffuse in its origin but will become more localized as the intensity increases. The joints most often affected are the knees, shoulder, and elbows.
- Symptomatic relief may be obtained by splinting the extremity or by applying pressure over the affected joint.
- The decompression illness that affects the pulmonary system is referred to as the **chokes**. It is caused by arterial or venous nitrogen gas embolization that obstructs the pulmonary vasculature. The symptoms may begin immediately after a dive but often take up to 12 h to develop. They last between 12 and 48 h but can progress to a rapid deterioration. The classic triad of symptoms includes shortness of breath, cough, and substernal chest pain or chest tightness.

Neurologic Decompression Sickness

- Nitrogen gas embolism is the most serious decompression sickness. As with air embolus, the brain is most commonly affected.
- The onset of symptoms, however, will usually be delayed, with symptoms developing within 1 to 6 h after a dive is concluded.
- These victims require aggressive care, which includes 100 percent oxygen, intravenous fluids, and hyperbaric treatment. They are placed in the Trendelenburg or left lateral decubitus position to minimize the embolization to the brain.

Decompression Shock

- Decompression shock may be secondary to hypovolemia or due to vasovagal responses.
- Aggressive and timely management with intravenous fluids, 100 percent oxygen, and recompression therapy should be initiated as quickly as possible.

Cutaneous Decompression Sickness

- Rashes, with or without pruritus, can present with any of the following patterns: scarlatiniform, mottling (cutis marmorata), and erysipeloid.
- The release of nitrogen gas bubbles can cause subcutaneous emphysema, often involving the neck and other sites.
- Treatment of individuals with subcutaneous emphysema begins with 100 percent oxygen. The patient is then carefully examined for more serious dysbarisms and admitted.

Treatment of Decompression Sickness and Air Embolus

- The treatment of choice for most air emboli and decompression illnesses is hyperbaric (recompression) therapy. This is initiated as soon as possible, ideally within 6 h of the onset of symptoms.
- Before hyperbaric treatment is initiated, certain procedures should be followed. Endotracheal tube cuffs and Foley catheter balloons should be filled with saline rather than air. It is essential to identify any pneumothorax and insert a chest tube prior to recompression.
- Special precautions should also be taken for victims who must be transported by helicopter or airplane. In some cases, even the slightest elevation that results in exposure to a decreased ambient pressure, may compromise the victim by causing further gas expansion.
- Victims of type I decompression sickness are advised to abstain from any further scuba diving for at least 4 to 6 weeks, and type II victims must wait at least 4 to 6 months.

DYSBARISMS CAUSED BY ABNORMAL GAS CONCENTRATION

Nitrogen Narcosis

- The inhalation of nitrogen gas at elevated partial pressures may cause an interference with nerve conduction. As a result, nitrogen narcosis can produce a narcotic or intoxicating effect during a dive.
- The greatest risk of nitrogen narcosis is drowning. With any evidence or suspicion of confusion, disorientation, or altered mental status, the dive should be terminated.
- *For assistance with scuba diving-related injuries, contact:* **Divers Alert Network (DAN)**
  ○ 24-Hour Diving Emergencies: 919-684-8111 or 1-919-684-4DAN (collect)
  ○ Information Line: 1-800-446.2671 or 1-919-684-2948, Mon through Fri, 9 AM to 5 PM (EST)
  ○ Http://*www.diversalertnetwork.org/*

BIBLIOGRAPHY

HIGH-ALTITUDE ILLNESS

Carpenter TC, Niermeyer S, Durmowicz AG: Altitude-related illness in children. *Curr Probl Pediatr* 28:177–198, 1998.

DeHart RL (ed): *Fundamentals of Aerospace Medicine*, 2d ed. Baltimore, MD: Williams & Wilkins; 1996.

Hackett PH, Roach RC: High-altitude illness. *N Engl J Med* 345:107–114, 2001.

DYSBARIC INJURIES

Bove A, Davis J (eds): *Diving Medicine*, 3d ed. Philadelphia: Saunders, 1997.

Hardy KR: Diving-related emergencies. *Emerg Med Clin North Am* 15:223, 1997.

Kizer K: Scuba diving and dysbarisms. In: Auerbach P, ed. *Wilderness Medicine, Management of Wilderness and Environmental Emergencies.* St. Louis: Mosby, 2001.

QUESTIONS

1. Which of the following is **NOT** a factor in the development of high-altitude illness?
   A. Rate of ascent
   B. Time of ascent
   C. Altitude achieved
   D. Length of stay
   E. Pharmacologic agents

2. Which of the following is a critical element in an individual's ability to acclimatize?
   A. Hypoxic hypoventilation
   B. Selective vasoconstriction
   C. Erythropoietin output
   D. Increased cerebral blood flow
   E. Compensatory metabolic acidosis

3. Signs and symptoms of acute mountain sickness (AMS) are typically seen in what time period following a rapid ascent?
   A. 1 to 3 h
   B. 4 to 8 h
   C. 9 to 12 h
   D. 24 h
   E. 36 h

4. A 15-year-old child is brought by paramedics for evaluation of a headache. You learn that the patient is visiting his grandmother in the mountains. The headache has persisted throughout the night and the patient reports difficulty sleeping. Which of the following additional signs or symptoms would be consistent with a diagnosis of AMS?

A. Increased urine output
B. Peripheral edema
C. Leg cramps
D. Pulmonary edema
E. Visual disturbances

5. Which of the following should **NOT** be used in treatment of acute mountain sickness (AMS)?
   A. Prochlorperazine
   B. Dexamethasone
   C. Acetaminophen
   D. Morphine
   E. Acetazolamide

6. You are staffing a medical station when an adolescent is brought for evaluation of severe headaches, nausea, and vomiting. You learn that the patient was treated 12 h ago for AMS. On examination, the patient appears confused and exhibits truncal ataxia. Which of the following is **NOT** part of the first line treatment for high-altitude cerebral edema (HACE)?
   A. Rapid descent
   B. High-flow oxygen
   C. Dexamethasone
   D. Furosemide
   E. Hyperbaric therapy with Gamow bag

7. Which of the following signs and symptoms would be concerning and consistent with disease progression in a patient suspected of having high-altitude pulmonary edema (HAPE)?
   A. Dyspnea on exertion
   B. Dyspnea at rest
   C. Clear, productive cough
   D. Fatigue
   E. Dry cough

8. Which of the following measures would **NOT** be recommended as prevention for barotitis?
   A. Topical vasoconstrictor nasal spray
   B. Pseudoephedrine
   C. Clearing ears every 2 to 3 ft during diving descent
   D. Frequent swallowing during airplane descent
   E. Acetayolamide

9. A member of a diving class is brought to the emergency department following the conclusion of a dive. The patient complains of diffuse sharp, throbbing pain involving his knees, shoulder, and elbows. He also reports mild parasthesias. You suspect decompression sickness. Which of the following would **NOT** be recommended to provide symptomatic relief for this patient?
   A. Splinting the extremity
   B. Applying pressure over the joint
   C. Oxygen
   D. Intravenous fluids
   E. Placement in Trendelenburg

ANSWERS

1. B. High-altitude illness most often affects young and otherwise healthy individuals. The major factors that influence the incidence, onset, and severity of high-altitude illness are the rate of ascent, altitude achieved, and length of stay. A slow, graded ascent is the key to acclimatization. Pharmacologic agents are beneficial adjuncts to acclimatization.

2. C. The hematopoietic response to high altitude is a critical element in an individual's ability to acclimatize. Within hours of ascent, erythropoietin output is increased in response to hypoxia. The hypoxic ventilatory response (HVR) attempts to compensate for the decrease in arterial P_{O_2}. An inadequate HVR has been suggested as the etiology for AMS.

3. B. The onset of AMS symptoms is usually within 4 to 8 h of a rapid ascent. In some cases, symptoms can be delayed for up to 4 days. Symptoms develop following strenuous activity or sleeping at high altitude.

4. B. The clinical presentation of AMS includes the following symptoms: headache, sleep disturbance, fatigue, shortness of breath, dizziness, anorexia, nausea, and vomiting. Signs on physical examination include fine rales and peripheral edema consistent with fluid retention in AMS.

5. D. Treatment of acute mountain sickness is descent. If descent is not an option, there are various pharmacologic agents that can be beneficial including dexamethasone, acetazolamide, prochloroperazine, and acetaminophen. Narcotics, such as morphine, should be avoided because of depression of the hypoxic ventilatory response (HVR).

6. D. HACE is the most severe, life-threatening form of high-altitude illness. HACE commonly begins with symptoms of AMS and progresses to diffuse neurologic dysfunction. Definitive treatment for HACE is immediate descent. Other first-line therapies include high-flow oxygen, dexamethasone, and hyperbaric therapy with the Gamow bag. Furosemide and mannitol are considered second-line treatments.

7. B. HAPE is a life-threatening manifestation of high-altitude illness and represents a unique form of non-cardiogenic pulmonary edema. Early symptoms include dry cough, fatigue, and dyspnea on exertion. As HAPE progresses, the patient will have a productive, clear cough. This intensifies to severe dyspnea at rest, a cardinal sign of HAPE.

8. D. Barotitis is the most common diving-related barotraumas. Preventive measures include topical vasoconstrictor nasal spray, pseudoephedrine, and clearing ears every 2 to 3 ft during descent. Valsalva maneuvers are also effective but can cause permanent injury to the structures of the inner ear. Acetazomide has no effect.

9. E. Symptoms of decompression sickness usually develop within 6 to 12 h after the conclusion of a dive. A sharp, throbbing pain is a common presentation. Symptomatic relief can be obtained by splinting the extremity or by applying pressure over the affected joint. Patients who exhibit signs and symptoms consistent with neurologic decompression sickness require aggressive care and placement in Trendelenburg or left lateral decubitus position to minimize the embolization to the brain.

117 RADIATION EMERGENCIES

Gary R. Strange
Ira J. Blumen
Valerie A. Dobiesz

TYPES OF RADIATION

IONIZING RADIATION

- Ionizing radiation interacts with matter, converting atoms to ions as a result of gain or loss of electrons. Ionizing radiation is more dangerous than non-ionizing radiation because such reactions lead to breaks in both DNA and RNA, damaging important biologic functions at the cellular level.
- Types of ionizing radiation include particulate radiation such as α-particles, β-particles, and neutrons and non-particulate forms of radiation such as X-rays and gamma-rays.

NON-IONIZING RADIATION

- Non-ionizing radiation is relatively low energy in nature and does not result in acute radiation injuries or contamination. Adverse effects are limited to local heat production.

RADIATION EXPOSURE

- The clinical effects of radiation exposure are related to the:
  - Type of radiation
  - Amount of radiation
  - Nature of the exposure (continuous or intermittent)

- Total time of the exposure
- Distance from the radiation source
- Presence of any shielding (amount and type).

RADIATION INJURIES

- There are two categories of radiation injuries with which the emergency physician should be familiar. The first type is an *exposure* injury, which generally represents no threat to emergency care providers. *Contamination*, the second type of radiation injury, may represent a potential risk to emergency personnel.

EXPOSURE

LOCALIZED RADIATION INJURIES
- Localized radiation injuries most commonly affect the upper extremities, with the buttocks and thighs representing the next most common sites. Typically, these injuries occur in the occupational setting but adults or children may unknowingly come into contact with a radiation source by handling an unknown object and putting it into their pockets.
- Initial localized radiation injury looks like thermal injury to the skin. However, appearance is delayed. Radiation injury should be considered in the differential diagnosis for any patient who presents with a painless "burn" but who does not remember a thermal or chemical insult.

WHOLE-BODY EXPOSURE
- *Acute radiation syndrome* may develop following a whole-body exposure of 100 rad or more that occurs over a relatively short period of time. Organ systems with rapidly dividing cells (bone marrow, gastrointestinal tract) are the most vulnerable to radiation injury.
- A progressive sequence of signs and symptoms following a whole-body exposure can be divided into four stages.
  - Prodromal
  - Latent
  - Manifest illness
  - Recovery
- The prodromal stage can begin within minutes to hours after exposure and is dose-dependent. The most common symptoms of this stage include nausea, vomiting, and fatigue.
- In a lower-dose exposure, the prodromal symptoms will resolve over a period of days to weeks, followed by a latent stage. Progressively higher radiation doses will prolong the prodromal stage while limiting the

latent period until a point is reached when it appears that the prodromal stage proceeds directly to the manifest illness stage without any resolution of the prodromal symptoms.
- During the manifest illness stage, specific organ symptoms develop and the patient is at the greatest risk for infection and bleeding. Three syndromes may develop during this stage, depending on the total amount of radiation exposure:
  - The hematopoietic syndrome (220 to 600 rad)
  - The gastrointestinal syndrome (600 to 1000 rad)
  - The neurovascular syndrome (over 1000 rad).
- Although the effect of radiation on the hematopoietic system is characterized by pancytopenia, the absolute lymphocyte count is the best hematologic way to estimate exposure (Fig. 117-1). Leukocyte counts may be elevated initially due to demargination, but the lymphocyte portion of the differential will quickly start to decrease.
- With intermediate levels of exposure, gastrointestinal illness will be evident with abrupt onset of severe vomiting and diarrhea. The latent stage may be quite short and is followed by continued GI symptoms, leading to relentless fluid loss, fever, and prostration.
- Total-body irradiation with more than 1000 rad affects even cells that are relatively resistant to injury and results in a neurovascular syndrome. Ataxia and confusion quickly develop and there is direct vascular damage, with resultant circulatory collapse. The patient usually expires within hours.

CONTAMINATION

- If the patient's condition permits, decontamination should begin in the pre-hospital setting. This will reduce the potential spread of radioactive material and will decrease the potential contamination of hospital workers or other rescuers. If appropriate management steps are taken, the radiation-contaminated patient should present little danger to hospital staff, even if decontamination was incomplete.

MANAGEMENT

GENERAL CONCEPTS

- While both prehospital and hospital workers may be at risk, it is the prehospital personnel and other rescuers who respond to the site of a radiation accident who are more often exposed to significant radiation. A threshold of 5000 mrem (5 rem) should be the exposure limit, except to save a life. A once-in-a-lifetime exposure to

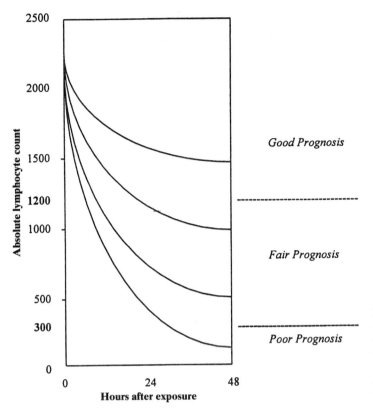

FIG. 117-1 A 48-h check of the absolute lymphocyte count suggesting the severity of the exposure to radiation. Good prognosis: a lymphocyte count greater than 1200/mm³. 100- to 200-rad exposure. Fair prognosis: an absolute lymphocyte count of 300 to 1200/mm³. 200- to 400-rad exposure. Poor prognosis: lymphocyte count below 300/mm³. More than 400-rad exposure.

100,000 mrem (100 rem) to save a life has been established by the National Council on Radiation Protection as acceptable and will not result in any undue morbidity.

RADIATION ACCIDENT PLAN

- The Joint Commission on Accreditation of Healthcare Organizations (JCAHO) requires each emergency department to have a radiation accident plan. In the event of a medically significant radiation accident, a well-prepared and practiced plan will supply emergency care providers with an appropriate knowledge base, management protocols, and additional resources that can be called upon.
- The U.S. Department of Energy also is available to coordinate a federal response and provide assistance through the Radiological Assistance Program (RAP). RAP is managed at eight regional coordinating offices across the country.
- The Radiation Emergency Assistance Center/Training Site (REAC/TS) in Oak Ridge, Tennessee, is also available to provide treatment and medical consultation for injuries resulting from radiation exposure and contamination. REAC/TS can be contacted by calling (865) 576-1005.

GENERAL PROCEDURES

- When exposed solely to irradiation from gamma-rays, X-rays, β-particles, and neutrons, patients do not usually become radioactive. However, the radiation accident plan must assume that there will be external contamination.

EXTERNAL CONTAMINATION

- Victims of radiation exposure who show no signs of injury and are otherwise healthy may be best served at designated decontaminated facilities. In general, hospital resources should be used for radiation victims who also require medical management.
- The process of decontamination, or cleaning the patient of particulate radioactive debris, should be initiated as soon as possible following the event. Rescue personnel must wear protective clothing, including rubber gloves, shoe covers, masks, and film badges. This protective clothing does not reduce the exposure to penetrating radiation. Rather, it serves to prevent any radioactive particles from coming in contact with the personnel or their clothing and to facilitate cleanup and disposal.

- Initially, any open wounds are covered and the patient's clothing is removed; all articles are placed in clearly labeled plastic bags. Up to 70 to 90 percent of external contamination can be eliminated by this action alone.
- The use of damp washcloths, rather than rinsing with running water, may be more practical for some emergency departments. The disposal of contaminated washcloths in plastic bags may be easier than the collection of contaminated wash water.
- Open, uncontaminated wounds are covered with sterile dressings and contaminated wounds are then cleaned aggressively. Whenever possible, a dosimeter should be used to determine the completeness of the decontamination.

INTERNAL CONTAMINATION

- Radioactive particles that are ingested or inhaled or that contaminate open wounds can cause significant cellular damage. These particles will continue to irradiate tissues until they are eliminated, neutralized, or blocked, or until they decay naturally. In general, there is a 1 to 2-hour window of time during which absorption of these particles occurs.
- Ideally, chelating agents are administered within 1 hour of exposure. Chelating agents provide an ion-exchange matrix that binds metals. This prevents tissue uptake and promotes urinary excretion of a stable complex containing the radioactivity. Diethylenetriaminepentaacetic acid (DTPA) is an effective chelating agent for many heavy metals.
- A blocking agent reduces radioactive uptake by saturating the tissues with a non-radioactive element. Lugol's solution (potassium iodide) is a blocking agent that reduces the uptake of radioactive iodine (^{131}I) by the thyroid gland by as much as 90 percent if administered within 1 hour of exposure. If treatment is delayed until 6 hours after exposure, the uptake is reduced by approximately 50 percent. An exposure of 10 to 30 rem warrants the initiation of this treatment.

BIBLIOGRAPHY

Aghababian RV: *Emergency Medical Response Plan for Radiation Accidents.* February 22, 1999. <http://www.bumc.bu.edu/Departments/PageMain.asp?Page=1880&Department-ID=286>

American Academy of Pediatrics: Risk of ionizing radiation exposure to children: A subject review. *Pediatrics* 101:717, 1998.

Durante M, Manti L: Estimates of radiological risk from a terrorist attack using plutonium. *Radiat Environ Biophys* 41: 125–130, 2002.

Fong G, Schrader DC: Radiation disasters and emergency department preparedness. *Emerg Med Clin North Am* 14:349–370, 1996.

Guidance for Radiation Accident Management. Radiation Emergency Assistance Center/Training Site (REAC/TS), Oak Ridge Institute for Science and Education, Oak Ridge, TN <http://www.orau.gov/reacts/manage.htm>.

Illinois Department of Nuclear Safety: *Evaluating and Treating Patients Accidentally Exposed to Radiation or Contaminated with Radioactive Materials.* Illinois Dept. of Nuclear Safety, Illinois, October, 1995.

Mettler FA, Williamson SL: Pediatric radiation injuries. In: Behrman RE, Kliegman RM, Jenson HB, eds. *Nelson Textbook of Pediatrics*, 16th ed. Philadelphia: Saunders, 2148–2152, 2000.

QUESTIONS

1. Which of the following does not relate to the clinical effects seen in radiation exposure?
   A. Type of radiation
   B. Total time of exposure
   C. Distance from the radiation source
   D. State of hydration at time of exposure
   E. Presence of shielding
2. A 10-year-old girl has an accidental whole-body exposure to ionizing radiation during a school field trip. The exposure is deemed significant at over 200 rads. What initial prodromal symptoms do you anticipate in this patient?
   A. No symptoms
   B. Nausea, vomiting, and fatigue
   C. Pancytopenia especially lymphocyte counts
   D. Severe vomiting, diarrhea, and fever
   E. Ataxia and confusion
3. What is the best hematologic marker to estimate the amount of radiation exposure?
   A. The absolute lymphocyte count
   B. The absolute neutrophil count
   C. Eosinophilia
   D. Hematocrit levels
   E. Peripheral smears
4. Which of the following is true regarding radiation injuries?
   A. Hospitals do not need to develop management protocols and can contact appropriate agencies in times of need
   B. Decontamination is not needed in these injuries
   C. Specific antidotes are available for treatment of acute radiation syndromes from whole-body irradiation

D. Time from exposure to symptom onset is inversely related to dose in external irradiation

E. A protracted exposure causes more harm than a quickly delivered dose in external irradiation

5. Which of the following is a true statement regarding radiation injuries?

A. Non-ionizing radiation causes acute radiation injuries and contamination

B. Localized radiation injuries most commonly affect the buttocks and thighs

C. Types of ionizing radiation include alpha particles, beta particles, X rays, and gamma rays

D. The cardiovascular and CNS are most vulnerable to radiation injury

E. Rescue personnel need not wear any protective clothing

ANSWERS

1. D. The clinical effects of radiation exposure are related to the type of radiation, amount of radiation, nature of the exposure (continuous or intermittent), total time of exposure, distance from radiation source, and presence of any shielding (amount and type).

2. B. A progressive sequence of signs and symptoms develop after whole-body exposure and are divided into four stages; prodromal, latent, manifest illness, and recovery. The prodromal stage can begin within minutes to hours after exposure and is dose dependent. The most common symptoms in the prodromal stage are nausea, vomiting, and fatigue. It is during the manifest illness stage that the patient develops pancytopenia, GI symptoms of severe vomiting, diarrhea, dehydration, electrolyte abnormalities, and fever, and at higher levels cardiovascular and CNS symptoms such as ataxia, confusion, hypotension, and death.

3. A. The effect of radiation on the hematopoietic system is characterized by pancytopenia and can occur at levels of 220 to 600 rads. The best hematologic way to estimate exposure is the absolute lymphocyte count. A lymphocyte count greater than 1200/mL indicates a good prognosis 24 h after exposure. A lymphocyte count below 500/mL predicts severe illness. If lymphocytes are depleted within 6 h, death is likely.

4. D. The Joint Commission on Accreditation of Healthcare Organizations (JCAHO) requires each ED to have a radiation accident plan. Decontamination should be done in these injuries and should begin in the pre-hospital setting to reduce potential spread of radioactive material and potential contamination of hospital and rescue workers. Treatment for acute radiation syndrome from whole-body irradiation is primarily supportive. The time from exposure to symptom onset is inversely related to the dose in external irradiation and a quickly delivered dose causes more harm than a protracted exposure.

5. C. Non-ionizing radiation is relatively low energy and does not result in acute radiation injuries or contamination. Localized radiation injuries most commonly affect the upper extremities and typically occur in the occupational setting. Types of ionizing radiation include particulate radiation such as alpha particles, beta particles, and neutrons, and non-particulate forms of radiation such as X-rays and gamma-rays. Organ systems with rapidly dividing cells (bone marrow, gastrointestinal tract) are the most vulnerable to radiation injury. Rescue personnel must wear protective clothing, including rubber gloves, shoe covers, masks, and film badges.

118 CHILD MALTREATMENT

Veena Ramaiah
Jill Glick
Gary R. Strange
Patricia Lee

PHYSICAL ABUSE

- The history is vital in distinguishing inflicted from noninflicted injury. The key component to making a diagnosis of physical abuse is the compatibility of the history and mechanism given by the caretaker to explain the injuries sustained.

CUTANEOUS LESIONS

- Bruises, marks, bites, and burns are the most common and most recognizable signs of maltreatment. When documenting these lesions, it is important to note the location, size, shape, and number. If possible, an estimation of age is also helpful. Multiple cutaneous lesions in various stages of healing are highly suspicious for abuse.
- Bruises are common in active, healthy children. Noninflicted bruises tend to be on prominent bony areas, such as elbows/forearms, knees/shins, and forehead. Bruises in relatively protected areas of the body, such as eyes, cheeks, neck, trunk, genitals, and buttocks, are suspicious for abuse. The developmental age of the patient is important. Bruising in a non-ambulatory child is suspicious for abuse.
- Determining the age of a bruise is both difficult and inaccurate. Studies have shown that color change and healing time vary with age of the patient, location on the body, and depth of injury.
- An immersion burn caused by holding a child in hot water leaves a characteristic stocking or glove pattern on the extremities with well-demarcated edges, uniform burn depth, and few satellite splash lesions. The buttocks may be burned, with central sparing where the buttocks are in contact with the tub.

FRACTURES

- The mechanism of injury must be consistent with the type of fracture. Red flags include inappropriate delay in seeking medical care, multiple fractures in various stages of healing, and metaphyseal or rib fractures. Any child under the age of 2 years with a fracture suspicious for abuse should have a complete skeletal survey to detect occult or healing fractures.
- Overall, long bone fractures in children are less specific and less suspicious for child abuse. However, spiral fractures of the femur and humerus in nonambulatory children **ARE** very suspicious for abuse.

HEAD INJURY

- Head injuries are the leading cause of death and morbidity from child maltreatment.
- Shaken baby/shaken impact syndrome occurs in children under 2 years old. Violent shaking causes a shearing acceleration and deceleration injury within the brain. The relatively large head and weak neck muscles in children contribute to the problem. The shearing results in subdural/subarachnoid hemorrhage, often with diffuse axonal injury and cerebral edema.

- The classic triad in shaken baby/shaken impact syndrome is:
  ○ Subdural hematoma
  ○ Retinal hemorrhages
  ○ Skeletal injury

VISCERAL INJURY

- Visceral injuries account for only 2 percent of inflicted injuries. However, they are the second leading cause of death from physical abuse.

SEXUAL ABUSE

- The most important factor in diagnosing sexual abuse is an awareness that sexual abuse occurs. It is estimated that 3 per 1000 children are sexually abused per year, although the true incidence is unknown.
- The history is the key to establishing the diagnosis of sexual abuse. Sexually abused children can present to the emergency department with various complaints, including a disclosure of sexual abuse, abdominal or urogenital symptoms, genital injuries, sexual behavior inappropriate for the child's age, or medical reasons unrelated to abuse.
- Whenever possible, the child is interviewed separately from the caregiver and other family members. The questioner's responses must be supportive and empathetic, without expressions of shock or unrealistic promises. Interview the family separately from the child to ascertain their knowledge of the abuse, as well as to assess the child's safety.
- The physical examination leaves the genital and perianal examination for last. Document any signs of trauma. External inspection of the vaginal and peri-anal areas is usually sufficient. The prepubertal child is examined in the supine frog leg, supine knee-chest, and prone knee-chest positions, whereas pubertal and postpubertal females are examined in lithotomy position.
- There are two main visualization techniques for females, the separation and the traction views. The separation view involves separating the labia majora outward in both directions. The traction view involves grasping the labia majora and pulling outward and downward. This dilates the introitus and provides a clear view of the hymen, the posterior fourchette, and anterior vagina.
- The most common finding in sexual abuse is a normal physical examination. In well over half of all sexual abuse cases, there are no signs of trauma.
- Forensic evidence is collected if the sexual abuse or assault occurred within 72 h of the child's presentation to the emergency department. Collection of the underwear and linens for evidence improves recovery of forensic evidence.

NEGLECT

- Neglect is the most common type of maltreatment reported. From the point of view of the emergency department, neglected children can be categorized as medical, supervisional, educational, physical, and nutritional.

CHILD PROTECTION SERVICES AND THE LEGAL SYSTEM

- In all 50 states, child protection laws require all professionals who interact with children to notify the state child protection services if there is a suspicion of child maltreatment. Suspicion is defined as having reasonable cause to believe a child may be harmed.
- The physician has an obligation to inform the parents or caretakers of concerns about the child's well being and to explain to them the mandated requirement to notify state child protection services. As an advocate for the child, the physician must refrain from angry or accusatory statements when talking with the family.

BIBLIOGRAPHY

Brodeur AE (ed): *Child Maltreatment: A Clinical Guide and Reference.* St. Louis: Medical Publishing, Inc., 1994.

Christian CW, Lavelle JM, De Jong AR, et al: Forensic evidence findings in prepubertal victims of sexual assault. *Pediatrics* 106:100–104, 2000.

Reece RM (ed): *Child Abuse, Medical Diagnosis and Management.* Philadelphia: Lea & Febiger, 1994.

Wang C, Harding K: *Current Trends in Child Abuse Reporting and Fatalities: The Results of the 1998 Annual Fifty State Survey.* Chicago: National Center on Child Abuse Prevention Research, 1999.

QUESTIONS

1. A 2-year-old child is brought in by the parents for burns to buttock area. Parents state that the child climbed into a bathtub of hot water and sustained the burns. On examination, you notice a well-demarcated, second degree burn to buttocks of uniform burn depth and few splash lesions. In addition, buttocks

demonstrate a central area of spared burn. Appropriate treatment for these lesions is:

A. Apply silvadene cream to burns and bandage and discharge home with follow-up in 24 h

B. Contact child protective services for suspicion of child abuse, file a report, and discharge home with follow-up in 1 to 2 days

C. Assume protective custody, treat the burns, contact child protective services, and detain the child until safety is assured

D. Debride wounds and discharge home on appropriate antibiotics

E. Confront the parents about your suspicion of child abuse and if adequate explanation is provided, discharge home with follow-up arranged by child protective services

2. A 3-month-old infant is brought by the parents for repeated emesis. On examination, the child is lethargic. A septic workup is initiated and the chest radiograph reveals a right rib fracture. When questioned, the parents state that the child might have sustained this injury when he rolled off the bed last night. The most appropriate course of management should be:

A. Begin IV hydration, obtain a CBC and blood culture; begin ceftriaxone and admit for antibiotics therapy

B. Perform skeletal survey and CT brain

C. Contact child protective services and arrange for home visit in 24 h

D. Obtain pulse oximetry and administer medication for pain; discharge home if no evidence of hypoxia

E. If septic workup, including lumbar puncture, is negative, and child is improved after IV hydration, discharge home with follow-up to pediatrician in 24 h

3. A 3-year-old child is brought by the parents with a right lower extremity deformity. Radiographs reveal a nondisplaced spiral fracture to the tibia. According to the parents, the child was jumping on the bed immediately prior to arrival and fell off onto the floor, sustaining the above injury. Physical examination also reveals multiple, small bruises in various stages of resolution located on bilateral anterior tibias and a small, ecchymotic area to the right forehead. When questioned, the parents state that the child is very active and has occasional falls, which resulted in the bruising. Appropriate management of this injury should be:

A. Consult orthopedics for immediate management

B. Contact child protective services and arrange for protective custody

C. Confront the parents that spiral fractures are pathognomonic for child abuse

D. Perform skeletal survey

E. Discharge home with follow-up by child protective services

4. A 3-year-old female is brought by her mother with complaints of burning with urination and concerns about sexual abuse. Physical examination is normal. Urinalysis is also normal. Your response should be:

A. Tell the mother that a negative physical examination to include an intact hymen rules out sexual abuse

B. Attempt to question the child and parents together about the possibility of sexual abuse

C. Explain that the most common finding of sexual abuse is a negative physical examination

D. Contact child protective services and assume protective custody

E. Explain that no further investigation is warranted

ANSWERS

1. C. An immersion burn is caused by holding a child in hot water. This burn leaves a characteristic stocking or glove pattern on the extremities with well-demarcated edges, uniform burn depth, and few satellite splash lesions. The buttocks may be burned, with central sparing where the buttocks are in contact with the tub. In all 50 states, child protection laws require all professionals who interact with children to notify the state child protection services if there is a suspicion of child maltreatment. Suspicion is defined as having reasonable cause to believe a child may be harmed.

2. B. Rib fractures in a 3-month-old child are consistent with child abuse. Familiarity of developmental milestones is essential in assessing the historical facts. Three-month-old infants do not roll off beds!! In addition, lethargy and vomiting are suggestive of an intracerebral injury. Head injuries are the leading cause of death and morbidity from child maltreatment. Shaken baby syndrome is characterized by finding a subdural hematoma, retinal hemorrhages, and skeletal injury. Any child under the age of 2 years with a fracture suspicious for abuse should have a complete skeletal survey to detect occult or healing fractures.

3. A. Long bone fractures in children are less specific and less suspicious for child abuse. Spiral fractures of the femur and humerus in nonambulatory children are very suspicious for abuse. Bruises are common in healthy, active children. Noninflicted bruises tend to be on prominent bony areas, such as elbows/ forearms, knees/shins, and forehead. Bruises in relatively protected areas of the body, such as eyes, cheeks, neck, trunk, genitals, and buttocks, are suspicious for abuse.

4. C. The most common finding in sexual abuse is a normal physical examination. In well over half of all sexual abuse cases, there are no signs of trauma. The history is the key to the diagnosis of sexual abuse. Sexually abused children can present to the emergency department with various complaints, including a disclosure of sexual abuse, abdominal or urogenital symptoms, genital injuries, sexual behavior inappropriate for the child's age, or medical reasons unrelated to abuse. Whenever, possible, the child should be interviewed by a trained professional separately from the caregiver and other family members.

119 PSYCHIATRIC EMERGENCIES

Heather M. Prendergast
Tanya R. Anderson
Gary R. Strange

PRINCIPLES OF MANAGEMENT

- Psychiatric assessment of the pediatric patient centers on evaluating safety concerns and the need for hospitalization. Decision-making will usually be based on information obtained from multiple collateral sources.
- The first priority is determining whether in the current state the child poses a threat to self or others.
- Issues regarding the medical stability of the patient must be addressed immediately.
- Management of the aggressive or violent child may require the use of physical or chemical restraints, but these measures should be viewed as a last resort. Children often respond to simple situational interventions, such as placement in a quiet room with minimal external stimulation; speaking with the child in a calm, reassuring tone; acknowledgment of the child's distress; and offering the child an opportunity to participate in the immediate decision making.
- If the child does not respond favorably and continues to pose a threat, the use of physical restraints may be required. For legal as well as ethical reasons, it is important that the physician and emergency department staff be familiar with the proper technique for applying physical restraints (Table 119-1).
- In the emergency setting, there are two vital components of the pediatric psychiatric interview: the history and the mental status evaluation.

TABLE 119-1 ABCDs of Physically Restraining a Child

A	Assistance in applying restraints. At least 4 members of the ED or security staff are needed
B	Be careful to avoid contact with bodily fluids
C	Communicate with the patient and family Constantly monitor the patient
D	Document reason for restraints, time placed, reassessments of the patient, and the time removed

- Information obtained during the history should include:
  - Details of the current crisis situation
  - Apparent triggers
  - Timeline
  - Previous episodes
  - Psychiatric history
  - Symptoms of depression
  - Presence of suicidal or homicidal ideation
  - Home environment
- Specific components of the mental status examination include:
  - Orientation
  - Appearance
  - Memory
  - Cognition
  - Relatedness
  - Speech
  - Affect
  - Thought content
  - Thought process
- Table 119-2 lists some important areas to address in evaluating the suicidal risk of a patient.
- The physician must perform a directed but thorough physical examination prior to medically clearing the child. A careful search for signs or symptoms of poisoning, self-inflicting wounds, and abuse should be undertaken.
- A child psychiatric consultation should be obtained whenever there is uncertainty about the assessment, safety, or diagnosis, or if there are treatment dilemmas. Treatment plans are best formulated in conjunction with a child psychiatry consultant and the family.
- It is important to be familiar with the indications for hospitalization (Table 119-3), as well as the resources available in the area.

THE SUICIDAL PATIENT

- The incidence of suicide among patients under 18 years of age is increasing in epidemic proportions. A number of risk factors have been identified:
  - Presence of a psychiatric disorder
  - Substance abuse

TABLE 119-2   Assessing Suicidal Risks in Children

Suicidal Fantasies or Actions
Have you ever thought of hurting yourself?
Have you ever threatened or attempted to hurt yourself?
Have you ever wished to or threatened to commit suicide?
Consequences/Concepts of What Would Happen
What did you think would happen if you tried to hurt or kill yourself?
What did you want to have happen?
Did you think you would die?
Did you think you would have severe injuries?
Circumstances at the Time of the Child's Suicidal Behavior
What was happening at the time you thought about killing yourself or tried to kill yourself?
Was anyone else with you or near you when you thought about suicide or tried to kill yourself?
Previous Experiences With Suicidal Behavior
Have you ever thought about killing yourself or tried to kill yourself before?
Do you know of anyone who thought about, attempted, or committed suicide?
How did this person carry out his or her suicidal ideas or action? When did this occur?
Motivations for Suicidal Behaviors
Open-ended questions:
Why do you want to kill yourself?
Why did you try to kill yourself?
Closed-ended questions (if patient does not provide enough information):
Did you want to frighten someone?
Did you want to get even with someone?
Did you hear voices telling you to kill yourself?
Did you wish someone would rescue you before you tried to hurt yourself?
Experiences and Concepts of Death
What happens when people die?
Can they come back again?
Do they go to a better place?
What will happen when you die?
Depression
Do you cry a lot?
Do you ever feel sad, upset, angry, or bad?
Do you ever feel that you are not worthwhile?
Do you have difficulty sleeping, eating, and concentrating on schoolwork?
Do you blame yourself for things that happen?
Family and Environmental Situations
Do you have difficulty in school?
Do you worry that your parents will punish you for doing poorly in school?
Do your parents fight a lot?
Is anyone in your family sad, depressed, and very upset? Who?
Does anyone in your family talk about suicide or try to kill themselves?

SOURCE: Reproduced with permission from Pfeffer CR: *The Suicidal Child.* New York: Guilford, 1986.

TABLE 119-3   Indications for Hospitalization or Removal From Current Environment

- Danger to self
- Danger to others
- Family unable to care for the child
- Physical or sexual abuse
- Failure of outpatient treatment
- Need for stabilization on or adjustment of medication

- Male gender
- High parental stress
- Presence of a firearm in the home
- Dysfunctional family relationships

ASSESSMENT

- The focus should be on the lethality of the act, the true suicidal intent of the child, and the family support system. Depending on the developmental stage, children have different perceptions of the concept of death (Table 119-4) and often miscalculate the lethality of acts.
- Because of the high correlation between depression and suicide, the interview should be structured to uncover signs or symptoms of depression, such as:
  - Insomnia (or hypersomnia)
  - Crying spells
  - Poor appetite (or increased appetite)
  - Fatigue
  - Poor concentration
  - Decreased attention to personal hygiene
  - Flat effect
  - Poor eye contact

MANAGEMENT

- Any history of ingestion must be taken seriously and thoroughly investigated with appropriate toxicology screening.
- If the patient requires medical admission, it is important that an observer be placed with the patient for the duration of the medical portion of the hospital stay. Once the patient is medically cleared, a determination of the need for inpatient psychiatric hospitalization is made. Indications for inpatient psychiatric management include the following:
  - Inability to maintain a no-suicide contract
  - Active suicidal ideation (plan and intent)
  - High intent or lethality of attempt
  - Psychosis

TABLE 119-4   Developmental Concepts of Death

CONCEPT OF DEATH	PERCEPTION
Up to age 5	Death viewed as a reversible process
Ages 5 to 9	Death tends to be internalized; begins to understand the concept of irreversibility
Age 9 and older	Death viewed as irreversible, final

○ Previous history of suicide attempts
○ Family incapable or unwilling to monitor and protect patient

THE PSYCHOTIC PATIENT

ASSESSMENT

- Psychosis in the pediatric patient may be either organically or psychiatrically based.
- It is important to identify patients belonging to the organic group, since the treatment options are different. In the younger child, the etiology is often organically based. Organic precipitants include:
  ○ Central nervous system lesions
  ○ Infections
  ○ Trauma
  ○ Hypoxia
  ○ Toxins
  ○ Vitamin deficiencies
  ○ Metabolic disorders
  ○ Endocrine disorders
  ○ Rheumatic diseases
  ○ Reye's syndrome
  ○ Wilson's disease
- Functional causes of childhood psychosis include:
  ○ Pervasive developmental disorders, such as autism
  ○ Schizophrenia
  ○ Posttraumatic stress disorder
  ○ Mood disorders
- Acute disorientation, fluctuations in consciousness, disruption in intellectual functioning, and impairment in recent memory suggest an organic etiology. A more insidious onset is consistent with a functional etiology.

MANAGEMENT

- It is important to alleviate a child's fear and anxiety. This requires use of supportive statements, specific instructions, and repetition. Many patients will require physical or chemical restraints.
- First-line pharmacologic agents for agitation include:
  ○ Diphenhydramine: 25 mg orally or intramuscularly
  ○ Droperidol: 0.625 to 2.5 mg intramuscularly
  ○ Haloperidol:
    - Ages 6 to 12 years, 1 to 3 mg/dose intramuscularly
    - Over age 12, 2 to 5 mg/dose intramuscularly
    - Doses can be repeated every 30 min up to a maximum dose of 40 mg
- Side effects of neuroleptics include extrapyramidal symptoms, which respond to anticholinergics:
  ○ Benzotropine: 1 to 2 mg orally or intramuscularly
  ○ Diphenhydramine: 25 mg orally or intramuscularly
- Benzodiazepines should be avoided since they may have a paradoxical effect, and can exacerbate underlying organic causes.

SCHIZOPHRENIA

- Childhood schizophrenia is a rare disorder in which children exhibit abnormalities in reality testing, perception, behavior, and social relatedness. The incidence of schizophrenia increases steadily after the onset of puberty.
- Many of the symptoms exhibited are the direct result of the impaired thought content:
  ○ Delusions
  ○ Loose associations
  ○ Catatonic states
  ○ Inappropriate affect
  ○ Auditory hallucinations (usually persecutory or commanding)
- Psychotic patients may become dangerous when command hallucinations tell them to hurt self or others, when they exhibit poor impulse control, poor contact with reality, or poor decision making.
- It is not infrequent for a child to present to the ED with a first psychotic episode. Admission must be considered when the conditions listed in Table 119-3 are met. Cooperative patients with good family support who do not meet those criteria can be referred for outpatient treatment.

MANIA

- Manic episodes can be seen in late adolescence and are characterized by an expansive or irritable mood and a pattern of excessive indulgence. Patients exhibit inflated self-esteem, grandiosity, and erratic and disinhibited behaviors. They are prone to excessive spending, promiscuity, and reckless behavior. There is a decreased need for sleep, increased negative energy, exaggerated euphoria, racing thoughts, and pressured speech. Patients can experience delusions and sometimes become aggressive and combative.
- There is often a family history of bipolar disorder.
- When evaluating a manic patient, it is important to keep a broad differential because many organic and psychiatric disorders can have similar presentations. Collateral history is very important in making an accurate assessment.
- The mainstay of treatment for bipolar disorder is a mood stabilizer. Lithium and valproic acid are the most commonly prescribed. They may not be particularly

useful in the emergency setting because of the time necessary to reach therapeutic levels. For this reason, patients may require hospitalization, often involuntarily. For the acutely agitated patient, low-dose neuroleptics may be required.

POSTTRAUMATIC STRESS DISORDER (PTSD)

- At-risk children include those who have:
  - Endured physical, sexual, or emotional abuse
  - Been threatened with serious injury
  - Witnessed violent acts
- The exposure is internalized and manifested in several ways. Children continually relive the trauma through recurrent nightmares, flashbacks, and repetitive play involving aspects of the trauma. They exhibit intense distress during events that resemble the ordeal. Another possible response is to exhibit generalized numbness to certain stimuli and people.
- PTSD is more likely to be the cause when the stress has been severe, there has been parental distress, and when there is temporal proximity to the traumatic event.
- Problems arise when children are not provided with a supportive and protective environment following traumatic events.

THE SUBSTANCE ABUSER

- To intervene effectively with the substance abuse patient, the emergency physician has to be familiar with the risk factors, stages of abuse, and treatment options (Table 119-5).

ASSESSMENT

- Children are not likely to be forthcoming with information about substance abuse. The emergency department presentation is usually the result of either concerned caregivers or problems caused by the substance abuse. It is important to be direct in questioning and to speak in a calm, nonjudgmental tone.

MANAGEMENT

- Patients found to be acutely intoxicated but receptive to treatment should be referred or admitted for detoxification. It is mandatory that patients and their families be provided with information about referrals to outpatient treatment centers. Arranging an intake

TABLE 119-5 Stages of Substance Abuse

STAGE	DESCRIPTION
1	Potential for abuse Decreased impulse control Need for immediate gratification Availability of tobacco, drugs, alcohol, inhalants Need for peer acceptance
2	Experimentation: learning the euphoria Use of inhalants, tobacco, marijuana, and alcohol with friends Few consequences May increase to regular use Little change in behavior
3	Regular use: seeking the euphoria Use of other drugs, such as stimulants, LSD, sedatives Behavioral changes and some consequences Increased frequency of use Use alone Buying or stealing drugs
4	Regular use: preoccupation with the "high" Daily use of drugs Loss of control Multiple consequences and risk-taking Estrangement from family and "straight" friends
5	Burnout: use of drugs begins to feel normal Use of multiple substances; cross-addiction Guilt, withdrawal, shame, remorse, depression Physical and mental deterioration Increased risk-taking, self-destructive behavior, suicidal behavior

SOURCE: Reproduced with permission from the American Academy of Pediatrics Committee on Substance Abuse: Indications for management and referral of patients involved in substance abuse. *Pediatrics* 106:143–148, 2000.

prior to discharge from the emergency department increases the compliance rate.

PSYCHOTROPIC MEDICATIONS

- Psychotropic medications should generally not be initiated in an emergency department. Referral to an outpatient child mental health clinic is usually necessary to obtain thorough evaluation, diagnosis, treatment planning, and appropriate follow-up care.

BIBLIOGRAPHY

American Academy of Pediatrics Committee on Substance Abuse: Indications for management and referral of patients involved in substance abuse. *Pediatrics* 106:143–148, 2000.

Halamandaris PV, Anderson TR: Children and adolescents in the psychiatric emergency setting. *Psychiatr Clin North Am* 22:865–874, 1999.

Labellarte M, Ginsburg G, Walkup J: The treatment of anxiety disorder in children and adolescents. *Biol Psychiatry* 46:1567–1578, 1999.

Olshaker JS, Browne B, Jerrard DA, et al: Medical clearance and screening of psychiatric patients in the emergency department. *Acad Emerg Med* 4:124–128, 1997.

Peterson B, Zhang H, Lucia S, et al: Risk factors for presenting problems in child psychiatric emergencies. *J Am Acad Child Adolesc Psychiatry* 35:1162–1173, 1996.

Sater N, Constantino J: Psychiatric emergencies in children with psychiatric conditions. *Pediatr Emerg Care* 14:42–50, 1998.

Schulz SC, Findling RL, Wise A, et al: Child and adolescent schizophrenia. *Psychiatr Clin North Am* 21:43–56, 1998.

Sills MR, Bland SD: Summary statistics for pediatric psychiatric visits to US emergency departments, 1993–1999. *Pediatrics* 110: e40, 2002.

Ulloa R, Birmaher B, David A, et al: Psychosis in a pediatric mood and anxiety disorders clinic: Phenomenology and correlates. *J Am Acad Child Adolesc Psychiatry* 39:337–345, 2000.

QUESTIONS

1. A 6-year-old child is brought to the emergency department for evaluation of aggressive behavior. The child is well known to your institution and is followed by Child Psychiatry. Upon entering the examination room, you observe the child kicking and arguing with his sibling. You are worried about the child's safety. The most appropriate intervention at this time would be:
   A. Place the child in soft restraints
   B. Place the child in leather restraints
   C. Administer Haldol at 1 mg/dose intramuscularly
   D. Have the sibling leave the room with one of the parents
   E. Immediately contact the child's psychiatrist

2. A 16-year-old adolescent is brought to the emergency department for evaluation of ingestion of extra strength Tylenol tablets (#5) following a breakup with his girlfriend. You note that the patient seems a bit withdrawn. The patient denies being suicidal and dismisses his actions by stating, "It was a simple oversight." Which of the following would **NOT** place this patient at a higher risk for suicide?
   A. Daily use of marijuana
   B. Presence of a firearm in home
   C. Susceptible to peer pressure
   D. Frequent family conflicts
   E. History of bipolar disorder

3. As the treating physician, you are aware of the high correlation between depression and suicide. Which of the following would heighten your index of suspicion for depression in an adolescent patient?
   A. Repeatedly falling asleep during evaluation
   B. Crying while discussing the recent death of a family member
   C. Preoccupation with hairstyle and clothing
   D. Focused on completion of crossword puzzles instead of the interview
   E. Inappropriate laughing

4. A teenager is brought to the emergency department for evaluation of a suicidal gesture that included a handwritten, hand-delivered note stating his intentions at 1 PM that afternoon. Upon further evaluation, you determine that there was no true suicidal intent of the child. You discuss the options with the family and the psychiatrist on call. Which of the following would be an indication for inpatient hospitalization?
   A. No previous history of suicidal gestures
   B. Expression of remorse by patient
   C. Family unwilling to monitor and protect patient
   D. History of depression
   E. Patient reluctantly agrees to maintain a no-suicide contract

5. An 8-year-old boy is brought to the emergency department for acute agitation. Parents note that over the last week, the patient has gradually deteriorated. Which of the following would be more consistent with a functional etiology?
   A. Family history of schizophrenia
   B. Traumatic death of sibling 6 months ago
   C. History of cerebral palsy following hypoxia at birth
   D. Low-grade temperature
   E. History of juvenile rheumatoid arthritis currently in remission

ANSWERS

1. D. Management of the aggressive or violent child with physical or chemical restraints should be viewed as a last resort. The most appropriate actions would be to attempt to minimize external stimulation by removing the sibling from the room.

2. C. Most adolescents are very susceptible to peer pressure, but there is no association with an increased risk for suicidal behavior. All the other factors listed have been identified as risk factors for suicidal behavior.

3. A. Insomnia or hypersomnia is often a symptom of depression. Other signs and symptoms include: poor concentration, decreased attention to personal hygiene, and inappropriate crying spells.

4. C. If the patient's family demonstrates an inability or unwillingness to monitor and protect the patient; this is an indication for admission. Other indications for inpatient hospitalizations would include a patient that is actively suicidal with a plan, psychosis, previous history of suicidal attempts, and inability to maintain a no-suicide contract.

5. B. This patient may be suffering from posttraumatic stress disorder. Other functional causes of childhood psychosis include pervasive developmental disorders, schizophrenia, and mood disorders. Functional etiologies tend to have a more insidious onset.

120 PEDIATRIC PREHOSPITAL CARE

Ronald A. Dieckmann
Robert W. Schafermeyer
Gary R. Strange
Valerie A. Dobiesz

INTRODUCTION

- Emergency medical services for children (EMSC) is now an important ingredient of American EMS systems. EMSC refers to an entire EMS-EMSC continuum of pediatric emergency care, critical care, and trauma services (Fig. 120-1). EMSC is fully within the general EMS system and only works well when the general EMS system is effective.
- *Clinical features* include prevention of illness and injury, pediatric equipment, pediatric treatment protocols, transportation, emergency departments, specialized pediatric centers, and pediatric rehabilitation.
- *Operational features* include EMS system adaptations for children, communications, medical direction and education, data and information management, public information and education, and research.

FEDERAL EMSC PROGRAM

- EMSC had its birth in 1984, with the passage of the Emergency Medical Services for Children (EMSC) Act. This act established funding for state and local pediatric components for EMS systems through the Maternal and Child Health Division within the Health Resources and Services Administration. It also established the Federal EMSC Program, which is now an active partner with the EMS Division of the National Highway Traffic Safety Administration (NHTSA) in improving emergency medical services for children.
- The diverse products of EMSC-funded projects, all readily available on-line or through the federal EMSC program, include the following:
  - A national clearinghouse, the EMSC National Resource Center, in Washington, DC. Its website (*www.ems-c.org*) provides detailed information on EMSC products, including the EMSC Five Year Plan.
  - An EMSC data center, the National EMSC Data Analysis Resource Center (NEDARC), in Salt Lake City. The mission of NEDARC is to help EMS

Five components
Prevention
Medical home/primary physician
Prehospital system
ED and hospital
Rehabilitation

Clinical features
Prevention programs
Pediatric equipment
Pediatric treatment protocols and practice guidelines
Transportation
Emergency departments
Specialized pediatric centers
Pediatric rehabilitation

Operational features
EMS system adaptations for children
Communications
Medical direction
Human resources education
Data and information management
Public information and education
Research

FIG. 120-1 EMS-EMSC continuum.

agencies develop their own capabilities to formulate and answer research questions and to effectively convert available data into informative reports with appropriate statistical analyses (website: *www. nedarc.med.utah.edu*).

○ A comprehensive booklet entitled "EMSC Model," published by the California EMS Authority, with nine different sets of EMSC guidelines and five sets of EMSC recommendations for integration of EMSC into state and local EMS systems.

○ Model EMSC legislation. Many states have enacted EMSC bills to mandate and help fund EMSC within state EMS agencies. The American Academy of Pediatrics (AAP) has a template for EMSC legislation that can be easily modified for individual states (website: *www.aap.org*).

○ A national standard curriculum (NSC) for emergency medical technician (EMT) basics, and most recently for EMT paramedics and EMT intermediates, sponsored by NHTSA and the Maternal and Child Health Bureau (MCHB). These curricula outline comprehensive educational objectives for prehospital professionals (website: *www.nhtsa.dot. gov/people/injury/ems*).

EMSC IN STATE EMS SYSTEMS

• One mechanism for highlighting EMSC within state EMS systems is through the ongoing NHTSA program for EMS system assessments. This standardized evaluation process provides an excellent opportunity for states to review their current EMSC capabilities and to plan and implement improvements.

EPIDEMIOLOGY

• Injuries account for half of pediatric ambulance transports and illnesses account for the other half (Table 120-1).

• The leading causes of childhood death are both age- and geography-related. In some states, fires and burns are the leading causes of death in children under 5 years of age. In other states, motor vehicle incidents are the leading cause. In some sun-belt states, drowning is first. In rural areas, motor vehicle incidents are the leading cause of death, but homicide and suicide are more common for urban males.

• Children with special health care needs are a diverse group of patients who frequently need out-of-hospital emergency assessment and treatment. The American College of Emergency Physicians (ACEP) and the AAP have recently published an Emergency Information Form for CSHCN (Fig. 120-2).

TABLE 120-1   Epidemiology of Pediatric Illnesses and Injuries for Ambulance Transports

INJURIES	ILLNESSES
Mechanism	*CNS*
Automobile incidents	Seizures
Occupant	Altered level of consciousness
Pedestrian	*Respiratory*
Bicyclist	Wheezing
Falls	Choking
Burns	Apnea
Frequency of anatomic areas	*Metabolic/toxic*
of injury	Ingestions
Head	Fever
Limbs/pelvis	*Gastrointestinal*
Back	Abdominal pain
Chest	Vomiting
Abdomen	

CLINICAL COMPONENTS OF EMS-EMSC

PREVENTION

• Prehospital professionals, emergency nurses, and physicians have participated as educators and advocates in many injury and illness prevention programs and community strategies for patients and families (Table 120-2).

PEDIATRIC EQUIPMENT

• Prehospital professionals require special pediatric equipment and supplies for BLS and ALS ambulances (Tables 120-3 and 120-4). Equipment and supplies must be logically organized, routinely checked, and readily available.

PREHOSPITAL TREATMENT AND TRANSPORTATION

• Treatment policies or protocols are fundamental to pediatric prehospital care. Recently, the National Association of EMS Physicians developed pediatric field treatment protocols for prehospital professionals. They are available on-line (*www.naemsp.org*).

EMERGENCY DEPARTMENTS

• ALL hospital EDs in every community must have the appropriate equipment, staff, and policies to provide appropriate care for children (Tables 120-5a, b). This is especially true since automobile transport to the

Emergency Information Form for Children With Special Needs

American College of
Emergency Physicians®

American Academy
of Pediatrics

Date form completed	Revised	Initials
By Whom	Revised	Initials

Last name:

Name:	Birth date: Nickname:
Home Address:	Home/Work Phone:
Parent/Guardian:	Emergency Contact Names & Relationship:
Signature/Consent*:	
Primary Language:	Phone Number(s):

Physicians:

Primary Care Physician:	Emergency Phone:
	Fax:
Current Specialty Physician: Specialty:	Emergency Phone:
	Fax:
Current Specialty Physician: Specialty:	Emergency Phone:
	Fax:
Anticipated Primary ED:	Pharmacy:
Anticipated Tertiary Care Center:	

Diagnoses/Past Procedures/Physical Exam:

1.

2.

3.

4.

Synopsis:

Baseline physical findings:

Baseline vital signs:

Baseline neurological status:

*Consent for release of this form to health care providers

FIG. 120-2 The emergency information form for children with special needs.

Last name:

Diagnoses/Past Procedures/Physical Exam continued:

Medications:

Significant baseline ancillary findings (lab, x-ray, ECG):

1.

2.

3.

4.

Prostheses/Appliances/Advanced Technology Devices:

5.

6.

Management Data:

Allergies: Medications/Foods to be avoided   **and why:**

1.

2.

3.

Procedures to be avoided   **and why:**

1.

2.

3.

Immunizations

Dates						Dates					
DPT						Hep B					
OPV						Varicella					
MMR						TB status					
HIB						Other					

Antibiotic prophylaxis: Indication: Medication and dose:

Common Presenting Problems/Findings With Specific Suggested Managements

Problem	Suggested Diagnostic Studies	Treatment Considerations

Comments on child, family, or other specific medical issues:

Physician/Provider Signature: **Print Name:**

FIG. 120-2 (*Continued*)

TABLE 120-2   Examples of Common Injuries and Possible Prevention Strategies

Vehicle Trauma	Infant and child restraint seats Seat belts and air bags Pedestrian safety programs Motorcycle helmets
Cycling	Bicycle helmets Bicycle paths separate from motor vehicle traffic
Recreation	Appropriate safety padding and apparel Cyclist/skateboard/skater safety programs Soft, energy-absorbent playground surfaces
Drowning	Four-sided locked pool enclosures Pool alarms Immediate adult supervision Caretaker CPR training Swimming lessons Pool/beach safety instruction Personal flotation device
Poisoning and Household	Proper storage of chemicals and medications Child safety packaging
Burns	Proper maintenance and monitoring of electrical appliances and cords Fire/smoke detectors Proper placement of cookware on stovetop
Other	Discouragement of infant walker use Gated stairways Babysitter first aid training Child care worker first aid training

TABLE 120-3   Pediatric Basic Life Support Ambulance Equipment, Medications, and Supplies

1. Oropharyngeal airways: infant, child
2. Bag-valve resuscitator, child reservoir[a]
3. Clear masks for resuscitator: infant, child, adult
4. Nasal cannulas: child and adult sizes
5. Oxygen masks: child, adult
6. Blood pressure cuffs: infant, child, adult
7. Backboard
8. Cervical immobilization device[b]
9. Extremity splints
10. Burn dressings[c]
11. Sterile scissors or equivalent umbilical cord cutting device[d]
12. Thermal blanket
13. Portable suction unit[e]
14. Suction catheters: infant, child, adult
15. Tonsil suction tip
16. Bulb syringe
17. Obstetric pack
18. Car seat

[a]Ventilation bags used for resuscitation should be self-refilling without a pop-off valve. The child and adult bags are suitable for supporting adequate tidal volumes for the entire pediatric age range. A child bag is defined as one that has at least a 45-mL reservoir. An adult bag has at least a 1-L reservoir.
[b]A cervical immobilization device should be a soft device that can immobilize the neck of an infant, child, or adult. It may be towel rolls or a commercially available neck-cradling device. Cervical immobilization of a small infant can be achieved by use of towel rolls and tape rather than a cervical collar or sandbags. (Infants may need support under the shoulders to keep a neutral spine position.)
[c]Burn dressings may include commercially available packs and/or clean sheets and dressings.
[d]Sterile scissors or equivalent devices are for cutting the umbilical cord during childbirth and may be stocked separate from the obstetrical pack carried by the EMS provider to assure sterility.
[e]This may include a motorized suction device or a hand-driven device.

nearest hospital, regardless of designation, is common, particularly when the problem is acute illness as opposed to injury.

SPECIALIZED PEDIATRIC CENTERS

- Specialized centers are frequently children's hospitals, but general hospitals may also provide such services. Some local EMS systems have a two-tiered plan for children, involving identification of hospitals with minimal capabilities and hospitals with specialized pediatric capabilities.

REHABILITATION

- Rehabilitation services are crucial for selected patients who sustain critical illnesses and injuries. Systematic identification of suitable rehabilitation services and facilities and implementation of referral procedures are key elements in the EMS-EMSC continuum.

OPERATIONAL COMPONENTS OF EMS-EMSC

EMS SYSTEM

- Permanent state EMSC leadership within the state EMS system is essential for the development and maintenance of strong EMSC. A state EMSC office may be created through legislation or implemented by state EMS regulation.

MEDICAL DIRECTION

- Effective medical direction includes review and modification of treatment and nontreatment policies, procedures, and protocols for children.
- Medical direction entails both real time on-line (direct) elements, as well as off-line (indirect) elements.
  - On-line issues may include questions about treatment, field triage (Table 120-6), scene control, transport, destination, transport refusals, and consent.
  - Off-line medical direction includes prospective and retrospective components.

TABLE 120-4 Pediatric Advanced Life Support Ambulance Equipment, Medications, and Supplies

ALS units should have all the equipment listed on the BLS list plus the following additional items:

1. Monitor defibrillator[b]
2.[a] Laryngoscope with straight blades 0 through 4 and curved blades 2, 3, and 4
3.[a] Pediatric and adult size stylets for endotracheal tubes
4.[a] A pediatric Magill forceps
5.[a] Endotracheal tubes: uncuffed sizes 2.5 through 6.0 and cuffed 6.0 through 8.0
6. Arm boards: infant, child
7. Intravenous catheters 14–24 gauge
8. Microdrip and macrodrip IV devices[c]
9.[a] Intraosseous needles
10. Drug dose chart or tape[d]

[a]These items are required only if the skill to use them is part of the scope of practice of the local EMS providers.
[b]All defibrillators should be able to deliver 5 to 400 J. The addition of pediatric paddles may give the responding unit enhanced capabilities, but they may not be essential for units that rarely use this equipment. The defibrillator may be equipped with only adult paddles/pads or pediatric and adult paddles/pads. Units carrying only adult paddles/pads should ensure that providers are trained in the proper use of adult paddles in infants and children. When the defibrillator cannot deliver lower power, shock at lowest possible energy level.
[c]These may include burettes, microdrip tubing, or in-line volume controllers.
[d]This may include charts giving the drug doses in milliliters or milligrams per kilogram, with precalculated doses based on weight, or a tape that determines the proper dose based on the length of the patient.

- Prospective medical direction includes development of treatment protocols, transport policies, procedural policies (eg, intraosseous infusions, endotracheal intubation), destination policies, personnel education, data collection, and quality improvement programs.
- Retrospective components include reviews of run sheets, focused audits, and analyses of nontransport cases, deaths, and any unusual occurrences or untoward events, as well as medicolegal problems.

COMMUNICATIONS

- Training of dispatchers is currently highly variable. In advanced EMS systems, dispatchers may have an extensive role in providing prearrival instructions to scene bystanders and appropriate prioritization of vehicle dispatch.

EDUCATION

- Education of prehospital professionals is essential for optimal pediatric prehospital care. Both BLS and ALS services require unique pediatric adaptations to teach knowledge and skills.

TABLE 120-5a Pediatric Medications for Emergency Departments

RESUSCITATION MEDICATIONS	OTHER DRUG GROUPS
Atropine	Activated charcoal
Adenosine	Analgesics
Calcium chloride	Antibiotics (parenteral)
Dextrose	Anticonvulsants
Epinephrine (1:1000, 1:10,000)	Antidotes (common antidotes should be available), prostaglandin E_1[a]
Lidocaine	
Naloxone hydrochloride	Antipyretics
Sodium bicarbonate (4.2%)	Bronchodilators
	Corticosteroids
	Inotropic agents
	Neuromuscular blocking agents
	Oxygen
	Sedatives

[a]For less frequently used antidotes and medications, a procedure for obtaining them should be in place.
SOURCE: Adapted from Committee on Pediatric Equipment and Supplies for Emergency Departments, National Emergency Medical Services for Children Resource Alliance: Guidelines for pediatric equipment and supplies for emergency departments. *Ann Emerg Med.* 31:54–57, 1998.

- Continuing education is also essential because skills decay is rapid. The Pediatric Education for Prehospital Professionals (PEPP) course was recently developed through a national consensus process orchestrated by the AAP. The course is a 2-day interactive, assessment-oriented, case-based continuing education program in pediatrics with both BLS and ALS versions that are fully consistent with the NSC curricula. The PEPP course has a website (*www.PEPPsite.com*), which allows ongoing on-line education and communication between the AAP, the national steering committee, and EMS professionals.

DATA AND INFORMATION MANAGEMENT

- Information management involves monitoring, evaluating, and modifying the education, patient care, and regional care protocols based on patient outcome. Information management mechanisms must identify not only performance problems, but also system deficiencies that affect children and families.

PUBLIC INFORMATION AND EDUCATION

- The need for public education on the proper use of EMS persists in spite of much play in the media. Many injured or seriously ill children still end up being transported to EDs by private vehicles instead of activating the EMS system and taking advantage of the full range of EMSC services.

TABLE 120-5b   Pediatric Equipment and Supplies for Emergency Departments

Monitoring Equipment
- Cardiorespiratory monitor with strip recorder
- Defibrillator with pediatric and adult paddles (4.5 cm and 8 cm) or corresponding adhesive pads
- Pediatric and adult monitor electrodes
- Pulse oximeter with sensors and probe sizes for children
- Thermometer or rectal probe[a]
- Sphygmomanometer
- Doppler blood pressure device
- Blood pressure cuffs (neonatal, infant, child, and adult arm and thigh cuffs)
- Method to monitor endotracheal tube and placement[b]
- Stethoscope

Airway Management
- Portable oxygen regulators and canisters
- Clear oxygen masks (standard and nonrebreathing: neonatal, infant, child, and adult)
- Oropharyngeal airways (sizes 0–5)
- Nasopharyngeal airways (12F through 30F)
- Bag-valve-mask resuscitator, self-inflating (450 and 1000 mL sizes)
- Nasal cannulas (child and adult)
- Endotracheal tubes: uncuffed (2.5, 3.0, 3.5, 4.0, 4.5, 5.0, 5.5, and 6.0 mm) and cuffed (6.5, 7.0, 7.5, 8.0, and 9.0 mm)
- Stylets (infant, pediatric, and adult)
- Laryngoscope handle (pediatric and adult)
- Laryngoscope blades: straight or Miller (0, 1, 2, and 3) and Macintosh (2 and 3)
- Magill forceps (pediatric and adult)
- Nasogastric/feeding tubes (5F through 18F)
- Suction catheters: flexible (6F, 8F, 10F, 12F, 14F, and 16F)
- Yankauer suction tip
- Bulb syringe
- Chest tubes (8F through 40F)[c]
- Laryngeal mask airway (sizes 1, 1.5, 2, 2.5, 3, 4, and 5)

Vascular Access
- Butterfly needles (19–25 gauge)
- Catheter-over-needle devices (14–24 gauge)
- Rate limiting infusion device and tubing
- Intraosseous needles (may be satisfied by standard bone marrow aspiration needles)
- Arm board
- Intravenous fluid and blood warmers[c]
- Umbilical vein catheters[c,e] (size 5F feeding tube may be used)
- Seldinger technique vascular access kit[c]

Miscellaneous
- Infant and standard scales
- Infant formula and oral rehydrating solutions[c]
- Heating source (may be met by infrared lamps or overhead warmer)[c]
- Towel rolls, blanket rolls, or equivalent
- Pediatric restraining devices
- Resuscitation board
- Sterile linen[f]
- Length-based resuscitation tape or precalculated drug or equipment list based on weight

Specialized Pediatric Trays
- Tube thoracotomy with water seal drainage capability[b]
- Lumbar puncture
- Pediatric urinary catheters
- Obstetric pack
- Newborn kit[c]
- Umbilical vessel cannulation supplies[c]
- Venous cutdown[c]
- Needle cricothyrotomy tray
- Surgical airway kit (may include a tracheostomy tray or a surgical cricothyrotomy tray)[c]

Fracture Management
Cervical immobilization equipment[g]
Extremity splints[c]
Femur splints[c]

Medical Photography Capability

---

[a]Suitable for hypothermic and hyperthermic measurements with temperature capability from 25°C to 44°C.

[b]May be satisfied by a disposable CO_2 detector of appropriate size for infants and children. For children 5 years or older who are ≥20 kg in body weight, an esophageal detection bulb or syringe may be used additionally.

[c]Equipment that is essential but may be shared with the nursery, pediatric ward, or other inpatient service and is readily available to the ED.

[d]To regulate rate and volume.

[e]Ensure availability of pediatric sizes within the hospital.

[f]Available within hospital for burn care.

[g]Many types of cervical immobilization devices are available, including wedges and collars. The type of device chosen depends on local preferences and policies and procedures. Chosen device should be stocked in sizes to fit infants, children, adolescents, and adults. Use of sandbags to meet this requirement is discouraged, because they may cause injury if the patient has to be turned.

SOURCE: Adapted from Committee on Pediatric Equipment and Supplies for Emergency Departments, National Emergency Medical Services for Children Resource Alliance: Guidelines for pediatric equipment and supplies for emergency departments. *Ann Emerg Med.* 31:54–57, 1998.

TABLE 120-6   Examples of Field Treatment Protocols

Respiratory distress and failure
Airway obstruction
Bradycardia and tachycardia
Cardiopulmonary arrest
Trauma
Child maltreatment
Seizures
Toxic ingestions and exposures
Altered mental status and seizures
Newborn care

BIBLIOGRAPHY

American Academy of Pediatrics, Committee on Pediatric Emergency Medicine: Guidelines for pediatric emergency care facilities. *Pediatrics* 96:526–537, 1995.

American Academy of Pediatrics, Committee on Pediatric Emergency Medicine, and American College of Emergency Physicians, Pediatric Committee: Care of children in the emergency department: Guidelines for preparedness: *Ann of Emerg Med* 37:423–427, 2001.

American College of Emergency Physicians: Emergency care guidelines. *Ann Emerg Med* 29:564–571, 1997.

Committee on Pediatric Equipment and Supplies for Emergency Departments, National Emergency Medical Services for Children Resource Alliance: Guidelines for pediatric equipment and supplies for emergency departments. *Ann Emerg Med* 31:54–57, 1998.

Dieckmann R, Brownstein D, Gausche-Hill M, American Academy of Pediatrics: *Textbook of Pediatric Education for Prehospital Professionals.* Sudbury, MA: Jones & Bartlett, 2000.

Eckstein M, Jantos T, Kelly N, Cardillo A: Helicopter transport of pediatric trauma patients in an urban emergency medical services system: A critical analysis. *J Trauma* 53:340–344, 2002.

Foltin G, Tunik M, Cooper A, et al: *Teaching Resources for Instructors in Prehospital Pediatrics*, Version 2.0. New York: Center for Pediatric Emergency Medicine, 1998.

Gausche-Hill M, Brownstein D, Dieckmann R, American Academy of Pediatrics: *Resource Manual for Pediatric Education for Prehospital Professionals.* Sudbury, MA: Jones & Bartlett, 2001.

Institute of Medicine, Committee on Pediatric Emergency Medical Services: Durch JS, Lohr KN (eds): *Institute of Medicine Report: Emergency Medical Services for Children.* Washington, DC: National Academy Press, 1993.

National Emergency Medical Services for Children Resource Alliance, Committee on Pediatric Equipment and Supplies for Emergency: Guidelines for pediatric equipment and supplies for emergency departments. *Ann Emerg Med* 31:54–57, 1998.

U.S. Health Resources and Services Administration, Maternal and Child Health Bureau: *Five-Year Plan: Midcourse Review: Emergency Medical Services for Children, 1995–2000.* Washington, DC: Emergency Medical Services for Children, National Resource Center, 1997.

QUESTIONS

1. Which of the following is the most accurate description of emergency medical services for children (EMSC)?
   A. A separate and distinct EMS system for children with little overlap or coordination with the adult EMS system.
   B. An entire system of pediatric emergency care, critical care, and trauma services within the general EMS system.
   C. A federally funded organization devoted solely to the prehospital care of children.
   D. A legislative proposal being developed to coordinate care of pediatric patients.
   E. A subcommittee of the American College of Emergency Physicians for those interested in pediatric emergency services.

2. Which of the following is true regarding pediatric EMS patients?
   A. The majority (>90 percent) of pediatric ambulance transports are injuries.
   B. The majority (>90 percent) of pediatric ambulance transports are illnesses.
   C. The leading cause of childhood deaths is motor vehicle crashes in all states.
   D. The leading cause of childhood deaths is both age- and geography-related and varies accordingly.
   E. Children with special health care needs do not generally access the EMS system.

3. Clinical components of EMS-EMSC include all of the following except:
   A. Prevention programs
   B. Requirements for special pediatric equipment on ambulances
   C. Treatment policies and protocols for pediatric prehospital care
   D. Stipulating that all hospital EDs have appropriate equipment, staff, and policies to care for children
   E. Mandating and regulating specialized pediatric training on all staff treating children

ANSWERS

1. B. Emergency medical services for children (EMSC) is an important ingredient of the EMS system and refers to an entire EMS-EMSC continuum of pediatric emergency care, critical care, and trauma services. EMSC is fully within the general EMS system and not a separate system. The two ideally should be integrated and coordinated in their efforts to be effective.

2. D. Injuries account for half of pediatric ambulance transports and illnesses account for the other half. The leading cause of death is both age- and geography-related. For example, in some states, fires and burns are the leading cause of death in children under 5 years of age and motor vehicle collision is the leading cause in others.

3. E. Clinical components of EMS-EMSC include prevention programs, pediatric equipment requirements on ambulances, developing treatment policies and protocols for pediatric prehospital care, as well as mandating that all hospital EDs in every community have appropriate equipment, staff, and policies to provide appropriate care for children. They also include designating specialized pediatric centers and systematic identification of suitable rehabilitation services.

121 INTERFACILITY TRANSPORT

Ira J. Blumen
Howard Rodenberg
Thomas J. Abramo
Gary R. Strange
Heather M. Prendergast

INTRODUCTION

- Many critically ill pediatric and neonatal patients are transported miles from one hospital to another. The process of interfacility transport includes:
  ○ Stabilizing the patient
  ○ Identifying the need for transfer
  ○ Selecting the most appropriate method of transport
  ○ Communicating the pertinent information to the receiving hospital
  ○ Transporting the patient while maintaining appropriate monitoring and therapy

STABILIZING THE PATIENT

- A stable airway must be assured prior to transfer. Endotracheal intubation is required if the child is at risk for deteriorating and losing the airway en route.
- Adequate fluids or blood products should be administered to assure perfusion of vital tissues. Ongoing volume loss, such as hemorrhage, should be controlled prior to transport whenever possible.
- Definitive management of some disease processes should be started prior to transport. For example, antibiotics should be started when infectious processes are involved.
- Endotracheal tubes, intravenous lines, and other life-saving equipment should be meticulously secured. Sedation alone or in combination with paralysis may be required to control the patient and to prevent dislodgment of the endotracheal tube, vascular access, Foley catheter, and other equipment.

REFERRING HOSPITAL RESPONSIBILITIES

- Transfer agreements that include specific criteria are preferably worked out beforehand. Such agreements should address the special medical services available at potential receiving facilities and admission criteria for each of these services.

- The referring physician must determine the most appropriate receiving physician and hospital for the patient. A more distant institution may be considered more appropriate than a closer one if the referring institution has a specialized transport team able to perform advanced care during transport.
- Initial contact with the accepting physician should take place as early in the case as possible.
- Detailed institution- and patient-specific information must be relayed. Appropriate records and transfer forms that comply with EMTALA regulations must be completed and sent with the patient.
- The referring physician should also discuss the rationale for transport with the family and explain the risks and benefits of transfer and the mode of transport to be used.

RECEIVING FACILITY RESPONSIBILITIES

- A requirement of EMTALA is that hospitals with specialized facilities shall not refuse to accept appropriate transfers if they have the capacity to treat the individual. The receiving facility should have appropriate mechanisms in place to assure that referring hospitals can access their capabilities quickly.
- The receiving physician may make further recommendations regarding evaluation and management. The receiving physician also should be aware of the availability of hospital resources for management of the case and the current availability of bed space for the patient.
- The receiving physician should also be familiar with available transport options, and the referring and receiving physicians should agree on the mode of transport, the transport team's composition, and the equipment needed for the transport.

MODE OF TRANSPORT

- The mode of transport selected will depend on a number of factors including:
  ○ Condition of the patient
  ○ Distance to the receiving hospital
  ○ Cost
  ○ Availability of alternatives
  ○ Weather conditions
- The ground ambulance is the vehicle most commonly used for pediatric and neonatal transport. Its advantages include:
  ○ Relatively large and stable working environment

○ Resistance to most weather-related problems

○ Ability to stop if a patient requires further resuscitation

• Helicopters can quickly deliver a team and return the patient and team to the receiving hospital. Unfortunately, air travel may be prohibited by weather conditions. Noise and vibrations in helicopters make it difficult to auscultate and to hear monitor alarms. This environment may also have very limited working space and some procedures may be impossible to perform.

• Fixed-wing aircraft are generally available and practical only for very long-distance transports. In many cases, the advantages of speed and a better working environment are offset by the dependence on an airport for landing, which then requires an additional vehicle for transport from the airport to the hospital.

• According to EMTALA, the transfer must be effected by qualified personnel and requires the use of necessary and medically appropriate life-support measures during the transfer. Whenever possible, the individual needs of the patient should be matched with appropriate transport personnel and equipment.

• All patient transports require both direct and indirect physician medical control. Unless it is assumed by the accepting specialist or the medical director for the transport service, medical responsibility for the transfer remains with the referring physician until the patient arrives at the receiving facility.

BIBLIOGRAPHY

American Academy of Pediatrics Task Force on Interhospital Transport: *Guidelines for Air and Ground Transportation of Neonatal and Pediatric Patients.* Elk Grove Village, IL: American Academy of Pediatrics, 1993.

American College of Emergency Physicians: Appropriate interhospital patient transfer policy statement. *Ann Emerg Med* 22:768, 1993.

Bitterman RA (ed): *Providing Emergency Care Under Federal Law: EMTALA.* Dallas: American College of Emergency Physicians, 2001.

Nieman CT, Merlino JI, Kovach B, et al: Intubated pediatric patients requiring transport: A review of patients, indications, and standards. *Air Med* J 21:22–25, 2002.

Woodward GA, Insoft RM, Pearson-Shaver AL, et al: The state of interfacility transport: Consensus of the second National Pediatric and Neonatal Interfacility Transport Medicine Leadership Conference. *Pediatr Emerg Care* 18:38–43, 2002.

QUESTIONS

1. A 9-year-old child is brought to the Emergency Department for right lower quadrant (RLQ) abdominal pain, low-grade fever, and anorexia for 3 days. The vital signs are all within normal limits. The examination is consistent with appendicitis. Your facility does not have a pediatric surgeon-on-call. The child will need to be transferred to the nearest pediatric tertiary care center located 5 miles away. Which of the following would be **MOST** appropriate in management of this child **PRIOR** to transfer?
   A. No intervention is necessary.
   B. Intravenous bolus of normal saline
   C. Foley catheter to monitor urine output
   D. Intravenous antibiotics
   E. Intubation tray in the event of acute deterioration

2. A 6-year-old child is brought to the ED for evaluation of a forearm fracture that may need operative intervention. Your facility does not have orthopedic services. You contact the orthopedic surgeon-on-call at the nearest tertiary care facility; however, he is refusing to accept the patient because the patient has no insurance. The orthopedist suggests that you transfer the patient to the county hospital that is located 25 miles away. The **MOST** appropriate action would be?
   A. Arrange transfer to the county hospital
   B. Go ahead and transfer the patient anyway to the nearest hospital without an accepting physician
   C. Transfer the patient to the county hospital without an accepting physician
   D. Admit the patient to the medical service at your hospital
   E. Inform the consultant that he is in violation of EMTALA by refusing the patient on the basis of insurance status and contact your hospital administrator

3. A 2-year-old toddler is brought to your community hospital for an asthma exacerbation. After several hours of treatment, the child has significantly improved. However, you feel the child would benefit from a 23-h admission. Your facility does not have inpatient pediatric beds. The receiving hospital is 8 miles away. Which mode of transportation would be **MOST** appropriate for this child?
   A. Helicopter to ensure rapid transport
   B. Ground ambulance with ACLS capabilities
   C. Ground ambulance with BLS capabilities
   D. Discharge the patient and have parents transport by private vehicle
   E. Mode of transportation depends upon weather conditions.

ANSWERS

1. D. Intravenous antibiotics would be the most appropriate for this patient considering the working diagnosis of appendicitis. The choice of antibiotics should be made in conjunction with the receiving physician. The decision to institute more aggressive stabilizing measures depends upon the condition of the patient and the risk for deterioration.

2. E. A requirement of EMTALA is that a hospital with specialized facilities should not refuse to accept appropriate transfers if they have the capacity to treat the patient. It is unacceptable to transfer a patient without an accepting physician and would be a violation of EMTALA by the referring physician.

3. B. The patient appears to be relatively stable and does not require rapid transport via helicopter. Ground ambulance with ACLS capabilities would be most appropriate considering the reason for admission.

Section 21
ETHICAL AND LEGAL ISSUES

122 MEDICOLEGAL CONSIDERATIONS

Gary R. Strange
Steven Lelyveld
Heather M. Prendergast

CONSENT

- There are two basic legal principles regarding consent in a pediatric emergency department:
  - In whom is ultimate responsibility vested?
  - What are the conditions by which that responsibility is breached?
- Implied consent to treat becomes operative when two conditions are met:
  - The patient lacks competence to make an independent decision. In the pediatric emergency department, with a few exceptions, this criterion is met by the state's definition of a minor and the lack of presence of a responsible adult.
  - A true emergency exists, for which delay in treatment would endanger life or cause permanent disability to the patient.
- For illnesses that are not life- or limb-threatening, a parent or legal guardian must give consent to treat.
- The **emancipated minor** may give consent to treat. This person is defined as below the stated statutory age, lives away from parents, is self-supporting, and not subject to parental control. In most states, the adolescent meets these criteria by being married, pregnant, or in the armed forces.
- An increasing number of states recognize a **mature minor**. While not fully emancipated, the adolescent can give consent if between the ages of 14 and 18 years, understands the risks, the physician believes the patient can make an informed decision, and the treatment does not involve serious risk of harm.
- Often, a child will present with an adult who is not a parent or, in the case of divorce, a noncustodial parent. The rules for implied consent apply to serious illness. The consent for less-serious problems should be obtained from the responsible adult "in locum parentis" and, when applicable, the mature minor. An attempt should be made to contact the parent or legal guardian.
- Most states have laws dictating that parental consent need not be obtained for minors in detention facilities or foster homes. Consult your legal department for the state agency responsible for these wards of the state.
- No parent has the right to refuse treatment if such refusal will result in harm to the child. The state's obligation to protect the child supersedes the parent's right to religious expression.

MALPRACTICE

- Malpractice is based on liability stemming from negligence. The plaintiff must prove four things:
  - The physician had a **duty** to the plaintiff based on a physician–patient relationship.
  - An applicable **standard of care** was violated.
  - An **injury** occurred that is compensable.
  - The violation of the standard of care **caused** the injury.
- As emergency physicians cannot refuse care, duty to treat is present for all patients presenting to an emergency department.
- The standard of care is defined as what a reasonable physician, with similar training and experience,

practicing in a like setting, presented with the same type of patient, would be expected to do. It is not defined as what the best physician with the best resources can do.

- Most potential suits will not occur if patients feel that the physician truly cares about his or her health and is doing his or her best to help. Always explain your actions to those patients who can understand.

BIBLIOGRAPHY

Annas GJ: Scientific evidence in the courtroom. *N Engl J Med* 330:1018, 1994.

Committee on Medical Liability: Guidelines for expert witness testimony in medical liability cases. *Pediatrics* 94:755, 1994.

Forster G, Robinson A, Rogstad K: National guideline for the management of suspected sexually transmitted infections in children and young people. *Sex Transm Infect* 78:314–315, 2002.

Garner BA (ed): *Black's Law Dictionary*, 7th ed. St. Paul: West Publishing Company, 1999.

Sullivan DJ: Minors and emergency medicine. *Emerg Med Clin North Am* 11:841, 1993.

QUESTIONS

1. A 16-year-old pregnant teenager (G1P0) presents to the emergency department for evaluation of a 3-day history of dysuria and flank pain. Her temperature is 101°F, with a pulse of 110. Physical examination is notable for mild suprapubic tenderness and left costovertebral angle tenderness. Which of the following would be the most appropriate next course of action?
   A. Administer antipyretics and wait until a parent or guardian is contacted before continuing care.
   B. Obtain urinalysis, but delay antipyretics until parent or guardian is contacted.
   C. Delay both urinalysis and antipyretics until parent or guardian is contacted.
   D. Proceed with antipyretics and urinalysis while attempting to contact the parents or guardian.
   E. Proceed with antipyretics and urinalysis and contact parents or guardian according to the patient's wishes.

2. A 14-year-old boy is brought to the emergency department by his custodial parent for an acute forearm injury. Physical examination reveals an obvious deformity and decreased capillary refill. Which of the following principles would apply to treatment of this child?
   A. In-locum parentis
   B. Implied consent
   C. Mature minor
   D. Emancipated minor
   E. Direct consent

3. A 15-year-old teenager presents by herself to the emergency department for evaluation of a vaginal discharge. Although she lives with her parents, she is requesting that her parents not be notified. The patient admits to being sexually active but denies pregnancy. An obligation to treat this patient would be based on which of the following principles?
   A. Emancipated minor
   B. Mature minor
   C. Patient confidentiality
   D. Implied consent
   E. Substituted judgment

4. A 2-year-old toddler is brought to the ED for evaluation of burns to both legs. You believe the child needs to be transferred to the only available pediatric burn facility, which is 20 miles away. The mother objects because of the distance. The best course of action would be the following:
   A. Address the mother's concern and transfer to a nearer hospital without a burn center.
   B. Attempt to address the mother's concern, but still transfer the child to the pediatric burn center.
   C. Ignore the mother's concern and transfer the patient to the pediatric burn center.
   D. Take custody of the child and transfer to the pediatric burn center.
   E. Contact the father and attempt to get his consent for transfer.

5. A 10-year-old boy is brought to a rural community hospital for evaluation of an acute abdominal pain, persistent vomiting, and anorexia. Physical examination reveals a dehydrated patient with a low-grade fever and right lower quadrant abdominal pain with rebound and guarding. Several attempts to reach the on-call surgeon are unsuccessful and 3 to 4 h go by. In spite of IV hydration and antibiotics ordered by the ED physician, the child continues to deteriorate. When the surgeon finally answers, he does not want to take care of the child since there is no insurance. You are able to reach a surgeon at another institution, and the patient is transferred and taken directly to the operating room. On the arrival to the other facility, the child is in shock and suffers a long, complicated hospital course. A successful malpractice suit against the on-call surgeon could be based on which of the following principles?
   A. Duty to treat
   B. Violation of standard of care
   C. Compensable injury
   D. Cause-effect relationship
   E. All of the above.

ANSWERS

1. E. The patient is an emancipated minor because of her pregnancy; therefore, may give her own consent to treat. Other criteria for emancipated minors include: marriage, service in armed forces, self-supporting, and not subject to parental control.

2. B. Based on the physical examination, a true limb-threatening emergency exists and implied consent would be operative. The patient presents with the custodial parent, therefore, in-locum parentis would not be applicable. There is no indication that the patient is an emancipated or mature minor. Direct consent may be obtained from the custodial parent but is not required in an emergency situation.

3. B. Patients between the ages of 14 and 18 years of age can give consent to treatment in certain states. It is necessary that the patient understands the risks of treatment and appears competent. In addition, the treatment cannot pose any risk of serious harm to the patient. This patient lives with her parents, and does not meet any other criteria for emancipation. Substituted judgment is a concept applied to situations when a patient is not competent to make decisions for himself or herself.

4. B. Taking the time to address a parent's concerns is always a good practice in medicine. In addition, you must explain to the mother that she cannot refuse treatment for her child if such refusal will result in harm of the child. This patient meets criteria for transfer to a burn center and should be transferred for optimal management. Delay from seeking consent from others is not appropriate. Taking custody of the child is an option to be used only if the mother cannot be convinced to comply with appropriate medical care.

5. E. On-call physicians are required to be accessible within a reasonable period of time. Failure to be reasonably available to the ED is a violation of the standard of care. Duty to treat by the emergency physician was met, but the hospital and its medical staff have a further duty to treat emergency medical conditions within the scope of their ability without regard for ability to pay. In this case, there was an emergency medical condition that required operative intervention for stabilization. The receiving hospital also has an obligation to report a case like this as a violation of EMTALA regulations.

123 ETHICAL CONSIDERATIONS

John D. Lantos
Gary R. Strange
Patricia Lee

- In pediatric emergency care, the central ethical issue is the relationship between physicians and parents in determining what is or is not in a child's best interest. In settings where treatment must be provided quickly for patients who may be unstable, standard medical treatment is generally considered to be best for children. If the child is in imminent danger of loss of life or limb, treatment should be provided, even over parental objections

- First, it must be decided from whom to obtain consent. For young children, except in an emergency, parents or legal guardians must consent. In a true emergency (defined in most states as a situation in which there is an immediate threat of loss of life or limb), parental consent is not necessary and physicians must initiate treatment immediately. For older children, parental consent may not be necessary for particular diseases, such as those related to reproductive health or for psychiatric conditions.

- Some states have mature minor statutes, which apply to younger patients who demonstrate decisional capacity and may be able to give informed consent or decline treatment despite their parents' wishes.

- Both physicians and parents are held to a high standard, namely, to do what is best for the child. If physicians think that parents' failure to consent to a procedure places the child at imminent risk of harm, emergency protective custody is taken and the procedure is performed anyway.

- In the United States, the Child Abuse Prevention and Treatment Act of 1974 defines abuse and neglect as "the physical and mental injury, sexual abuse, negligent treatment or maltreatment of a child under the age of 18 by a person who is responsible for the child's welfare under circumstances which indicate that the child's health and welfare are harmed or threatened thereby." State definitions based on this law vary. Arguments about whether a particular act constitutes abuse may focus on:
  - The nature of the act itself
  - Whether the act caused harm
  - Whether there was or should have been prior recognition that the act would cause harm
  - Whether the caretaker might have prevented the harm

- Cultural or religious differences may also play a role in evaluating what constitutes medical neglect. Christian Scientists, for example, may claim that it is appropriate not to take their sick children to a doctor, while courts may determine that such behavior constitutes neglect.
- State statutes generally require reporting if someone "has reasons to believe that a child has been subjected to abuse." Such laws do not even attempt to quantify the degree of suspicion, the quality of the evidence, or the likelihood of abuse that must be present to compel a report.
- An apparent consensus about child abuse masks profound disagreements about the proper boundaries of family privacy, parental obligations, and governmental responsibility to oversee the care and nurturing of children. These disagreements are reflected in difficulties in defining child abuse, in enforcing compliance with mandatory reporting requirements, and in evaluating the effects of interventions. Thus, while the law requires that child abuse be reported if it is suspected, health professionals can create their own index of suspicion.

BIBLIOGRAPHY

Jacobstein CR, Baren JM: Emergency treatment of minors. *Emerg Med Clin North Am* 17:341–352, 1999.

Perkin RM: Ethical issues in pediatric emergency medicine: children's rights and health. *Emerg Med Specialty Reports Suppl* 5372:1–12, 2002.

QUESTIONS

1. A 14-year-old female presents with vaginal bleeding and missed menses. The most appropriate next action would be which of the following?
   - A. Contact the girl's parents for permission to treat prior to beginning treatment
   - B. Begin treatment and attempt to contact parents later
   - C. Contact child protective services and assume protective custody
   - D. Begin treatment.
   - E. Call the parents and fully inform them of the patient's condition

2. A 2-week-old male is brought to the emergency department with a fever of 103°F. Physical examination reveals a lethargic infant. You explain to the parents the need to perform a septic work-up, including a lumbar puncture, but they refuse all care. They attempt to leave the emergency department with their son. Your appropriate action should be:
   - A. Assume emergency protective custody and perform work-up. Contact child protective services.
   - B. Contact their private physician and allow the child to be transported to the private physician office for evaluation. Contact child protective services.
   - C. Contact child protective services and allow child to be discharged home with parents.
   - D. Restrain the parents and perform the septic workup.
   - E. Contact child protective services and request that they come to the hospital to perform a complete evaluation.

3. A 12-year-old is brought by his babysitter and presents to the emergency department with abdominal pain, which is determined to be the result of appendicitis. When the parents arrive, they state that they are Christian Scientists and do not wish their child to receive any further care. Appropriate action should be which of the following?
   - A. Perform appendectomy against parents wishes
   - B. Contact court and assume protective custody
   - C. Allow parents to sign out child against medical advice
   - D. Discharge child to custody of parents
   - E. Restrain parents and contact legal authorities

ANSWERS

1. D. For young children, except in an emergency, parents or legal guardians must consent. For older children, parental consent may not be necessary for diseases of reproductive health or for psychiatric conditions.

2. A. In a true emergency (defined in most states as a situation in which there is an immediate threat of loss of life or limb), parental consent is not necessary and physicians must initiate treatment immediately. In this case of a febrile lethargic 2-week-old infant, an emergency evaluation and treatment is mandatory. If a physician thinks that the parents' failure to consent to a procedure places the child at imminent risk of harm, emergency protective custody is taken and the procedure is performed anyway. In this case, the physician must assume protective custody and treat appropriately.

3. B. Cultural or religious differences may also play a role in evaluating what constitutes medical neglect. Christian Scientists may claim that it is appropriate not to take their sick children to a doctor, while courts may determine that such behavior constitutes neglect.

INDEX

Page numbers followed by the letters *f* and *t* indicate figures and tables, respectively.